# Monitoring and Surveillance of Veterinary Antimicrobial Use and Antibiotic Resistance in Animals

# Monitoring and Surveillance of Veterinary Antimicrobial Use and Antibiotic Resistance in Animals

Editor

**Clair L. Firth**

MDPI • Basel • Beijing • Wuhan • Barcelona • Belgrade • Manchester • Tokyo • Cluj • Tianjin

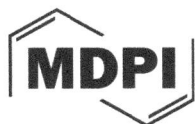

*Editor*
Clair L. Firth
Unit of Veterinary Public Health and Epidemiology
Institute of Food Safety, Food Technology
and Veterinary Public Health
University of Veterinary Medicine
Vienna
Austria

*Editorial Office*
MDPI
St. Alban-Anlage 66
4052 Basel, Switzerland

This is a reprint of articles from the Special Issue published online in the open access journal *Antibiotics* (ISSN 2079-6382) (available at: www.mdpi.com/journal/antibiotics/special_issues/veterinary_antimicrobial).

For citation purposes, cite each article independently as indicated on the article page online and as indicated below:

LastName, A.A.; LastName, B.B.; LastName, C.C. Article Title. *Journal Name* **Year**, *Volume Number*, Page Range.

**ISBN 978-3-0365-4082-5 (Hbk)**
**ISBN 978-3-0365-4081-8 (PDF)**

© 2022 by the authors. Articles in this book are Open Access and distributed under the Creative Commons Attribution (CC BY) license, which allows users to download, copy and build upon published articles, as long as the author and publisher are properly credited, which ensures maximum dissemination and a wider impact of our publications.

The book as a whole is distributed by MDPI under the terms and conditions of the Creative Commons license CC BY-NC-ND.

# Contents

**About the Editor** . . . . . . . . . . . . . . . . . . . . . . . . . . . . . . . . . . . . . . . . . . . vii

**Preface to "Monitoring and Surveillance of Veterinary Antimicrobial Use and Antibiotic Resistance in Animals"** . . . . . . . . . . . . . . . . . . . . . . . . . . . . . . . . . . . . . . ix

**Cassandra Eibl, Ricardo Bexiga, Lorenzo Viora, Hugues Guyot, José Félix and Johanna Wilms et al.**
The Antibiotic Treatment of Calf Diarrhea in Four European Countries: A Survey
Reprinted from: *Antibiotics* **2021**, *10*, 910, doi:10.3390/antibiotics10080910 . . . . . . . . . . . . . . . 1

**Andrea Feuerstein, Nelly Scuda, Corinna Klose, Angelika Hoffmann, Alexander Melchner and Kerstin Boll et al.**
Antimicrobial Resistance, Serologic and Molecular Characterization of *E. coli* Isolated from Calves with Severe or Fatal Enteritis in Bavaria, Germany
Reprinted from: *Antibiotics* **2021**, *11*, 23, doi:10.3390/antibiotics11010023 . . . . . . . . . . . . . . 19

**Clair L. Firth, Reinhard Fuchs and Klemens Fuchs**
National Monitoring of Veterinary-Dispensed Antimicrobials for Use on Pig Farms in Austria: 2015–2020
Reprinted from: *Antibiotics* **2022**, *11*, 216, doi:10.3390/antibiotics11020216 . . . . . . . . . . . . . . 35

**María Dávalos-Almeyda, Agustín Guerrero, Germán Medina, Alejandra Dávila-Barclay, Guillermo Salvatierra and Maritza Calderón et al.**
Antibiotic Use and Resistance Knowledge Assessment of Personnel on Chicken Farms with High Levels of Antimicrobial Resistance: A Cross-Sectional Survey in Ica, Peru
Reprinted from: *Antibiotics* **2022**, *11*, 190, doi:10.3390/antibiotics11020190 . . . . . . . . . . . . . . 49

**Blaž Cugmas, Miha Avberšek, Teja Rosa, Leonida Godec, Eva Štruc and Majda Golob et al.**
How Accurate Are Veterinary Clinicians Employing Flexicult Vet for Identification and Antimicrobial Susceptibility Testing of Urinary Bacteria?
Reprinted from: *Antibiotics* **2021**, *10*, 1160, doi:10.3390/antibiotics10101160 . . . . . . . . . . . . . 63

**Charlotte Doidge, Helen West and Jasmeet Kaler**
Antimicrobial Resistance Patterns of *Escherichia coli* Isolated from Sheep and Beef Farms in England and Wales: A Comparison of Disk Diffusion Interpretation Methods
Reprinted from: *Antibiotics* **2021**, *10*, 453, doi:10.3390/antibiotics10040453 . . . . . . . . . . . . . . 73

**Clair L. Firth, Annemarie Käsbohrer, Peter Pless, Sandra Koeberl-Jelovcan and Walter Obritzhauser**
Analysis of Antimicrobial Use and the Presence of Antimicrobial-Resistant Bacteria on Austrian Dairy Farms—A Pilot Study
Reprinted from: *Antibiotics* **2022**, *11*, 124, doi:10.3390/antibiotics11020124 . . . . . . . . . . . . . . 91

**Do Kyung-Hyo, Byun Jae-Won and Lee Wan-Kyu**
Antimicrobial Resistance Profiles of *Escherichia coli* from Diarrheic Weaned Piglets after the Ban on Antibiotic Growth Promoters in Feed
Reprinted from: *Antibiotics* **2020**, *9*, 755, doi:10.3390/antibiotics9110755 . . . . . . . . . . . . . . . 107

**Mayu Horie, Dongsheng Yang, Philip Joosten, Patrick Munk, Katharina Wadepohl and Claire Chauvin et al.**
Risk Factors for Antimicrobial Resistance in Turkey Farms: A Cross-Sectional Study in Three European Countries
Reprinted from: *Antibiotics* **2021**, *10*, 820, doi:10.3390/antibiotics10070820 . . . . . . . . . . . . . . 119

**Natcha Dankittipong, Egil A. J. Fischer, Manon Swanenburg, Jaap A. Wagenaar, Arjan J. Stegeman and Clazien J. de Vos**
Quantitative Risk Assessment for the Introduction of Carbapenem-Resistant Enterobacteriaceae (CPE) into Dutch Livestock Farms
Reprinted from: *Antibiotics* **2022**, *11*, 281, doi:10.3390/antibiotics11020281 . . . . . . . . . . . . . . **139**

**Alexander Melchner, Sarah van de Berg, Nelly Scuda, Andrea Feuerstein, Matthias Hanczaruk and Magdalena Schumacher et al.**
Antimicrobial Resistance in Isolates from Cattle with Bovine Respiratory Disease in Bavaria, Germany
Reprinted from: *Antibiotics* **2021**, *10*, 1538, doi:10.3390/antibiotics10121538 . . . . . . . . . . . . . **169**

**Karin Sjöström, Rachel A. Hickman, Viktoria Tepper, Gabriela Olmos Antillón, Josef D. Järhult and Ulf Emanuelson et al.**
Antimicrobial Resistance Patterns in Organic and Conventional Dairy Herds in Sweden
Reprinted from: *Antibiotics* **2020**, *9*, 834, doi:10.3390/antibiotics9110834 . . . . . . . . . . . . . . **187**

**Andrea Micke Moreno, Luisa Zanolli Moreno, André Pegoraro Poor, Carlos Emilio Cabrera Matajira, Marina Moreno and Vasco Túlio de Moura Gomes et al.**
Antimicrobial Resistance Profile of *Staphylococcus hyicus* Strains Isolated from Brazilian Swine Herds
Reprinted from: *Antibiotics* **2022**, *11*, 205, doi:10.3390/antibiotics11020205 . . . . . . . . . . . . . . **205**

**Vanessa Silva, Manuela Caniça, Eugénia Ferreira, Madalena Vieira-Pinto, Cândido Saraiva and José Eduardo Pereira et al.**
Multidrug-Resistant Methicillin-Resistant Coagulase-Negative Staphylococci in Healthy Poultry Slaughtered for Human Consumption
Reprinted from: *Antibiotics* **2022**, *11*, 365, doi:10.3390/antibiotics11030365 . . . . . . . . . . . . . . **217**

**Giorgia Schirò, Delia Gambino, Francesco Mira, Maria Vitale, Annalisa Guercio and Giuseppa Purpari et al.**
Antimicrobial Resistance (AMR) of Bacteria Isolated from Dogs with Canine Parvovirus (CPV) Infection: The Need for a Rational Use of Antibiotics in Companion Animal Health
Reprinted from: *Antibiotics* **2022**, *11*, 142, doi:10.3390/antibiotics11020142 . . . . . . . . . . . . . . **229**

**Deepthi Vijay, Jasbir Singh Bedi, Pankaj Dhaka, Randhir Singh, Jaswinder Singh and Anil Kumar Arora et al.**
Knowledge, Attitude, and Practices (KAP) Survey among Veterinarians, and Risk Factors Relating to Antimicrobial Use and Treatment Failure in Dairy Herds of India
Reprinted from: *Antibiotics* **2021**, *10*, 216, doi:10.3390/antibiotics10020216 . . . . . . . . . . . . . . **249**

**Shawn Ting, Abrao Pereira, Amalia de Jesus Alves, Salvador Fernandes, Cristina da Costa Soares and Felix Joanico Soares et al.**
Antimicrobial Use in Animals in Timor-Leste Based on Veterinary Antimicrobial Imports between 2016 and 2019
Reprinted from: *Antibiotics* **2021**, *10*, 426, doi:10.3390/antibiotics10040426 . . . . . . . . . . . . . . **265**

# About the Editor

**Clair L. Firth**

Clair L. Firth is a veterinarian and animal scientist. She holds a veterinary research doctorate in antimicrobial use and resistance on dairy farms from the University of Veterinary Medicine, Vienna, Austria. A British citizen, she gained a Bachelor of Science degree with honours from the University of Nottingham (UK) in Animal Science with European Studies (German) and a Master of Science degree in Agricultural Development from the University of London's Imperial College, before relocating to Austria. After spending more than a decade in pharmaceutical research and development, she now divides her time between working as a farm veterinarian in first opinion clinical practice in the Austrian countryside and teaching students at the University of Veterinary Medicine in Vienna.

# Preface to "Monitoring and Surveillance of Veterinary Antimicrobial Use and Antibiotic Resistance in Animals"

Antimicrobial resistance is a global One Health topic that affects us all, whether we are working in human or veterinary medicine. Although antibiotic use in farm animals is decreasing in many countries, other nations are still using these essential medical resources as growth promoters to boost economic gains. As veterinarians responsible for animal welfare, it is vital that we are permitted to treat sick animals effectively, but we must learn to be more prudent in our use of these drugs. It is essential that we, as responsible clinicians, policy makers, and researchers, develop methods of quantifying, monitoring, benchmarking, and reporting antibiotic use in both farm and companion animals, so that antimicrobial stewardship schemes can be implemented and their successes or failures analysed. This Special Issue includes research on antibiotic use and resistance in a variety of animal species, covering cattle, sheep, pigs, poultry, and pets. The relationship between antimicrobial use and resistance in animals is investigated on a global scale, with authors from Austria, Australia, Brazil, Germany, Italy, India, the Netherlands, Peru, Portugal, Slovenia, and the United Kingdom.

**Clair L. Firth**
*Editor*

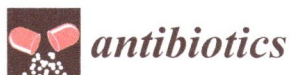

*Article*

# The Antibiotic Treatment of Calf Diarrhea in Four European Countries: A Survey

Cassandra Eibl [1], Ricardo Bexiga [2], Lorenzo Viora [3], Hugues Guyot [4], José Félix [2], Johanna Wilms [5], Alexander Tichy [6] and Alexandra Hund [1,7,*]

[1] University Clinic for Ruminants, Department for Farm Animals and Veterinary Public Health, University of Veterinary Medicine Vienna, 1210 Vienna, Austria; Cassandra.Eibl@vetmeduni.ac.at
[2] Centro de Investigação Interdisciplinar em Sanidade Animal, Faculdade de Medicina Veterinária, Universidade de Lisboa, 1300-477 Lisbon, Portugal; ricardobexiga@fmv.ulisboa.pt (R.B.); jose_duarte_felix@hotmail.com (J.F.)
[3] School of Veterinary Medicine, College of Medical, Veterinary and Life Sciences, University of Glasgow, Glasgow G61 1GH, UK; Lorenzo.Viora@glasgow.ac.uk
[4] Clinical Department of Production Animals, Fundamental and Applied Research for Animals and Health, University of Veterinary Medicine, 1210 Vienna, Austria; Hugues.Guyot@uliege.be
[5] Tierarztpraxis Geisenhausen, 84144 Geisenhausen, Germany; johanna.wilms@gmx.de
[6] Platform Bioinformatics and Biostatistics, Department for Biomedical Sciences, University of Veterinary Medicine, 1210 Vienna, Austria; Alexander.Tichy@vetmeduni.ac.at
[7] Agricultural Center for Cattle, Grassland, Dairy, Game and Fisheries of Baden-Württemberg (LAZBW), 88326 Aulendorf, Germany
* Correspondence: Alexandra.Hund@lazbw.bwl.de

**Abstract:** Neonatal calves are commonly affected by diarrhea caused by different pathogens, but not always bacteria. Yet, antibiotics are routinely used as a treatment to an unknown extent. It was our goal to survey antibiotic use for the treatment of neonatal calf diarrhea in different countries and to identify influencing factors. A total of 873 farmers and veterinarians in Austria, Belgium, Portugal, and Scotland participated in a voluntary online survey. The data were analyzed using classification and regression tree analyses and chi$^2$ tests. Overall, 52.5% of the participants stated that they use antibiotics when treating neonatal calf diarrhea. Of those, 27% use them always, and 45% use highest priority critically important antibiotics. The most important factor differentiating antibiotic use practices was the country the participants were from, which could be due to regulatory differences between the countries. All antibiotic products stated were licensed for use in cattle, but several were not licensed for the treatment of diarrhea in calves. Our study shows that there is an urgent need for more scientific evidence to define best practices for the treatment of neonatal calf diarrhea. Furthermore, consensual criteria for antibiotic therapy must be defined, and targeted training for farmers and veterinarians must be provided.

**Keywords:** neonatal calf diarrhea; survey; antibiotics; HPCIA

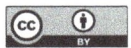

## 1. Introduction

### 1.1. Regulatory Basis

Neonatal calf diarrhea (NCD) is the most commonly treated disease in cattle [1,2]. In Europe, the approach to treating sick calves is determined by law to a certain extent: Any calf, which appears to be ill or injured, must be treated appropriately without delay, and veterinary advice must be obtained as soon as possible for any calf that is not responding to the stock keeper's care [3]. Choosing medical treatment is the responsibility of the attending veterinarian and, depending on the legal situation, the responsibility of the farmer. To which extent farmers can get involved in the treatment of sick animals is regulated at the country level [3–6]. All antibiotics licensed for use in food-producing animals are prescription-only medicines that may only be administered following a clinical assessment of the animal or group of animals, diagnosis, and prescription by a veterinarian [7]. Ideally and according to best practice, the choice of antibiotic drug is determined by appropriate laboratory tests such as culture and sensitivity testing [8,9]. The veterinarian must weigh the benefits and risks for animals, humans, and the environment based on her or his knowledge and considering the current state of knowledge in veterinary medicine. The veterinarian can then recommend the most appropriate therapeutic treatment by use of the optimal drug, dosage, and duration of treatment [7,10]. Ensuring responsible antibiotic use on-farm is an essential part of a veterinarian's role, even though they may not be directly administering the medicines [10].

There are no legal regulations governing antibiotic use in detail. However, several national veterinary organizations have developed antibiotic use principles, programs, and algorithms (Table 1). These guidelines are intended to be a practical benchmark for a careful, medically justified use of antibiotics. Both animal and human health could benefit by minimizing the risks associated with the emergence and spread of antimicrobial resistance [11]. Prudent use of antibiotics should lead to more rational and targeted use.

Table 1. Summary of guidelines for antibiotic use.

| Country | Guideline |
| --- | --- |
| Austria | Leitlinien für den sorgfältigen Umgang mit antibakteriell wirksamen Tierarzneimitteln des Bundesministeriums für ASGK (BMASGK-74330/0008-IX/B/15/2018, AVN Nr. 2018/11a) Umgang mit antibakteriell wirksamen Tierarzneimitteln- Leitfaden für die tierärztliche Praxis, Bundesministeriums für ASGK und Österreichische Tierärztekammer 2019 |
| Belgium | AMCRA- Kenniscentrum inzake antibioticagebruik en -resistentie bij dieren: Richtlijnen voor goed Gebruik van antibiotica, June 2016 Royal Decree, July 2016 (conditions of use of drugs for veterinarians and farmers) |
| Portugal | No such guidelines have been published by official or professional bodies |
| United Kingdom | British Veterinary Association: BVA policy position on the responsible use of antimicrobials in food-producing animals, May 2019 British Veterinary Association: Responsibly use of antimicrobials in veterinary practice: the 7-point plan, 2019 British Cattle Veterinary Association: AMR Statement, December 2016 RUMA (Responsible use of medicines in agriculture alliance) guidelines for farmers and veterinarians: Responsible use of antimicrobials in cattle production, May 2015 |
| International | EU: Guidelines for the prudent use of antimicrobials in veterinary medicine (2015/C 299/04) WHO guidelines on use of medically important antimicrobials in food-producing animals 2017 WHO list of Critically Important Antimicrobials for Human Medicine (WHO CIA list) 2017 |

*1.2. Antibiotic Use in Calves with Diarrhea*

There are several issues with the antibiotic treatment of calves with NCD, as the correct indication for treatment and choice of drug is often problematic. The etiological diagnosis is the first important pitfall [12]; Viral and parasitic pathogens are more likely to be involved as primary causes of NCD than bacterial pathogens. Therefore, the majority of antibiotic treatments may not be justified [12–14].

The decision to administer antibiotics should not be based only on the clinical signs and type of diarrhea or the veterinarian's clinical experience but on diagnostic testing as well. The detection of *Escherichia coli* (*E. coli*) F5 (K99) or of bacteremia, for example, may warrant the use of an antibiotic. For rapid animal-side testing of fecal pathogens, several point-of-care tests have been described [15–17]. A test for the detection of bacteremia in connection with bacteriuria in newborn calves has been validated but is not widely used in practice to date [18].

Aside from *E. coli*, treatment of NCD with oral or injectable antibiotics may only be necessary in cases where the calves show signs of systemic illness such as fever and depression or in calves that have blood or mucosal shreds in their feces, as it marks a breakdown of the blood-gut barrier [19]. The treatment of the concomitant Gram-negative septicemia and bacteremia and the decrease in numbers of coliform bacteria in the proximal small intestine and abomasum is the most important goal of antibiotic therapy in NCD [19,20]. Therefore, the antibiotic must be excreted in bile and reach an effective level in the gastrointestinal tract [21].

Antibiotics may have an impact on the microbiome in the gastrointestinal tract. There are significant differences in microbial diversity between healthy and diarrheic calves within a farm [22,23]. Such microbiome changes in sick calves usually return to the pre-diarrheal stage after a week [24]. It is uncertain if the reduction in microbial diversity occurs due to the disease itself or the antibiotic treatment [22]. A very limited number of studies show that therapeutic antibiotics delay the temporal development of diversity [25]. As an example, the use of tulathromycin for treatment appeared to have a negative impact on the richness and diversity of the gut microbiome [26]. A study in 2009 showed that calves treated with antibiotics or fed with medicated milk replacer had 70% and 31% more days with diarrhea, respectively, compared to calves with NCD that only received antibiotics in cases with fever and depression [27].

The Belgian Knowledge Center for the Use of Antibiotics and Antibiotic Resistance in Animals (AMCRA) does not advise the use of antibiotics as the first-line treatment of NCD. Second choice drugs are sulfonamides with trimethoprim, amoxicillin, amoxicillin and clavulanic acid, colistine, gentamicine, and paromomycin. As the third choice, quinolones and flumequine are recommended, but diagnostic testing (culture and sensitivity) is mandatory beforehand. For septicemia, the drugs of choice are penicillin or sulfonamides with trimethoprim. The second- and third-choice antibiotics for this indication are the same as listed for NCD treatment [28]. In Switzerland, official treatment guidelines for NCD do not recommend antibiotic treatment in simple cases. However, in NCD due to *E. coli* K99, amoxicillin as the first choice and sulfonamides with trimethoprim as the second choice for oral and parenteral treatment are recommended. Neomycin and amoxicillin with clavulanic acid can be used as the third choice for oral treatment. Colistine and quinolones are recommended for restricted use only after culture and sensitivity, and the use of cephalosporins is strictly discouraged due to their low concentrations in the intestinal tract [29].

Outside the EU, Berchtold and Constable (2008) and Constable (2009) propose amoxicillin, ampicillin, and potentiated sulfonamides as first-choice antibiotics for parenteral administration in patients suffering from NCD. For oral administration, amoxicillin or amoxicillin/clavulanate potassium has been recommended. The second choice of antibiotics is third- and fourth-generation cephalosporins, such as ceftiofur and cefquinome. The last-choice antibiotics are fluoroquinolones, which should only be used for the treatment of *E. coli* diarrhea and salmonellosis in calves [19–21].

The British Veterinary Association (BVA, London, United Kingdom) has recommended minimal use of third and fourth-generation cephalosporins, fluoroquinolones, and colistin [10]. These drugs should only be used where they have been demonstrated by sensitivity testing to be the only suitable choice to avoid unnecessary suffering.

Unfortunately, even in the absence of known disease, antibiotics are used extensively in calves for both therapeutic and prophylactic purposes worldwide [14,30]. Although selling milk replacer containing antibiotics has been prohibited in the European Union for almost 30 years, it is still common practice in many countries to feed calves prophylactically with medicated milk replacers containing antibiotic agents such as oxytetracycline and neomycin [1,31–35]. In 2012, a Belgian study reported that a reduction in oral antibiotic group treatments for prophylactic and metaphylactic reasons would be the simplest and probably the most efficient way to achieve a reduction in antibiotic use in the veal industry [36].

There is a potential misuse of antibiotics occurring in extra-label use, including with highest priority critically important antimicrobials (HPCIA). These HPCIA contain the antibiotic classes fluoroquinolones, cephalosporins (third and higher generations), macrolides and ketolides, glycopeptides, and polymyxin [37]. Each antibiotic preparation is labeled for certain therapeutic indications. Any deviation and thus extra-label use has to be dictated by a veterinarian and must be justified [10]. It is only allowed in the event of a therapeutic emergency and must not result in violative usage in food-producing animals [38]. According to several international guidelines [10,39,40], extra-label use must be reserved for exceptional circumstances, following appropriate sensitivity testing, and the usage of HPCIA must be restricted for use as a last resort under veterinary direction. However, the extra-label use of antibiotics administered by the farmer and mandated by the veterinarians is reported [1]. Although several antibiotic classes are labeled for treatment of diarrhea in calves [21], extra-label use such as the use of spectinomycin solely or in combination with oxytetracycline in calves is observed quite often as this combination is widely used on farms to prevent diarrhea [1,41,42]. Other recommend antibiotics include ceftiofur hydrochloride for the treatment of diarrhea [31,34]. Macrolides were used in 11% of the cases, where oral antibiotics were administered as treatment [43]. In Sweden, streptomycin is occasionally used to treat diarrhea in calves [44]. Constable et al. (2009) propose that the extra-label use is justified for the treatment of calf diarrhea due to the lack of published studies documenting the clinical efficacy of antibiotics with a label claim for the treatment of calf diarrhea and because of the life-threatening situations that can occur in calves with diarrhea [19]. According to Mohler et al. (2019), most of the drugs effective against Gram-negative bacteria are not labeled for the dose rate that provides therapeutic drug concentrations [45].

It is also reported that calves treated for diarrhea frequently received more than one type of antibiotic agent [14]. Additionally, there is a tendency to rely on personal experience for antibiotic usage and dosage [34,46].

*1.3. Aim of the Study*

There is little information available about decision-making processes concerning the use of antibiotics in treating calves with diarrhea. The aim of our study was to describe the treatment of neonatal calf diarrhea in the four different European countries, Austria, Belgium, Portugal, and Scotland, as part of the United Kingdom, using an online survey. In this part of the study, we focused on specifying factors influencing decision-making in veterinarians and farmers concerning the use of antibiotics. We also compare antibiotic treatment regimens to scientific best practices and national guidelines.

## 2. Results

*2.1. Respondent Characteristics*

A total of 873 questionnaires (Austria: 547, Belgium: 92, Portugal: 163, Scotland: 71) were included in the analysis. Of those, 597 were answered by farmers (female: 138, male: 458, N/A: 1) and 276 by veterinarians (female: 83, male: 192, N/A: 1). Based on the results of Vetsurvey 2018 (total numbers of veterinarians in each country), 17.6% of the veterinarians in Austria, 1.4% in Belgium, 2.6% in Portugal, and 0.3% in the United Kingdom participated in our study [47]. The age of the participants ranged from 18 to 75 years ($n = 870$, $32.9 \pm 13.3$; 30 years; mean $\pm$ SD; median). Most of the participants were Austrian farmers ($n = 446$) with a median age of 25 years. In terms of experience, 23.1% of the participants were working with both dairy and beef cattle (called mixed in the following text), 55.5% were mainly working with dairy cattle, and 21.2% with beef cattle only ($n = 872$).

*2.2. Use of Antibiotics for the Treatment of NCD*

As shown in Figure 1, 458 participants out of 873 stated that they used antibiotics in calves suffering from NCD. Country was the most important variable (normalized weight 100%) for the differentiation of antibiotic use in calves with NCD, followed by occupation and age (91.1% and 46.1%). Experience only accounted for 10.9% and sex for 0.3% in normalized weight. Austrian veterinarians and farmers used significantly fewer antibiotics than participants from the other countries. Based on occupation, Austrian farmers administered fewer antibiotics compared to veterinarians.

Logistic regression analysis showed a significant impact of age on the probability of antibiotic use for the treatment of NCD in veterinarians (Figure 2, intercept = 2.45; slope = $-0.026$; $p = 0.031$). The younger the veterinarians were, the higher the probability of using antibiotics. However, even in older veterinarians, the probability was still over 60%. Regarding the use of HPCIA, there was no significant relation with age in veterinarians.

*2.3. Situations Where Antibiotics Are Being Used*

Of the 458 respondents using antibiotics for the treatment of NCD, 404 participants provided more information in the question "if you usually use antibiotics-please state when" and "please state approximate %". Of those, 30.7% ($n = 124$) stated that they used antibiotics always and 69.3% ($n = 277$) in some situations (Figure S1), namely in an average of 48.5% ± 28.7% (median 50%). CART analysis resulted in the country as the most important factor to classify the frequency of antibiotic use, followed by experience with normalized importance of 68.6%, age (42.3%), occupation (7.1%), and sex (4.5%). Participants from Portugal and Scotland used antibiotics significantly more frequently in every case without differentiating further (in some situations: 54.1%, $n = 92$; always: 45.9%, $n = 78$) compared to respondents from Austria and Belgium (in some situations: 80.3%, $n = 188$; always: 19.7%, $n = 46$). Out of the total of 88 respondents working with beef cattle in Scotland and Portugal, 65 (farmers and veterinarians) used antibiotics for the treatment of NCD, and 44% of those ($n = 39$) stated that they used them always when treating NCD. Participants younger than 41.5 years working with dairy cattle and mixed cattle used antibiotics significantly more often in every case of NCD compared to older participants (>41.5 years).

A total of 227 participants specified the situations when they used antibiotics in treating NCD. Most of the participants ($n = 183$) said that they used them in calves with NCD when their body temperatures were above normal (>39.5 °C) or when they had blood in the feces (hematochezia, $n = 164$). Calves suffering from NCD that had very watery diarrhea or were not able to stand were treated with antibiotics by 157 and 137 participants, respectively. Absence of suckling reflex ($n = 101$), sunken eyes ($n = 82$), cold mouth ($n = 79$), and an internal temperature below normal (hypothermia, <38.0 °C, $n = 65$) were used less frequently as indication to use antibiotics.

The question "specify the situation: others" was a free text answer and was answered by 22 participants. They stated that they used antibiotics in the following situations: dehydration, mucosal shreds in the feces or signs of sepsis (e.g., increased episcleral vascular injection), if homeopathy does not help, when the duration of diarrhea is longer than two days, another organ is affected (e.g., bronchitis), a negative result of rota- and coronavirus rapid test, based on the appearance of the stool, if *E. coli* or *Salmonella* infection are suspected and one participant stated that this depended on the calf's age.

Pearson chi-square test revealed that, compared to veterinarians, farmers administered significantly more often antibiotics when calves had watery feces ($p = 0.016$), whereas veterinarians chose to administer antibiotics when the calves were not suckling ($p = 0.014$), had sunken eyes ($p = 0.001$), a body temperature above or below normal ($p < 0.001$ and $p = 0.017$, respectively) and blood in the feces ($p = 0.001$). Based on CART analysis, body temperature above normal was the most important factor comparing veterinarians and farmers: 114 of 132 (86.3%) veterinarians and 69 of 154 farmers (44.8%) said that they used antibiotics in this case.

Women stated significantly more often that they would use antibiotics when body temperature was above normal compared to men ($p = 0.007$). Participants working with beef cattle administered significantly more antibiotics compared to participants working with dairy cattle or in the mixed sector ($p < 0.0001$); regarding the use of HPCIA, there was no difference. Participants working with dairy used significantly fewer antibiotics in calves with a body temperature above normal ($p = 0.003$).

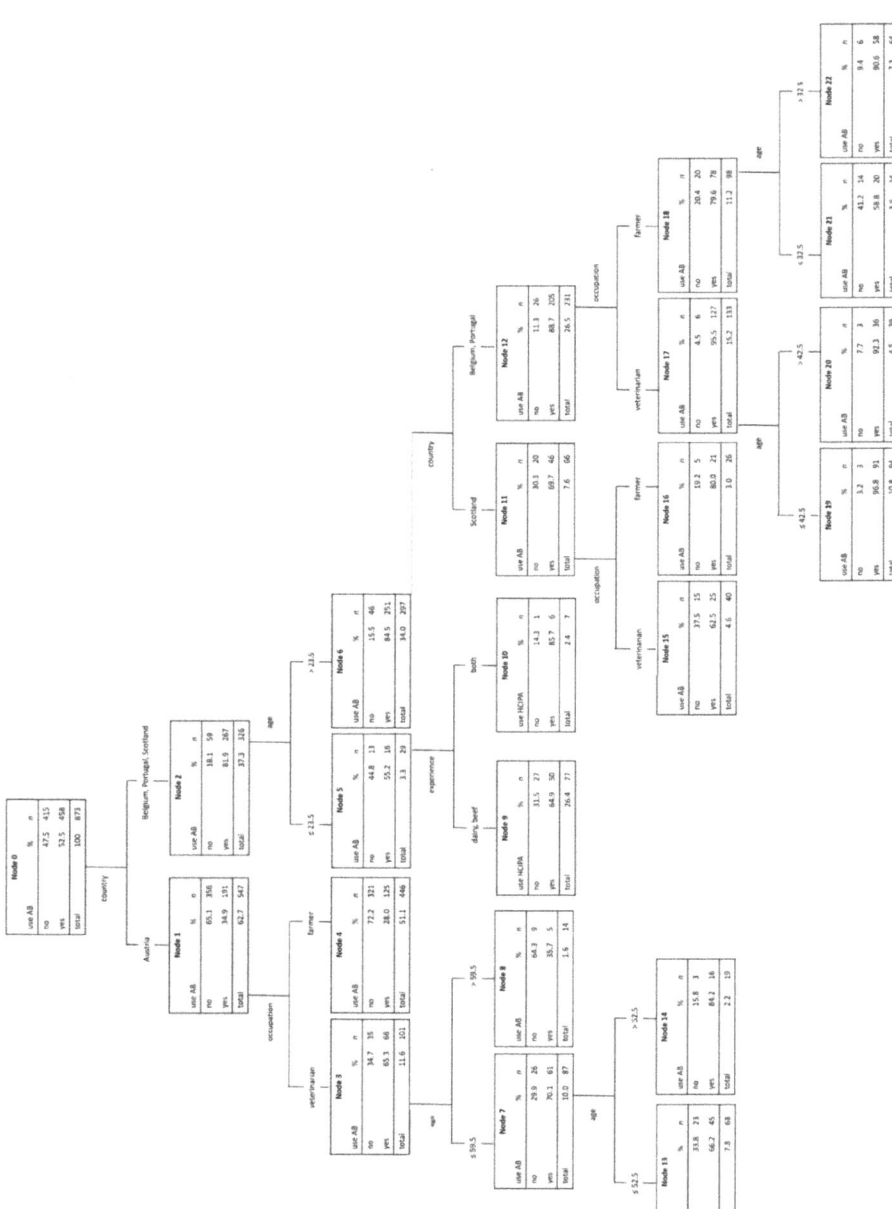

**Figure 1.** CART: Association of different factors on the use of antibiotics for the treatment of NCD.

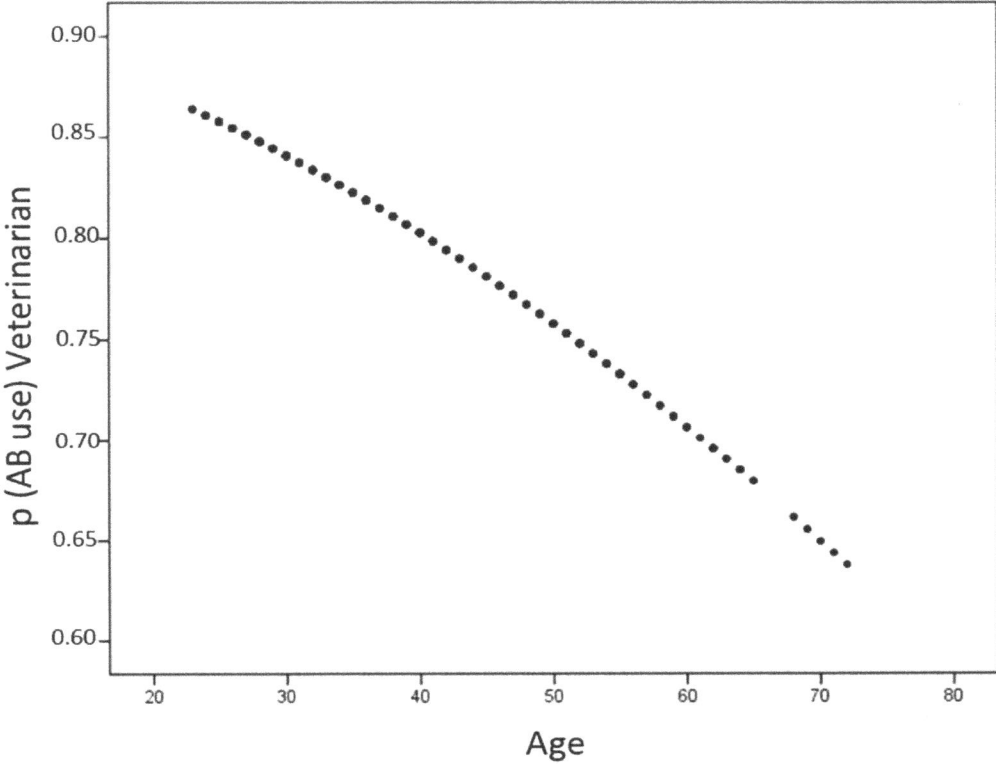

**Figure 2.** The probability of veterinarians using an antibiotic for the treatment of NCD depended on their age.

*2.4. Antibiotic Classes as First, Second, or Third Choice*

When farmers and veterinarians were asked, "Which antibiotic do you use as first, second, and third choice for the treatment of calves with diarrhea?", quinolones, sulfonamides, and penicillins were the three antibiotic classes most frequently named in all three choice categories (Figure 3). All antibiotics that were stated in this questionnaire were licensed for use in cattle, but several were not licensed for the treatment of diarrhea in calves specifically, including ceftiofur and cefoperazon (third generation cephalosporins), tulathromycin and tilmicosin (macrolids), as well as florfenicol (fenicoles). All used quinolones were licensed for cattle and most of them for treatment of infections of the gastrointestinal tract caused by enrofloxacin, danofloxacin, or flumequin susceptible strains of *E. coli* (e.g., Advocid®, Enrosleecol®, Fluyesyva inyectable®). However, several marbofloxacin drugs (e.g., Marbocyl®, Marbosyva®, Marbox®, Ubiflox®) were stated as well, although they were only licensed for the treatment of mastitis and respiratory infections.

Some participants stated registered trade names that did not contain antibiotics but could be used for treating calves with NCD, for example, NSAIDs (Tolfedine®), parasympatholytics (Buscopan®), oral rehydration solutions (Elektrydal®, Nutrivet total®) and antiparasitic drugs (Baycox®, Halocur®).

## 2.5. Use of Oral and Injectable Antibiotics

In questions 6 and 7, participants were asked if they used oral and/or injectable antibiotics as treatment in calves with diarrhea. The highest proportions of respondents stated they would use injectable antibiotics (Table 2).

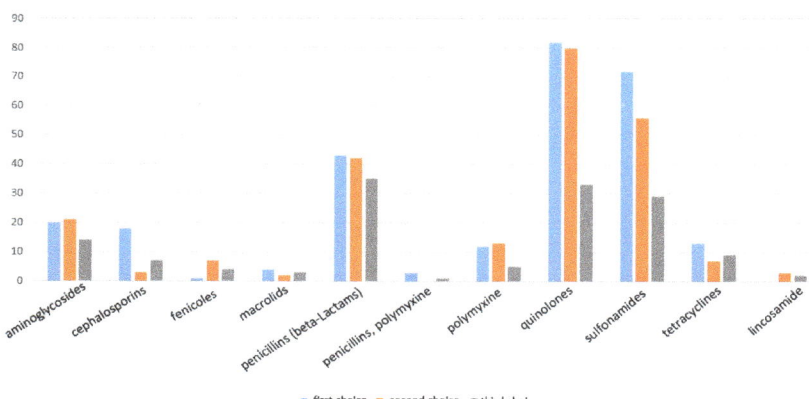

**Figure 3.** Use of antibiotic classes as first, second, or third choice.

**Table 2.** Number of participants using oral and injectable antibiotics by occupation and experience.

| Professional Group | Oral Antibiotic | Injectable Antibiotic | Total Answers |
|---|---|---|---|
| Beef veterinarians | 21 | 56 | 67 |
| Dairy veterinarians | 36 | 67 | 98 |
| Mixed veterinarians | 43 | 76 | 110 |
| Beef farmer | 18 | 54 | 118 |
| Dairy farmer | 47 | 116 | 387 |
| Mixed farmer | 17 | 18 | 91 |

## 2.6. Use of HPCIA for Treatment of NCD

The majority (206 out of 291) of participants who answered questions on the type of antibiotic they were giving to calves with NCD named at least one class of HPCIA as their choice (Figure 4). Again, country was by far the most important factor for differentiating the use of HPCIA. In relation to country, the normalized importance of sex, age, experience, and occupation accounted for only 27.6%, 21.0%, 20.5%, and 16.8%, respectively. Veterinarians and farmers in Scotland named significantly fewer brands of HPCIA drugs compared to participants in Austria, Belgium, and Portugal. Based on sex, Scottish women used HPCIA significantly more often than men.

## 2.7. Use of HPCIA According to Situation

Almost 70% of the participants named at least one HPCIA as the drug of choice for the treatment of NCD when they also chose "calves had a body temperature above normal" as the reason for antibiotic treatment. Approximately 60% named HPCIA and chose calves suffering from watery diarrhea as reason, whereas 50% named HPCIA as the drug of choice and chose calves that were not standing or had bloody feces as a reason to administer antibiotics. Based on CART results, "body temperature above normal" received the highest importance for the decision to administer HPCIA, followed by watery feces (19.1%) and sunken eyes (11.1%). The absence of a suckling reflex (84.3%), blood in the feces (65.2%), body temperature below normal (54.9%), and cold mouth (16.4%) were chosen as a reason for antibiotic treatment by more participants who did not name an HPCIA as the drug of choice.

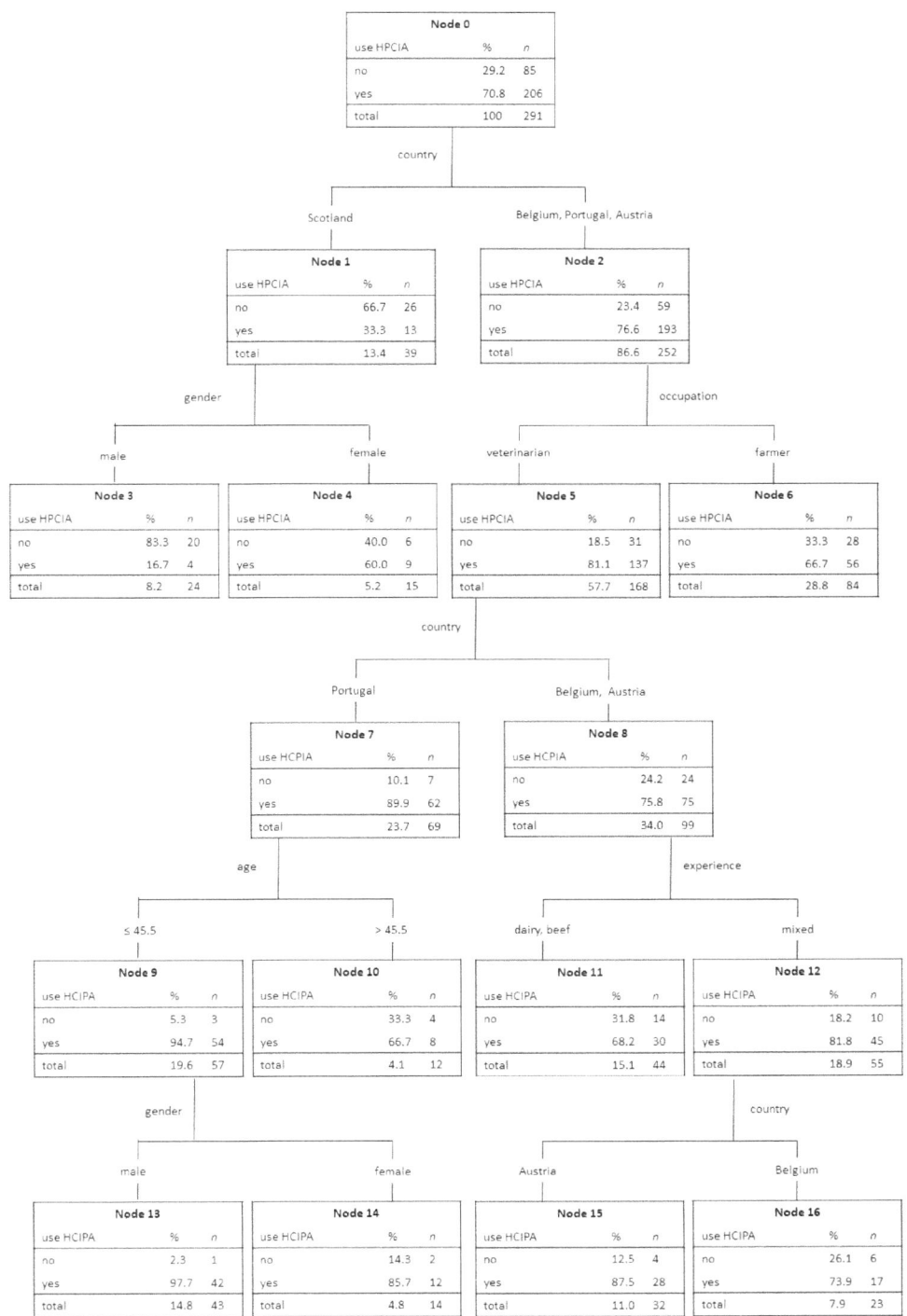

**Figure 4.** CART: Association of different factors on the use of HPCIA for the treatment of NCD.

## 3. Discussion

This survey was carried out to gain insight into the factors that would influence the decision of veterinarians and farmers in four different European countries on whether or not to use antibiotics for the treatment of NCD. The survey was conducted with veterinarians and farmers volunteering to answer the questionnaire, thus yielding different amounts of participants from each country.

Over 50% of respondents of the survey stated that they used antibiotics in calves affected by NCD. Some people even stated that they use them always, and others used them about half of the time. The use of antibiotics to treat NCD might not be necessary: most cases of NCD are caused by viral and parasitic pathogens, with *E. coli* K99 being the third most prevalent infectious agent in NCD worldwide [48–50]. Therefore, blanket antibiotic treatment of NCD should be strongly discouraged.

Aside from bacterial pathogens as a cause of NCD, calves that are affected by septicemia as a result of NCD must be treated using antibiotics. Studies have shown that severely ill calves may be bacteremic and, as a result, septic, especially if they are very young (<5 days) and affected by the failure of passive transfer of immunity [50–53]. Bacteremia cannot be diagnosed based on clinical signs; it may be detectable if it occurs in connection with constant bacteriuria using a catalase-based calf-side urine test [18]. However, septicemia, the systemic inflammatory response (SIRS), can be diagnosed by performing a thorough clinical examination [53–55]. Trefz et al. (2016) based clinical evidence of septicemia on marked hyperaemia of mucous membranes, congestion/injection of episcleral vessels, mucosal or subscleral bleeding, or hypopyon. The authors assumed the presence of SIRS in calves with two of the clinical criteria hyperthermia or hypothermia (reference interval, 38.5–39.5 °C), tachycardia (>120 beats/min), and tachypnoea (>36 breaths/min) [56]. Constable (2004) stated that potential *E. coli* bacteremia should be treated in calves with diarrhea that have a reduced suckle reflex, marked dehydration, weakness, inability to stand, or clinical depression [21]. Most participants of our study specified fever and hematochezia as an indication to administer antibiotics to calves suffering from NCD. Both could be signs of sepsis and the disruption of the blood-gut barrier and are therefore reasonable choices [13,53,54]. The same two clinical signs, fever and hematochezia, were used to develop a simple algorithm for the treatment of calves affected by NCD, which lead to a significant reduction in antibiotic use with no changes in morbidity and mortality [13].

Interestingly, hypothermia, or cold mouth as a sign of it, was chosen by the fewest participants as reasons for antibiotic treatment [13]. Of course, those signs, such as sunken eyes and very watery diarrhea, could be related to dehydration and do not necessarily warrant the use of antibiotics, along with the inability to stand or suckle, which could be due to D-lactic acidosis [57]. Some participants even pointed out that factors such as the duration of sickness or color of feces play a significant role as well. Such findings show the urgent need for implementing an algorithm for treating NCD and restricting antibiotic use to calves with defined clinical symptoms.

Using the above-mentioned clinical signs as guidance for treatment decisions in calves with NCD together with commercially available rapid/point-of-care tests would be a valuable contribution to the reduction in antibiotic use in calves [15–17]. In the authors' opinion, there is a real need for well-constructed intervention studies testing treatments alongside recorded clinical signs and secondary factors. Additionally, the impact of antibiotic treatment and the consequences for the gastrointestinal microbiome need to be characterized further.

To the authors' knowledge, there are no studies investigating clinical signs in calves with NCD and benefits from antibiotic treatment. It has been observed that veterinarians use several factors to make the decision to use a certain antibiotic drug. Clinical factors such as clinical signs, expected pathogen, the spectrum of activity of the drug, experience using the drug on own farm, response to previous therapy, ease of administration, the farmer's ability to administer the drug, recommended frequency of treatment, and drugs cost were their main reasons for choosing an antibiotic drug over another [58–60].

However, non-clinical drivers such as the veterinarian-farmer relationship were just as relevant [58,61,62] and could play a further role in the increased use of antibiotics by veterinarians. Fear of unsuccessful treatment, lack of confidence in the diagnosis, and dairy farmer's demands are the major influencers for veterinarians' antibiotic use even in conditions not requiring antibiotic use. An increased workload can also play an important role, as veterinarians fear to revisit when the animal did not improve after the first treatment, and they are called again [58]. Furthermore, veterinarians fear they will be blamed if antibiotics later prove necessary [58,63]. Similar results are reported in a Dutch study in 2015, where veterinarians confirmed that the perceived pressure from clients can be a driver for antibiotic use [61].

Farmers from Austria, Belgium, and Portugal administered significantly fewer antibiotics and HPCIA compared to veterinarians. This could be due to legislation in Austria, with the largest proportion of farmers participating, where veterinarians must see an animal before prescribing antibiotics for this specific animal only. Therefore, it would be common for farmers not to have antibiotics in stock because they would not be allowed to make treatment decisions without a veterinarian. In a study from New Zealand, farmers stated that the most important factor (besides the veterinarian's advice) for the selection of antibiotics was their own experience [59]. Meanwhile, apart from themselves, veterinarians identified farmers as the people having the most important role in responsible antibiotic use, especially as it is often farmers who make the treatment decisions on-farm. Therefore, it is necessary to make sure they are sufficiently informed about the etiology of calf diarrhea and the use of HPCIA, and they understand antibiotics classes, indications, and dosages [43]. However, some farmers in our study named drugs such as butylscopolamine bromide and metamizole, as well as oral electrolytes as antibiotic agents in questions 19 to 21. This may occur because some farmers do not know the pharmacological properties of drugs they use for treating sick calves or because they misunderstood the question. According to Sawant et al. (2005), the main reasons for farmer's misuse of antibiotics on-farm are failure to consult a veterinarian for treating sick animals, absence of antibiotic treatment records, and lack of written protocols for treating sick animals [1]. Such often simple and cost-effective treatment protocols or algorithms for antibiotic selection for diarrhoeic calves have been proved successful as means of a reduction in antibiotics usage as these guidelines lead to a more rational use [13,27].

In several European countries, national and international bodies have developed and issued a variety of recommendations and treatment guidelines in recent years to reduce inappropriate prescribing and antibiotic use [7,10,11]. However, there is no widely agreed simple guide for farmers and vets for NCD treatment to help reduce antimicrobial resistance. An example of such a guide can be found in the Teagasc Calf Rearing Manual [64].

The effectiveness of such guidelines is questionable: although 90% of bovine veterinarians stated that they read cattle-related journals regularly, official reports were considered less popular information sources [65]. Instead, practitioners said they value training/literature, experience, label, sensitivity testing results, and universities as the most important information sources, which influenced their antibiotic prescribing behaviors. Almost 80% of the veterinarians frequently participated in cattle medicine-trainings such as meetings, workshops, and congresses [65]. Therefore, continuing veterinary education of veterinarians, who are the first line of information to farmers, is a key to reducing antibiotic use and, particularly, those HPCIA [13].

Besides country, age was the second most important factor regarding normalized weight. The median age of 30 years of all participants in our study may be because younger people were more likely to fill out an online survey than older people, who prefer paper and pencil surveys [66]. We suspect that older farmers asked their more technology-experienced children for help filling in the online questionnaire, who then stated their own data (e.g., age, sex).

The probability of using an antibiotic for the treatment of NCD decreased with increasing age in veterinarians. Krupat et al. (2000) found out that human patients were more satisfied with physicians whose orientation was congruent with theirs than those who had a different opinion [67]. However, older and more experienced physicians were better able to refuse patients' demands [68,69]. Although those studies apply to human medicine, it is reasonable to assume that veterinarians are subject to the same mechanisms in the veterinarian-client interaction and that older veterinarians are more likely to follow treatment plans that they consider most appropriate.

One of the most important factors in veterinarians governing the selection of an antibiotic for treatment is their own experience [46,59,63]. The lack of experience and confidence might be a reason for a higher amount of antibiotics used for the treatment of NCD carried out by younger colleagues. A small survey including staff of a veterinary teaching hospital in the U.S. showed that veterinarians who graduated after 1999 were less concerned about antibiotic resistance and judicious use of antibiotics than older colleagues [60]. Such an attitude could reflect an inadequate emphasis on training of our younger graduates in some schools more focused on small animal cases [60,70].

Fluoroquinolones, sulfonamides, and penicillins were the most frequently specified classes for the antibiotic treatment of NCD in our study. This outcome is similar to previous studies [31,34], including an Italian survey, where quinolones were quoted by 54% of the surveyed veterinarians as their first choice and by 38% as their second choice for the treatment of diarrhea in calves [65]. A study carried out in Switzerland showed that the common treatment of calf diarrhea consisted of fluoroquinolones, which were used in 47% of the parenteral treatments [43]. These results indicate that there is a variety of antibiotics and HPCIA that are used for the treatment of NCD, despite questionable efficacy [57]. Antibiotics should only be used in calves suffering from NCD that are also affected by Gram-negative septicemia, mainly caused by *E. coli* [19,21]. As mentioned previously, studies differentiating infectious agents responsible for NCD show that *E. coli* only affects a small proportion of calves, making it only the third most prevalent cause of NCD worldwide [48,49]. Aggravatingly, as already mentioned, there is a lack of well design studies to determine the most effective antibiotic treatment for Gram-negative septicemia in calves suffering from NCD.

Several antibiotics that are not licensed for use in NCD treatment were cited from veterinarians and farmers as first, second, or third choice in this study. The reason for this is probably be found in the lack of knowledge on licensed indications. This leads to extra-label use and treatment decisions, which are based on beliefs of efficacy rather than science [71]. Many practices adopted in the field are not evidence-based. A reason for the frequent choice of quinolones as the second or third choice may be based on the fear of septicemia when a non-HPCIA does not work as a drug of first choice.

Veterinarians from Scotland stated less HPCIA as drugs of choice in calves with NCD. This could be due to a better understanding of the prudent use of antibiotics, as implemented in the Red Tractor program [72]. Herein, among other measures, the use of HPCIA is only allowed as a last resort under veterinary direction, backed up by sensitivity or diagnostic testing. Antibiotic failures must be discussed. Staff, which is responsible for medicine administration, is instructed to attend training courses (handling, correct administration storage conditions, purchasing routes). In the case of non-conformance, including repeated use of HPCIA without testing, there is an impact on certification.

Our study shows clearly that similar programs need to be implemented in all European countries to increase the awareness of prudent antibiotic use in the farming and veterinary community.

## 4. Materials and Methods

### 4.1. Questionnaire

A questionnaire (http://biosegur.fmv.ulisboa.pt/index.php/356164/lang-en) (access date 25 June 2021) was designed by RB for collecting information on the treatment of neonatal calf diarrhea (NCD). The questionnaire was translated and made available to veterinarians and dairy and beef farmers in Portugal (RB), Belgium (HG), Scotland (LV), Austria, and adjacent German-speaking countries (summarized to Austria in the following text; AH). The surveys were conducted for a limited number of weeks per country from February 2016 until January 2019. The veterinarians and farmers were informed via newsletters and through e-mails from various organizations (e.g., vet board) or during conferences. The survey was available online, and some questionnaires were filled out during farm visits or by veterinarians at a conference or over the phone. The entire questionnaire covered many aspects of medical treatment of NCD and husbandry practices regarding sick calves. The part applying to antibiotic treatment consisted of a maximum of 21 questions (Table 2). The questionnaire included 'yes' or 'no' questions, single- and multiple-choice questions, as well as open-ended questions. For questions 19 to 21 (first-, second-, and third-choice antibiotics), commercial names or drug names were accepted as possible answers. To decrease reactance, the forced-choice answer format was avoided; therefore, the number of responses per question varies.

All questionnaires were individually examined for aberrant results and plausibility before statistical analyses. In order for questionnaires to be included in the study, 2 out of 4 personal questions (Table 3 question 1–4) and at least one technical question had to be answered.

Table 3. Questions of the survey relevant for the use of antibiotics in treating NCD.

| Number | Question | Answer Options |
|---|---|---|
| 1 | Country | Individual answer |
| 2 | Profession | Veterinarian/farmer |
| 3 | Age | Individual answer |
| 4 | Sex | Female/male |
| 5 | Type of animal you have more experience with | Dairy/beef |
| 6 | In your approach to calves with diarrhea, do you usually use as treatment: oral antibiotic | Yes/no |
| 7 | In your approach to calves with diarrhea, do you usually use as treatment: injectable antibiotic | Yes/no |
| 8 | If you usually use antibiotics, please state when | Individual answer |
| 9 | Please state approximate % | Individual answer |
| 10 | Specify the situations: calf is not standing | Yes/no |
| 11 | Specify the situations: calf has no sucking reflex | Yes/no |
| 12 | Specify the situations: calf has sunken eyes | Yes/no |
| 13 | Specify the situations: calf has watery diarrhea | Yes/no |
| 14 | Specify the situations: calf has rectal temperature below normal (<38.0 °C) | Yes/no |
| 15 | Specify the situations: cold mouth/cold extremities | Yes/no |
| 16 | Specify the situations: calf has rectal temperature above normal (>39.5 °C) | Yes/no |
| 17 | Specify the situations: calf has blood in the faces | Yes/no |
| 18 | Specify the situations: other | Individual answer |
| 19 | What are the brand names of the antibiotics you most frequently use: 1st choice | Individual answer |
| 20 | What are the brand names of the antibiotics you most frequently use: 2nd option | Individual answer |
| 21 | What are the brand names of the antibiotics you most frequently use: 3rd option | Individual answer |

### 4.2. Data Analysis

All statistical analyses were performed using IBM SPSS v24. Differences in frequency distributions were analyzed using Pearson's chi-square test. Logistic regression analysis was performed to model the impact of age on the probability of antibiotic use. Classification and regression tree (CART) analyses were carried out to predict the use of antibiotics, HPCIA, and the frequency of antibiotics use based on the given information's about participants (country, occupation, experience, sex, and age) or signs (e.g., bloody feces, sucking reflex, temperature above or below normal). Every factor that is added to the model receives a value for its importance within the classification process. The importance is calculated using the GINI-Index. As a result, the importance of each factor is given in percentages in relation to the most important factor (normalized importance). Trees were pruned to avoid too complex trees. As a stopping rule, the minimal size for parent nodes was set to 25, the minimal size for child nodes was set to 10. For all analyses a $p$-value below 5% ($p < 0.05$) was seen as significant.

## 5. Conclusions

This study illustrates that there may be excessive use of antibiotics and HPCIA for the treatment of NCD. The younger the veterinarians were, the higher the probability of using antibiotics. Even in older veterinarians, the probability of using antibiotics was still over 60%. Most respondents stated that they would choose to administer antibiotics in calves with fever and bloody feces, which could be indicators for sepsis and indeed warrant antibiotic use. However, it is very likely that antibiotic use could be substantially decreased in the treatment of calves with NCD implementing specific guidelines and targeted training for veterinarians and farmers. Even without better scientific evidence, it is clear that many veterinarians and associated farmers are not applying best practice and agreed overall guidance similar to that seen in SCOPs (Sustainable Control of Parasites in Sheep) for anthelmintics in the U.K. is sorely needed.

**Supplementary Materials:** The following are available online at https://www.mdpi.com/article/10.3390/antibiotics10080910/s1, Figure S1: CART: Association of different factors on the use of antibiotics according to the question "If you usually use antimicrobials, please state when".

**Author Contributions:** Conceptualization, R.B., L.V., H.G., J.F., J.W., and A.H.; methodology, R.B., L.V., H.G., J.F., J.W., and A.H.; software, R.B.; validation, R.B., L.V., H.G., J.F., J.W., and A.H.; formal analysis, C.E., A.T., and A.H.; investigation, C.E. and A.H.; resources, R.B., L.V., H.G., and A.H.; data curation, C.E. and A.T.; writing—original draft preparation, C.E. and A.H.; writing—review and editing, R.B., L.V., H.G., C.E., and A.H.; visualization, C.E., A.T., and A.H.; supervision, A.H.; project administration, C.E., R.B., L.V., H.G., and A.H. All authors have read and agreed to the published version of the manuscript.

**Funding:** Open Access Funding by the University of Veterinary Medicine Vienna, the Universidade de Lisboa, the University of Glasgow and the University of Liège.

**Institutional Review Board Statement:** Not applicable.

**Informed Consent Statement:** Not applicable.

**Data Availability Statement:** The data presented in this study are available upon request.

**Acknowledgments:** We want to thank all the participating veterinarians and farmers in Austria, Belgium, Portugal, and Scotland. Furthermore, we are very grateful for the help of Sarah Michel, Niall Boyd, and David Logue for their precious contribution.

**Conflicts of Interest:** The authors declare no conflict of interest.

## References

1. Sawant, A.A.; Sordillo, L.M.; Jayarao, B.M. A Survey on Antibiotic Usage in Dairy Herds in Pennsylvania. *J. Dairy Sci.* **2005**, *88*, 2991–2999. [CrossRef]
2. Klein-Jöbstl, D.; Iwersen, M. Farm characteristics and calf management practices on dairy farms with and without diarrhea: A case-control study to investigate risk factors for calf diarrhea. *J. Dairy Sci.* **2014**, *97*, 5110–5119. [CrossRef] [PubMed]
3. Council Directive 2008/119/EC Laying Down Minimum Standards for the Protection of Calves. Available online: https://eur-lex.europa.eu/legal-content/EN/TXT/PDF/?uri=CELEX:32008L0119&from=EN (accessed on 30 April 2021).
4. Veterinär-Arzneispezialitäten-Anwendungsverordnung 2010BGBl. II Nr. 137/2017. Available online: https://www.ris.bka.gv.at/eli/bgbl/II/2017/137 (accessed on 30 April 2021).

5. Royal Decree. Available online: http://www.ejustice.just.fgov.be/cgi_loi/change_lg.pl?language=fr&la=F&cn=2016072106&table_name=loi (accessed on 30 April 2021).
6. RCVS, Code of Professional Conduct for Veterinary Surgeon, Veterinary Care. Available online: https://www.rcvs.org.uk/setting-standards/advice-and-guidance/code-of-professional-conduct-for-veterinary-surgeons/supporting-guidance/veterinary-medicines/ (accessed on 30 April 2021).
7. Leitlinien Für Den Sorgfältigen Umgang Mit Antibakteriell Wirksamen Tierarzneimitteln (BMASGK-74330/0008-IX/B/15/2018, AVN Nr. 2018/11a). Available online: https://www.ris.bka.gv.at/Dokumente/Avn/AVN_20181129_AVN_2018_11a_2/201811a_AntibiotokaLL_Beilage.pdfsig (accessed on 30 April 2021).
8. Commission Notice—Guidelines for the Prudent Use of Antimicrobials in Veterinary Medicine (2015/C 299/04). Available online: https://ec.europa.eu/health/sites/health/files/antimicrobial_resistance/docs/2015_prudent_use_guidelines_en.pdf (accessed on 30 April 2021).
9. Weese, J.; Giguère, S.; Guardabassi, L.; Morley, P.; Papich, M.; Ricciuto, D.; Sykes, J. ACVIM Consensus Statement on Thera-peutic Antimicrobial Use in Animal. *J. Vet. Intern. Med.* **2015**, *29*, 487–498. [CrossRef] [PubMed]
10. BVA Position on the Responsible Use of Antimicrobials in Food Producing Animals. Available online: https://www.bva.co.uk/media/1161/bva-policy-position-on-the-responsible-use-of-antimicrobials-in-food-producing-animals-1.pdf (accessed on 30 April 2021).
11. Ungemach, F.R.; Müller-Bahrdt, D.; Abraham, G. Guidelines for prudent use of antimicrobials and their implications on antibiotic usage in veterinary medicine. *Int. J. Med. Microbiol.* **2006**, *296*, 33–38. [CrossRef] [PubMed]
12. Hässig, M.; Kretschmar, S. Evidence-based use of antimicrobials in veal calves with diarrhea. *Open J. Vet. Med.* **2016**, *6*, 28–39. [CrossRef]
13. Gomez, D.E.; Arroyo, L.G.; Poljak, Z.; Viel, L.; Weese, J.S. Implementation of an algorithm for selection of antimicrobial therapy for diarrhoeic calves: Impact on antimicrobial treatment rates, health and faecal microbiota. *Vet. J.* **2017**, *226*, 15–25. [CrossRef]
14. Walker, W.L.; Epperson, W.B.; Wittum, T.E.; Lord, L.K.; Rajala-Schultz, P.J.; Lakritz, L. Characteristics of dairy calf ranches: Morbidity, mortality, antibiotic use practices, and biosecurity and biocontainment practices. *J. Dairy Sci.* **2012**, *95*, 2204–2214. [CrossRef]
15. Cho, Y.I.; Sun, D.; Cooper, V.; Dewell, G.; Schwartz, K.; Yoon, K.J. Evaluation of a commercial rapid test kit for detecting bovine enteric pathogens in feces. *J. Vet. Diagn. Investig.* **2012**, *24*, 559–562. [CrossRef]
16. Lichtmannsperger, K.; Hinney, B.; Joachim, A. Molecular characterization of Giardia intestinalis and Cryptosporidium parvum from calves with diarrhoea in Austria and evaluation of point-of-care tests. *Comp. Immunol. Microbiol. Infect. Dis.* **2019**, *66*. [CrossRef] [PubMed]
17. Luginbühl, A.; Reitt, K.; Metzler, A.; Kollbrunner, M.; Corboz, L.; Deplazes, P. Field study of the prevalence and diagnosis of diarrhea-causing agents in the newborn calf in a Swiss veterinary practice area. *Schweiz. Arch. Tierheilkd.* **2005**, *14*, 245–252. [CrossRef]
18. Raboisson, D.; Clement, J.; Queney, N.; Lebreton, P.; Schelcher, F. Detection of bacteriuria and bacteremia in newborn calves by a catalase-based urine test. *J. Vet. Intern. Med.* **2010**, *24*, 1532–1536. [CrossRef]
19. Constable, P.D. Treatment of Calf Diarrhea: Antimicrobial and Ancillary Treatments. *Vet. Clin. Food Anim.* **2009**, *25*, 101–120. [CrossRef] [PubMed]
20. Berchtold, J.F.; Constable, P.D. Antibiotic Treatment of Diarrhea in Preweaned Calves. *Food Ani. Prac.* **2009**, 520–525. [CrossRef]
21. Constable, P.D. Antimicrobial Use in the Treatment of Calf Diarrhea. *J. Vet. Intern. Med.* **2004**, *18*, 8–17. [CrossRef] [PubMed]
22. Gomez, D.E.; Arroyo, L.G.; Costa, M.C.; Viel, L.; Weese, J.S. Characterization of the Fecal Bacterial Microbiota of Healthy and Diarrheic Dairy Calves. *J. Vet. Intern. Med.* **2017**, *31*, 928–939. [CrossRef] [PubMed]
23. Zeineldin, M.; Aldridge, B.; Lowe, J. Dysbiosis of the fecal microbiota in feedlot cattle with hemorrhagic diarrhea. *Microb. Pathog.* **2018**, *115*, 123–130. [CrossRef] [PubMed]
24. Kim, E.T.; Lee, S.J.; Kim, T.Y.; Lee, H.G.; Atikur, R.M.; Gu, B.H.; Kim, D.H.; Park, B.Y.; Son, J.K.; Kim, M.H. Dynamic Changes in Fecal Microbial Communities of Neonatal Dairy Calves by Aging and Diarrhea. *Animals* **2021**, *11*, 1113. [CrossRef] [PubMed]
25. Ma, T.; Villot, C.; Renaud, D.; Skidmore, A.; Chevaux, E.; Steele, M.; Guan, L.L. Linking perturbations to temporal changes in diversity, stability, and compositions of neonatal calf gut microbiota: Prediction of diarrhea. *ISME J.* **2020**, *14*, 2223–2235. [CrossRef] [PubMed]
26. Martin, C.C.; Baccili, C.C.; Avila-Campos, M.; Hurley, D.J.; Gomez, V. Effect of prophylactic use of tulathromycin on gut bacterial populations, inflammatory profile and diarrhea in newborn Holstein calves. *Vet. Sci. Res. J.* **2021**, *136*, 268–276. [CrossRef]
27. Berge, A.B.C.; Moore, D.A.; Besser, T.E.; Sischo, W.M. Targetin therapy to minimize antimicrobial use in preweaned calves: Effects on health, growth, and treatment costs. *J. Dairy Sci.* **2009**, *92*, 4707–4714. [CrossRef]
28. AMCRA. Available online: https://formularium.amcra.be/i/15 (accessed on 30 April 2021).
29. Therapieleitfaden für Tierärztinnen und Tierärzte—Rinder. Available online: https://www.blv.admin.ch\T1\guilsinglrightblv\T1\guilsinglrighttherapieleitfaden-de (accessed on 30 April 2021).
30. Gorbach, S.L. Antimicrobial Use in Animal feed-time to stop. *N. Engl. J. Med.* **2001**, *345*, 1202–1203. [CrossRef]
31. Berge, A.C.B.; Lindeque, P.; Moore, D.A.; Sischo, W.M. A Clinical Trial Evaluating Prophylactic and Therapeutic Antibiotic Use on Health and Performance of Preweaned Calves. *J. Dairy Sci.* **2005**, *88*, 2166–2177. [CrossRef]

32. Donovan, D.C.; Franklin, S.T.; Chase, C.C.L.; Hippen, A.R. Growth and Health of Holstein Calves Fed Milk Replacers Supplemented with Antimicrobials or Enteroguard. *J. Dairy Sci.* **2002**, *85*, 947–950. [CrossRef]
33. Radostits, O.M.; Rhodes, C.S.; Mitchell, M.E.; Spotswood, T.P.; Wenkoff, M.S. A clinical evaluation of antimicrobial agents and temporary starvation in the treatment of acute undifferentiated diarrhea in newborn calves. *Can. Vet. J.* **1975**, *16*, 219–227. [PubMed]
34. Zwald, A.G.; Ruegg, P.L.; Kaneene, J.B.; Warnick, L.D.; Wells, S.J.; Fossler, C.; Halbert, L.W. Management Practices and Reported Antimicrobial Usage on Conventional and Organic Dairy Farms. *J. Dairy Sci.* **2004**, *87*, 191–201. [CrossRef]
35. Thames, C.H.; Pruden, A.; James, R.E.; Ray, P.P.; Knowlton, K.F. Excretion of antibiotic resistance genes by dairy calves fed milk replacers with varying doses of antimicrobials. *Front. Microbiol.* **2012**, *139*, 139. [CrossRef]
36. Pardon, B.; Catry, B.; Dewulf, J.; Persoons, D.; Hostens, M.; De Bleecker, K.; Deprez, P. Prospective study on quantitative and qualitative antimicrobial and anti-inflammatory drug use in white veal calves. *J. Antimicrob. Chemother.* **2012**, *67*, 1027–1038. [CrossRef]
37. WHO List of Critically Important Antimicrobials for Human Medicine (WHO CIA List). Available online: https://www.who.int/foodsafety/publications/cia2017.pdf (accessed on 26 April 2021).
38. Tierarzneimittelkontrollgesetz, Fassung 16.05.2021 (§ 1 Abs 2 Z 2 TAKG). Available online: https://www.ris.bka.gv.at/GeltendeFassung/Bundesnormen/20001741/TAKG%2c%20Fassung%20vom%2016.05.2021.pdf (accessed on 30 April 2021).
39. BVA Policy Position on the Responsible Use of Antimicrobials in Food Producing Animals, Responsibly Use of Antimicrobials in Veterinary Practice: The 7-Point Plan. Available online: https://www.bva.co.uk/resources-support/medicines/responsible-use-of-antimicrobials-in-veterinary-practice-poster/ (accessed on 30 April 2021).
40. Bundes Tierärztekammer: Leitlinien für den Sorgfältigen Umgang Mit Antibakteriell Wirksamen Tierarzneimitteln—Mit Erläuterungen—Beilage Zum Deutschen Tierärzteblatt 3/2015. Available online: https://www.bundestieraerztekammer.de/tieraerzte/leitlinien/ (accessed on 30 April 2021).
41. Barnett, S.; Sischo, W.; Moore, D.; Reynolds, J. Evaluation of flunixin meglumine as an adjunct treatment for diarrhea in dairy calves. *J. Am. Vet. Med. Assoc.* **2003**, *223*, 1329–1333. [CrossRef]
42. Berge, A.B.C.; Moore, D.; Sischo, W. Field Trial Evaluating the Influence of Prophylactic and Therapeutic Antimicrobial Administration on Antimicrobial Resistance of Fecal Escherichia coli in Dairy Calves. *Appl. Environ. Microbiol.* **2006**, *72*, 3872–3878. [CrossRef] [PubMed]
43. Pipoz, F.; Meylan, M. Gesundheit und Antibiotikaverbrauch bei Aufzuchtkälbern in Milchviehbetrieben: Managementfaktoren, Prävalenz und Behandlung von Kälberkrankheiten. *Schweiz. Arch. Tierheilkd.* **2016**, *158*, 389–396.
44. de Verdier, K.; Nyman, A.; Greko, C.; Bengtsson, B. Antimicrobial Resistance and Virulence Factors in Escherichia coli from Swedish Dairy Calves. *Acta Vet. Scan.* **2012**, *54*, 2. [CrossRef]
45. Mohler, V.L.; Izzo, M.M.; House, J.K. Salmonella in Calves. *Vet. Clin. Food Anim.* **2009**, *25*, 37–54. [CrossRef] [PubMed]
46. De Briyne, N.; Atkinson, J.; Pokludová, L.; Borriello, S.P.; Price, S. Factors influencing antibiotic prescribing habits and use of sensitivity testing amongst veterinarians in Europe. *Vet. Rec.* **2013**, *19*, 475. [CrossRef]
47. Vetsurvey 2018. Available online: https://fve.org/publications/european-veterinary-survey-2018-future-veterinarians-younger-and-female/ (accessed on 12 July 2021).
48. Wei, X.; Wang, W.; Dong, Z.; Cheng, F.; Zhou, X.; Li, B.; Zhang, J. Detection of Infectious Agents Causing Neonatal Calf Diarrhea on Two Large Dairy Farms in Yangxin County, Shandong Province, China. *Front. Vet. Sci.* **2021**, *7*, 1256. [CrossRef]
49. Caffarena, R.D.; Casaux, M.L.; Schild, C.O.; Fraga, M.; Castells, M.; Colina, R.; Corbellini, L.G.; Riet-Correa, F.; Giannitti, F. Causes of neonatal calf diarrhea and mortality in pasture-based dairy herds in Uruguay: A farm-matched case-control study. *Braz. J. Microbiol.* **2021**, *52*, 977–988. [CrossRef]
50. Brunauer, M.; Roch, F.F.; Conrady, B. Prevalence of Worldwide Neonatal Calf Diarrhoea Caused by Bovine Rotavirus in Combination with Bovine Coronavirus, *Escherichia coli* K99 and *Cryptosporidium* spp.: A Meta-Analysis. *Animals* **2021**, *11*, 1014. [CrossRef]
51. Fecteau, G.; Van Metre, D.C.; Pare, J.; Smith, B.P.; Higgins, R.; Holmberg, C.A.; Jang, S.; Guterbock, W. Bacteriological culture of blood from critically ill neonatal calves. *Can. Vet. J.* **1997**, *38*, 95–100.
52. Lofstedt, J.; Dohoo, I.R.; Duizer, G. Model to predict septicemia in diarrheic calves. *J. Vet. Int. Med.* **1999**, *13*, 81–88. [CrossRef]
53. Fecteau, G.; Pare, J.; Van Metre, D.C.; Smith, B.P.; Holmberg, C.A.; Guterbock, W.; Jang, S. Use of a clinical sepsis score for predicting bacteremia in neonatal dairy calves on a calf rearing farm. *Can. Vet. J.* **1997**, *38*, 101–104.
54. Jones, G.R.; Lowes, J.A. The systemic inflammatory response syndrome as a predictor of bacteraemia and outcome from sepsis. *QJM* **1996**, *89*, 515–522. [CrossRef] [PubMed]
55. Bonelli, F.; Meucci, V.; Divers, T.J.; Boccardo, A.; Pravettoni, D.; Meylan, M.; Belloli, A.G.; Sgorbini, M. Plasma procalcitonin concentration in healthy calves and those with septic systemic inflammatory response syndrome. *Vet. J.* **2018**, *234*, 61–65. [CrossRef] [PubMed]
56. Trefz, F.M.; Feist, M.; Lorenz, I. Hypoglycaemia in hospitalised neonatal calves: Prevalence, associated conditions and impact on prognosis. *Vet. J.* **2016**, *217*, 103–108. [CrossRef] [PubMed]
57. Trefz, F.M.; Lorch, A.; Feist, M.; Sauter-Louis, C.; Lorenz, I. Construction and validation of a decision tree for treating metabolic acidosis in calves with neonatal diarrhea. *Vet. Res.* **2012**, *8*, 238. [CrossRef] [PubMed]

58. Gibbons, J.F.; Boland, F.; Buckley, J.F.; Butler, F.; Egan, J.; Fanning, S.; Markey, B.K.; Leonard, F.C. Influences on antimicrobial prescribing behaviour of veterinary practitioners in cattle practice in Ireland. *Vet. Rec.* **2013**, *172*, 14. [CrossRef]
59. McDougall, S.; Compton, C.W.R.; Botha, N. Factors influencing antimicrobial prescribing by veterinarians and usage by dairy farmers in New Zealand. *N. Z. Vet. J.* **2017**, *65*, 84–92. [CrossRef] [PubMed]
60. Ekakoro, J.E.; Okafor, C.C. Antimicrobial use practices of veterinary clinicians at a veterinary teaching hospital in the United States. *Vet. Anim. Sci.* **2019**, *7*. [CrossRef]
61. Speksnijder, D.C.; Jaarsma, D.A.C.; Verheij, T.J.M.; Wagenaar, J.A. Attitudes and perceptions of Dutch veterinarians on their role in the reduction of antimicrobial use in farm animals. *Prev. Vet. Med.* **2015**, *121*, 365–373. [CrossRef]
62. Coyne, L.A.; Pinchbeck, G.L.; Williams, N.J.; Smith, R.F.; Dawson, S.; Pearson, R.B.; Latham, S.M. Understanding antimicro-bial use and prescribing behaviours by pig veterinary surgeons and farmers: A qualitative study. *Vet. Rec.* **2014**, *175*, 593. [CrossRef]
63. Vijay, D.; Bedi, J.S.; Dhaka, P.; Singh, R.; Singh, J.; Arora, A.K.; Gill, J.P.S. Knowledge, Attitude, and Practices (KAP) Survey among Veterinarians, and Risk Factors Relating to Antimicrobial Use and Treatment Failure in Dairy Herds of India. *Anti-biotics* **2021**, *10*, 2016.
64. Teagasc Calf Rearing Manual. Available online: https://www.teagasc.ie/publications/2017/teagasc-calf-rearing-manual.php (accessed on 30 April 2021).
65. Busani, L.; Graziani, C.; Franco, A.; Di Egidio, A.; Binkin, N.; Battisti, A. Survey of the knowledge, attitudes and practice of Italian beef and dairy cattle veterinarians concerning the use of antimicrobials. *Vet. Rec.* **2004**, *155*, 733–738. [CrossRef]
66. Mulder, J.; de Bruijne, M. Willingness of Online Respondents to Participate in Alternative Modes of Data Collection. *Surv. Pract.* **2019**, *12*. [CrossRef]
67. Krupat, E.; Rosenkranz, S.L.; Carter, M.Y.; Barnard, K.; Putnam, S.M.; Inui, T.S. The practice orientations of physicians and patients: The effect of doctor–patient congruence on satisfaction. *Patient Educ. Couns.* **2000**, *39*, 49–59. [CrossRef]
68. Stewart, M. Effective physician–patient communication and health outcomes: A review. *Can. Med. Assoc. J.* **1995**, *152*, 1423–1433.
69. Laine, C.; Davidoff, F. Patient-centered medicine. A professional evolution. *J. Am. Med. Assoc.* **1996**, *275*, 152–156. [CrossRef]
70. Prescott, J.F.; Boerlin, P. Antimicrobial use in companion animals and Good Stewardship Practice. *Vet. Rec.* **2016**, *179*, 486–488. [CrossRef]
71. Olsen, A.; Sischo, W.M.; Berge, A.C.B.; Adams-Progar, A.; Moore, D.A. A retrospective cohort study comparing dairy calf treatment decisions by farm personnel with veterinary observations of clinical signs. *J. Dairy Sci.* **2019**, *102*, 6391–6403. [CrossRef]
72. Red Tractor Program. Available online: https://assurance.redtractor.org.uk/contentfiles/Farmers-6910.pdf?_=636585120315070190; https://assurance.redtractor.org.uk/contentfiles/Farmers-6935.pdf?_=636643269105341095 (accessed on 26 April 2021).

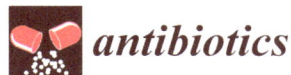

Article

# Antimicrobial Resistance, Serologic and Molecular Characterization of *E. coli* Isolated from Calves with Severe or Fatal Enteritis in Bavaria, Germany

Andrea Feuerstein [1], Nelly Scuda [1], Corinna Klose [1], Angelika Hoffmann [1], Alexander Melchner [2], Kerstin Boll [1], Anna Rettinger [1], Shari Fell [3], Reinhard K. Straubinger [4] and Julia M. Riehm [2,*]

[1] Bavarian Health and Food Safety Authority, 91058 Erlangen, Germany; heubeck.a95@gmail.com (A.F.); Nelly.Scuda@lgl.bayern.de (N.S.); Corinna.klose@lgl.bayern.de (C.K.); Angelika.Hoffmann@lgl.bayern.de (A.H.); Kerstin.Boll@lgl.bayern.de (K.B.); anna.Rettinger@lgl.bayern.de (A.R.)
[2] Bavarian Health and Food Safety Authority, 85764 Oberschleissheim, Germany; alexander.melchner@t-online.de
[3] Chemical and Veterinary Investigation Office, 72488 Sigmaringen, Germany; Shari.Fell@web.de
[4] Department of Veterinary Sciences, Faculty of Veterinary Medicine, Institute of Infectious Diseases and Zoonoses, Ludwig-Maximilians-University, 80539 Munich, Germany; R.Straubinger@lmu.de
* Correspondence: Julia.Riehm@lgl.bayern.de

**Abstract:** Worldwide, enterotoxigenic *Escherichia coli* (ETEC) cause neonatal diarrhea and high mortality rates in newborn calves, leading to great economic losses. In Bavaria, Germany, no recent facts are available regarding the prevalence of virulence factors or antimicrobial resistance of ETEC in calves. Antimicrobial susceptibility of 8713 *E. coli* isolates obtained from 7358 samples of diseased or deceased diarrheic calves were investigated between 2015 to 2019. Considerably high rates of 84.2% multidrug-resistant and 15.8% extensively drug-resistant isolates were detected. The resistance situation of the first, second and third line antimicrobials for the treatment, here amoxicillin-clavulanate, enrofloxacin and trimethoprim-sulfamethoxazole, is currently acceptable with mean non-susceptibility rates of 28.1%, 37.9% and 50.0% over the investigated 5-year period. Furthermore, the ETEC serotypes O101:K28, O9:K35, O101:K30, O101:K32, O78:K80, O139:K82, O8:K87, O141:K85 and O147:K89, as well as the virulence factors F17, F41, F5, ST-I and stx1 were identified in a subset of samples collected in 2019 and 2020. The substantially high rates of multi- and extensively drug-resistant isolates underline the necessity of continuous monitoring regarding antimicrobial resistance to provide reliable prognoses and adjust recommendations for the treatment of bacterial infections in animals.

**Keywords:** *E. coli*; calves; enteritis; antimicrobial resistance; serotypes; virulence; multidrug-resistant; extensively drug-resistant

## 1. Introduction

*Escherichia coli* account to the major enteric and systemic pathogens of the Gram-negative rods within the family Enterobacteriaceae. Most of the *E. coli* colonizing the intestinal tract of animals and humans are commensal, but facultative pathogenic strains may cause intestinal disorder or even severe and life-threatening extraintestinal disease [1,2]. In calves, enterotoxigenic *E. coli* (ETEC) pose a leading cause of intestinal disease, especially within the first four days of life [3–5]. ETEC encode lipopolysaccharide structures (LPS) that may act as endotoxins, fimbrial adhesins and finally enterotoxins. The endotoxins within the blood stream cause fever, damage of endothelial cells and disseminated intravascular coagulation (DIC), that leads to acute shock and sudden death [1]. The serological LPS characterization in calves comprise the *E. coli* serogroups O8, O9 and O101, and respective serotypes O9:K35 and O101:K30, as these are known for endotoxin effect [6]. Further, the serotype O78:K80 plays a major role in systemic disease, septicemia and endotoxic shock of newborn calves [1,6,7]. In piglets, the serotype O141:K85 in combination with F4 fimbria is specific for the postweaning diarrhea syndrome [6]. As well, three further serotypes O139:K82, O8:K87 and O147:K89 play an important role as pathogens for swine [6,8]. Proteinaceous fimbrial adhesins precipitate the bacterial attachment to the enteric mucosa that avert the mechanical shedding of virulent strains from the gut by peristalsis [1,4,9]. Former studies showed that the fimbrial adhesins F5, F17 and F41 are associated with calf diarrhea [4]. For ETEC, two different types of enterotoxins contribute to diarrhea in calves, the heat-stable toxin (ST) and heat-labile toxin (LT), respectively [1,10,11]. On a molecular level, the toxins increase the second messengers cyclic adenosine/ guanosine monophosphate (cAMP/cGMP), that effect an active secretion of fluid and electrolytes in the small intestine leading to extreme loss of fluid within the organism [11,12]. Further, ruminants are known to be a major reservoir of human pathogenic Shiga toxin-producing *E. coli* (STEC) [13–16]. Shiga toxins (stx1, stx2) may lead to enterocyte damage, subsequent bloody diarrhea and endothelial damage leading to internal hemorrhages and septicemia in susceptible neonatal calves [1,17,18]. Enterohemorrhagic *E. coli* (EHEC), a subset of STEC, further include intimin, an adhesin coded from the enterocyte effacement pathogenicity island (eaeA) [19,20] and enterohemolysin, a toxin encoded by the ehxA gene [21]. As published in several case reports, a majority of human EHEC disease outbreaks are caused by the serotype O157:H7 originating from contaminated ground beef [13,22,23]. This serotype is responsible for the hemorrhagic colitis and the life-threatening hemolytic uremic syndrome with the occurrence of thrombocytopenia, hemolytic anemia and thrombotic microangiopathy that may lead to acute renal failure and death [23–26].

Worldwide, neonatal diarrhea is still a major economic problem on cattle farms and the therapy with antimicrobials is crucial in routine practice [27]. However, the medication with bactericide antibiotics is solely, but highly indicated exclusively in the case of life-threatening sepsis [28,29]. The Swiss antibiotic therapy guidelines for veterinarians recommend amoxicillin-clavulanate as a first line, sulfonamide-trimethoprim as a second line and fluoroquinolones as a third line choice, here enrofloxacin [29]. A study from 2014 revealed that veterinarians in Europe mainly used polymyxins (44%), (fluoro)quinolones (18%), penicillins (13%), aminoglycosides (9%) and third and fourth generation cephalosporins (8%) in calves with diarrhea emphasizing the problem of an inappropriate use of antibiotics [30]. This contributes to a higher level of antimicrobial resistant bacteria in young animals compared to adults [31–33]. In addition, the emergence of multidrug- and pandrug-resistant *E. coli* in fecal samples of diarrheic calves has been recently and repeatedly reported [33,34]. According to the expert proposal for standard definitions for acquired resistance from the European Centre for Disease Prevention and Control (ECDC), strains are classified as "multidrug-resistant" if these are non-susceptible (resistant or intermediate) to at least one antimicrobial agent in more than three categories. Isolates meet the definition "extensively drug-resistant" if these are non-susceptible in all agents but two or fewer categories. Finally, isolates non-susceptible to all agents in all antimicrobial categories are ranked as "pandrug-resistant" [35].

Previous data show that the prevalence of extended-spectrum β-lactamase (ESBL)-producing *E. coli* in calves increased from 7% to 29% between 2006 and 2013 in Germany [27]. ESBL-producing strains do encode for numerous resistance genes and may transduce these to other, even commensal, bacteria [36]. Animals hosting these *E. coli* bacteria constitute a resistance gene reservoir that may affect the health of man and animals [36,37].

Only few data are available on the identification of ETEC from calves in Bavaria. However, the discrimination between the physiological intestinal flora and pathogenic *E. coli* is crucial [1,6,38]. The aim of the present study was to provide recent information about the most prevalent pathotypes of *E. coli*. These include the investigation of the current virulence factors, serotypes and trends in antimicrobial resistance [9,39–42].

## 2. Results

### 2.1. Antimicrobial Susceptibility

Within the study period 8713 *E. coli* were isolated from 7358 diarrheic calves at the federal state veterinary laboratory in Bavaria, Germany (Table S1). This number matches an average count of 1740 isolates per year that is in accordance with previous years (data not shown). The results on antimicrobial susceptibility testing revealed mean non-susceptibility values of 28.1% for amoxicillin-clavulanate, 37.9% for enrofloxacin and 50% for trimethoprim-sulfamethoxazole (Figures 1 and 2, Table S1). The highest non-susceptibility value of a substance within each antimicrobial class revealed 11.9% for tulathromycin (macrolides), 18.3% for colistin (polymixins), 61.9% for tetracycline (tetracyclines), 62.2% for spectinomycin (aminoglycosides), 69.7% for ampicillin (penicillins), 80.5% for cephalothin (cephalosporins) and 96.8 % for florfenicol (phenicols) (Figure 1). A 5-year tendency from 2015 to 2019, evaluated for amoxicillin-clavulanate, enrofloxacin and trimethoprim-sulfamethoxazole, revealed a statistically significant decrease of the non-susceptibility rates for amoxicillin-clavulanate and enrofloxacin ($p < 0.05$) (Figure 2, Table 1). Regarding trimethoprim-sulfamethoxazole a significant decrease was assessed from 51.9% to 47.8% between 2015 and 2017 regarding the non-susceptible *E. coli* isolates ($p < 0.05$). A subsequent increase was further revealed from 47.8% to 52.5% in the years 2017 to 2019 ($p < 0.05$) (Figure 2, Table 1). Categorizing the 8713 isolates according to the ECDC expert proposal, 84.2% of the isolates (7336/8713) were multidrug-resistant, 15.7% (1368/8713) were extensively drug-resistant, eight isolates (0.1%) were pandrug-resistant and one isolate was susceptible to all antimicrobials tested. As we only tested antimicrobials licensed for the veterinary use, and none of the latest antimicrobials available on the market, we rededicated the eight presumably pandrug-resistant as extensively drug-resistant summing up to 1376 isolates in this specification (Figure 3).

**Table 1.** Statistic parameters regarding the increase or decrease of resistance values within the five-year period for the three clinically relevant antimicrobials (Figure 2).

| Antimicrobial | Years | OR | CI (95%) |
|---|---|---|---|
| amoxicillin-clavulanate | 2015–2019 | 0.95 | 0.92–0.98 [1] |
| enrofloxacin | 2015–2019 | 0.91 | 0.88–0.94 [1] |
|  | 2015–2017 | 0.92 | 0.85–1.0 [1] |
| trimethoprim-sulfamethoxazole | 2015–2019 | 1.0 | 0.97–1.03 |
|  | 2017–2019 | 1.11 | 1.03–1.19 [1] |

OR: odds ratio, CI: confidence interval, [1] $p$-value (Wald test) < 0.05.

| Treatment choice | Antimicrobial agent | Antimicrobial class | 0.02 | 0.03 | 0.05 | 0.06 | 0.13 | 0.25 | 0.5 | 1 | 2 | 4 | 8 | 16 | 32 | 64 | 128 | Susceptible % | Intermediate % | Resistant % | Non-susceptible % | No result % | MIC$_{50}$ [µg/ml] | MIC$_{90}$ [µg/ml] |
|---|---|---|---|---|---|---|---|---|---|---|---|---|---|---|---|---|---|---|---|---|---|---|---|---|
| 1st line | Amoxicillin-clavulanic acid[1] | Betalactam combination agents | | | | | | | | | | | | 1614 | 2182 | 2468 | 1701 | 746 | | 71,9 | 19,5 | 8,6 | 28,1 | 0,01 | 8 | 16 |
| 1st line | Enrofloxacin | Fluoroquinolones | 909 | 2937 | - | 546 | 228 | 790 | 272 | 54 | 2971 | | | | | | | 62,1 | 3,8 | 34,1 | 37,9 | 0,07 | 0,06 | 4 |
| 1st line | Trimethoprim-sulfamethoxazole[2] | Folate pathway inhibitors | | | 2 | | | 4119 | 141 | 47 | 47 | 4353 | | | | | | 50,0 | | 50,0 | 50,0 | 0,05 | 2 | 8 |
| 2nd line | Gentamicin | Aminoglycosides | | | | | | 2186 | 3119 | 875 | 660 | 138 | 449 | 1260 | | | 16 | 80,4 | 5,1 | 14,5 | 19,6 | 0,10 | 0,5 | 16 |
| 2nd line | Spectinomycin | Aminoglycosides | | | | | | | | | 5 | | 4 | 219 | 3064 | 1159 | 4262 | 37,8 | 13,3 | 48,9 | 62,2 | 0,00 | 64 | 128 |
| 2nd line | Cephalothin | Cephalosporins I & II | | | | | | | | 7 | 32 | 159 | 1505 | 2997 | 4013 | | | 19,5 | 34,4 | 46,1 | 80,5 | 0,00 | 16 | 32 |
| 3rd line | Ceftiofur | Cephalosporins III & IV | | | | 81 | 2519 | 2588 | 1152 | 350 | 241 | 1778 | | | | | | 76,8 | 2,8 | 20,4 | 23,2 | 0,05 | 0,5 | 8 |
| 3rd line | Ampicillin | Penicillins | | | | 2 | 2 | 2 | 5 | 150 | 1375 | 1063 | 45 | 21 | | 6050 | | 30,3 | 0,2 | 69,5 | 69,7 | 0,00 | 32 | 64 |
| 3rd line | Florfenicol | Phenicols | | | | | | | | | 263 | 3154 | 5281 | | | | | 3,2 | 36,2 | 60,6 | 96,8 | 0,00 | 8 | 16 |
| 3rd line | Colistin | Polymyxins | | | | | | 7116 | 1352 | 15 | 82 | 159 | | | | | | 81,7 | 16,5 | 1,8 | 18,3 | 0,05 | 0,5 | 1 |
| 3rd line | Tetracycline | Tetracyclines | | | | 6 | | 5 | 188 | 1943 | 1061 | 112 | 44 | 5352 | | | | 38,1 | 0,5 | 61,4 | 61,9 | 0,02 | 16 | 16 |
| 3rd line | Tulathromycin[3] | Macrolides | | | | | | | 15 | | 778 | 2428 | 2942 | 882 | 373 | 579 | | 88,1 | 4,7 | 7,2 | 11,9 | 8,22 | 8 | 32 |

**Figure 1.** Minimum inhibitory concentration (MIC) distribution of 8713 *E. coli* isolates on 12 antimicrobial agents from 11 antimicrobial classes. The three first lines represent the clinically relevant substances, first to third treatment choices in buiatrics. The red line demarcates the breakpoint towards resistance, the green line a breakpoint towards intermediate. Regarding the two combination compounds, only the concentration of the former substance is presented; the ratio of amoxicillin:clavulanic acid is 2:1 (1), concentration ratio of trimethoprim:sulfamethoxazole is 1:19 (2). Tulathromycin has not been tested in the first quarter of 2015 (3). The summation of intermediate and resistant isolates was named non-susceptible (4). Some results were not evaluable (5).

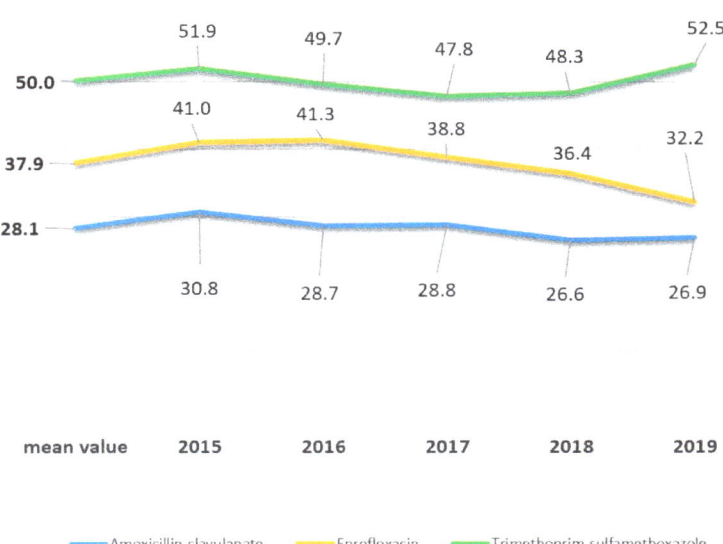

**Figure 2.** The mean value (bold) and the five-year trend on non-susceptible *E. coli* isolated from calves revealed the highest proportion of isolates against trimethoprim-sulfamethoxazole, followed by enrofloxacin and amoxicillin-clavulanate. The trends regarding enrofloxacin and amoxicillin-clavulanate remain at a stable level and rather tend towards a decrease regarding the number of non-susceptible isolates. The graph of non-susceptible isolates regarding trimethoprim-sulfamethoxazole reveals a decrease, 2016–2017, followed by a steep increase of non-susceptible isolates in 2019. The corresponding statistic parameters are presented in Table 1.

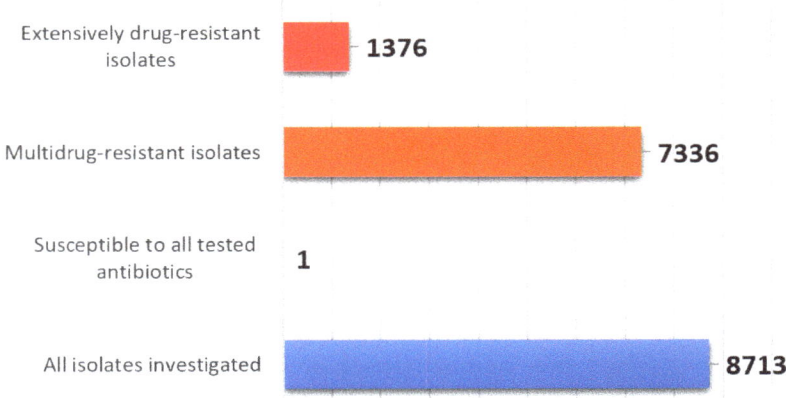

**Figure 3.** The classification of 8713 *E. coli* into extensively drug-resistant and multi drug-resistant isolates was carried out according to the expert proposal for standard definitions for acquired resistance. We categorized eight potential pandrug-resistant isolates in the category extensively drug resistant, as we only tested antimicrobials licensed for the veterinary use and did not include the latest antimicrobials available on the market.

### 2.2. Serologic Characterization

Serotyping of a randomly chosen subset of 108 *E. coli* isolated in 2019 and 2020 revealed 38 unequivocally typeable (35.2%), 29 untypeable (26.8%) and 41 seronegative (38%) strains

(Tables 2 and S2). The most frequently detected serotypes were O101:K28 (8.3%; $n = 9$), O9:K35 and O139:K82 (6.5%; $n = 7$), O101:K30 (3.7%; $n = 4$), O101:K32, O78:K80 and O8:K87 (2.8%; $n = 3$). The serotypes O141:K85 and O147:K89 were detected once each (Tables 2 and S2). Finally, the serotypes O138:K81, O149:K91 and O157:H7 were not detected at all.

The fimbrial antigen F5 agglutinated in 6.5% of the isolates ($n = 7$) in combination with the serotypes O101:K30, O101:K28 and O9:K35. The fimbrial antigen F4 agglutinated in 4.6% of the isolates ($n = 5$), and exclusively combined with the serotype O139:K82 (Tables 2 and S2).

**Table 2.** The serologic and molecular characterization revealed 13 different serotypes known to be pathogenic for cattle and other species. Furthermore, four different genotypes were detected with five different coding sequences for fimbria and/or toxins in one or more isolates. Some of the isolates were untypeable/ seronegative and did not reveal any of the investigated virulence factors (green box).

| Serotype | Additionally Known for Pathogenicity in | Number of Isolates | Non-Virulent | Molecular Results | | | |
|---|---|---|---|---|---|---|---|
| | | | | F17 | F5ST-I | F5F41ST-I | stx1 |
| O9:K35 | | 6 | 5 | 1 | | | |
| O9:K35/F5 | | 1 | | | | 1 | |
| O101:K28 | | 6 | 6 | | | | |
| O101:K28/F5 | | 3 | | | 3 | | |
| O101:K30 | | 1 | | 1 | | | |
| O101:K30/F5 | | 3 | | | | 3 | |
| O101:K32 | | 3 | 3 | | | | |
| O78:K80 | Human/sheep | 3 | 3 | | | | |
| O8:K87 | Swine | 3 | 3 | | | | |
| O139:K82 | Swine | 2 | 2 | | | | |
| O139:K82/F4 | Swine | 5 | 4 | 1 | | | |
| O141:K85 | Swine | 1 | 1 | | | | |
| O147:K89 | Swine | 1 | | 1 | | | |
| untypeable | | 29 | 20 | 7 | | | 2 |
| seronegative | | 41 | 37 | 4 | | | |
| Total | | 108 | 84 | 15 | 3 | 4 | 2 |

### 2.3. Molecular Characterization

Within the molecular characterization, 14 PCR assays targeted genes for the expression of fimbria, adhesin, hemolysin and toxins. A positive result was obtained for 24 isolates and 35 single assays, respectively (Tables 2 and S2). The most frequently detected genes coded for the fimbria F17 (13.9%; 15/108), F41 (3.7%; 4/108) and F5. The latter was always detected in combination with the toxin gene coding for ST-I (6.5%; 7/108). Finally, the gene coding for stx1 was detected in two of 108 isolates (1.9%). Seven of 108 isolates (6.5%) carried more than one type of virulence-associated genes (Tables 2 and S2). The fimbrial antigens F4, F6, F18, O157, adhesin eaeA, hemolysin ehxA and the toxins LT, ST-II and stx2 were not detected in any isolate. The occurrence of F4 fimbria in the serotyping assays could not be confirmed in the PCR investigation (Tables 2 and S2). In all, 84 of 108 isolates were negative in all PCR assays (Tables 2 and S2).

### 3. Discussion

Antibiotic treatment is the fundamental therapy regarding serious or life-threatening bacterial infections in man and animals [28,29]. Records regarding antimicrobial susceptibility on single substances are collected in many countries all over the world [43]. Worldwide this is a critical topic in line with the One Health issue [44]. Monitoring on the application and more important efficacy of antimicrobials regarding bacterial infections of farm animals is possible on principle in industrial countries. However, it is costly and difficult to standardize [36]. Published data from Canada in 2018 revealed a 51.6% susceptibility rate of 489 *E. coli* against trimethoprim-sulfamethoxazole, which is in consensus with our data (50%) (Figures 1 and 2) [45]. Tetracycline was accounted to be effective in 36.8% and resembles our findings at 38.1% (Figure 1) [45]. Further, authors from the United States and Germany determined similar high resistance rates for tetracycline, with 71.1% and 70.9%. These data rather resemble the rate of 61.4% revealed in the present study (Figure 1) [46,47].

The antimicrobial class of fluoroquinolones includes enrofloxacin which is one of the substances of choice for the treatment of diarrhea in young cattle [29,48]. In Germany, the usage of fluoroquinolones has risen from 2011 to 2013 in human and veterinary medicine. This trend needs close monitoring to preserve the efficacy of the agent [27]. Fluoroquinolones are assessed as highest priority clinically important antimicrobials and as one of the few options for the treatment of serious *Salmonella* and *E. coli* infections in children recommended by the World Health Organization (WHO) [49]. The legislation reacted and passed a law in 2017 including obligatory antimicrobial susceptibility testing in case of the application of fluoroquinolones or third or fourth generation cephalosporines in Germany [50]. In the present study, the investigated *E. coli* isolated revealed a resistance rate of 34.1% regarding enrofloxacin (Figure 1). This finding correlates with published results from South America in 2017, with 36.4% [51].

Antimicrobial substances or closely related compounds may likewise be licensed for the use in man and animals. The application in an organism does trigger the development of antimicrobial resistance in present bacteria [49]. Legal restrictions regarding the use of cephalosporines, especially from the third and fourth generation, aim at a high prioritization of critically important antimicrobials in human medicine [49]. This is again in accordance with the terms of One Health [27,44]. The use of cephalosporines for the therapy of *E. coli* diarrhea in calves is a malpractice, as the effective therapeutic concentration is not reached within the gut [29]. Nonetheless, cephalosporin is the fifth-most commonly prescribed antimicrobial in the case of diarrhea with 8% according to a recent survey in Europe [30]. Regarding the third generation cephalosporine ceftiofur, a susceptibility rate of 86.4% could be determined in a study from Canada between 1994 and 2013 [45]. Significantly, our findings revealed 76.8% (Figure 1). Compared to data from the USA collected within the years 1960 until 2002 and in 2007, the resistance rate was at 7.4% and 11%, whereas in the present study the resistance rate of ceftiofur revealed 20.4% (Figure 1) [46,52]. This result is concerning, and the use of ceftiofur must be scrutinized critically, if not avoided completely. The resistance rates of the first generation cephalosporine, cephalothin, were lower in a comparable study regarding data within the period of 1960 to 2002, with 20.1%, in contrast to our results with an average rate at 46.1% from 2015 to 2019 (Figure 1) [46]. Currently, the standard antimicrobial therapy of mastitis in cows includes penicillins as well as first and second generation cephalosporines in the EU. Traces of antibiotics may reach the calves through the feeding of antibiotic contaminated waste milk [36]. To predict a reliable trend regarding the prevalence of ESBL-producing *E. coli*, PCR and sequencing methods should be applied to investigate the existence of ESBL- encoding genes as these are probably more accurate than the phenotypic characterization [53]. A study from 2013 revealed high rates (32.8%, 196 of 598 samples) of ESBL-encoding *E. coli* on dairy and beef cattle farms in Bavaria [54].

Completely inconsistent data are publicly available regarding the resistant rates for *E. coli* isolates and the substance florfenicol within the phenicol group. A 78% share of resistant isolates was determined in a study from the USA in 2006, only a 28% share from Canada in 2018, and a share of 35% from Bavaria, Germany, in 2002 [45,52,55]. In the present study, a rather higher resistance rate of 60.6% was determined for florfenicol (Figure 1). There was no information about ages of animals within the American and Canadian studies [45,52]. Since lower resistance rates were previously published in older animals for the substances ampicillin, tetracycline, streptomycin, sulfamethoxazole and chloramphenicol, this might accordingly apply for florfenicol [32]. This argument, however, still does not explain the diverse results of the Bavarian study from 2002 and the present study (Figure 1) [55].

With a 9% share of the most frequently listed antimicrobials, aminoglycosides remain at the fourth top position for the treatment of diarrhea in calves [30]. As these are almost solely used in the therapy of enterococcal endocarditis and multidrug-resistant tuberculosis in humans, they account to the high priority, clinically important antimicrobials in human medicine [49]. An application in veterinary medicine should therefore be prudent and well considered. Gentamicin belongs to the aminoglycoside antimicrobial class and has a withdrawal time for meat of more than 200 days in Germany for cattle and the indication of gastrointestinal disease. As this is economically hardly acceptable, the application of gentamicin is quite limited [48]. However, resistance to gentamicin among *E. coli* isolated from animals has been increasing from 0% to 40% between 1970 and 2002 within the United States [46]. Another long-term investigation from Germany revealed a further decrease of resistance rates including data from 2010 until 2013, and 2016 until 2017, respectively [47]. In the present study, the resistance rate of *E. coli* against Gentamicin was at 14.1% (Figure 1). Likewise, spectinomycin is an aminoglycoside antibiotic as well, and frequently used in combination with lincomycin for oral application in the treatment of simultaneous infection of the respiratory and the gastrointestinal tract in calves. The meat withdrawal time of 21 days is acceptable for farmers and practitioners and may be an explanation for the frequent prescription [48]. Within the present study and correspondingly a resistance rate of 48.9% was revealed in calves (Figure 1).

As stated by the WHO, the antimicrobial class of polymyxins accounts for the highest priority in critically important antimicrobials regarding the treatment of serious infections with Enterobacteriaceae and *Pseudomonas aeruginosa* in human medicine [49]. Despite rather frequent prescription of polymyxins in the treatment of diarrhea in animals, investigated *E. coli* isolates are still highly susceptible [30]. In the present study, the resistance rate against colistin revealed to be only 1.8% (Figure 1). Corresponding to this suggestion, another study revealed that only 3.8% of the isolates were resistant to colistin [47].

The aminopenicillin family, as well as the preparation amoxicillin-clavulanate, belong to the high priority critically important antimicrobials for the therapy of *Listeria* and *Enterococcus* spp. infections in humans according to the WHO [49]. For the aminopenicillin, ampicillin, an alarming resistance rate of 76.3% was determined in *E. coli* published in a most recent study from Germany [47]. Regrettably, a rate of 69.5% was determined in the present work as a similar result (Figure 1). Consequently, the recommendation on the usage of ampicillin for the treatment of calf diarrhea cannot further be continued. The amoxicillin-clavulanate susceptibility rate averaged at 57% in Germany in 2013 [27]. In the present study, the average susceptibility rate was 71.9%, and the resistance rate was 8.6% (Figure 1). Accordingly, a recently published study reported 7% of resistant *E. coli* isolates in Germany in 2018 [34]. Analogical to the report on the resistance monitoring study 2018 of the Federal Office of Consumer Protection and Food Safety, Germany, we determined decreasing non-susceptibility rates regarding the clinically important antimicrobial amoxicillin-clavulanate [34]. In conclusion, the resistance rates of *E. coli* against amoxicillin-clavulanate have decreased since 2013 and remained on a constant level within the years 2015 and 2019. This is a positive trend is beneficial for the One Health point of view [27].

Comparing data originating from other continents and collected over the last 60 years clearly reveals an increase of resistance regarding *E. coli* in nine out of the 12 tested drugs, namely gentamicin, cephalothin, ceftiofur, enrofloxacin, trimethoprim-sulfamethoxazole, ampicillin, amoxicillin-clavulanate, florfenicol and tetracycline [27,34,45–47,51,52,55]. Out of the 12 tested drugs in the present study, eight substances are similarly suitable for the treatment of human patients, namely gentamicin, spectinomycin, cephalothin, ampicillin, tetracycline, amoxicillin-clavulanate, colistin and trimethoprim-sulfamethoxazole (Figure 1) [49]. The application of these in veterinary medicine should be prudent due to the One Health aspect.

In a published study from Canada in 2018, 48.7% of multidrug-resistant *E. coli* were isolated from ruminants [45]. Within another study from the USA covering the years 1950 until 2002, a significantly increasing trend in resistance was observed for ampicillin, sulfonamide and tetracycline antibiotics regarding more than 1700 *E. coli* isolates. Two of these strains were identified as pandrug-resistant and originated from cattle in 2001 [46]. Further, multidrug resistance in *E. coli* increased from 7.2% to 63% between 1950 and 2002. Finally, 59.1% of the strains recovered form cattle were classified as multidrug resistant in the USA [46]. In the present study, we detected an even higher rate of 84.2% regarding multidrug resistance, 15.7% extensively drug-resistance and 0.1% pandrug-resistance (Figure 3). Furthermore, there were no exclusively susceptible isolates found amongst 108 isolates recovered in 2019 and 2020 from diarrheic calves in Bavaria (Table S2). Comparably high levels of antimicrobial resistance were published regarding the countries Brazil and Uruguay. Calves aged up to 60 days revealed a multidrug-resistance rate in *E. coli* at 78.7%, and at 61.6%, respectively [51]. As published, these bacteria occurred frequently in herds with high levels of diarrhea symptoms and subsequent antimicrobial therapy, as equally described in the present study [31].

Besides antimicrobial resistance, the determination of virulence regarding infectious agents is crucial in diagnostics. The discrimination from commensal *E. coli* was determined investigating virulence factors and evaluating the pathogenicity of isolates. As published, the *E. coli* serotypes O139:K82, O8:K87 and O147:K89 are pathogenic in swine [6]. However, in the present study, a fair amount of such isolates, six out of 108, were isolated from cattle, respectively (Tables 2 and S2). In laboratory diagnostics, implication of these serotypes should therefore be considered. Three isolates were identified as the serotype O78:K80, which frequently causes septicemia in calves (Table 2) [5,7,56]. However, more than one third, 38%, of the *E. coli* in this study revealed to be entirely seronegative (Tables 3 and S2), as it was as well published previously [57]. Preferably and in accordance with the One Health approach, the screening of *E. coli* isolated from diseased animals should always be of interest to identify zoonotic and human pathogenic serotypes [25]. As a matter of fact, formula associated with severe human syndromes included the serotypes O26, O103, O111, O117, O128, O145 and O146 respectively [13,22,23,58].

**Table 3.** In all, 16 different polyvalent and monovalent (mono) antisera were used for the agglutination and the characterization of *E. coli*. The listed serotypes are known for their pathogenicity in humans and farm animals.

| Antiserum for Initial Screening | Respective Follow Up Agglutination | Specific Serotypes Occur in Cattle, but Are Found as Well/Especially in |
|---|---|---|
| Polyvalent anti-*E. coli* C | | |
| | O9:K35, mono | |
| | O101:K28, mono | |
| | O101:K30, mono | |
| | O101:K32, mono | |
| | F5, mono | |
| O78:K80, mono | | Human, sheep |
| Polyvalent anti-*E. coli* P | | |
| | O8:K87, mono | |
| | O138:K81, mono | |
| | O139:K82, mono | |
| | O141:K85, mono | Swine |
| | O147:K89, mono | |
| | O149:K91, mono | |
| | F4, mono | |
| O157:H7, mono | | Association with food-poisoning |

In recent studies, the fimbrial adhesins F17, F41 and F5 were frequently and significantly correlated with diseased calves compared to healthy animals [4,9]. These findings clearly correspond to the results of the present study (Tables 2 and S2). Other selective fimbrial antigens, F4, F6 and F18, occur frequently in isolates from diarrheic piglets [1,10,59]. As to be expected, we did not detect these amongst our strains isolated from calves (Table S2). Even five serologically F4 positive isolates were not confirmed within our molecular investigation (Tables 2 and S2). We assume that none of these isolates carry the specific primer sites, or agglutination was non-specific [9]. However, working at a federal state laboratory, we do research cross species infections especially among farm animals [60]. Furthermore, we consider the One Health approach, here especially the idea from farm to fork, and therefore continuously consider possible correlations between food-borne human pathogens and isolates from farm animals [27,44].

As published, hemolysis in *E. coli* isolates from piglets is a reliable diagnostic marker for virulence and pathogenicity [61–63]. Within the present study, only few (3/108) isolates revealed a hemolytic phenotype that was not even confirmed within the molecular analysis (Table S2). We conclude that hemolysis is not a relevant marker for virulence of *E. coli* isolated from calves in the present study. This statement is in accordance with prior publications [64,65].

Regarding the present study, ST-I was found in similar prevalence at a rate of 6.5% (7/108) compared to published data (Tables 2 and S2) [4,66]. The enterotoxins LT and ST-II were not detected in the present study (Table S2) and this again resembles data of relevant previous studies [4,56]. Concluding published data, ETEC isolated from calves only produced ST-I, whereas ETEC isolated from pigs may encode varying combinations of the enterotoxins LT, ST-I and ST-II [11,67]. In the present study, the detection rate of stx1 was very low and stx2 as well as intimin were not detected at all among the diarrheic calves' isolates (Tables 2 and S2). This finding matches the results of previously published data to a high degree [9,51,68]. Obviously, the detection rate of Shiga toxins rose with the number of colonies isolated from each clinical sample, suggesting the selection of up to 35 colonies [69,70]. In the present investigation however, only up to three colonies were analyzed per clinical sample (Table S2). Other published results suggested a positive correlation between animal age and the amount of Shiga toxin, supporting our findings including animals of young age [69–71]. Targeted infection studies with STEC led to severe disease and bloody diarrhea in neonatal calves, but more recent studies disproved this observation revealing a still controversial discussion [4,72–74].

*Limits of the Study*

The antimicrobial susceptibility testing was carried out with a standard panel of antibiotics currently used in veterinary diagnostics in Germany. The results are therefore limited to substances only partially prescribed in human diagnostics and sometimes even in veterinary medicine regarding other countries of the world.

A thorough molecular investigation of single isolates is fairly time consuming and costly compared to the benefit that might be drawn from the results. In routine diagnostics, the molecular methods therefore can hardly be kept up.

## 4. Materials and Methods

*4.1. Study Design and Bacterial Isolates*

At the Bavarian Health and Food Safety Authority in Germany 7358 fecal samples of diseased or deceased calves with enteritis younger than six weeks of age were analyzed and included in the present study. Samples were collected between January 2015 and December 2019. Clinical symptoms ranged from low general condition, diarrhea, fever, sepsis and sudden death, respectively. A total of 8713 *E. coli* strains were isolated and confirmed through positive fluorescence on ECD agar (Merck Millipore, Burlington, MA, USA) and a positive Kovacs-Indole reaction (Merck Millipore, Burlington, MA, USA). All isolates were subject to antimicrobial resistance testing, further analysis and cryopreservation at the internal vaccine laboratory.

*4.2. Antimicrobial Susceptibility Testing*

Antimicrobial susceptibility testing was carried out according to the protocols published in CLSI VET01, 5th edition (Clinical and Laboratory Standards Institute, Wayne, PA, USA) [41]. Breakpoints were adopted from CLSI Vet01S, 5th edition, and national breakpoints for farm animals [41,42,75]. We used the microbroth dilution method on the following twelve different antimicrobial agents (antimicrobial class): Amoxicillin-clavulanic acid (betalactam combination agent), enrofloxacin (fluoroquinolone), Trimethoprim-sulfamethoxazole (folate pathway inhibitor), gentamicin and spectinomycin (aminoglycosides), cephalothin (cephalosporin I and II), ceftiofur (cephalosporin III and IV), ampicillin (penicillin), florfenicol (phenicol), colistin (polymyxin), tetracycline (tetracycline) and tulathromycin (macrolide). A commercially available set was used according to the manufacturer's instructions (Micronaut-S, Grosstiere 4, Merlin, Bruker, Bornheim, Germany). The minimum inhibitory concentration (MIC) of each isolate and antibiotic substance was metered using a photometric plate reader system (Micronaut Scan and MCN6 software, Merlin/ Sifin, Bruker, Bornheim, Germany). Subsequently, the MIC value was reconciled with supplemented CLSI breakpoints, to categorize the respective *E. coli* isolate into "susceptible", "intermediate" and "non-susceptible" for each antimicrobial substance tested [41,42,75,76]. *E. coli* ATCC 25922 was used as quality control strain [41].

*4.3. Phenotypic Analysis and Serotyping*

We deeper investigated a subset of 108 *E. coli* isolated in 2019 and 2020 originating from 66 diarrheic calves. The isolates were subcultured on Gassner agar (Oxoid Deutschland GmbH, Wesel, Germany) to differentiate specific colony morphology. The expression of potential virulent F5 fimbria was investigated by subculturing the isolates on pH 7.5 stabile, "minimum of casein" (Minca) agar (Sifin Diagnostics GmbH, Berlin, Germany) as previously published [76]. Finally, potential hemolytic properties of isolates were interpreted as described with subcultures on Columbia Sheep Blood Agar (Sifin Diagnostics GmbH, Berlin, Germany) [77]. Growth incubation was carried out for 18 to 24 h at 37 °C at all times. Serotyping for specific O-antigens was carried out using two polyvalent and 14 monovalent agglutination sera in a hierarchical approach according to the manufacturer's instructions (Sifin Diagnostics GmbH Berlin, Germany) (Table 3). If an isolate showed a positive agglutination reaction with a polyvalent serum, but none with any correspondent monovalent or several reactions with various correspondent monovalent sera, it was categorized as untypeable. If an isolate showed no positive agglutination with any serum, it was categorized as seronegative.

*4.4. Molecular Investigation*

The molecular characterization of the *E. coli* isolates in the present study aimed at surface antigens, toxins and virulence factors. In all, 14 different target genes were of interest. Amongst were seven fimbrial genes F4, F5, F6, F17, F18, F41 and the outer membrane protein O157:H-. Further, two virulence genes were included, here adhesin intimin (eaeA), and enterohemolysin (ehxA). Finally, PCR targets coding for five toxins were screened, including heat-labile toxin (LT), heat-stabile toxin I (ST-I) and II (ST-II), Shiga toxin 1 (stx1) and stx2 (Table 4). Primer sequences were adopted from published protocols [9,39,40]. All 14 qPCR assays were performed applying a singleplex high resolution melting method, using AccuMelt HRM SuperMix (Quantabio, Beverly MA, USA) in 20 µL volumes according to the manufacturer's instructions. DNA was extracted after thermolysis. The primers were added in a concentration of 0.2 µM each, and 3 µL of template DNA was used. Polymerase chain reaction assays were conducted on a Stratagene MX3000P device (Agilent Technologies, Waldbronn, Germany). The cycling protocol comprised an initial single denaturation step for 10 min at 95 °C, followed by 40 cycles of annealing and polymerization for 30 s at 60 °C and 10 s at 95 °C. After completing amplification, the melting curve analysis was performed. Specific melting temperatures were determined for each molecular target and all tested isolates. Reference strains were used as positive controls and kindly provided from Prof. R. Bauerfeind (Justus-Liebig-Universität, Gießen, Germany), and purchased from the German Collection of Microorganisms and Cell Cultures GmbH (DSMZ, Braunschweig, Germany) (Table 4).

Table 4. Targets and primers for the molecular characterization of *E. coli* isolated from calves.

| Target Protein | Gene(s) | Primer | Oligo Sequence (5′ -> 3′) | Size (bp) | Melting Temperature (°C) ± 0.2 °C | Reference | Reference Isolate |
|---|---|---|---|---|---|---|---|
| Fimbria/outer membrane protein | F4 | F4_F<br>F4_R | GGTGGAACCAAACTGACCATTAC<br>TCCATCTACACCACCAGTTACTGG | 102 | 81.0 | [9] | 7156 |
| | F5 | F5_F<br>F5_R | TTGGAAGCACCTTGCTTTAACC<br>TCACTTGAGGGTATATGCGATCTTT | 101 | 77.4 | [9] | 7159 |
| | F6 | F6_F<br>F6_R | GCGGATTAGCTCTTTCAGACCA<br>TGACAGTACCGGCCGTAACTC | 102 | 83.2 | [9] | 7155 |
| | F17 | F17_F<br>F17_R | ACTGAGGATTCTATGCRGAAAATTCAA<br>CCGTCATAAGCAAGCGTAGCAG | 83 | 79.7 | [9] | 5397 |
| | F18 | F18_F<br>F18_R | CCTGCTAAGCAAGAGAATATATCCAGA<br>AGAACATATACTCAGTGCCAACAGAGAT | 82 | 73.3 | [9] | 7160 |
| | F41 | F41_F<br>F41_R | CCTTTGTCATTTGGTGCGG<br>TCAAATACTGTACCAGCAGAACCAC | 101 | 81.5 | [9] | 7159 |
| | O157 (rfbE) | O157_F<br>O157_R | CGATGAGTTTATCTGCAAGGTGAT<br>TTTCACACTTATTGGATGGTCTCAA | 88 | 78.3 | [39] | DSMZ 19206 |
| Adhesin | intimin (eaeA) | Intimin_F<br>Intimin_R | CCAGCTTCAGTCGCGATCTC<br>GGCCTGCAACTGTGACGAA | 91 | 86.1 | [9] | 7158 |
| Hemolysin | enterohemolysin (ehxA) | ehec-F2<br>ehec-R | CGTTAAGGAACAGGAGGTGTCAGTA<br>ATCATGTTTTCCGCCAATGAG | 142 | 79.5 | [40] | DSMZ 19206 |
| Toxin | heat-labile toxin (LT) | LT_F<br>LT_R | CTGCCATCGATTCCGTATATGAT<br>CAGAACTATGTTCGGAATATCGCA | 81 | 75.3 | [9] | 7157 |
| | heat-stabile toxin (ST-I) | ST-I_F<br>ST-I_R | TACCTCCCGTCATGTTGTTTCAC<br>CCTCGACATATAACATGATGCAACTC | 101 | 76.1 | [9] | 7155 |
| | heat-stabile toxin (ST-II) | St-II_F<br>St-II_R | TTTTTCTATTGCTACAAATGCCTATGC<br>AACCTTTTTTACAACTTTCCTTGGC | 101 | 75.9 | [9] | 7156 |
| | Shiga toxin 1 (stx1) | Stx1_F<br>Stx1_R | TCCCCAGTTCAATGTAAGATCAAC<br>TTTCGTACAACACTGGATGATCTCA | 81 | 79.0 | [9] | 7158 |
| | Shiga toxin 2 (stx2) | Stx2_F<br>Stx2_R | GAGTGACGACTGATTTGCATTCC<br>CCATGACAACGGACAGCAGTT | 82 | 84.6 | [9] | 7158 |

*4.5. Statistical Analysis*

All statistical analyses were performed using the free software R Studio version 1.2.5033 (RStudio, Inc., Boston, MA, USA). Resistance trends of three clinically relevant antimicrobials amoxicillin-clavulanate, enrofloxacin and trimethoprim-sulfamethoxazole were evaluated by calculating a logistic regression model. The respective year was set as a continuous variable. The resulting odds ratio (OR) > 1 indicated an increased resistance trend, whereat an OR < 1 indicated a decreased antimicrobial resistance. The Wald test was used to determine the statistical significance of the year-antimicrobial trend. A value of $p < 0.05$ was considered significant (Table 1).

## 5. Conclusions

We conclude that an extensive monitoring, characterization and the analysis of antimicrobial resistance regarding enteritis causing *E. coli* is crucial to determine the currently raging serotypes, virulent genotypes and most important, the resistance situation. It is then possible to calculate reliable tendencies and prognoses from data collected over long terms in routine diagnostics. This is an important premise for objective and professional treatment recommendations regarding humans and animals within the scope of One Health. A further goal should be a slowdown of the increasing antimicrobial resistance situation that constitutes a global public health threat.

**Supplementary Materials:** The following supporting information can be downloaded at: https://www.mdpi.com/article/10.3390/antibiotics11010023/s1, Table S1: data set for all 8713 isolates from 2015–2019. Table S2: data set for a subset of 108 isolates in 2019–2020.

**Author Contributions:** Conceptualization, A.F., R.K.S. and J.M.R., methodology, A.F., A.H., K.B. and J.M.R.; software, A.F., A.M. and K.B.; validation, A.F., N.S., C.K., A.H., S.F. and J.M.R.; formal analysis, A.F., A.H., A.R., S.F., R.K.S. and J.M.R.; investigation, A.F., A.M., K.B., A.R. and S.F.; resources, C.K., K.B., A.R., S.F. and J.M.R.; data curation, A.F. and J.M.R.; writing—original draft preparation, A.F., N.S., A.M. and J.M.R.; writing—review and editing, N.S., C.K., K.B., A.R. and R.K.S.; visualization, A.F. and J.M.R.; supervision, R.K.S. and J.M.R.; project administration, J.M.R.; funding acquisition, K.B. and J.M.R. All authors have read and agreed to the published version of the manuscript.

**Funding:** This research received no external funding.

**Institutional Review Board Statement:** Not applicable.

**Acknowledgments:** The authors are grateful to the veterinary bacteriology staff members for technical support. Furthermore, the authors are grateful to the staff of the StabLab, Ludwig-Maximilians-University Munich, for a basic teaching class in statistical analyses.

**Conflicts of Interest:** The authors declare no conflict of interest.

## References

1. Quinn, P.J.; Markey, B.K.; Leonard, F.C.; Fitzpatrick, E.S.; Fanning, S.; Hartigan, P.J. *Veterinary Microbiology and Microbial Disease*; Wiley: Chichester, UK, 2011.
2. Kaper, J.B.; Nataro, J.P.; Mobley, H.L. Pathogenic Escherichia coli. *Nat. Rev. Genet.* **2004**, *2*, 123–140. [CrossRef] [PubMed]
3. Foster, D.M.; Smith, G.W. Pathophysiology of Diarrhea in Calves. *Veter Clin. North Am. Food Anim. Pract.* **2009**, *25*, 13–36. [CrossRef] [PubMed]
4. Kolenda, R.; Burdukiewicz, M.; Schierack, P. A systematic review and meta-analysis of the epidemiology of pathogenic Escherichia coli of calves and the role of calves as reservoirs for human pathogenic E. coli. *Front. Cell. Infect. Microbiol.* **2015**, *5*, 23. [CrossRef] [PubMed]
5. Cho, Y.-I.; Yoon, K.-J. An overview of calf diarrhea—Infectious etiology, diagnosis, and intervention. *J. Veter Sci.* **2014**, *15*, 1–17. [CrossRef]
6. Linton, A.H.; Hinton, M.H. Enterobacteriaceae associated with animals in health and disease. *Soc. Appl. Bacteriol. Symp. Ser.* **1988**, *65*, S71–S85. [CrossRef]
7. Ewers, C.; Schüffner, C.; Weiss, R.; Baljer, G.; Wieler, L.H. Molecular characteristics ofEscherichia coli serogroup O78 strains isolated from diarrheal cases in bovines urge further investigations on their zoonotic potential. *Mol. Nutr. Food Res.* **2004**, *48*, 504–514. [CrossRef]

8. Nagy, B.; Fekete, P.Z. Enterotoxigenic Escherichia coli in veterinary medicine. *Int. J. Med. Microbiol.* **2005**, *295*, 443–454. [CrossRef]
9. Sting, R.; Stermann, M. Duplex real-time PCr assays for rapid detection of virulence genes in E. coli isolated from post-weaning pigs and calves with diarrhoea Duplex Real-Time PCR-Assays für den raschen Nachweis von Virulenz-Genen in E. Coli-Isolaten durchfallerkrankter Absatzferkel und Kälber. *Dtsch. Tierärztliche Wochenschr.* **2008**, *115*, 231–238.
10. Dubreuil, J.D.; Isaacson, R.E.; Schifferli, D.M. Animal Enterotoxigenic Escherichia coli. *EcoSal Plus* **2016**, *7*. [CrossRef]
11. Gyles, C.L. Escherichia coli cytotoxins and enterotoxins. *Can. J. Microbiol.* **1992**, *38*, 734–746. [CrossRef]
12. Field, M.; Graf, L.H., Jr.; Laird, W.J.; Smith, P.L. Heat-stable enterotoxin of Escherichia coli: In vitro effects on guanylate cyclase activity, cyclic GMP concentration, and ion transport in small intestine. *Proc. Natl. Acad. Sci. USA* **1978**, *75*, 2800–2804. [CrossRef]
13. Gyles, C.L. Shiga toxin-producing Escherichia coli: An overview. *J. Anim. Sci.* **2007**, *85*, E45–E62. [CrossRef]
14. Beutin, L.; Geier, D.; Steinrück, H.; Zimmermann, S.; Scheutz, F. Prevalence and some properties of verotoxin (Shiga-like toxin)-producing Escherichia coli in seven different species of healthy domestic animals. *J. Clin. Microbiol.* **1993**, *31*, 2483–2488. [CrossRef]
15. Montenegro, M.A.; Bülte, M.; Trumpf, T.; Aleksić, S.; Reuter, G.; Bulling, E.; Helmuth, R. Detection and characterization of fecal verotoxin-producing Escherichia coli from healthy cattle. *J. Clin. Microbiol.* **1990**, *28*, 1417–1421. [CrossRef]
16. Blanco, M.; Blanco, J.; Blanco, J.E.; González, E.A.; Gomes, T.; Zerbini, L.; Yano, T.; de Castro, A. Genes coding for Shiga-like toxins in bovine verotoxin-producing Escherichia coli (VTEC) strains belonging to different O:K:H serotypes. *Veter Microbiol.* **1994**, *42*, 105–110. [CrossRef]
17. Wieler, L.H.; Bauernfeind, R. *E coli: Shiga Toxin Methods and Protocols*; Philpott, D., Ebel, F., Eds.; Humana Press Inc.: Totowa, NJ, USA, 2003; ISBN 978-1-59259-316-3. [CrossRef]
18. Dean-Nystrom, E.A.; Bosworth, B.T.; Moon, H.W. Pathogenesis of Escherichia Coli O157:H7 in Weaned Calves. *Adv. Exp. Med. Biol.* **1999**, *473*, 173–177. [CrossRef]
19. Dean-Nystrom, E.A.; Bosworth, B.T.; Cray, W.C., Jr.; Moon, H.W. Pathogenicity of Escherichia coli O157:H7 in the intestines of neonatal calves. *Infect. Immun.* **1997**, *65*, 1842–1848. [CrossRef]
20. Dean-Nystrom, E.A.; Bosworth, B.T.; Moon, H.W.; O'Brien, A.D. Escherichia coli O157:H7 requires intimin for enteropathogenicity in calves. *Infect. Immun.* **1998**, *66*, 4560–4563. [CrossRef]
21. Taneike, I.; Zhang, H.-M.; Wakisaka-Saito, N.; Yamamoto, T. Enterohemolysin operon of Shiga toxin-producingEscherichia coli: A virulence function of inflammatory cytokine production from human monocytes. *FEBS Lett.* **2002**, *524*, 219–224. [CrossRef]
22. Beutin, L.; Aleksic′, S.; Zimmermann, S.; Gleier, K. Virulence factors and phenotypical traits of verotoxigenic strains of Escherichia coli isolated from human patients in Germany. *Med. Microbiol. Immunol.* **1994**, *183*, 13–21. [CrossRef]
23. Boerlin, P.; McEwen, S.A.; Boerlin-Petzold, F.; Wilson, J.B.; Johnson, R.P.; Gyles, C.L. Associations between Virulence Factors of Shiga Toxin-Producing Escherichia coli and Disease in Humans. *J. Clin. Microbiol.* **1999**, *37*, 497–503. [CrossRef]
24. Nataro, J.P.; Kaper, J.B. Diarrheagenic Escherichia coli. *Clin. Microbiol. Rev.* **1998**, *11*, 142–201. [CrossRef]
25. Croxen, M.A.; Law, R.J.; Scholz, R.; Keeney, K.M.; Wlodarska, M.; Finlay, B.B. Recent Advances in Understanding Enteric Pathogenic Escherichia coli. *Clin. Microbiol. Rev.* **2013**, *26*, 822–880. [CrossRef]
26. Mayer, C.L.; Leibowitz, C.S.; Kurosawa, S.; Stearns-Kurosawa, D.J. Shiga Toxins and the Pathophysiology of Hemolytic Uremic Syndrome in Humans and Animals. *Toxins* **2012**, *4*, 1261–1287. [CrossRef] [PubMed]
27. Federal Office of Consumer Protection and Food Safety, Paul-Ehrlich-Gesellschaft für Chemotherapie e.V. Report on the Consumption of Antimicrobials and the Spread of Antimicrobial Resistance in Human and Veterinary Medicine in Germany. Available online: https://www.bvl.bund.de/SharedDocs/Downloads/05_Tierarzneimittel/germap2015_EN.pdf?__blob=publicationFile&v=5 (accessed on 23 December 2021).
28. Constable, P.D. Treatment of Calf Diarrhea: Antimicrobial and Ancillary Treatments. *Veter Clin. North Am. Food Anim. Pract.* **2009**, *25*, 101–120. [CrossRef] [PubMed]
29. Vetsuisse-Fakultät. *Umsichtiger Einsatz von Antibiotika bei Rindern, Schweinen und kleinen Wiederkäuern, Therapieleitfaden für Tierärztinnen und Tierärzte*; Gesellschaft Schweizer Tierärztinnen und Tierärzte; Bundesamt für Lebensmittelsicherheit und Veterinärwesen: Bern, Switzerland, 2019; Available online: https://www.blv.admin.ch/blv/de/home/tiere/tierarzneimittel/antibiotika/nationale-strategie-antibiotikaresistenzen--star--/sachgemaesser-antibiotikaeinsatz.html (accessed on 23 December 2021).
30. De Briyne, N.; Atkinson, J.; Borriello, S.P.; Pokludová, L. Antibiotics used most commonly to treat animals in Europe. *Vet. Rec.* **2014**, *175*, 325. [CrossRef] [PubMed]
31. De Verdier, K.; Nyman, A.; Greko, C.; Bengtsson, B. Antimicrobial resistance and virulence factors in Escherichia coli from swedish dairy calves. *Acta Veter Scand.* **2012**, *54*, 2. [CrossRef] [PubMed]
32. Khachatryan, A.R.; Hancock, D.D.; Besser, T.E.; Call, D.R. Role of Calf-Adapted Escherichia coli in Maintenance of Antimicrobial Drug Resistance in Dairy Calves. *Appl. Environ. Microbiol.* **2004**, *70*, 752–757. [CrossRef]
33. Cao, H.; Pradhan, A.K.; Karns, J.S.; Hovingh, E.; Wolfgang, D.R.; Vinyard, B.T.; Kim, S.W.; Salaheen, S.; Haley, B.J.; Van Kessel, J.A.S. Age-Associated Distribution of Antimicrobial-Resistant Salmonella enterica and Escherichia coli Isolated from Dairy Herds in Pennsylvania, 2013–2015. *Foodborne Pathog. Dis.* **2019**, *16*, 60–67. [CrossRef]
34. Federal Office of Consumer Protection and Food Safety. Report on the Resistance Monitoring Study 2018. 2020. Available online: https://www.bvl.bund.de/EN/Home/home_node.html (accessed on 23 December 2021).

35. Magiorakos, A.-P.; Srinivasan, A.; Carey, R.B.; Carmeli, Y.; Falagas, M.E.; Giske, C.G.; Harbarth, S.; Hindler, J.F.; Kahlmeter, G.; Olsson-Liljequist, B.; et al. Multidrug-resistant, extensively drug-resistant and pandrug-resistant bacteria: An international expert proposal for interim standard definitions for acquired resistance. *Clin. Microbiol. Infect.* **2012**, *18*, 268–281. [CrossRef]
36. Murphy, D.; Ricci, A.; Auce, Z.; Beechinor, J.G.; Bergendahl, H.; Breathnach, R.; Bureš, J.; Duarte Da Silva, J.P.; Hederová, J.; Hekman, P.; et al. EMA and EFSA Joint Scientific Opinion on measures to reduce the need to use antimicrobial agents in animal husbandry in the European Union, and the resulting impacts on food safety (RONAFA). *EFSA J.* **2017**, *15*, 4666. [CrossRef]
37. Astorga, F.; Navarrete-Talloni, M.J.; Miró, M.P.; Bravo, V.; Toro, M.; Blondel, C.J.; Hervé-Claude, L.P. Antimicrobial resistance in E. coli isolated from dairy calves and bedding material. *Heliyon* **2019**, *5*, e02773. [CrossRef]
38. Ørskov, F.; Ørskov, I. Escherichia coli serotyping and disease in man and animals. *Can. J. Microbiol.* **1992**, *38*, 699–704. [CrossRef]
39. Perelle, S.; Dilasser, F.; Grout, J.; Fach, P. Detection by 5′-nuclease PCR of Shiga-toxin producing Escherichia coli O26, O55, O91, O103, O111, O113, O145 and O157:H7, associated with the world's most frequent clinical cases. *Mol. Cell. Probes* **2004**, *18*, 185–192. [CrossRef]
40. Nielsen, E.M.; Andersen, M.T. Detection and Characterization of Verocytotoxin-Producing Escherichia coli by Automated 5′ Nuclease PCR Assay. *J. Clin. Microbiol.* **2003**, *41*, 2884–2893. [CrossRef]
41. CLSI. *Performance Standards for Antimicrobial Disk and Dilution Susceptibility Tests for Bacteria Isolated from Animals*, 5th ed.; CLSI standard Vet01; Clinical and Laboratory Standards Institute: Wayne, PA, USA, 2018.
42. CLSI. *Performance Standards for Antimicrobial Disk and Dilution Susceptibility Tests for Bacteria Isolated from Animals*, 4th ed.; CLSI supplement Vet08; Clinical and Laboratory Standards Institute: Wayne, PA, USA, 2018.
43. Franklin, A.; Acar, J.; Anthony, F.; Gupta, R.; Nicholls, T.; Tamura, Y.; Thompson, S.; Threlfall, E.; Vose, D.; Van Vuuren, M.; et al. Antimicrobial resistance: Harmonisation of national antimicrobial resistance monitoring and surveillance programmes in animals and in animal-derived food. *Rev. Sci. Tech.* **2001**, *20*, 859–870. [CrossRef]
44. German Federal Government. DART 2020—Fighting Antibiotic Resistance for the Good of Both Humans and Animals. Available online: https://www.bmel.de/SharedDocs/Downloads/EN/Publications/DART2020.html (accessed on 23 December 2021).
45. Awosile, B.B.; Heider, L.C.; Saab, M.E.; McClure, J.T. Antimicrobial resistance in mastitis, respiratory and enteric bacteria isolated from ruminant animals from the Atlantic Provinces of Canada from 1994-2013. *Can. Veter J.* **2018**, *59*, 1099–1104.
46. Tadesse, D.A.; Zhao, S.; Tong, E.; Ayers, S.; Singh, A.; Bartholomew, M.J.; McDermott, P.F. Antimicrobial Drug Resistance in Escherichia coli from Humans and Food Animals, United States, 1950–2002. *Emerg. Infect. Dis.* **2012**, *18*, 741–749. [CrossRef]
47. Tenhagen, B.-A.; Käsbohrer, A.; Grobbel, M.; Hammerl, J.; Kaspar, H. Antibiotikaresistenz von E. coli aus Rinderpopulationen in Deutschland. *Tierärztliche Prax. Ausg. G Großtiere Nutztiere* **2020**, *48*, 218–227. [CrossRef]
48. Insitute for Pharmacology, Pharmacy and Toxicology, Veterinary Faculty, University Leipzig. Vetidata Veterinary Information Service. Available online: https://www.vetidata.de/public/index.php (accessed on 19 February 2021).
49. World Health Organization. Critically Important Antimicrobials for Human Medicine, 5th Revision 2016. Available online: https://www.who.int/foodsafety/publications/antimicrobials-fifth/en/ (accessed on 10 October 2020).
50. Federal Ministry of Justice and Consumer Protection. Verordnung über tierärztliche Hausapotheken; 2018. Available online: https://www.gesetze-im-internet.de/t_hav/BJNR021150975.html (accessed on 23 December 2021).
51. Umpiérrez, A.; Bado, I.; Oliver, M.; Acquistapace, S.; Etcheverría, A.; Padola, N.L.; Vignoli, R.; Zunino, P. Zoonotic Potential and Antibiotic Resistance of Escherichia coli in Neonatal Calves in Uruguay. *Microbes Environ.* **2017**, *32*, 275–282. [CrossRef]
52. Sawant, A.A.; Hegde, N.V.; Straley, B.A.; Donaldson, S.C.; Love, B.C.; Knabel, S.J.; Jayarao, B.M. Antimicrobial-Resistant Enteric Bacteria from Dairy Cattle. *Appl. Environ. Microbiol.* **2007**, *73*, 156–163. [CrossRef] [PubMed]
53. Hoffmann, H.; Stürenburg, E.; Heesemann, J.; Roggenkamp, A. Prevalence of extended-spectrum β-lactamases in isolates of the Enterobacter cloacae complex from German hospitals. *Clin. Microbiol. Infect.* **2006**, *12*, 322–330. [CrossRef] [PubMed]
54. Schmid, A.; Hörmansdorfer, S.; Messelhäusser, U.; Käsbohrer, A.; Sauter-Louis, C.; Mansfeld, R. Prevalence of Extended-Spectrum β-Lactamase-Producing Escherichia coli on Bavarian Dairy and Beef Cattle Farms. *Appl. Environ. Microbiol.* **2013**, *79*, 3027–3032. [CrossRef] [PubMed]
55. Werckenthin, C.; Seidl, S.; Riedl, J.; Kiossis, E.; Wolf, G.; Stolla, R.; Kaaden, O.-R. Escherichia coli Isolates from Young Calves in Bavaria: In Vitro Susceptibilities to 14 Anti-microbial Agents. *J. Veter Med. Ser. B* **2002**, *49*, 61–65. [CrossRef]
56. Blanco, J.; Gonzalez, E.; Garcia, S.; Blanco, M.; Regueiro, B.; Bernardez, I. Production of toxins by Escherichia coli strains isolated from calves with diarrhoea in Galicia (North-western Spain). *Veter Microbiol.* **1988**, *18*, 297–311. [CrossRef]
57. Holland, R.E.; Wilson, R.A.; Holland, M.S.; Yuzbasiyan-Gurkan, V.; Mullaney, T.P.; White, D.G. Characterization of eae+ Escherichia coli isolated from healthy and diarrheic calves. *Veter Microbiol.* **1999**, *66*, 251–263. [CrossRef]
58. Bielaszewska, M.; Mellmann, A.; Bletz, S.; Zhang, W.; Köck, R.; Kossow, A.; Prager, R.; Fruth, A.; Orth-Höller, D.; Marejková, M.; et al. Enterohemorrhagic Escherichia coli O26:H11/H−: A New Virulent Clone Emerges in Europe. *Clin. Infect. Dis.* **2013**, *56*, 1373–1381. [CrossRef]
59. Casey, T.A.; Bosworth, B.T. Design and Evaluation of a Multiplex Polymerase Chain Reaction Assay for the Simultaneous Identification of Genes for Nine Different Virulence Factors Associated with Escherichia Coli that Cause Diarrhea and Edema Disease in Swine. *J. Veter Diagn. Investig.* **2009**, *21*, 25–30. [CrossRef]
60. Bavarian Health and Food Safety Authority. Available online: https://www.lgl.bayern.de/ (accessed on 16 December 2021).
61. Frydendahl, K. Prevalence of serogroups and virulence genes in Escherichia coli associated with postweaning diarrhoea and edema disease in pigs and a comparison of diagnostic approaches. *Veter Microbiol.* **2002**, *85*, 169–182. [CrossRef]

62. Khac, H.V.; Holoda, E.; Pilipcinec, E.; Blanco, M.; Blanco, J.E.; Mora, A.; Dahbi, G.; López, C.; González, E.A.; Blanco, J. Serotypes, virulence genes, and PFGE profiles of Escherichia coli isolated from pigs with postweaning diarrhoea in Slovakia. *BMC Veter Res.* **2006**, *2*, 10. [CrossRef]
63. Schierack, P.; Steinrück, H.; Kleta, S.; Vahjen, W. Virulence Factor Gene Profiles of Escherichia coli Isolates from Clinically Healthy Pigs. *Appl. Environ. Microbiol.* **2006**, *72*, 6680–6686. [CrossRef]
64. Coura, F.M.; Diniz, S.D.A.; Mussi, J.M.S.; Silva, M.X.; Lage, A.P.; Heinemann, M.B. Characterization of virulence factors and phylogenetic group determination of Escherichia coli isolated from diarrheic and non-diarrheic calves from Brazil. *Folia Microbiol.* **2016**, *62*, 139–144. [CrossRef]
65. Nguyen, T.D.; Vo, T.T.; Vu-Khac, H. Virulence factors in Escherichia coli isolated from calves with diarrhea in Vietnam. *J. Veter Sci.* **2011**, *12*, 159–164. [CrossRef]
66. Yadegari, Z.; Brujeni, G.N.; Ghorbanpour, R.; Moosakhani, F.; Lotfollahzadeh, S. Molecular characterization of enterotoxigenic Escherichia coli isolated from neonatal calves diarrhea. *Veter Res. Forum* **2019**, *10*, 73–78. [CrossRef]
67. World Health Organization. Escherichia coli diarrhoea. *Bull. World Health Organ.* **1980**, *58*, 23–36.
68. Mainil, J.G.; Duchesnes, C.J.; Whipp, S.C.; Marques, L.R.; O'Brien, A.D.; Casey, T.A.; Moon, H.W. Shiga-like toxin production and attaching effacing activity of Escherichia coli associated with calf diarrhea. *Am. J. Veter Res.* **1987**, *48*, 743–748.
69. Wieler, L.H.; Bauerfeind, R.; Baljer, G. Characterization of Shiga-like Toxin Producing Escherichia coli (SLTEC) Isolated from Calves with and without Diarrhoea. *Zent. Für Bakteriol.* **1992**, *276*, 243–253. [CrossRef]
70. Mainil, J.G.; Jacquemin, E.R.; Kaeckenbeeck, A.E.; Pohl, P.H. Association between the effacing (eae) gene and the Shiga-like toxin-encoding genes in Escherichia coli isolates from cattle. *Am. J. Veter Res.* **1993**, *54*, 1064–1068.
71. Wells, J.G.; Shipman, L.D.; Greene, K.D.; Sowers, E.G.; Green, J.H.; Cameron, D.N.; Downes, F.P.; Martin, M.L.; Griffin, P.M.; Ostroff, S.M. Isolation of Escherichia coli serotype O157:H7 and other Shiga-like-toxin-producing E. coli from dairy cattle. *J. Clin. Microbiol.* **1991**, *29*, 985–989. [CrossRef]
72. Chanter, N.; Morgan, J.H.; Bridger, J.C.; Hall, G.A.; Reynolds, D.J. Dysentery in gnotobiotic calves caused by atypical Escherichia coli. *Veter Rec.* **1984**, *114*, 71. [CrossRef]
73. Hall, G.A.; Reynolds, D.J.; Chanter, N.; Morgan, J.H.; Parsons, K.R.; Debney, T.G.; Bland, A.P.; Bridger, J.C. Dysentery Caused by Escherichia coli (S102-9) in Calves: Natural and Experimental Disease. *Veter Pathol.* **1985**, *22*, 156–163. [CrossRef]
74. Ngeleka, M.; Godson, D.; Vanier, G.; Desmarais, G.; Wojnarowicz, C.; Sayi, S.; Huang, Y.; Movasseghi, R.; Fairbrother, J.M. Frequency of Escherichia coli virotypes in calf diarrhea and intestinal morphologic changes associated with these virotypes or other diarrheagenic pathogens. *J. Veter Diagn. Investig.* **2019**, *31*, 611–615. [CrossRef]
75. Luhofer, G.; Böttner, M.; Hafez, H.; Kaske, M. Vorschläge der Arbeitsgruppe "Antibiotikaresistenz" für die Belegung von Mikrotiterplatten zur Empfindlichkeitsprüfung von Bakterien gegenüber antimikrobiellen Wirkstoffen in der Routinediagnostik—Mastitis- und Großtierlayouts. *Berl. Munch. Tierarztl. Wochenschr* **2004**, *117*, 245–251.
76. Guinée, P.A.; Jansen, W.H.; Agterberg, C.M. Detection of the K99 antigen by means of agglutination and immunoelectrophoresis in Escherichia coli isolates from calves and its correlation with entertoxigenicity. *Infect. Immun.* **1976**, *13*, 1369–1377. [CrossRef] [PubMed]
77. Pasayo, R.A.G.; Sanz, M.E.; Padola, N.L.; Moreira, A.R. Phenotypic and genotypic characterization of enterotoxigenic Escherichia coli isolated from diarrheic calves in Argentina. *Open Veter J.* **2019**, *9*, 65–73. [CrossRef] [PubMed]

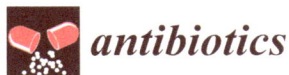

Article

# National Monitoring of Veterinary-Dispensed Antimicrobials for Use on Pig Farms in Austria: 2015–2020

Clair L. Firth [1], Reinhard Fuchs [2] and Klemens Fuchs [2,*]

[1] Unit of Veterinary Public Health & Epidemiology, University of Veterinary Medicine, 1210 Vienna, Austria; clair.firth@vetmeduni.ac.at
[2] Data, Statistics and Risk Assessment, Austrian Agency for Health and Food Safety (AGES), 8010 Graz, Austria; reinhard.fuchs@ages.at
* Correspondence: klemens.fuchs@ages.at

**Abstract:** Antimicrobial use in livestock production systems is increasingly scrutinised by consumers, stakeholders, and the veterinary profession. In Austria, veterinarians dispensing antimicrobials for use in food-producing animals have been required to report these drugs since 2015. Here, we describe the national monitoring systems and the results obtained for Austrian pig production over a six-year period. Antimicrobial dispensing is described using the mass-based metric, milligrams per population correction unit (mg/PCU) and the dose-based metric, Defined Daily Dose (DDDvet) per year and divided into the European Medicines Agency's prudent use categories. Pig production was divided into breeding units, fattening farms, farrow-to-finish farms, and piglet-rearing systems. Over all six years and all pig production systems, the mean amount of antimicrobials dispensed was 71.6 mg/PCU or 2.2 DDDvet per year. Piglet-rearing systems were found to have the highest levels of antimicrobial dispensing in DDDvet, as well as the largest proportion of Category B antimicrobials, including polymyxins. Although progress has been made in promoting a more prudent use of antimicrobials in veterinary medicine in Austria, further steps need to be taken to proactively improve animal health and prevent disease to reduce the need for antimicrobials, particularly those critically important for human medicine, in the future.

**Keywords:** antimicrobial use; pigs; veterinary; monitoring

## 1. Introduction

Globally, antimicrobial use in agriculture, particularly in food-producing animals, is increasingly seen critically by consumers [1]. Although the use of antimicrobials as growth promoters has been banned in the European Union (EU) since 2006, these medications are often still used for disease prophylaxis, and reductions in antimicrobial use (AMU) are both possible and necessary in order to ensure their continued effectiveness against bacterial infections. From 2022, the new Veterinary Medicinal Products Regulation (2019/6) in the EU will legislate new restrictions on AMU in veterinary medicine and requires all member states to monitor and record veterinary AMU in their countries, initially in food-producing animals, but eventually (from 2029) in pets as well [2].

The excessive use of antimicrobials in pig production initially came under criticism in Denmark in the 1990s, and the country was among the first to successively ban a variety of antimicrobials as growth promoters from 1995 onwards [1,3]. Denmark also led the way in benchmarking pig producers and introducing penalty schemes, such as the yellow card for excessive antimicrobial use in 2010 [3]. A number of other European countries, such as the Netherlands, also began to document their veterinary antimicrobial use, and the first EU report of veterinary antimicrobial sales (the ESVAC report) was published by the European Medicines Agency in 2011, using sales data from nine countries [4].

The Austrian health authorities began contributing data on veterinary antimicrobial sales from pharmaceutical companies/wholesale pharmacies to the European Union's

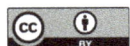

annual ESVAC report in 2010. To date, reported sales of veterinary antimicrobial drugs in Austria for food-producing animals have ranged from a maximum of 63 mg/population correction unit (PCU) in 2010 to a minimum of 42.6 mg/PCU in 2019 [5,6]. Since 2015, it has been required by local law for all veterinarians in Austria who dispense antimicrobials for use in food-producing animals to annually report the amounts dispensed to the relevant authorities [7]. In addition, antimicrobials are only available from veterinarians, and, since 2005, injectable (as well as intramammary and intrauterine) antimicrobials have been further restricted and can only be dispensed to farmers who are members of the Austrian Animal Health Service (*Tiergesundheitsdienst*, TGD) and have completed training courses in the use and administration of veterinary medications [8,9]. Antimicrobials administered directly by the veterinarians themselves do not currently have to be reported, although their use is documented in both veterinary practice and on-farm records [7].

Pig production in Austria is not an extremely large industry, when compared internationally. The average herd size is 133 head (ranging from 15,950 holdings keeping only 1–3 pigs to 12 units with more than 3000 pigs) [10,11]. Based on official data available with respect to the reference day of 1st June each year, the pig population included here ranged from a minimum of 2,773,225 pigs in 2019 to a maximum of 2,845,451 in 2015 (mean number of pigs from 2015–2020: 2,802,433; median: 2,799,632) [10]. Pig producers are primarily located in the federal states of Upper Austria (39.8% of total pig numbers in 2020), Lower Austria (27.0%), and Styria (26.8%) [10].

The most recent national data records in metric tonnes in 2020 reported that 73.4% of all veterinary antimicrobials dispensed in Austria were for use in pigs (ranging from 71.8–76.4% between 2016 to 2020), compared to 19.7% in cattle (beef and dairy) and 6.7% in poultry [12]. However, when comparing these figures to other countries, it is important to note that the Austrian national-monitoring system currently only includes antimicrobials dispensed by veterinarians to farmers and does not include those administered by the veterinarians themselves.

The data presented here represent the results of the national monitoring of veterinary antimicrobials dispensed between 2015 and 2020. To allow comparison with other countries and systems, the data analysis focuses on using international metrics, such as mg/PCU (population corrected unit) and Defined Daily Doses (DDDvet), as published by the European Medicines Agency and recommended by European expert groups [13,14].

## 2. Results
### 2.1. Study Population

Pig production in Austria is divided into farrow-to-finish farms, fattening farms, breeding units, and piglet-rearing units. Figure 1 shows the proportions of the different pig production systems in the study population over the years included here. The study population (i.e., farms where antimicrobials were dispensed and reported to the authorities by herd veterinarians) covers between 81% (in 2015) and 87% (in 2020) of the total national pig production.

Data are provided in standardised livestock units, as defined by the Austrian Ministry of Agriculture [15]. The vast majority of pigs included in this study population were kept in fattening and farrow-to-finish units (mean: 351,261 and 310,933 LSU; median 348,398 and 315,147 LSU, respectively). An extremely small number of pigs are reared in piglet-rearing systems (mean: 7809 LSU; median 7450 LSU) (Figure 1).

### 2.2. Overall Antimicrobials Dispensed
2.2.1. Mass-Based Metrics (mg/PCU)

All veterinarians treating farm animals and dispensing antimicrobials to farmers for use in such animals are required by Austrian law to report their annual dispensed amounts [7]. The data included here are taken from these national records of annual antimicrobial monitoring between 2015 and 2020 [12].

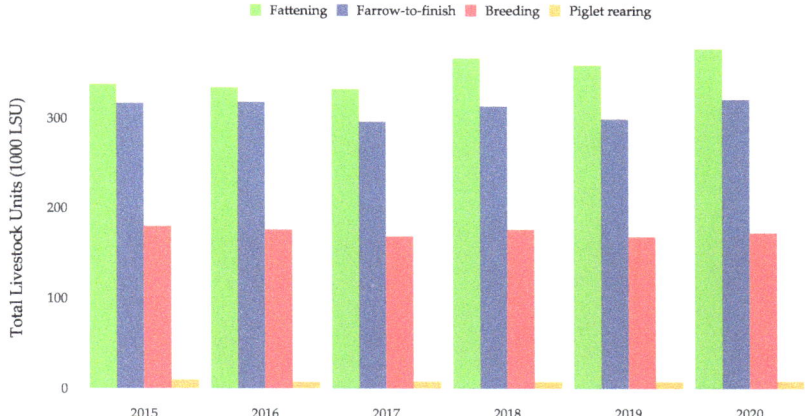

**Figure 1.** Comparative numbers of 1000 livestock units (LSU) in Austrian pig production systems (included in the study population, i.e., farms where antimicrobials were dispensed and reported) between 2015 and 2020.

Antimicrobials dispensed by herd veterinarians for use in pig production between 2015 and 2020 are shown in milligrams per population correction unit (mg/PCU, as defined in the European Medicines Agency's ESVAC report and calculated for the entire national pig herd [6]) in Figure 2. (NB. 1 PCU is approximately equivalent to 1 kg livestock biomass). For all pig production systems overall, the antimicrobial use ranged from a maximum of 79.3 mg/PCU in 2018 to a minimum of 66.5 mg/PCU in 2019.

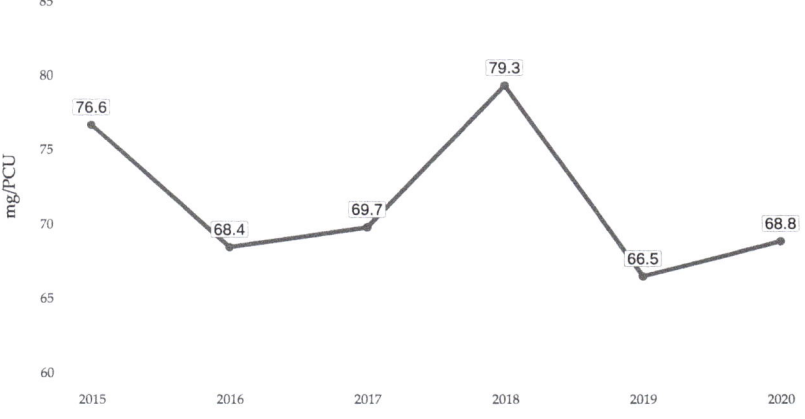

**Figure 2.** Amount of antimicrobials (mg/PCU) dispensed for use in pigs in Austria between 2015 and 2020.

Table 1 shows the proportions of antimicrobial dispensing by veterinarians for use in the various pig production systems. The vast majority of antimicrobial dispensing in mg/PCU over all six years was for use in farrow-to-finish and fattening farms. It is important to note that the decreasing proportion of pig production units that were "not assignable" to a specific production system has fallen dramatically (from 4.6% to 0.8%) since the monitoring system was first initiated in 2015. This is primarily due to improvements to the electronic-reporting system and the data-plausibility checks now in place.

**Table 1.** Proportion in percent per year of antimicrobials dispensed for use in Austrian pigs for different farm types, based on mg/PCU.

| Production System | 2015 | 2016 | 2017 | 2018 | 2019 | 2020 |
|---|---|---|---|---|---|---|
| Farrow-to-finish | 34.1 | 34.5 | 35.6 | 35.5 | 35.1 | 35.3 |
| Fattening | 36.0 | 38.0 | 36.6 | 37.6 | 38.7 | 40.0 |
| Piglet rearing | 1.5 | 1.2 | 0.9 | 1.1 | 1.1 | 0.8 |
| Breeding | 23.9 | 23.6 | 23.9 | 22.2 | 22.4 | 23.1 |
| Not assignable | 4.6 | 2.7 | 3.1 | 3.7 | 2.8 | 0.8 |

2.2.2. Comparison of Mass-Based and Dose-Based Metrics

A variety of antimicrobial monitoring guidelines and recommendations suggests the use of dose-based metrics, such as the European Medicines Agency's DDDvet, to allow for divergences in dosing to be accounted for within AMU records [14,16]. Recording antimicrobial dispensing in mg/PCU often leads to an overestimation of some antimicrobials and an underestimation of others [16,17].

Figure 3 demonstrates the proportions of the total antimicrobial-dispensing data collected in 2020 when analysed by mg/PCU or DDDvet. The differences between tetracyclines in mg/PCU (59.6% of all antimicrobials dispensed) compared to around 43.8% of all dispensed DDDvet are particularly striking. By contrast, aminoglycosides make up 8.3% of antimicrobials dispensed by DDDvet compared to just 1.9% by mg/PCU, and polymyxins make up a much higher proportion of overall use (9.5%) by DDDvet compared to under 5% as mg/PCU (Figure 3).

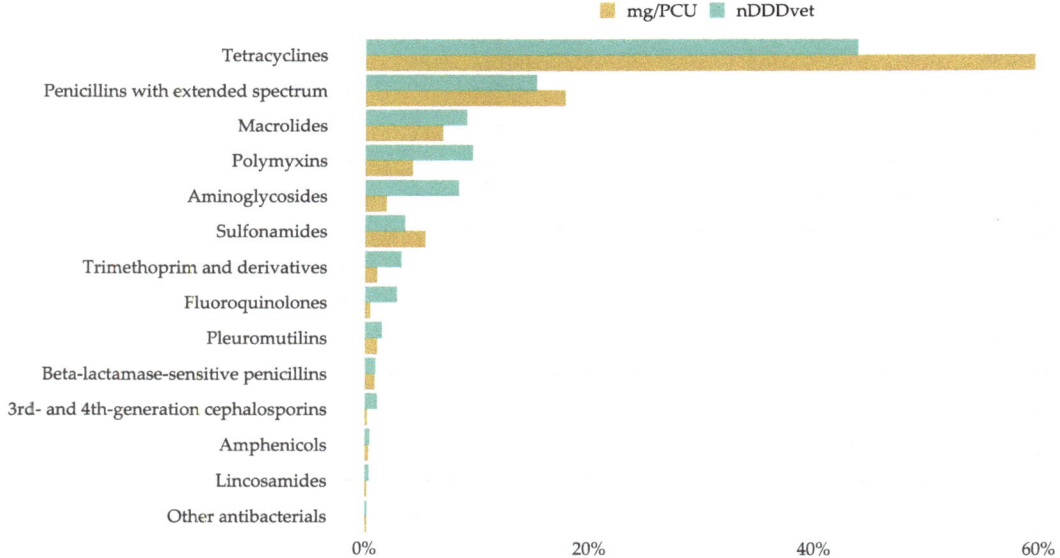

**Figure 3.** Comparison of the mean proportions of mass-based and dose-based metrics for antimicrobial classes dispensed for use in pigs in Austria in 2020.

When antimicrobial dispensing is presented by the proportion of DDDvet per year for the entire monitoring period (see Table 2), tetracyclines continue to make up the largest proportion each year (ranging from a maximum of 50.43% in 2018 to a minimum 39.77% in 2019). Extended-spectrum penicillins make up a much lower proportion (between 13.72–15.54%) and remain in second place over the study period, while polymyxins and macrolides alternate for the third most frequently dispensed antimicrobials. By contrast, when antimicrobial dispensing is presented by proportion of mg/PCU, although tetracyclines continue to make up the vast majority of antimicrobial use (generally > 60%), polymyxins have fallen to fifth place and make up only 2.77% to 4.19% of antimicrobial dispensing (compared to a much higher proportion of between 6.93–9.51% when analysed by DDDvet/year) (Table 3).

**Table 2.** Proportion in percent per year of antimicrobial classes dispensed for use in Austrian pigs, based on the European Medicines Agency's DDDvet.

| Antimicrobial Class | Proportion of Antimicrobials Dispensed in % per Year | | | | | |
|---|---|---|---|---|---|---|
|  | 2015 | 2016 | 2017 | 2018 | 2019 | 2020 |
| Tetracyclines | 44.68 | 45.33 | 46.57 | 50.43 | 39.77 | 43.79 |
| Penicillins with extend. spectrum | 13.72 | 13.88 | 15.43 | 14.02 | 15.54 | 15.22 |
| Polymyxins | 8.01 | 8.63 | 7.65 | 6.93 | 8.18 | 9.51 |
| Macrolides | 8.67 | 8.43 | 9.10 | 9.77 | 9.87 | 9.00 |
| Aminoglycosides | 1.46 | 1.20 | 1.21 | 3.66 | 10.83 | 8.30 |
| Sulfonamides | 3.99 | 3.94 | 4.72 | 4.24 | 4.34 | 3.55 |
| Trimethoprim and derivatives | 3.79 | 3.81 | 4.57 | 4.00 | 4.05 | 3.22 |
| Fluoroquinolones | 2.15 | 2.35 | 2.57 | 2.30 | 2.57 | 2.83 |
| Pleuromutilins | 0.94 | 1.17 | 0.98 | 1.42 | 1.58 | 1.53 |
| 3rd/4th-gen. cephalosporins | 0.96 | 1.05 | 1.03 | 0.95 | 1.09 | 1.10 |
| β-lactamase-sensitive penicillins | 0.94 | 0.96 | 0.93 | 0.82 | 0.90 | 0.94 |
| Amphenicols | 0.43 | 0.41 | 0.38 | 0.44 | 0.42 | 0.43 |
| Lincosamides | 5.43 | 4.74 | 2.78 | 0.48 | 0.47 | 0.37 |
| Other antibacterials | 4.82 | 4.10 | 2.10 | 0.54 | 0.39 | 0.21 |

**Table 3.** Proportion in percent per year of antimicrobial classes dispensed for use in Austrian pigs, based on mg/PCU.

| Antimicrobial Class | Proportion of Antimicrobials Dispensed in % per Year | | | | | |
|---|---|---|---|---|---|---|
|  | 2015 | 2016 | 2017 | 2018 | 2019 | 2020 |
| Tetracyclines | 63.91 | 63.61 | 61.88 | 64.37 | 56.40 | 59.58 |
| Penicillins with extend. spectrum | 14.25 | 14.54 | 16.23 | 14.73 | 18.51 | 17.76 |
| Macrolides | 6.36 | 6.20 | 6.47 | 7.02 | 7.63 | 6.86 |
| Sulfonamides | 5.92 | 5.78 | 6.84 | 6.07 | 6.91 | 5.34 |
| Polymyxins | 3.13 | 3.45 | 3.02 | 2.77 | 3.67 | 4.19 |
| Aminoglycosides | 1.14 | 1.08 | 0.96 | 1.10 | 2.17 | 1.90 |
| Pleuromutilins | 0.62 | 0.78 | 0.64 | 0.86 | 1.13 | 1.08 |
| Trimethoprim and derivatives | 1.13 | 1.15 | 1.37 | 1.21 | 1.38 | 1.07 |
| β-lactamase-sensitive penicillins | 0.78 | 0.80 | 0.77 | 0.69 | 0.85 | 0.87 |
| Fluoroquinolones | 0.32 | 0.36 | 0.38 | 0.36 | 0.43 | 0.46 |
| Amphenicols | 0.28 | 0.27 | 0.24 | 0.29 | 0.31 | 0.31 |
| 3rd/4th-gen. cephalosporins | 0.15 | 0.17 | 0.16 | 0.15 | 0.20 | 0.20 |
| Lincosamides | 0.84 | 0.76 | 0.46 | 0.13 | 0.17 | 0.19 |
| Other antibacterials | 1.19 | 1.06 | 0.58 | 0.26 | 0.23 | 0.19 |

### 2.3. Antimicrobials of Critical Importance to Human Medicine

Antimicrobial dispensing presented here is divided into categories as defined by the European Medicines Agency's Antimicrobial Expert Group (AMEG) [18,19]. Category A is not included, as antimicrobials in this category are not licensed for use in veterinary medicine in the EU (although they may be used off-label in nonfood-producing animal species). Categories B and C are critically important for human medicine and should be used restrictively (Category B: 3rd and 4th generation cephalosporins, fluoroquinolones, and polymyxins) or with caution (Category C includes e.g., macrolides, extended-spectrum penicillins, amongst others). Category D antimicrobials should be used prudently and include tetracyclines, sulfonamide/trimethoprim, beta-lactamase-sensitive penicillins, etc. With the exception of macrolides, Category B ("restrict") antimicrobials are comparable to the WHO's highest-priority, critically important antimicrobials (HPCIA) [18,19]. Further details are provided in the Section 5.

In all production systems, the majority of antimicrobials dispensed were in Category D, with the exception of piglet-rearing units, where a substantial proportion of antimicrobials dispensed were in Category B. For details, see Figure 4 and Sections 2.5 and 2.8 below. Again, the differences in mass-based versus dose-based metrics became apparent and can be seen very clearly when comparing Figure 4 (mg/PCU) with Figure 6d (DDDvet for piglet-rearing systems).

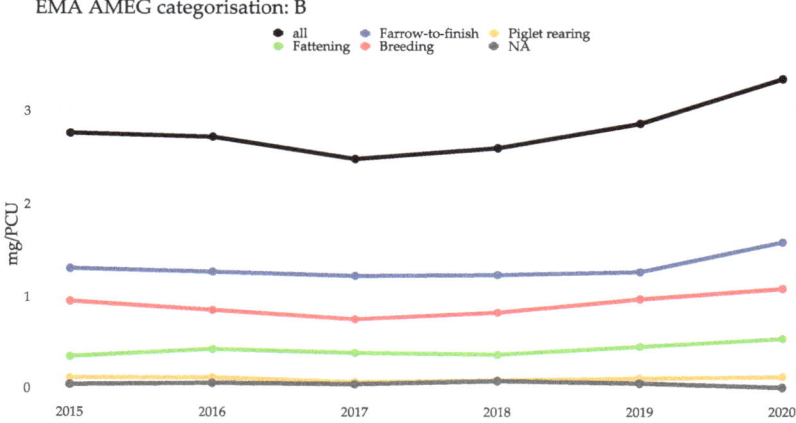

**Figure 4.** Antimicrobials (in mg/PCU) dispensed in Category B (the use of which should be "restricted") by pig production system over time.

### 2.4. Route of Administration for the Dispensed Antimicrobials

As would be expected, the vast majority of antimicrobials dispensed in all categories for use in Austrian pig production were for oral administration. Category D antimicrobials for oral use ranged from 53 mg/PCU in 2019 to around 66 mg/PCU in 2018, as shown in Figure 5. By mg/PCU, the most frequently dispensed antimicrobial class for oral use in Category D ("prudent use") were tetracyclines (37.2 mg/PCU (2019)–50.8 mg/PCU (2018)) followed by macrolides (4.0 mg/PCU (2016)–5.2 mg/PCU (2018)) in Category C ("use with caution") and polymyxins (2.1 mg/PCU (2017)–2.9 mg/PCU (2020)) ("restrict use") in Category B; for details see Supplementary Figure S1. Injectable antimicrobials were dispensed at very low levels ranging from 0.4–0.5 mg/PCU in Category B to 2.6–2.9 mg/PCU in Category D (Figure 5). Specifically, the most commonly dispensed injectable antimicrobials were found in the classes of aminoglycosides (0.60 mg/PCU (2016)–0.75 mg/PCU (2015), Category C), beta-lactamase-sensitive pencillins (0.54 mg/PCU (2017)–0.60 mg/PCU (2020), Category D), and macrolides (0.27 mg/PCU (2019)–0.31 mg/PCU (2020), Category C), amongst others (Supplementary Figure S1).

### 2.5. Antimicrobial Use on Piglet production/Breeding Units

Breeding (piglet production) units made up approximately 20.5% of pig-producing units in Austria from 2015–2020, on average, ranging from 19.6% to 21.3% of pig production by LSU. Antimicrobial use on breeding pig units is shown in Figure 6a. The mean number of pigs kept on breeding units was 173,251 LSU.

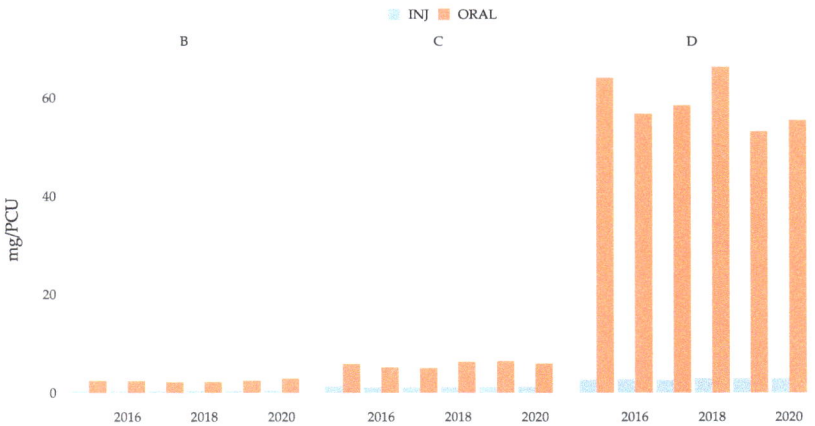

**Figure 5.** Antimicrobials (in mg/PCU) dispensed and divided by route of administration over time. INJ = systemic/injectable administration; ORAL = oral administration.

*2.6. Antimicrobial Use on Farrow-To-Finish Farms*

Farrow-to-finish farms made up approximately 36.9% of pig-producing units in Austria from 2015–2020, on average, ranging from 35.9% to 38.1% of pig production by LSU (a mean number of pig equivalent to 310,933 LSU). Antimicrobial use on farrow-to-finish farms is shown in Figure 6b

*2.7. Antimicrobial Use on Fattening Farms*

Fattening/finishing farms made up approximately 41.7% of pig-producing units in Austria from 2015–2020, on average, ranging from 40.0% to 43.1% of pig production by LSU. The mean number of pigs kept on Austrian fattening farms was 351,261 LSU. Antimicrobial use on fattening farms is shown in Figure 6c, divided by EMA category. The vast majority of antimicrobials dispensed for use on fattening farms fall into Category D (prudent use).

*2.8. Antimicrobial Use on Piglet-Rearing Farms*

Piglet-rearing farms made up only a very small proportion of Austrian pig production, with, on average, approximately 0.9% of pigs produced in Austria from 2015–2020 by LSU (with a mean number of pigs equivalent to 7809 LSU). Only 23.3 of such farms reported antimicrobial use to the authorities, on average, over the six-year period (median 23.5 farms). Antimicrobial use on piglet-rearing units is shown in Figure 6d. It is important to note that the antimicrobial use in DDDvet per year on piglet-rearing farms is substantially higher than in other production systems. Furthermore, antimicrobial use in Category B (antimicrobials which are critical for human medicine and should be avoided) increased in 2020 to the highest level recorded since 2016 (median: 1.44 DDDvet/year in 2016 compared to 1.34 DDDvet/year in 2020).

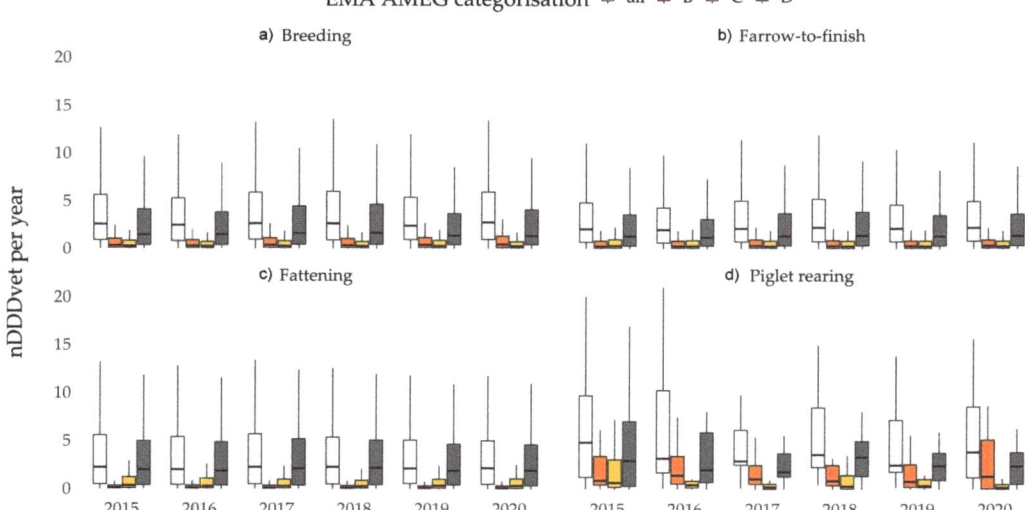

**Figure 6.** National recording of antimicrobials dispensed for use on a variety of pig production systems ((**a**) breeding units; (**b**) farrow-to-finish farms; (**c**) fattening farms; (**d**) piglet-rearing units) by European Medicines Agency antimicrobial category (B, C, D) and DDDvet/year.

## 3. Discussion

The data presented here provide a comprehensive overview of veterinary antimicrobial dispensing for use on Austrian pig farms over a six-year period. Given the mandatory nature of reporting and the fact that data were provided for between 81–87% of national pig production in Austria, these analyses can be considered an accurate representation of antimicrobial dispensing for use in pig production in the country. Nevertheless, it is important to note that antimicrobials administered directly by veterinarians themselves (rather than dispensed to farmers), while no doubt making up a small proportion of antimicrobial use in pig production overall, were not included in this dataset.

The most recent data available on total antimicrobial dispensing for all pig production systems in Austria were calculated to be 68.8 mg/PCU. (NB. 1 PCU is approximately equivalent to 1 kg livestock biomass). These figures are comparable with antimicrobial sales reported in a study of veterinary wholesale data in Switzerland in 2015 (77.4 mg/kg) [20], but are higher than those previously reported for a small convenience sample of 75 pig farms in Austria (mean over four years: 33.9 mg/kg) [21]. By contrast, the Austrian national figures are much lower than those recently reported for 67 Irish pig farms (161.9 mg/PCU) or the UK figures for the national pig herd in 2020 (namely 105 mg/kg) [22,23].

With respect to Defined Daily Doses (DDDvet), the mean value of the six-year median DDDvet per year (2.2 DDDvet/year) reported here and covering all pig production systems is difficult to compare with other dose-based metrics, as calculation methods vary. A recent study in Italy (using national DDD metrics) reported annual median values of between 6.24–7.57 DDDita/100 kg on 36 fattening farms [24], which is substantially higher than the Austrian national mean of the six-year median value of 2.17 DDDvet for fattening farms determined here. Meanwhile, a Swiss study of 227 pig farms reported a mean treatment of 4 DDDvet over a one-year period [25], which is also higher than that reported here in Austria.

When analysing antimicrobial use by substance, the Austrian data show that tetracyclines are dispensed in the greatest volumes by mass. However, it is important to note that mass-based calculations are often skewed with respect to older antimicrobial molecules which have higher dosage requirements in mg/kg than other newer drugs which may be more potent [14,16,26]. Oxytetracycline, for example, is licensed for use in pigs in Austria at a dosage of 40 mg/kg/d, which leads to a requirement of 2000 mg per day for a 50 kg pig. In contrast, the polymyxin, colistin, licensed at a dosage of 5 mg/kg/d, leads to a requirement of 250 mg per day for the same pig. This means that when comparing these antimicrobial drugs using mass-based metrics, oxytetracycline appears to be used at an eight-fold higher amount than colistin, which skews the overall proportions of antimicrobial classes in mg/kg. These discrepancies can be balanced out by using the defined daily dose (DDDvet), which refers to the daily dose as a whole, regardless of the amount of antimicrobial drug administered in milligrams.

For this reason, a comparison using dose-based metrics is essential [16]. Nevertheless, even when analysed by DDDvet metrics, tetracyclines still made up the majority (>55%) of antimicrobials dispensed for use in pig production in Austria between 2015–2020. Other studies have also reported that tetracyclines and penicillins are the most commonly used antimicrobials in pig production, such as a systematic review of 36 international papers [27] and a survey of 36 finishing pig farms in Italy [24]. In 2016, an Irish study of 67 farms, as well as Danish national reporting data, both demonstrated that tetracyclines were most frequently used [22,28], and similar findings have also been reported more recently from Japan [29]. The vast majority of tetracycline use in all these studies, as well as in the Austrian data presented here, was for oral administration. Whilst we do not have access to diagnoses data in Austria, tetracyclines are known to be commonly used for the treatment of gastrointestinal disorders and respiratory disease in pigs of all ages. Although tetracyclines are categorised by the EMA as the lowest level of caution (Category D, prudent use), some countries, such as Denmark, have seen increasing levels of antimicrobial resistance to this antibiotic and are now taking measures to reduce its routine use in pigs [28,30]. Similar resistance patterns have also been reported in studies in Austria, where tetracycline resistance was reported among 66% of *Streptococcus suis* isolates (increasing up to 88% of *Sc. suis* isolates obtained from joints) and 67.7% of *Escherichia coli* isolates obtained from piglets with diarrhoea [31,32].

Among piglet-rearing (and, to a much lesser extent, breeding) farms, a large proportion of antimicrobial dispensing was made up of polymyxins. This antimicrobial class contains the drug, colistin, which is commonly used to treat gastrointestinal disorders in young piglets (both pre- and post-weaning age), particularly disease caused by enterotoxigenic *Escherichia coli* (ETEC). While it is important to note that piglet-rearing farms make up only a very small proportion of Austrian pig producers (namely a mean number of pigs equivalent to 7809 LSU and between 0.8–1.5% of total antimicrobials dispensed for use in pigs by mg/PCU), polymyxins still made up a relatively large proportion (up to 9% by DDDvet, the third most frequently dispensed class in 2020) of antimicrobials dispensed in Austria overall. Polymyxins are classified by the European Medicines Agency as Category B antimicrobials, the use of which should be restricted as much as possible. Some countries, such as the UK and Denmark, have recently managed to avoid their use altogether among pig producers [23,28]. Although the most recent European Sales of Veterinary Antimicrobial Agents (ESVAC) report in 2021 stated that polymyxin use had fallen by 77% in 31 European countries since 2011, they are still sold at a higher level (based on mg/PCU metrics) in Germany, Poland, Hungary, Portugal, and Cyprus than in Austria [6]. The Netherlands has also reported a 7.3% increase in the use of colistin in all livestock production in 2020 and, as seen in the Austrian data, the vast majority of this use (91% of pig use) was for weaners [33]. Since plasmid-mediated colistin resistance was first detected in China in 2013, and the subsequent discovery of this resistance gene among pigs and humans throughout the world, recommendations have been made to reduce the use of this antimicrobial in livestock production wherever possible [34–36].

As would be expected, and as reported in many other studies [27,37,38], given the primarily intensive nature of pig production, the vast majority of antimicrobials were dispensed for oral administration. Systemically administered antimicrobials are generally used for the treatment of individual animals rather than entire groups and were dispensed at a very low level. Category D antimicrobials made up the largest proportion of antimicrobials dispensed for use by injection, namely 2.6 to 2.9 mg/PCU (compared to 53–66 mg/PCU for oral use). While dispensed at a much lower level than Category D antimicrobials for oral administration, Category B antimicrobials (including colistin) were more commonly dispensed for oral rather than systemic treatment, which is particularly concerning as a previous Austrian study of 75 pig farms demonstrated that oral treatments are frequently (in 75% of cases) underdosed and only 8% of cases were correctly dosed [21]. Furthermore, a number of studies have reported that the risk of antimicrobial resistance is substantially higher following oral antimicrobial treatment rather than parenteral administration of such drugs, and the European Medicines Agency also classes oral treatment, particular as a group treatment, to be the least preferable route of antimicrobial administration [19,39].

The data presented here have demonstrated that antimicrobials dispensed for use on pig units with a high number of young piglets make up the highest proportion of Category B antimicrobials, drugs which should be limited to restricted use. Here, it is particularly important for herd veterinarians to work together with pig producers to attempt to prevent disease, such as post-weaning diarrhoea, by improving hygiene and biosecurity, reducing stress, and vaccinating either breeding sows or young piglets whenever possible [40]. Given that colistin is critically important for human health (as the first-line drug for carbapenemase-producing *Enterobacteriaceae* infections), is primarily administered orally to pigs, and colistin-resistant bacteria have been isolated from wastewater from pig slaughterhouses in Germany, the use of this antimicrobial substance is an extremely relevant example of an essential One Health drug affecting human, animal, and environmental health [36,41,42]. For this reason, Austrian pig producers should attempt to learn from pig producers in other countries, where the use of colistin has been considerably reduced or stopped completely.

The implementation of the new EU Regulation 2019/6 will bring a number of changes to the use of veterinary antimicrobials in Austrian and European livestock production as a whole. Prophylactic use of antimicrobials will no longer be permitted, and only the metaphylaxis of a group will be allowed when one or more animal is proven to be infected. It is expected that the restrictions on the use of Category B antimicrobials will be tightened and enforced. For this reason, Austrian pig producers and their herd veterinarians will need to alter their antimicrobial use towards a more prudent use of these essential drugs in the future.

## 4. Conclusions

Based on mandatory veterinary reporting, antimicrobial dispensing in the pig sector in Austria has not decreased over the past six-year period. While the vast majority of antimicrobials dispensed are in the EU's least restrictive Category D, an alarming proportion of Category B antimicrobials (primarily polymyxins, namely colistin) are dispensed for use in young piglets. National-benchmarking schemes are already in place for herd veterinarians and are currently being rolled out to individual pig producers. In future, partly due to new EU legislation, changes will need to be made to improve pig health and prudent antimicrobial use in this sector.

## 5. Materials and Methods

In Austria, pharmaceutical companies, marketing authorisation holders (distributors), and pharmaceutical wholesalers are required by law to provide the authorities with details of the sales of veterinary drugs containing antimicrobials. Additionally, veterinarians with in-house pharmacies must also report the quantities of antibiotics that are dispensed for use in food-producing animals for each farm and livestock species. The legal basis for the collection of these data is the "Veterinary Antibiotics Volumetric Flows Regulation" (*Veterinär-Antibiotika Mengenströme Verordnung*), which was enacted in 2014 [7].

## 5.1. Pig Population Data

The number of animals reared on each farm, as well as animal movement and official veterinary authority data, and numbers of animals slaughtered were available from the official veterinary database, namely the "Veterinary Information System (VIS)".

Each farm was categorised into one farm type using the reported "production system type", and the number of pigs in each category (piglets, fattening pigs, breeding sows/boars) are from the VIS database. The categorisation was taken from official records and can broadly be defined as follows. Breeding units refers to farms where sows (and sometimes boars) are kept to produce piglets for sale (it is not known at the veterinary authority level whether these piglets then go on to fattening farms or piglet rearing units). Fattening farms rear grower/finisher pigs from 20–32 kg liveweight up to slaughter. Piglet-rearing units keep piglets from weaning (i.e., the sows are not present on this type of farm) until the beginning of the fattening period (approx. 20–32 kg). As the name would suggest, farrow-to-finish farms rear piglets from birth to slaughter.

## 5.2. Antimicrobial Use Data

Veterinarians with in-house practice pharmacies are required to provide the amount of dispensed antimicrobials for each marketing authorisation identification number (i.e., each licensed pharmaceutical product) for each farm and livestock species. This is used to calculate the total metric tonnes dispensed of each antimicrobial active ingredient each year. This metric was then converted into mg/PCU for pigs using the standardised method used by the Austrian authorities for the entire national pig herd and described for national reporting for the European Union's ESVAC report [6]. The standardised weight of a slaughtered pig as part of the PCU calculation is 65 kg; further details on the calculation of the PCU are provided elsewhere [6].

Furthermore, the number of Defined Daily Doses (DDDvet) for each antimicrobial substance, as defined by the European Medicines Agency, for the treatment of pigs was calculated as follows. The total number of milligrams of active ingredient dispensed for each antimicrobial substance was divided by the number of DDDvet for that antimicrobial substance with respect to pigs and the route of administration [13] to obtain the potential total number of Defined Daily Doses (DDDvet) for 1 kg animal biomass. To calculate the number of DDDvet per year, the following formula was used:

$$\text{DDDvet per year} = \frac{\text{Total annual number of DDDvet per 1 kg biomass}}{\text{Herd size of breeding animals (if present)} + \text{No. animals moved/slaughtered (in kg) for that year}}$$

Livestock numbers were estimated based on the number of reported animals on the farm combined with animal movement and slaughter data. To ensure uniformity, livestock numbers were converted into the Austrian Ministry of Agriculture's livestock units (LSU), e.g., piglets and weaners (up to 20 kg liveweight) are classified as 0.07 LSU, growers and young boars/sows (up to 50 kg liveweight) as 0.15 LSU, and breeding boars/sows as 0.30 LSU [15].

The data were also divided by route of drug administration, such as systemic or oral application, as well as by production group.

## 5.3. Classification into Prudent Use Categories

In addition, data were divided into groups based on the European Medicines Agency's classifications of B (restrict use), C (use with caution), and D (use prudently), as well as according to the World Health Organization category of "highest priority critically important antimicrobials" (HPCIAs) [18,43]. For details, see Table 4. (NB. The EMA classification A (avoid) was not included as it does not list any antimicrobial substances licensed for use in food-producing animals).

Table 4. Categorisation of veterinary antimicrobials according to the European Medicines Agency.

| European Medicines Agency Category | | | |
|---|---|---|---|
| A ("Avoid") Not authorised for veterinary use in the European Union | B ("Restrict") Critically important for human health | C ("Caution") Alternatives exist in human medicine | D ("Prudent use") First line treatments but only when medically necessary |
| • Carbapenems<br>• Glycopeptides<br>• Drugs used solely to treat tuberculosis<br>etc. | • Cephalosporins (3rd & 4th generation)<br>• Polymyxins<br>• Fluoroquinolones | • Aminoglycosides<br>• Aminopenicillins (in combination with beta-lactamase inhibitors)<br>• Cephalosporins (1st & 2nd generation)<br>• Amphenicols<br>• Lincosamides<br>• Pleuromutilins<br>• Macrolides<br>• Rifaximin | • Aminopenicillins<br>• Beta-lactamase sensitive penicillins<br>• Beta-lactamase resistant penicillins<br>• Sulphonamides (& combinations, incl. trimethoprim)<br>• Tetracyclines<br>• Nitrofuran derivatives<br>• Spectinomycin<br>• Bacitracin<br>• Fusidic acid<br>• Metronidazole |

Based on the EMA AMEG infographic [18].

*5.4. Statistical Analyses*

All statistical analyses were carried out using the statistical programming language R [44]. The data were prepared and plots were created using the tidyverse package [45].

**Supplementary Materials:** The following are available online at https://www.mdpi.com/article/10.3390/antibiotics11020216/s1, Figure S1: Antimicrobial classes (in mg/PCU) dispensed, divided by route of administration over time.

**Author Contributions:** Conceptualization, C.L.F., R.F. and K.F.; methodology, R.F. and K.F.; validation, K.F.; formal analysis, R.F.; investigation, C.L.F., R.F. and K.F.; resources, K.F.; data curation, R.F.; writing—original draft preparation, C.L.F.; writing—review and editing, C.L.F., R.F. and K.F.; visualization, R.F. and C.L.F.; supervision, K.F.; project administration, K.F.; funding acquisition, K.F. All authors have read and agreed to the published version of the manuscript.

**Funding:** This research received no external funding.

**Institutional Review Board Statement:** Not applicable.

**Informed Consent Statement:** Not applicable.

**Data Availability Statement:** The data included in this analysis were collated as part of a mandatory national monitoring programme and are not freely available in the public domain.

**Conflicts of Interest:** The authors declare no conflict of interest.

# References

1. O'Neill, J. *Antimicrobials in Agriculture and the Environment: Reducing Unnecessary Use and Waste*; The Wellcome Trust: London, UK, 2015. Available online: https://amr-review.org/ (accessed on 14 January 2022).
2. EU Regulation (EU) 2019/6 of the European Parliament and of the Council of 11 December 2018 on Veterinary Medicinal Products and Repealing Directive 2001/82/EC. Available online: https://eur-lex.europa.eu/eli/reg/2019/6/oj (accessed on 3 December 2021).
3. Jensen, H.H.; Hayes, D.J. Impact of Denmark's ban on antimicrobials for growth promotion. *Curr. Opin. Microbiol.* **2014**, *19*, 30–36. [CrossRef]

4. EMA Trends in the Sales of Veterinary Antimicrobial Agents in Nine European Countries: Reporting Period 2005–2009. Available online: www.ema.europa.eu/docs/en_GB/document_library/Report/2011/09/WC500112309.pdf (accessed on 30 June 2018).
5. European Medicines Agency. *Sales of Veterinary Antimicrobial Agents in 19 EU/EEA Countries in 2010-Second ESVAC Report*; European Medicines Agency: Amsterdam, The Netherlands, 2012.
6. European Medicines Agency. *Sales of Veterinary Antimicrobial Agents in 31 European Countries in 2019 and 2020 (11th ESVAC Report)*; European Medicines Agency: Amsterdam, The Netherlands, 2021.
7. BMG. Verordnung des Bundesministers für Gesundheit, mit der ein System zur Überwachung des Vertriebs und Verbrauchs von Antibiotika im Veterinärbereich eingerichtet wird (Veterinär-Antibiotika-Mengenstr. 2014. Available online: https://www.ris.bka.gv.at/Dokumente/BgblAuth/BGBLA_2014_II_83/BGBLA_2014_II_83.html (accessed on 14 January 2022).
8. BMGF Tierarzneimittelkontrollgesetz-TAKG [Control of Veterinary Medicinal Products Law]. Available online: https://www.ris.bka.gv.at/GeltendeFassung/Bundesnormen/20001741/TAKG,Fassungvom06.10.2016.pdf (accessed on 1 June 2017).
9. BMG. *Verordnung des Bundesministers für Gesundheit über die Anerkennung und den Betrieb von Tiergesundheitsdiensten (Tiergesundheitsdienst-Verordnung 2009-TGD-VO 2009)*; Bundesministerium für Gesundheit: Vienna, Austria, 2009; pp. 1–26.
10. Statistik Austria Table: Livestock 2011 to 2021 (Dated 3 September 2021). Available online: https://www.statistik.at/web_en/statistics/Economy/agriculture_and_forestry/livestock_animal_production/livestock/index.html (accessed on 12 January 2022).
11. BMLRT Tabelle 2.2.2.4-Struktur viehhaltender Betriebe Laut Veterinärinformationssystem (VIS) (Structure of Livestock-Keeping Agricultural Holdings according to Official Veterinary Authorities (VIS)). Available online: https://j1dev.agrarforschung.at/index.php?option=com_rsfiles&folder=Gruener_Bericht&Itemid=477&lang=de&limitstart=20 (accessed on 12 January 2022).
12. Fuchs, R.; Fuchs, K. *Bericht über den Vertrieb von Antibiotika in der Veterinärmedizin in Österreich 2016–2020 (Report on Veterinary Antimicrobial Sales/Dispensing in Austria 2016–2020)*; AGES: Graz, Austria, 2021.
13. EMA Defined Daily Doses for Animals (DDDvet) and Defined Course Doses for Animals (DCDvet): European Surveillance of Veterinary Antimicrobial Consumption (ESVAC). Available online: http://www.ema.europa.eu/docs/en_GB/document_library/Other/2016/04/WC500205410.pdf (accessed on 1 July 2021).
14. Sanders, P.; Vanderhaeghen, W.; Fertner, M.; Fuchs, K.; Obritzhauser, W.; Agunos, A.; Carson, C.; Borck Høg, B.; Dalhoff Andersen, V.; Chauvin, C.; et al. Monitoring of Farm-Level Antimicrobial Use to Guide Stewardship: Overview of Existing Systems and Analysis of Key Components and Processes. *Front. Vet. Sci.* **2020**, *7*, 540. [CrossRef]
15. BMLRT. Table 6.3.3—Umrechnungsschlüssel für landwirtschaftliche Nutztiere (Conversion table for farm animals (LSU). In *Grüner Bericht 2021*; Bundesministerium für Landwirtschaft, Regionen und Tourismus (BMLRT): Vienna, Austria, 2021; p. 243.
16. Sanders, P.; Mevius, D.; Veldman, K.; van Geijlswijk, I.; Wagenaar, J.A.; Bonten, M.; Heederik, D. Comparison of different antimicrobial use indicators and antimicrobial resistance data in food-producing animals. *JAC-Antimicrob. Resist.* **2021**, *3*, 1–4. [CrossRef]
17. O'Neill, L.; Rodrigues da Costa, M.; Leonard, F.; Gibbons, J.; Calderón Díaz, J.A.; McCutcheon, G.; Manzanilla, E.G. Does the Use of Different Indicators to Benchmark Antimicrobial Use Affect Farm Ranking? *Front. Vet. Sci.* **2020**, *7*, 558793. [CrossRef]
18. European Medicines Agency Categorisation of Antibiotics Used in Animals Promotes Responsible Use to Protect Public and Animal Health. Available online: https://www.ema.europa.eu/en/news/categorisation-antibiotics-used-animals-promotes-responsible-use-protect-public-animal-health (accessed on 23 June 2021).
19. European Medicines Agency Categorisation of Antibiotics in the European Union. Available online: https://www.ema.europa.eu/en/documents/report/categorisation-antibiotics-european-union-answer-request-european-commission-updating-scientific_en.pdf (accessed on 29 December 2021).
20. Stebler, R.; Carmo, L.P.; Heim, D.; Naegeli, H.; Eichler, K.; Muentener, C.R. Extrapolating Antibiotic Sales to Number of Treated Animals: Treatments in Pigs and Calves in Switzerland, 2011–2015. *Front. Vet. Sci.* **2019**, *6*, 318. [CrossRef]
21. Trauffler, M.; Griesbacher, A.; Fuchs, K.; Köfer, J. Antimicrobial drug use in Austrian pig farms: Plausibility check of electronic on-farm records and estimation of consumption. *Vet. Rec.* **2014**, *175*, 402. [CrossRef]
22. O'Neill, L.; Rodrigues da Costa, M.; Leonard, F.C.; Gibbons, J.; Calderón Díaz, J.A.; McCutcheon, G.; Manzanilla, E.G. Quantification, description and international comparison of antimicrobial use on Irish pig farms. *Porc. Health Manag.* **2020**, *6*, 30. [CrossRef]
23. Veterinary Medicines Directorate. *UK Veterinary Antibiotic Resistance and Sales Surveillance Report*; Veterinary Medicines Directorate: Addlesone, UK, 2021.
24. Tarakdjian, J.; Capello, K.; Pasqualin, D.; Santini, A.; Cunial, G.; Scollo, A.; Mannelli, A.; Tomao, P.; Vonesch, N.; Martino, G. Di Antimicrobial use on Italian Pig Farms and its Relationship with Husbandry Practices. *Animals* **2020**, *10*, 417. [CrossRef]
25. Echtermann, T.; Muentener, C.; Sidler, X.; Kümmerlen, D. Antimicrobial Drug Consumption on Swiss Pig Farms: A Comparison of Swiss and European Defined Daily and Course Doses in the Field. *Front. Vet. Sci.* **2019**, *6*, 240. [CrossRef]
26. Collineau, L.; Belloc, C.; Stärk, K.D.C.; Hémonic, A.; Postma, M.; Dewulf, J.; Chauvin, C. Guidance on the Selection of Appropriate Indicators for Quantification of Antimicrobial Usage in Humans and Animals. *Zoonoses Public Health* **2017**, *64*, 165–184. [CrossRef]
27. Lekagul, A.; Tangcharoensathien, V.; Yeung, S. Patterns of antibiotic use in global pig production: A systematic review. *Vet. Anim. Sci.* **2019**, *7*, 100058. [CrossRef]
28. Attauabi, M.; Borck Høg, B.; Müller-Pebody, B. *DANMAP 2020*; DTU, Statens Serum Institut: Copenhagen, Denmark, 2021.
29. Abe, R.; Takagi, H.; Fujimoto, K.; Sugiura, K. Evaluation of the antimicrobial use in pigs in Japan using dosage-based indicators. *PLoS ONE* **2020**, *15*, e0241644. [CrossRef] [PubMed]

30. Græsbøll, K.; Larsen, I.; Clasen, J.; Birkegård, A.C.; Nielsen, J.P.; Christiansen, L.E.; Olsen, J.E.; Angen, Ø.; Folkesson, A. Effect of tetracycline treatment regimens on antibiotic resistance gene selection over time in nursery pigs. *BMC Microbiol.* **2019**, *19*, 269. [CrossRef] [PubMed]
31. Renzhammer, R.; Loncaric, I.; Ladstätter, M.; Pinior, B.; Roch, F.F.; Spergser, J.; Ladinig, A.; Unterweger, C. Detection of Various *Streptococcus* spp. and Their Antimicrobial Resistance Patterns in Clinical Specimens from Austrian Swine Stocks. *Antibiotics* **2020**, *9*, 893. [CrossRef]
32. Renzhammer, R.; Loncaric, I.; Roch, F.; Pinior, B.; Käsbohrer, A.; Spergser, J.; Ladinig, A.; Unterweger, C. Prevalence of Virulence Genes and Antimicrobial Resistances in *E. coli* Associated with Neonatal Diarrhea, Postweaning Diarrhea, and Edema Disease in Pigs from Austria. *Antibiotics* **2020**, *9*, 208. [CrossRef]
33. SDA. *Usage of Antibiotics in Agricultural Livestock in The Netherlands in 2020-Trends and Benchmarking of Livestock Farms and Veterinarians*; The Netherlands Veterinary Medicines Institute: Utrecht, The Netherlands, 2021.
34. Rhouma, M.; Beaudry, F.; Letellier, A. Resistance to colistin: What is the fate for this antibiotic in pig production? *Int. J. Antimicrob. Agents* **2016**, *48*, 119–126. [CrossRef]
35. Liu, Y.-Y.; Wang, Y.; Walsh, T.R.; Yi, L.-X.; Zhang, R.; Spencer, J.; Doi, Y.; Tian, G.; Dong, B.; Huang, X.; et al. Emergence of plasmid-mediated colistin resistance mechanism MCR-1 in animals and human beings in China: A microbiological and molecular biological study. *Lancet Infect. Dis.* **2016**, *16*, 161–168. [CrossRef]
36. Al-Tawfiq, J.A.; Laxminarayan, R.; Mendelson, M. How should we respond to the emergence of plasmid-mediated colistin resistance in humans and animals? *Int. J. Infect. Dis.* **2017**, *54*, 77–84. [CrossRef]
37. van Rennings, L.; von Münchhausen, C.; Ottilie, H.; Hartmann, M.; Merle, R.; Honscha, W.; Käsbohrer, A.; Kreienbrock, L. Cross-Sectional Study on Antibiotic Usage in Pigs in Germany. *PLoS ONE* **2015**, *10*, e0119114. [CrossRef]
38. Burow, E.; Käsbohrer, A. Risk Factors for Antimicrobial Resistance in *Escherichia coli* in Pigs Receiving Oral Antimicrobial Treatment: A Systematic Review. *Microb. Drug Resist.* **2017**, *23*, 194–205. [CrossRef]
39. Burow, E.; Simoneit, C.; Tenhagen, B.A.; Käsbohrer, A. Oral antimicrobials increase antimicrobial resistance in porcine E. coli – A systematic review. *Prev. Vet. Med.* **2014**, *113*, 364–375. [CrossRef]
40. Collineau, L.; Backhans, A.; Dewulf, J.; Emanuelson, U.; Grosse Beilage, E.; Lehébel, A.; Loesken, S.; Okholm Nielsen, E.; Postma, M.; Sjölund, M.; et al. Profile of pig farms combining high performance and low antimicrobial usage within four European countries. *Vet. Rec.* **2017**, *181*, 657. [CrossRef]
41. Savin, M.; Bierbaum, G.; Blau, K.; Parcina, M.; Sib, E.; Smalla, K.; Schmithausen, R.; Heinemann, C.; Hammerl, J.A.; Kreyenschmidt, J. Colistin-Resistant Enterobacteriaceae Isolated From Process Waters and Wastewater From German Poultry and Pig Slaughterhouses. *Front. Microbiol.* **2020**, *11*, 2699. [CrossRef]
42. Rhouma, M.; Beaudry, F.; Thériault, W.; Letellier, A. Colistin in pig production: Chemistry, mechanism of antibacterial action, microbial resistance emergence, and one health perspectives. *Front. Microbiol.* **2016**, *7*, 1789. [CrossRef]
43. WHO. *Critically Important Antimicrobials for Human Medicine—5th Revision 2016*; WHO: Geneva, Switzerland, 2017.
44. R Core Team R: A Language and Environment for Statistical Computing. Available online: https://www.r-project.org/ (accessed on 5 January 2021).
45. Wickham, H.; Averick, M.; Bryan, J.; Chang, W.; D', L.; Mcgowan, A.; François, R.; Grolemund, G.; Hayes, A.; Henry, L.; et al. Welcome to the Tidyverse. *J. Open Source Softw.* **2019**, *4*, 1686. [CrossRef]

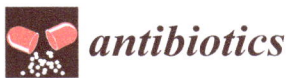

Article

# Antibiotic Use and Resistance Knowledge Assessment of Personnel on Chicken Farms with High Levels of Antimicrobial Resistance: A Cross-Sectional Survey in Ica, Peru

María Dávalos-Almeyda [1], Agustín Guerrero [1], Germán Medina [1], Alejandra Dávila-Barclay [2], Guillermo Salvatierra [2], Maritza Calderón [3], Robert H. Gilman [4] and Pablo Tsukayama [2,5,*]

1. School of Veterinary Medicine, Universidad Nacional San Luis Gonzaga, Ica 11004, Peru; maria.davalos@unica.edu.pe (M.D.-A.); agustingcanelo@gmail.com (A.G.); gemegir1@hotmail.com (G.M.)
2. Microbial Genomics Laboratory, Department of Cellular and Molecular Sciences, Faculty of Sciences and Philosophy, Universidad Peruana Cayetano Heredia, Lima 15102, Peru; alejandra.davila.b@upch.pe (A.D.-B.); guillermo.salvatierra@upch.pe (G.S.)
3. Infectious Diseases Research Laboratories, Department of Cellular and Molecular Sciences, Faculty of Sciences and Philosophy, Universidad Peruana Cayetano Heredia, Lima 15102, Peru; maritza.calderon.s@upch.pe
4. Department of International Health, Bloomberg School of Public Health, Johns Hopkins University, Baltimore, MD 21218, USA; gilmanbob@gmail.com
5. Parasites and Microbes, Wellcome Sanger Institute, Hinxton, Saffron Walden CB10 1RQ, UK
* Correspondence: pablo.tsukayama@upch.pe

**Abstract:** Poultry farming represents Peru's primary food animal production industry, where antimicrobial growth promoters are still commonly used, exerting selective pressure on intestinal microbial populations. Consumption and direct animal-to-human transmission have been reported, and farmworkers are at high risk of colonization with resistant bacteria. We conducted a cross-sectional survey among 54 farmworkers to understand their current antimicrobial resistance (AMR) awareness in Ica, Peru. To gain insight into the potential work-related risk of exposure to bacteria, we also measured the AMR rates in *Escherichia coli* isolated among 50 broiler chickens. Farmworkers were unaware of antimicrobial resistance (31.5%) or antibiotic resistance (16.7%) terms. Almost two-thirds (61%) consumed antibiotics during the previous month, and only 42.6% received a prescription from a healthcare professional. A total of 107 *E. coli* chicken isolates were obtained, showing a high frequency of multidrug-resistant (89.7%) and extended-spectrum beta-lactamase (ESBL) production (71.9%). Among ESBL-producer isolates, 84.4% carried the $bla_{CTX-M}$ gene. Results identified gaps in knowledge that reflect the need for interventions to increase antimicrobial awareness among poultry farmworkers. The high AMR rates among *E. coli* isolates highlight the need to reduce antimicrobial use in poultry farms. Our findings reveal a critical need for effective policy development and antimicrobial stewardship interventions in poultry production in Ica, Peru.

**Keywords:** AMR; public awareness; farmworkers; ESBL; chicken; growth promoters

## 1. Introduction

Peru records one of the largest per capita consumption rates of chicken meat in South America. Poultry farming represents the country's primary food animal production [1]. The widespread intensive systems of broiler chicken rearing, aimed to meet the high national demand, commonly use antimicrobials as growth promoters [2] to allow for more gut nutrient absorption [3]. The constant exposure to antimicrobials ultimately exerts selective pressure on the chicken's intestinal microbial populations [4]. In turn, these bacteria select and acquire antimicrobial resistance genes (ARGs) to adapt to their environment.

Consumption of animal products is one of the most common vehicles for introducing resistant *E. coli* strains into human populations [5–7]. Direct animal to human transmission of AMR has been reported, and farmworkers are at risk of colonization with resistant bacteria from animals [8–10] by various routes, including ingestion, inhalation, and dermal contact [11]. A lack of knowledge and awareness of appropriate antimicrobial use among farm owners and workers may worsen this problem [12,13]. Previous surveys applied to poultry farmworkers [14–17], drug vendors [18,19], and the general public [20–23] have exposed a poor understanding of the problem encompassing antibiotic resistance and the misuse of such drugs in livestock systems and human health. The emergence of multidrug-resistant (MDR) bacteria in animal populations and their potential carriage and gene exchange into clinical settings represent an emerging risk to global public health [24].

The World Health Organization's Global Action Plan on AMR addresses the need to strengthen knowledge and evidence-based practices through surveillance and research [25]. Accordingly, current national strategies designed to tackle the problem from all aspects of One Health have been proposed, starting with food chain surveillance [26]. In many low and middle-income countries (LMIC), antimicrobial use in poultry is not regulated, leading to misuse and facilitating the emergence and spread of AMR [27]. Baseline information and surveillance studies are scarce in Peru compared to other LMICs [28]. However, the potential dissemination of ARGs of gut bacteria from commercial chicken meat to humans with different degrees of exposure has recently been described [29].

Based on the lack of data concerning knowledge and awareness of AMR and antibiotic use among Peruvian poultry farmworkers, we surveyed individuals working in broiler chicken farms in Ica, one of the main poultry producing regions in Peru, to help understand the current state of awareness and common behaviors related to antimicrobial use in the workplace. Additionally, based on their potential work-related exposure to AMR transmission, we aimed to measure AMR rates in *E. coli* isolated from broiler chickens belonging to farms in the same area. We focused on the phenotypic and genotypic determinants of extended-spectrum beta-lactamase (ESBL) production, an important resistance mechanism associated with severe infections in hospital and community settings [30–32].

## 2. Results

Farmworker cross-sectional survey: The adapted antimicrobial knowledge and awareness survey was applied to 54 workers from various farms in Chincha Province, Ica, Peru. The mean age was 38.9 (range 21–66 years), and only 5.6% (three in 54) of the participants were women, two of which were veterinarians and one a vaccinator. Most male respondents were farm operators whose activities involved close contact with the feed mill and the birds, either as handlers or vaccinators, including veterinarians. According to their educational level, most participants only had an early or primary education (77.8%). A total of 61% reported taking antibiotics during the last month for personal use, and 68.5% incorrectly agreed with the statement that it was adequate to take antibiotics prescribed for friends or family as long as they were used to treat the same illness. In all, 42.6% said that they used antibiotics only when they received a prescription from a healthcare professional, and 20.4% stopped antibiotic treatment once they felt better (Table 1).

**Table 1.** Cross-sectional survey results of a sample of 54 farm workers from Ica poultry farms.

| Results | n (%) |
|---|---|
| Q1. When did you last take antibiotics? | |
| In the last month | 33 (61.0) |
| In the last 6 months | 19 (35.2) |
| In the last year | 1 (1.9) |
| More than a year ago | 1 (1.9) |
| Q2. On that occasion, did you get the antibiotics (or a prescription for them) from a doctor or nurse? | |
| Yes | 23 (42.6) |
| Q3. On that occasion, where did you get the antibiotics? | |
| Medical store or pharmacy | 36 (66.7) |

Table 1. Cont.

| Results | n (%) |
|---|---|
| I had them saved up from a previous time | 18 (33.3) |
| **Q4. When do you think you should stop taking antibiotics once you've begun treatment?** | |
| When you feel better | 11 (20.4) |
| When you've taken all of the antibiotics as directed | 42 (77.8) |
| Don't know | 1 (1.9) |
| **Q5. "It's okay to use antibiotics that were given to a friend or family member, as long as they were used to treat the same illness" (TRUE)** | |
| Yes | 37 (68.5) |
| **Q6. "It's okay to buy the same antibiotics, or request these from a doctor, if you're sick and they helped you get better when you had the same symptoms before" (TRUE)** | |
| Yes | 25 (46.3) |
| **Q7. Do you think these conditions can be treated with antibiotics?** | |
| Diarrhoea | 42 (77.8) |
| Bladder infection or urinary tract infection | 40 (74.1) |
| HIV/AIDS | 37 (68.5) |
| Gonorrhoea | 30 (55.6) |
| Fever | 28 (51.9) |
| Measles | 22 (40.7) |
| Cold and flu | 15 (27.8) |
| Sore throat | 10 (18.5) |
| Headaches | 10 (18.5) |
| Skin or wound infection | 8 (14.8) |
| Body aches | 8 (14.8) |
| Malaria | 5 (9.3) |
| **Q8. Have you ever heard of any of the following terms?** | |
| Antibiotic resistance | 45 (83.3) |
| Superbugs | 11 (20.4) |
| Antimicrobial resistance | 37 (68.5) |
| AMR | 5 (9.3) |
| Drug resistance | 38 (70.4) |
| Antibiotic-resistant bacteria | 18 (33.3) |
| **Q9. Do you agree that the following actions would help address the problem of antibiotic resistance? (Yes)** | |
| People should use antibiotics only when they are prescribed by a doctor or nurse | 48 (88.9) |
| Farmers should give fewer antibiotics to food-producing animals | 23 (42.6) |
| People should not keep antibiotics and use them later for other illnesses | 33 (61.1) |
| Parents should make sure all of their children's vaccinations are up-to-date | 21 (38.9) |
| People should wash their hands regularly | 13 (24.1) |
| Doctors should only prescribe antibiotics when they are needed | 50 (92.6) |
| Governments should reward the development of new antibiotics | 18 (33.3) |
| Pharmaceutical companies should develop new antibiotics | 22 (40.7) |

A total of 61.1% (33 in 54) of the participants had taken antibiotics during the previous month (Table 1, Q1), from which all were male. Participants between 34 and 43 years (39.4%, 13 out of 33) and with an early/primary educational level (78.8%, 26 out of 33) presented the highest frequency of antibiotic consumption during the last month. However, no significant differences were found ($p > 0.05$, Fisher's exact test, see Table 2). One question proposed a list of different illnesses and medical conditions, asking if they could be treated with antibiotics (Table 1, Q7). Among the listed diseases, only skin infection, gonorrhea, and bladder/urinary tract infection should be treated with antibiotics. The majority of respondents (74.1%, $n = 40$) correctly indicated bladder/urinary tract infections as pathologies treatable with antibiotics. Overall, 55.6% correctly selected gonorrhea and only 14.8% skin infections. Several farmworkers were unaware of infectious agents involved in the listed diseases, suggesting a treatment based on antibiotics for diarrhea (77.8%), HIV/AIDS (68.5%), fever (51.9%), measles (40.7%), cold/flu (27.8%), headaches (18.5%), sore throat (18.5%), body aches (14.8%), and malaria (9.3%). Results by educational level and age category are detailed in Figure 1.

**Table 2.** Participant's characteristics and use of antibiotics within the previous month.

| Characteristics | Total | Antibiotics Consumed during the Previous Month | | $p$-Value * |
|---|---|---|---|---|
| | | Yes ($n$ = 33) | No ($n$ = 21) | |
| Age (tertiles) | | | | |
| <34 | 18 (33.3) | 8 (24.2) | 10 (47.6) | 0.296 |
| 34–43 | 18 (33.3) | 13 (39.4) | 5 (23.8) | |
| >43 | 18 (33.3) | 12 (36.4) | 6 (28.6) | |
| Education level | | | | |
| Early/Primary | 42 (77.8) | 26 (78.8) | 16 (76.2) | 1.000 |
| Secondary | 12 (22.2) | 7 (21.2) | 5 (23.8) | |

* Fisher exact test, 95% confidence level.

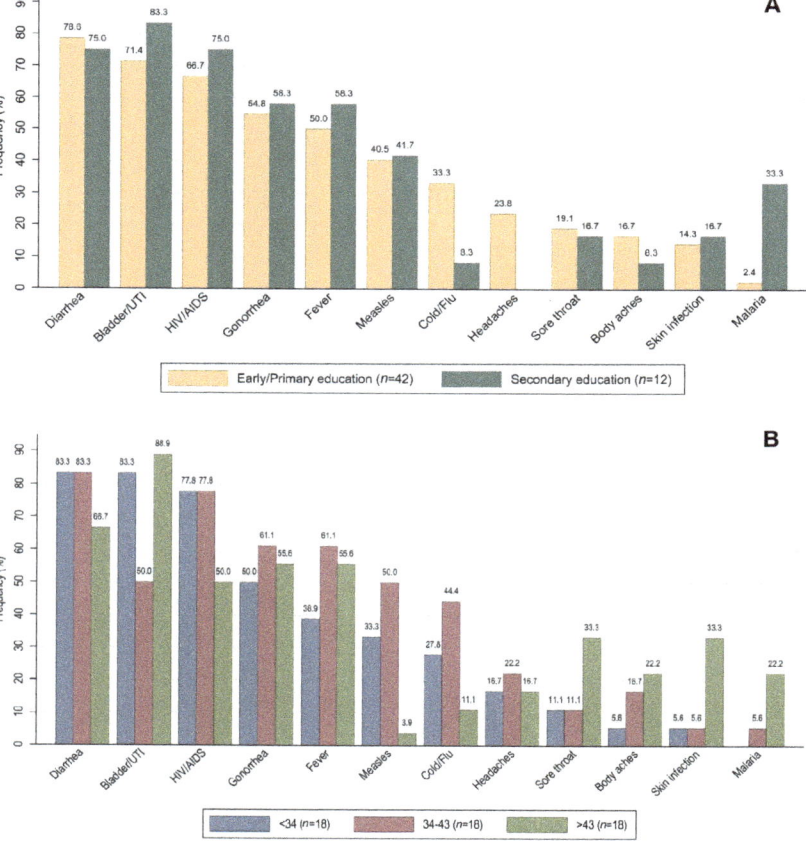

**Figure 1.** Frequency of responses to question: "Do you think these conditions can be treated with antibiotics?" Medical conditions to be treated with antibiotics: Gonorrhea, Bladder/UTI and Skin infection. (**A**) results by educational level, (**B**) results by age category in years.

A total of 31.5% of participants were unaware of the term antimicrobial resistance and 16.7% of antibiotic resistance. Moreover, only 33.3% had heard about antibiotic-resistant bacteria. The respondents answered eight queries regarding AMR with true or false answers (Table 1, Q9). A total of 88.9% correctly identified the statement that people should use antibiotics only when a doctor or nurse prescribes them. Most farmworkers (92.6%) responded that doctors should only prescribe antibiotics when needed, and 61.1% agreed not to keep antibiotics from one treatment and use them for other later illnesses. Additionally, 42.6% thought that farmers should give fewer antibiotics to food-producing animals. A group of respondents incorrectly agreed that having child vaccinations up to date (38.9%) and washing hands (24.1%) are good ways to help address the problem of antibiotic resistance.

The calculated knowledge score regarding antibiotic use resulted in a mean of 7.3 (SD:2.2) out of 14 points among all participants. The score of participants with a secondary educational level was higher than early/primary school graduates (Figure 2A). The oldest age group (>43 years) had the highest knowledge level on good antibiotic use, followed by the younger participants (<34 years) (Figure 2B). Participants who had taken antibiotics during the previous month showed better knowledge of antibiotics than those who reported not having taken any antibiotics (Figure 2C). However, no significant differences were found for educational level ($p > 0.05$, $t$-test), antibiotic consumption during the last month ($p > 0.05$, $t$-test), and age category ($p > 0.05$, one-way ANOVA).

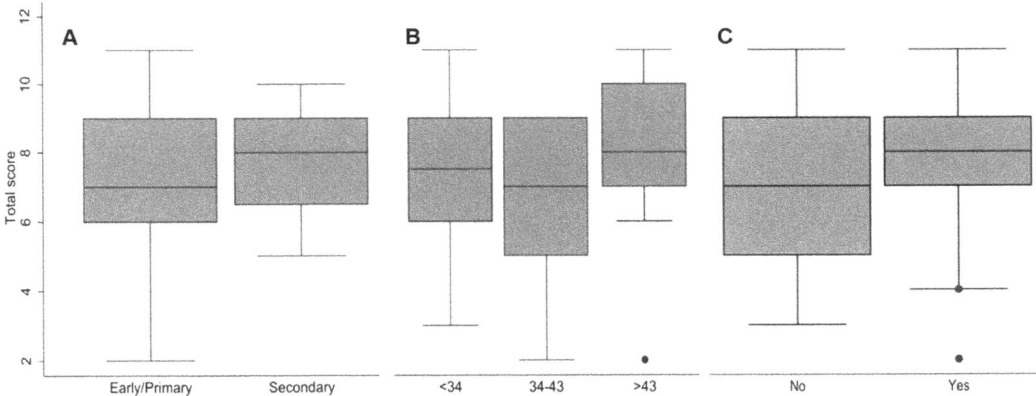

**Figure 2.** Calculated knowledge score regarding antibiotic use among participants. (**A**) educational level ($p = 0.420$, $t$-test), (**B**) age category in years ($p = 0.276$, one-way ANOVA), (**C**) antibiotic consumption during the last month ($p = 0.432$, $t$-test).

Determination of antibiotic resistance in commensal *E. coli* from chickens: *Escherichia coli* isolates ($n = 107$) were obtained from cloacal swabs of 50 broiler chickens from three different poultry farms (Farm A = 32, Farm B = 37, Farm C = 38) from three districts in Chincha, Ica. Susceptibility results for all isolates revealed an 89.7% multidrug-resistant (MDR) phenotype, with no statistical difference between the three farms ($p > 0.05$, Fisher's exact test). High resistance levels were found for trimethoprim/sulfamethoxazole (95.3%), amoxicillin (86.9%), nalidixic acid (85.1%), tetracycline (80.4%), and cefalotin (78.5%). No resistance to meropenem was found among isolates (see Table 3).

Table 3. Antimicrobial resistance rates of *E. coli* from chickens among sampled farms.

| Results | Total (n = 107) | Farm A (n = 32) | Farm B (n = 37) | Farm C (n = 38) | p-Value * |
|---|---|---|---|---|---|
| MDR | | | | | |
| Yes | 96 (89.7) | 28 (87.5) | 36 (97.3) | 32 (94.2) | 0.147 |
| ESBL | | | | | |
| Yes | 77 (71.9) | 20 (62.5) | 33 (89.2) | 24 (63.2) | 0.012 |
| Amphenicols | | | | | |
| Chloramphenicol | 72 (67.3) | 22 (68.8) | 21 (56.8) | 29 (76.3) | 0.200 |
| Tetracyclines | | | | | |
| Tetracycline | 86 (80.4) | 27 (84.4) | 23 (62.2) | 36 (94.7) | 0.002 |
| Sulfonamides | | | | | |
| Trimethoprim/sulfamethoxazole | 102 (95.3) | 31 (96.9) | 37 (100.0) | 34 (89.5) | 0.078 |
| Aminoglycosides | | | | | |
| Gentamicin | 64 (59.8) | 23 (71.9) | 21 (56.8) | 20 (52.6) | 0.246 |
| Macrolides | | | | | |
| Azithromycin | 2 (1.9) | 0 (0.0) | 1 (2.7) | 1 (2.6) | 1.000 |
| Penicillins | | | | | |
| Amoxicillin | 93 (86.9) | 29 (90.6) | 35 (94.6) | 29 (76.3) | 0.067 |
| Cephalosporins | | | | | |
| Cefalotin | 84 (78.5) | 21 (65.6) | 35 (94.6) | 28 (73.7) | 0.007 |
| Cefepime | 12 (11.2) | 4 (12.5) | 5 (13.5) | 3 (7.9) | 0.742 |
| Carbapenems | | | | | |
| Meropenem | 0 (0.0) | 0 (0.0) | 0 (0.0) | 0 (0.0) | N.A. |
| Quinolones | | | | | |
| Nalidixic Acid | 91 (85.1) | 26 (81.3) | 36 (97.3) | 29 (76.3) | 0.021 |
| Ciprofloxacin | 72 (67.3) | 15 (46.9) | 32 (86.5) | 25 (65.8) | 0.002 |

* Fisher exact test, 95% confidence level. N.A.: Not applicable.

Farm B had the highest frequency of resistant isolates to several antimicrobials, including nalidixic acid, amoxicillin, cefalotin, ciprofloxacin, and chloramphenicol. A high percentage of ESBL-producing *E. coli* (71.9%, 77/107) was identified, specifically in Farm B (89.2%, 33/37), compared to the other two ($p = 0.012$, Fisher's exact test). Moreover, all ESBL-producing isolates were identified as MDR, and 84.4% (65/77) carried $bla_{CTX-M}$, with no statistical difference between farms ($p > 0.05$, Fisher's exact test).

## 3. Discussion

The survey utilized an adaptation of a WHO questionnaire on AMR to investigate antibiotic use practices and knowledge among 54 farmworkers from broiler chicken farms. Several respondents were unaware of which pathologies should be treated with antibiotics and evidenced misconceptions about AMR. Participants had insufficient awareness of antibiotic-related terms, such as antimicrobial resistance or antibiotic-resistant bacteria. Moreover, some participants incorrectly correlated that having child vaccinations up to date and washing hands are good ways to address the problem of antibiotic resistance.

Participants who obtained a better antibiotic knowledge score of antibiotic use had a higher educational level. This finding matches with an observation described in the WHO survey that people with a lower education level are more likely to incorrectly use antibiotics than people with higher educational levels [33]. Older participants (>43 years) showed better antibiotic knowledge than the youngest age group (<34 years). However, younger cohorts often show good knowledge about antibiotics and antibiotic use [34,35]. In rural areas, people dealing with poultry are relatively older people, and their results could be associated with work experience or previous interactions with veterinarians.

Participants who had taken antibiotics during the last month obtained a better antibiotic knowledge score. Apparently, farmworkers with a recent exposure gain sufficient yet not comprehensive knowledge about antibiotics. Similar results have been previously reported among the general population [36,37]. Our findings highlight the need to train farmworkers on AMR as a potential measure to reduce the unregulated use of antimicrobials on farm animals. Actions that effectively build an understanding of how and when to take antimicrobials are critical among farmworkers in poultry settings. Effective interventions and educational programs delivered by health care professionals are needed to train farmworkers to raise awareness about AMR, as those part of the National Multisectoral Action Plan to Combat Antimicrobial Resistance, which include workshops and information dissemination on AMR through social media [26].

To gain insight regarding the potential work-related risk of exposure to AMR bacteria through chickens, our study measured, over a year, the rates of antimicrobial resistance in *E. coli* isolated from broiler chickens in a high-producing region in Peru. We found high levels of resistance and MDR phenotypes in most isolates. Our findings showed high resistance rates to antimicrobials commonly used in poultry farms, including trimethoprim/sulfamethoxazole, amoxicillin, nalidixic acid, tetracycline, and cefalotin. The use of antimicrobials in poultry production increases the selective pressure for commensal bacteria such as *E. coli* [4]. The increasing AMR rates in *E. coli* from poultry constitute a significant threat to human and animal health, with animals serving as zoonotic reservoirs of resistant bacteria [38]. Farm B showed the highest rates of ESBL phenotypes at 89.2%. Plasmids that encode ESBLs tend to carry genes giving resistance to antimicrobials such as quinolones, aminoglycosides, and sulfonamides [39]. While the same animal density was reported for the three farms, Farm B had a greater flock size. Pathogens can be introduced to a flock through various routes, including workers, feed, water, fomites, and other animals [40–42]. The high frequency of MDR *E. coli* in Farm B might be explained by a larger farm involving more workers, increasing potential contamination routes.

We observed a higher frequency of MDR ESBL-producing *E. coli* in Farm B than the others. Farm B reported using Zinc Bacitracin and Colistin Sulfate as growth promotors. However, we did not test susceptibility against those antibiotics, and we could not establish an association between the growth promotors used and the high levels of MDR isolates found. Based on previous reports, we hypothesize that a high prevalence of resistance in Farm B could be linked to a greater flock size and elevated temperature and humidity levels inside the houses, resulting in heat stress and consequent watery droppings that increase bedding humidity, which facilitates bacterial survival and colonization [43]. However, housing environmental conditions were not measured in this study. Among ESBL-producing isolates, 12 (15.6%) were negative for $bla_{CTX-M}$. This may be explained by the presence of other ESBL genes, such as $bla_{TEM}$ or $bla_{SHV}$ [44].

Dispensing therapeutic or prophylactic antibiotic doses in feed or water for mass administration and flock treatment is common in local and rural farms [45]. All farms reported administering Zinc Bacitracin to the birds during the pilot study period. Moreover, Farm B also administered colistin sulfate in feedstuff. Colistin is considered a last-resort drug for treating severe human clinical infections caused by MDR Gram-negative bacteria [36] and has been widely used in local animal production for decades. Even though a ban on polymyxin E import and trade in the country was established in 2019, local commerce still allows its use until stock depletion [46]. Supplementation with commercially available premixes containing sub-inhibitory amounts of antimicrobials, also a common local practice, is regarded to positively affect growth and aid with feed conversion [47]. However, antibiotics used as growth promoters alter the microbiota and generate a selective pressure that increases the rate of AMR in the microbiota of farm animals [48]. The elevated frequency of MDR *E. coli* isolates obtained in this study highlights the potential consequences of AGPs in poultry production and warrants further investigation of their impact as a feed additive in local settings.

This study had limitations. The cross-sectional survey focused on a small set of questions targeted at general knowledge and antimicrobial drugs usage. It was applied to a limited number of farmworkers in three farms. Future research should include more participants to address the full complexity of antibiotic knowledge and use and expand on questions specific to animal agriculture relating to current practices and beliefs concerning the antibiotic supplementation and treatment of food animals. Notably, efforts should be directed towards understanding the directionality of current practices [17] and the main drivers [49–51] of AMR in local poultry systems, as well as quantifying antibiotic use [52]. Temperature and humidity levels inside the poultry houses would have helped explain some of the data more accurately. Peru's poultry production model usually reuses bedding across the year, which could serve as a vehicle for MDR bacteria and ARGs from previous batches. In that sense, the frequency of bedding change could affect our results and should be considered in future studies, including manure management and its impact on other agricultural systems [53]. Our results may not represent the AMR situation in the poultry industry in Peru. However, they provide evidence of highly resistant *E. coli* in animal production. They should alert veterinary and public health stakeholders to control and limit antibiotic use in poultry production. The data could serve as a baseline for future qualitative AMR risk assessment frameworks [54]. A study of AMR clustering among farmworkers, chickens, and farm environments [55] integrating novel genomic techniques [56] could provide detailed insight into AMR transmission in foodborne pathogens and exposure risks in poultry farms in the region. Although it was not measured, these results hint at the possible work-related risk of exposure to highly resistant bacteria. Due to the nature of our results and considering the scarce publicly available data on AMR in the studied area, the results will be translated to Spanish and shared amongst the local agrarian and environmental health services, farmworkers, and owners.

## 4. Material and Methods

### 4.1. Farmworker Cross-Sectional Survey

Fifty-four workers from broiler chicken farms in Chincha province, northern Ica, Peru, were recruited after consenting to be surveyed on their knowledge and personal use of antibiotics. The World Health Organization (WHO) questionnaire: "Antibiotic resistance: multi-country awareness survey" [33], was translated into Spanish and modified in some sections to accommodate its application (see Supplementary Materials S1 and S2). The survey included nine questions with multiple-choice and true/false responses. It was applied by the face-to-face method, conducted by trained researchers for the answers to remain anonymous, and included demographic information, such as age, gender, and educational level. We generated a knowledge score based on Q5, Q6, and Q7. To calculate the score, all participants had to indicate whether Q5 and Q6 statements were false and correctly specify in Q7 which of the 12 different illnesses and medical conditions should be treated with antibiotics. Thus, we generated a total score of 14 points.

### 4.2. Study Farms

Three broiler chicken farms from the same region in Ica (Supplementary), were included (Figure 3A). The farms share market and biosecurity characteristics of Sector 2 of the FAO/OIE (2007) classification of poultry production systems [57], consisting of intensive semi-technified commercial productions with moderate to high biosecurity levels (Figure 3B). Flock sizes varied: Farm A had approximately 16,000 birds, Farm B 75,000, and Farm C 42,000. Yet, the three farms reported the same animal density of 8.5 chicken/m$^2$. All farms are located near roads leading to rural populated areas where other poultry and livestock productions also converge. We recorded information on the health status and antimicrobial drugs supplied to the flocks during the sampling period. All three farms reported zinc-bacitracin use as an antibiotic growth promoter (AGP) during the sampling periods. The use of colistin sulfate was reported in Farm B only.

### 4.3. Chicken Samples

We sampled 35-day old healthy broiler chickens ($n$ = 50) from the three farms during April, July, and December 2018. The sampling did not interfere with the way birds were raised. Chickens were randomly selected from each flock every time. Sterile swabs were inserted inside each bird's cloaca and rotated clockwise, securing contact with the mucosal surface. Cloacal swabs were transported in sterile saline solution tubes at 4 °C within 2 h to the laboratory for bacterial culture.

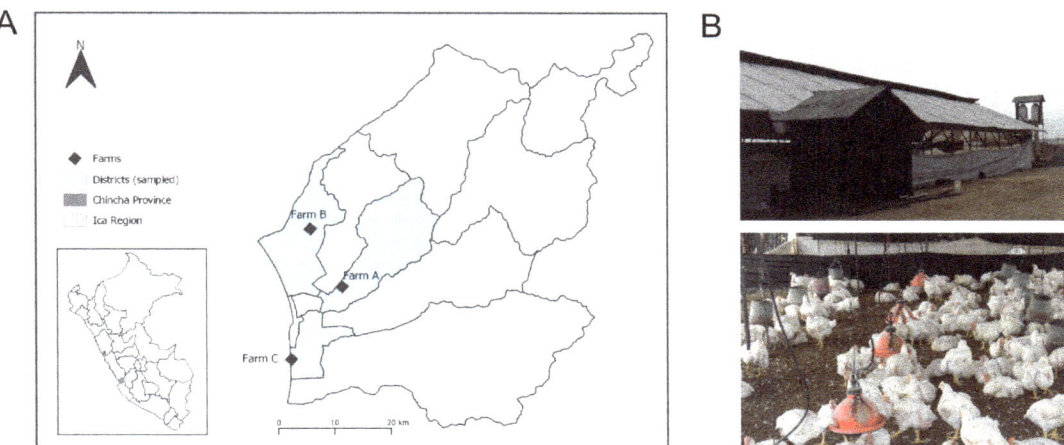

**Figure 3.** (**A**) Geographical location of the sampled farms along Chincha Province in Ica region, Peru. (**B**) Exterior and interior views of the chicken farms. The provincial map of Ica was created using QGIS v3.16.0 (https://qgis.org) (accessed on 23 February 2021).

*4.4. Bacterial Culture and Antibiotic Susceptibility Testing*

Samples were streaked in MacConkey agar (Becton Dickinson, Heidelberg, Germany) and incubated at 37 °C for 24 h. Three presumptive colonies per plate were selected for identification with a biochemical profiling panel, including Simmons Citrate, Triple Sugar Iron Agar, MIO medium (Motility, Indole, Ornithine), Lysine Iron Agar, and Methyl Red Voges-Proskauer Broth (Becton Dickinson). Those confirmed as *Escherichia coli* were included in the study and stored at −20 °C in Tryptic soy broth (TSB, Becton Dickinson) with 10% glycerol. Disk diffusion tests were performed for chloramphenicol (30 µg), meropenem (10 µg), nalidixic acid (30 µg), ciprofloxacin (5 µg), gentamicin (10 µg), azithromycin (15 µg), sulfa-trimethoprim (1.25 µg + 23.75 µg), tetracycline (30 µg), amoxicillin (20 µg), cefalotin (30 µg), and cefepime (30 µg) according to CLSI standards [58], using susceptible, intermediate, and resistant definitions. Extended-spectrum β-lactamase (ESBL) detection was performed using the cefotaxime-ceftazidime-cefepime-aztreonam and amoxicillin with clavulanic acid test [59].

*4.5. DNA Extraction*

We adapted a protocol based on heat treatment followed by boiling to release bacterial DNA [60]. Three to four colonies were picked from each isolate grown in Trypticase Soy Agar plates and diluted 1:4 in 200 µL of Tris-EDTA Buffer solution in 1.5 mL sterile tubes and vortexed. The tubes were then placed in a dry-heat plate at 100 °C for 10 min and centrifuged at 14,000 rpm for 5 min. The supernatant was transferred to a sterile tube for use in PCR assays.

*4.6. Detection of bla$_{CTX-M}$ Gene*

All positive isolates for phenotypic ESBL production were tested for the presence of the *bla*$_{CTX-M}$ gene. The primers used were 5′-TTTGCGATGTGCAGTACCAGTAA-3′ and 5′-CGATATCGTTGGTGGTGCCATA-3′, as previously described [61]. These amplify a conserved 544 bp fragment common to most *bla*$_{CTX-M}$ genes. PCR was carried out in a 25 µL reaction containing the following concentrations: 2 mM MgCl$_2$, 150 µM dNTPs, 1 µM of each primer, 1 Unit of Taq polymerase, 1× PCR buffer (10 mM Tris-HCl, 50 mM KCl), and 2 μL DNA template (20–50 ng). Reactions were performed with a 5-min denaturation at 94 °C, 35 annealing cycles at 94 °C, 58 °C, and 72 °C of 30 s each, and a final extension of 5 min at 72 °C on a PTC-150 thermocycler (MJ Research, Inc., Watertown, MA, USA). Amplification products were resolved on a 2% agarose gel with ethidium bromide. As positive controls, we used isolates with at least one of the $bla_{CTX-M}$ genes, confirmed by whole-genome sequencing (WGS) from a previous study [29].

*4.7. Data Analysis*

A bivariate analysis to compare antibiotic consumption during the last month between gender, educational level, and age category was performed using Fisher's exact test. The calculated knowledge score about antibiotics was compared for educational level and age category using a *t*-test and one-way analysis of variance (ANOVA), respectively. The Clinical & Laboratory Standards Institute (CLSI) guidelines were used to categorize isolates as susceptible, resistant, or intermediate. Multidrug resistance (MDR) was defined as an isolate expressing phenotypic resistance to three or more antibiotics classes [62]. A bivariate analysis to compare resistance results between sampled farms was performed using Fisher's exact test. Statistical analysis was performed with a 95% confidence level using STATA 16 (Stata Corp., College Station, TX, USA).

## 5. Conclusions

This study's survey results indicate insufficient knowledge amongst farmworkers regarding the antimicrobial resistance problem and the appropriate and prudent use of antimicrobial drugs for treating human diseases. *E. coli* isolates from chickens raised for human consumption showed high resistance rates to various antimicrobials used in human clinical settings. Our results highlight the need to (1) promote antibiotic knowledge and awareness among farmworkers, (2) implement measures to reduce the use of antimicrobials in poultry systems in Peru, and (3) establish surveillance systems to monitor the rates of antimicrobial-resistant bacteria in local chicken populations.

**Supplementary Materials:** The following supporting information can be downloaded at: https://www.mdpi.com/article/10.3390/antibiotics11020190/s1, S1: Study survey in English, S2: Study survey in Spanish.

**Author Contributions:** Conceptualization, M.D.-A., A.G., G.M., M.C., R.H.G. and P.T.; methodology, M.D.-A., A.G. and G.M.; validation, A.D.-B. and M.C.; formal analysis, G.S.; investigation, A.G. and A.D.-B.; resources, M.D.-A., A.G., G.M. and R.H.G.; data curation, A.D.-B. and G.S.; writing—original draft preparation, M.D.-A., A.G., G.M., A.D.-B. and G.S.; writing—review & editing, M.D.-A., A.G., G.M., A.D.-B., G.S., M.C., R.H.G. and P.T.; visualization, G.S.; supervision, R.H.G.; project administration, M.D.-A.; funding acquisition, R.H.G. and P.T. All authors have read and agreed to the published version of the manuscript.

**Funding:** The study was supported by the National Institutes of Health under Award Number D43 TW010074 grant and the Microbiology Laboratory of the School of Veterinary Medicine at Universidad Nacional San Luis Gonzaga. G.S. and P.T. were supported by the Fogarty International Center of the National Institutes of Health under Award Number D43TW009343 and the University of California Global Health Institute. G.S. was supported by the CONCYTEC-FONDECYT-World Bank Group contract number E033-01-08-2018-FONDECYT/Banco Mundial-Programas de Doctorado en Áreas Estratégicas y Generales.

**Institutional Review Board Statement:** Ethical approval was obtained from the Institutional Review Board of Servicio Nacional de Sanidad y Calidad Agroalimentaria from Ica, Peru (N°0042-2018-MINAGRI-SENASA-DEICA).

**Informed Consent Statement:** Requirements for informed consent for the survey were waived by the Research Office of the School of Veterinary Medicine and Zootechnics from Universidad Nacional San Luis Gonzaga de Ica (N°01-DICT-FMVZ-UNICA-2018).

**Data Availability Statement:** Non applicable.

**Acknowledgments:** We thank farm personnel for their participation in the survey and assistance during sampling; UNICA and UPCH field and laboratory personnel for data collection and sample processing.

**Conflicts of Interest:** The authors declare no conflict of interest.

# References

1. Statistics | Food and Agriculture Organization of the United Nations. Available online: http://www.fao.org/statistics/en (accessed on 11 May 2020).
2. Alkhalf, A.; Alhaj, M.; Al-Homidan, I. Influence of probiotic supplementation on blood parameters and growth performance in broiler chickens. *Saudi J. Biol. Sci.* **2010**, *17*, 219–225. [CrossRef] [PubMed]
3. Evans, M.C.; Wegener, H.C. Antimicrobial growth promoters and Salmonella spp., Campylobacter spp. in poultry and swine, Denmark. *Emerg. Infect. Dis.* **2003**, *9*, 489–492. [CrossRef] [PubMed]
4. Woolhouse, M.; Ward, M.; Van Bunnik, B.; Farrar, J. Antimicrobial resistance in humans, livestock and the wider environment. *Philos. Trans. R. Soc. B Biol. Sci.* **2015**, *370*. [CrossRef] [PubMed]
5. Hashempour-Baltork, F.; Hosseini, H.; Shojaee-Aliabadi, S.; Torbati, M.; Alizadeh, A.M.; Alizadeh, M. Drug resistance and the prevention strategies in food borne bacteria: An update review. *Adv. Pharm. Bull.* **2019**, *9*, 335–347. [CrossRef]
6. Liu, C.M.; Stegger, M.; Aziz, M.; Johnson, T.J.; Waits, K.; Nordstrom, L.; Gauld, L.; Weaver, B.; Rolland, D.; Statham, S.; et al. Escherichia coli ST131-H22 as a foodborne uropathogen. *MBio* **2018**, *9*, e00470-18. [CrossRef]
7. Davis, G.S.; Waits, K.; Nordstrom, L.; Grande, H.; Weaver, B.; Papp, K.; Horwinski, J.; Koch, B.; Hungate, B.A.; Liu, C.M.; et al. Antibiotic-resistant Escherichia coli from retail poultry meat with different antibiotic use claims. *BMC Microbiol.* **2018**, *18*, 174. [CrossRef]
8. Ho, B.T.; Dong, T.G.; Mekalanos, J.J. A view to a kill: The bacterial type VI secretion system. *Cell Host Microbe* **2014**, *15*, 9–21. [CrossRef]
9. Abdi, R.D.; Mengstie, F.; Beyi, A.F.; Beyene, T.; Waktole, H.; Mammo, B.; Ayana, D.; Abunna, F. Determination of the sources and antimicrobial resistance patterns of Salmonella isolated from the poultry industry in Southern Ethiopia. *BMC Infect. Dis.* **2017**, *17*, 352. [CrossRef]
10. Sun, J.; Liao, X.P.; D'Souza, A.W.; Boolchandani, M.; Li, S.H.; Cheng, K.; Luis Martínez, J.; Li, L.; Feng, Y.J.; Fang, L.X.; et al. Environmental remodeling of human gut microbiota and antibiotic resistome in livestock farms. *Nat. Commun.* **2020**, *11*, 1427. [CrossRef]
11. Neyra, R.C.; Vegosen, L.; Davis, M.F.; Price, L.; Silbergeld, E.K. Antimicrobial-resistant bacteria: An unrecognized work-related risk in food animal production. *Saf. Health Work* **2012**, *3*, 85–91. [CrossRef]
12. Oluwasile, B.; Agbaje, M.; Ojo, O.; Dipeolu, M. Antibiotic usage pattern in selected poultry farms in Ogun state. *Sokoto J. Vet. Sci.* **2014**, *12*, 45. [CrossRef]
13. Boamah, V.E.; Odoi, H.; Dalsgaard, A. Practices and Factors Influencing the Use of Antibiotics in Selected Poultry Farms in Ghana. *J. Antimicrob. Agents* **2016**, *2*, 120. [CrossRef]
14. Awogbemi, J.; Adeye, M.; Olugbenga, A.E. A Survey of Antimicrobial Agents Usage in Poultry Farms and Antibiotic Resistance in Escherichia Coli and Staphylococci Isolates from the Poultry in Ile-Ife, Nigeria. *J. Infect. Dis. Epidemiol.* **2018**, *4*, 4–11. [CrossRef]
15. Ozturk, Y.; Celik, S.; Sahin, E.; Acik, M.N.; Cetinkaya, B. Assessment of farmers' knowledge, attitudes and practices on antibiotics and antimicrobial resistance. *Animals* **2019**, *9*, 653. [CrossRef] [PubMed]
16. Al-Mustapha, A.I.; Adetunji, V.O.; Heikinheimo, A. Risk perceptions of antibiotic usage and resistance: A cross-sectional survey of poultry farmers in Kwara State, Nigeria. *Antibiotics* **2020**, *9*, 378. [CrossRef]
17. Caudell, M.A.; Dorado-Garcia, A.; Eckford, S.; Creese, C.; Byarugaba, D.K.; Afakye, K.; Chansa-Kabali, T.; Fasina, F.O.; Kabali, E.; Kiambi, S.; et al. Towards a bottom-up understanding of antimicrobial use and resistance on the farm: A knowledge, attitudes, and practices survey across livestock systems in five African countries. *PLoS ONE* **2020**, *15*, e0220274. [CrossRef]
18. Bâtie, C.; Kassie, D.; Randravatsilavo, D.N.R.M.; Baril, L.; Waret Szkuta, A.; Goutard, F.L. Perception of Drug Vendors and Pig and Poultry Farmers of Imerintsiatosika, in Madagascar, Toward Risks Related to Antibiotic Usage: A Q-Method Approach. *Front. Vet. Sci.* **2020**, *7*, 490. [CrossRef]
19. Kalam, M.A.; Alim, M.A.; Shano, S.; Nayem, M.R.K.; Badsha, M.R.; Al Mamun, M.A.; Hoque, A.; Tanzin, A.Z.; Khan, S.A.; Islam, A.; et al. Knowledge, attitude, and practices on antimicrobial use and antimicrobial resistance among commercial poultry farmers in Bangladesh. *Antibiotics* **2021**, *10*, 784. [CrossRef]
20. Prigitano, A.; Romanò, L.; Auxilia, F.; Castaldi, S.; Tortorano, A.M. Antibiotic resistance: Italian awareness survey 2016. *J. Infect. Public Health* **2018**, *11*, 30–34. [CrossRef]
21. Chukwu, E.E.; Oladele, D.A.; Awoderu, O.B.; Afocha, E.E.; Lawal, R.G.; Abdus-Salam, I.; Ogunsola, F.T.; Audu, R.A. A national survey of public awareness of antimicrobial resistance in Nigeria. *Antimicrob. Resist. Infect. Control* **2020**, *9*, 72. [CrossRef]
22. Effah, C.Y.; Amoah, A.N.; Liu, H.; Agboyibor, C.; Miao, L.; Wang, J.; Wu, Y. A population-base survey on knowledge, attitude and awareness of the general public on antibiotic use and resistance. *Antimicrob. Resist. Infect. Control* **2020**, *9*, 105. [CrossRef] [PubMed]

23. Michaelidou, M.; Karageorgos, S.A.; Tsioutis, C. Antibiotic use and antibiotic resistance: Public awareness survey in the republic of cyprus. *Antibiotics* **2020**, *9*, 759. [CrossRef] [PubMed]
24. Sastry, S.; Doi, Y. Fosfomycin: Resurgence of an old companion. *J. Infect. Chemother.* **2016**, *22*, 273–280. [CrossRef] [PubMed]
25. WHO. *Global Action Plan on Antimicrobial Resistance*; WHO: Geneva, Switzerland, 2017.
26. MINSA Plan Nacional para Enfrentar la Resistencia a los Antimicrobianos 2017–2021. Available online: http://www.digemid.minsa.gob.pe/UpLoad/UpLoaded/PDF/Acceso/URM/GestionURMTrabSalud/ReunionTecnica/VIII/Dia2/Antimicrobianos/PlanNacionalATM-2017-2021.pdf (accessed on 11 May 2020).
27. Usui, M.; Ozawa, S.; Onozato, H.; Kuge, R.; Obata, Y.; Uemae, T.; Ngoc, T.; Heriyanto, A.; Chalemchaikit, T.; Makita, K.; et al. Antimicrobial Susceptibility of Indicator Bacteria Isolated from Chickens in Southeast Asian Countries (Vietnam, Indonesia and Thailand). *J. Vet. Med. Sci.* **2014**, *76*, 685–692. [CrossRef]
28. Van Boeckel, T.P.; Pires, J.; Silvester, R.; Zhao, C.; Song, J.; Criscuolo, N.G.; Gilbert, M.; Bonhoeffer, S.; Laxminarayan, R. Global trends in antimicrobial resistance in animals in low- and middle-income countries. *Science* **2019**, *365*. [CrossRef]
29. Murray, M.; Salvatierra, G.; Dávila-Barclay, A.; Ayzanoa, B.; Castillo-Vilcahuaman, C.; Huang, M.; Pajuelo, M.J.; Lescano, A.G.; Cabrera, L.; Calderón, M.; et al. Market Chickens as a Source of Antibiotic-Resistant Escherichia coli in a Peri-Urban Community in Lima, Peru. *Front. Microbiol.* **2021**, *12*, 635871. [CrossRef]
30. Nadimpalli, M.; Vuthy, Y.; de Lauzanne, A.; Fabre, L.; Criscuolo, A.; Gouali, M.; Huynh, B.T.; Naas, T.; Phe, T.; Borand, L.; et al. Meat and fish as sources of extended-spectrum β-Lactamase– producing Escherichia coli, Cambodia. *Emerg. Infect. Dis.* **2019**, *25*, 126–131. [CrossRef]
31. Day, M.J.; Hopkins, K.L.; Wareham, D.W.; Toleman, M.A.; Elviss, N.; Randall, L.; Teale, C.; Cleary, P.; Wiuff, C.; Doumith, M.; et al. Extended-spectrum β-lactamase-producing Escherichia coli in human-derived and foodchain-derived samples from England, Wales, and Scotland: An epidemiological surveillance and typing study. *Lancet Infect. Dis.* **2019**, *19*, 1325–1335. [CrossRef]
32. Doi, Y.; Iovleva, A.; Bonomo, R.A. The ecology of extended-spectrum b-lactamases (ESBLs) in the developed world. *J. Travel Med.* **2017**, *24*, S45–S50. [CrossRef]
33. WHO. *Antibiotic Resistance: Multi-Country Public Awareness Survey*; WHO Press: Geneve, Switzerland, 2015; pp. 1–51.
34. Sørensen, K.; Pelikan, J.M.; Röthlin, F.; Ganahl, K.; Slonska, Z.; Doyle, G.; Fullam, J.; Kondilis, B.; Agrafiotis, D.; Uiters, E.; et al. Health literacy in Europe: Comparative results of the European health literacy survey (HLS-EU). *Eur. J. Public Health* **2015**, *25*, 1053–1058. [CrossRef]
35. Sadiq, M.B.; Syed-Hussain, S.S.; Ramanoon, S.Z.; Saharee, A.A.; Ahmad, N.I.; Noraziah, M.Z.; Khalid, S.F.; Naseeha, D.S.; Syahirah, A.A.; Mansor, R. Knowledge, attitude and perception regarding antimicrobial resistance and usage among ruminant farmers in Selangor, Malaysia. *Prev. Vet. Med.* **2018**, *156*, 76–83. [CrossRef] [PubMed]
36. Singer, R.S.; Patterson, S.K.; Meier, A.E.; Gibson, J.K.; Lee, H.L.; Maddox, C.W. Relationship between phenotypic and genotypic florfenicol resistance in Escherichia coli. *Antimicrob. Agents Chemother.* **2004**, *48*, 4047–4049. [CrossRef] [PubMed]
37. Salm, F.; Ernsting, C.; Kuhlmey, A.; Kanzler, M.; Gastmeier, P.; Gellert, P. Antibiotic use, knowledge and health literacy among the general population in Berlin, Germany and its surrounding rural areas. *PLoS ONE* **2018**, *13*, e0193336. [CrossRef] [PubMed]
38. Marshall, B.M.; Levy, S.B. Food Animals and Antimicrobials: Impacts on Human Health. *Clin. Microbiol. Rev.* **2011**, *24*, 718–733. [CrossRef]
39. Gupta, K.; Bhadelia, N. Management of urinary tract infections from multidrug-resistant organisms. *Infect. Dis. Clin. N. Am.* **2014**, *28*, 49–59. [CrossRef]
40. Maciorowski, K.G.; Herrera, P.; Jones, F.T.; Pillai, S.D.; Ricke, S.C. Effects on poultry and livestock of feed contamination with bacteria and fungi. *Anim. Feed Sci. Technol.* **2007**, *133*, 109–136. [CrossRef]
41. Skóra, J.; Matusiak, K.; Wojewódzki, P.; Nowak, A.; Sulyok, M.; Ligocka, A.; Okrasa, M.; Hermann, J.; Gutarowska, B. Evaluation of microbiological and chemical contaminants in poultry farms. *Int. J. Environ. Res. Public Health* **2016**, *13*, 192. [CrossRef]
42. Pearson, A.D.; Greenwood, M.; Healing, T.D.; Rollins, D.; Shahamat, M.; Donaldson, J.; Colwell, R.R. Colonization of broiler chickens by waterborne Campylobacter jejuni. *Appl. Environ. Microbiol.* **1993**, *59*, 987–996. [CrossRef]
43. Dhanarani, T.S.; Shankar, C.; Park, J.; Dexilin, M.; Kumar, R.R.; Thamaraiselvi, K. Study on acquisition of bacterial antibiotic resistance determinants in poultry litter. *Poult. Sci.* **2009**, *88*, 1381–1387. [CrossRef]
44. D'Andrea, M.M.; Arena, F.; Pallecchi, L.; Rossolini, G.M. CTX-M-type β-lactamases: A successful story of antibiotic resistance. *Int. J. Med. Microbiol.* **2013**, *303*, 305–317. [CrossRef]
45. Vermeulen, B.; De Backer, P.; Remon, J.P. Drug administration to poultry. *Adv. Drug Deliv. Rev.* **2002**, *54*, 795–803. [CrossRef]
46. Diario Oficial del Bicentenario. *Resolución Directoral No 0091-2019-MINAGRI-SENASA-DIAIA*; Diario El Peruano: Lima, Peru, 2019.
47. Cardinal, M.K.; Kipper, M.; Andretta, I.; Machado Leal Ribeiro, A. Withdrawal of antibiotic growth promoters from broiler diets: Performance indexes and economic impact. *Poult. Sci.* **2019**, *98*, 6659–6667. [CrossRef] [PubMed]
48. Nadimpalli, M.; Delarocque-Astagneau, E.; Love, D.C.; Price, L.B.; Huynh, B.-T.; Collard, J.-M.; Lay, K.S.; Borand, L.; Ndir, A.; Walsh, T.R.; et al. Combating Global Antibiotic Resistance: Emerging One Health Concerns in Lower-and Middle-Income Countries. *Clin. Infect. Dis.* **2018**, *66*, 963–969. [CrossRef] [PubMed]
49. Al Masud, A.; Rousham, E.K.; Islam, M.A.; Alam, M.U.; Rahman, M.; Al Mamun, A.; Sarker, S.; Asaduzzaman, M.; Unicomb, L. Drivers of Antibiotic Use in Poultry Production in Bangladesh: Dependencies and Dynamics of a Patron-Client Relationship. *Front. Vet. Sci.* **2020**, *7*, 78. [CrossRef]

50. Redding, L.E.; Brooks, C.; Georgakakos, C.B.; Habing, G.; Rosenkrantz, L.; Dahlstrom, M.; Plummer, P.J. Addressing Individual Values to Impact Prudent Antimicrobial Prescribing in Animal Agriculture. *Front. Vet. Sci.* **2020**, *7*, 297. [CrossRef]
51. Elmi, S.A.; Simons, D.; Elton, L.; Haider, N.; Hamid, M.M.A.; Shuaib, Y.A.; Khan, M.A.; Othman, I.; Kock, R.; Osman, A.Y. Identification of risk factors associated with resistant escherichia coli isolates from poultry farms in the east coast of peninsular malaysia: A cross sectional study. *Antibiotics* **2021**, *10*, 117. [CrossRef]
52. Wongsuvan, G.; Wuthiekanun, V.; Hinjoy, S.; Day, N.P.J.; Limmathurotsakul, D. Antibiotic use in poultry: A survey of eight farms in Thailand. *Bull. World Health Organ.* **2018**, *96*, 94–100. [CrossRef]
53. Jiang, W.; Paudel, S.K.; Amarasekara, N.R.; Zhang, Y.; Etienne, X.; Jones, L.; Li, K.W.; Hansen, F.; Jaczynski, J.; Shen, C. Survey of small local produce growers' perception of antibiotic resistance issues at farmers markets. *Food Control* **2021**, *125*, 107997. [CrossRef]
54. Chereau, F.; Opatowski, L.; Tourdjman, M.; Vong, S. Risk assessment for antibiotic resistance in South East Asia. *BMJ* **2017**, *358*, 2–8. [CrossRef]
55. Braykov, N.P.; Eisenberg, J.N.S.; Grossman, M.; Zhang, L.; Vasco, K.; Cevallos, W.; Muñoz, D.; Acevedo, A.; Moser, K.A.; Marrs, C.F.; et al. Antibiotic Resistance in Animal and Environmental Samples Associated with Small-Scale Poultry Farming in Northwestern Ecuador. *mSphere* **2016**, *1*, e00021-15. [CrossRef]
56. Moser, A.I.; Kuenzli, E.; Campos-Madueno, E.I.; Büdel, T.; Rattanavong, S.; Vongsouvath, M.; Hatz, C.; Endimiani, A. Antimicrobial-Resistant Escherichia coli Strains and Their Plasmids in People, Poultry, and Chicken Meat in Laos. *Front. Microbiol.* **2021**, *12*, 2106. [CrossRef] [PubMed]
57. FAO Animal Production and Health Division. *Poultry Sector Country Review: India*; FAO Animal Production and Health Division: Rome, Italy, 2008.
58. CLSI. *M100: Performance Standards for Antimicrobial Susceptibility Testing*, 28th ed.; Clinical and Laboratory Standards Institute: Wayne, PA, USA, 2018.
59. European Committee on Antimicrobial Susceptibility Testing. *Breakpoint Tables for Interpretation of MICs and Zone Diameters Version 7.1*; European Committee on Antimicrobial Susceptibility Testing: Växjö, Sweden, 2017.
60. Dashti, A.A.; Jadaon, M.M.; Abdulsamad, A.M.; Dashti, H.M. Heat Treatment of Bacteria: A Simple Method of DNA Extraction for Molecular Techniques. *Kuwait Med. J.* **2009**, *41*, 117–122.
61. Edelstein, M.; Pimkin, M.; Palagin, I.; Edelstein, I.; Stratchounski, L. Prevalence and Molecular Epidemiology of CTX-M Extended-Spectrum β-Lactamase-Producing Escherichia coli and Klebsiella pneumoniae in Russian Hospitals. *Antimicrob. Agents Chemother.* **2003**, *47*, 3724–3732. [CrossRef] [PubMed]
62. Magiorakos, A.P.; Srinivasan, A.; Carey, R.B.; Carmeli, Y.; Falagas, M.E.; Giske, C.G.; Harbarth, S.; Hindler, J.F.; Kahlmeter, G.; Olsson-Liljequist, B.; et al. Multidrug-resistant, extensively drug-resistant and pandrug-resistant bacteria: An international expert proposal for interim standard definitions for acquired resistance. *Clin. Microbiol. Infect.* **2012**, *18*, 268–281. [CrossRef]

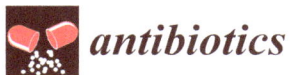

Article

# How Accurate Are Veterinary Clinicians Employing Flexicult Vet for Identification and Antimicrobial Susceptibility Testing of Urinary Bacteria?

Blaž Cugmas [1,2,*], Miha Avberšek [1], Teja Rosa [1], Leonida Godec [1], Eva Štruc [3], Majda Golob [4] and Irena Zdovc [4]

[1] Veterinary Clinic Zamba, Vets4science d.o.o., 3000 Celje, Slovenia; miha@vets4science.com (M.A.); teja.rosa@gmail.com (T.R.); leonida.kajdic@gmail.com (L.G.)
[2] Biophotonics Laboratory, Institute of Atomic Physics and Spectroscopy, University of Latvia, 1586 Riga, Latvia
[3] Vetamplify SIA, Veterinary Services, 1009 Riga, Latvia; eva@vetamplify.com
[4] Institute of Microbiology and Parasitology, Veterinary Faculty, University of Ljubljana, 1000 Ljubljana, Slovenia; majda.golob@vf.uni-lj.si (M.G.); irena.zdovc@vf.uni-lj.si (I.Z.)
* Correspondence: blaz.cugmas@lu.lv

**Citation:** Cugmas, B.; Avberšek, M.; Rosa, T.; Godec, L.; Štruc, E.; Golob, M.; Zdovc, I. How Accurate Are Veterinary Clinicians Employing Flexicult Vet for Identification and Antimicrobial Susceptibility Testing of Urinary Bacteria? *Antibiotics* **2021**, *10*, 1160. https://doi.org/10.3390/antibiotics10101160

Academic Editor: Albert Figueras

Received: 27 August 2021
Accepted: 22 September 2021
Published: 24 September 2021

**Publisher's Note:** MDPI stays neutral with regard to jurisdictional claims in published maps and institutional affiliations.

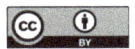

**Copyright:** © 2021 by the authors. Licensee MDPI, Basel, Switzerland. This article is an open access article distributed under the terms and conditions of the Creative Commons Attribution (CC BY) license (https://creativecommons.org/licenses/by/4.0/).

**Abstract:** Antibiotics are frequently used for treating urinary tract infections (UTI) in dogs and cats. UTI often requires time-consuming and expensive antimicrobial susceptibility testing (AST). Alternatively, clinicians can employ Flexicult Vet, an affordable chromogenic agar with added antibiotics for in-clinic AST. We investigated how well veterinary microbiologists and clinicians, without any prior experience, employ Flexicult Vet for the identification and AST of the most common canine and feline urinary pathogenic bacteria. We prepared 47 monoculture plates containing 10 bacterial species. The test's mean accuracy was 75.1% for bacteria identification (84.6% and 68.7% for microbiologists and clinicians, respectively) and 79.2% for AST (80.7% and 78.2%). All evaluators employed Flexicult Vet with the accuracies over 90% for the distinctively colored bacteria like *Escherichia coli* (red), *Enterococcus faecalis* (turquoise), and *Proteus* spp. (pale brown). However, the evaluators' experience proved important in recognizing lightly colored bacteria like *Staphylococcus pseudintermedius* (accuracies of 82.6% and 40.3%). Misidentifications of *E. faecium* additionally worsened AST performance since bacterial intrinsic resistance could not be considered. Finally, only 33.3% (3/9) of methicillin-resistant *S. pseudintermedius* (MRSP) were correctly detected. To conclude, Flexicult Vet proved reliable for certain urinary pathogens. In contrast, light-colored bacteria (e.g., *Staphylococcus*), often misidentified, require a standard AST.

**Keywords:** urinary tract infection; Flexicult Vet; antimicrobial susceptibility testing; pathogen identification; dogs; cats; veterinary microbiology

## 1. Introduction

Urinary tract infections (UTIs) are common in small animals since up to 27% of dogs, especially females, are affected during their lifetime. In cats, UTIs are rarer (<2%) and they usually appear in older cats (>10 years) [1–3]. Uncomplicated UTI can sporadically happen in otherwise healthy animals. In contrast, urinary infections in pets with anatomic or functional abnormalities may often persist, reoccur, or be insensitive to treatment. In 85% of cases, a single pathogen is the main cause of UTI. The most frequently isolated species are *Escherichia coli* (>50%), followed by *Staphylococcus* spp., *Enterococcus* spp., *Streptococcus* spp., *Proteus* spp., *Enterobacter* spp., *Pseudomonas* spp., and *Klebsiella* spp. [1,2,4–8].

Due to its high incidence, bacterial UTI is one of the main reasons for prescribing antibiotics in small animal medicine [9]. In contrast to human medicine, the range of available veterinary antibiotics is limited; thus, special care is required by veterinary clinicians to prevent misuse or overuse of antibiotics and to avoid the appearance of resistant strains. Resistant bacteria are an important but not the only undesirable outcome of improper use of antibiotics. Animal health (due to drug side effects, normal flora distortions [8,10,11]) and treatment costs (side effects and prolonged or recurrent UTIs) can all be directly impacted. Since antimicrobial resistance can also affect the health of humans (e.g., due to animal–human transmissions [12]), other animals, and environment, correct antibiotic use for UTI can contribute considerably to the One Health approach [13].

Therefore, managing UTI often requires antimicrobial susceptibility testing (AST) [1,3]. However, AST according to the CLSI standards [14] based on disc diffusion, broth dilution, or agar dilution methods in the certified microbiological laboratories can be time-consuming (up to a week) and expensive for some pet owners. Moreover, sample storage and shipping additionally contribute to the uncertainty of the final results [7]. Thus, empirical antimicrobial treatment is still the most comfortable for clinicians in small animal practice, who frequently opt even for second-line antibiotics (in 57% of UTI cases) [15].

Point-of-care (POC) tests have recently appeared to provide a faster and cheaper in-clinic AST, which might reduce the utilization of unnecessary or inappropriate antibiotics [16]. One of the most popular is Flexicult Vet, based on a chromogenic nonselective culture medium with added antibiotics in separate compartments (Figure 1). The test promises to provide data about bacteria species and sensitivity to the most common antibiotics in only 24 h. Existing studies indicated that the evaluator's experience plays an important role in the test's performance and accuracy. For example, one expert reached an accuracy of 100% using Flexicult Vet for bacterial identification [4]. On the other hand, less experienced evaluators achieved the lower accuracies of 53% [4], 58–77% [17], and 92–98% [18]. Furthermore, the test's AST performance resulted in accuracies between 39 and 99% [4,17,18].

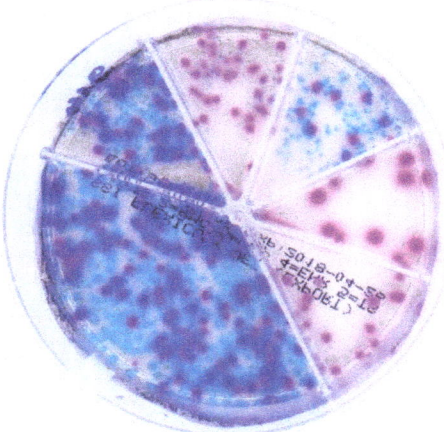

Figure 1. *Escherichia coli* (red colonies) and *Enterococcus faecalis* (turquoise) on Flexicult Vet agar.

Due to the reported large differences in Flexicult Vet performance, the aim of the present study was to evaluate how well the potential end-users, i.e., veterinary clinicians without a microbiological background, had employed Flexicult Vet for bacterial identification and AST interpretation. First, we inoculated Flexicult Vet with the monocultures of the most frequent canine and feline urinary pathogens. Furthermore, we compared how accurate bacteria were identified, and AST interpreted by experts (microbiologists and microbiological assistants) or veterinary practitioners, all without any prior Flexicult Vet experience. The results pointed out that veterinary clinicians can benefit from Flexicult Vet in some cases, but many limitations remain.

## 2. Results

On average, 75.1% of samples were identified correctly (Table 1). Experts outperformed clinicians with the mean bacteria species identification accuracies of 84.6% versus 68.7%, respectively. Moreover, clinicians seemed less confident in their evaluations due to the slightly wider 95% confidence interval (CI) (18.2 versus 14.7 percentage points, respectively). Surprisingly, not a single bacterium was identified perfectly. The highest identification accuracies were expectedly achieved for bacteria with distinct colors like red (*Escherichia coli*, 90.0%), turquoise (*Enterococcus faecalis*, 97.8%), and pale brown (*Proteus* spp., 90.0%) (Figure 2). Additionally, nine raters correctly identified a single isolate of *Pseudomonas aeruginosa* (an accuracy of 90.0%).

**Table 1.** Mean and 95% confidence intervals (CI, squared brackets) of identification accuracy (%) retrieved by experts (E) and clinicians (C). The most frequent misidentified bacteria are listed in the rounded brackets. Bacteria are abbreviated as *Enterobacter* spp. (Es), *Klebsiella* spp. (Ks), *S. canis* (Sc), *S. aureus* (Sa), and *P. aeruginosa* (Pa).

| | | Flexicult Vet | | | | | |
|---|---|---|---|---|---|---|---|
| **True Species** | Investigator | E. coli | S. pseudint. | E. faecium | E. faecalis | *Proteus* spp. | Other |
| *E. coli*, n = 13 | E | **98.1** [95.2–100.0] | 1.9 | | | | |
| | C | **84.6** [72.7–96.6] | 12.8 | 1.3 | | | 1.3 (Es, Ks) |
| | All | **90.0** [82.3–98.7] | 8.5 | 0.8 | | | 0.8 (Ea, Ks) |
| *S. pseudintermedius*, n = 11 | E | 8.3 | **82.6** [68.3–96.9] | 3.4 | | | 5.7 (Sc, Sa) |
| | C | 7.6 | **40.3** [22.8–57.7] | 21.6 | | | 30.6 (Sc, Pa) |
| | All | 7.9 | **57.2** [44.1–70.3] | 14.3 | | | 20.6 (Sc, Sa, Pa) |
| *E. faecium*, n = 6 | E | | 50.0 | **31.3** [15.2–47.3] | | | 18.8 (Sc) |
| | C | 1.6 | 25.0 | **27.6** [18.8–36.3] | 5.1 | | 40.8 (Sc, Pa, Ks) |
| | All | 1.0 | 35.0 | **29.0** [21.7–36.3] | 3.1 | | 32.0 (Sc, Pa, Ks) |
| *E. faecalis*, n = 9 | E | | | 1.4 | **98.6** [95.4–100] | | |
| | C | | | 0.9 | **97.2** [94.0–100] | | 1.9 (Pa) |
| | All | | | 1.1 | **97.8** [95.0–100] | | 1.1 (Pa) |
| *Proteus* spp., n = 4 | E | | | | | **93.8** [73.9–100] | 6.3 (Pa) |
| | C | | | | 8.3 | **87.5** [62.1–100] | 4.2 (Pa) |
| | All | | | | 5.0 | **90.0** [71.6–100] | 5.0 (Pa) |
| Other, n = 4 | E | 8.3 | | | 3.1 | | **88.5** [63.5–100] |
| | C | 2.1 | 4.9 | 3.5 | 9.7 | | **79.9** [52.0–100] |
| | All | 4.6 | 2.9 | 2.1 | 7.1 | | **83.3** [57.6–100] |
| All, n = 47 | | Experts: **84.6** [77.2–91.9] | | Clinicians: **68.7** [59.6–77.8] | | All: **75.1** [67.4–82.8] | |

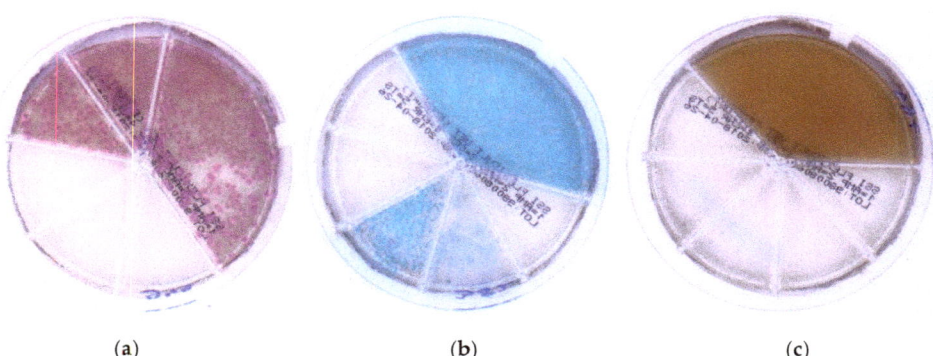

**Figure 2.** Bacteria of (**a**) *Escherichia coli* (red), (**b**) *Enetrococcus faecalis* (turquoise), and (**c**) *Proteus* spp. (brown), exhibiting distinct colors on the Flexicult Vet agar.

Oppositely, identification was more challenging for light-colored (pale) colonies (Figure 3). We found the lowest identification accuracy for *Enterococcus faecium* (29.0%), which was mostly misidentify for *Staphylococcus pseudintermedius* (35.0% of *E. faecium* samples) and *Streptococcus canis* (25.9%). Identifying *S. pseudintermedius* resulted in the highest discrepancy between experts and clinicians (82.6% vs. 40.3%), who had mistaken *S. pseudintermedius* for *E. faecium* and *S. canis* in 21.6% and 22.9% of cases, respectively.

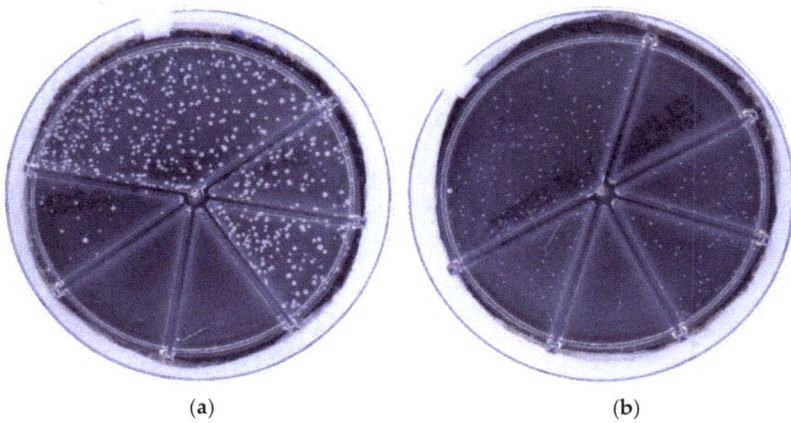

**Figure 3.** Pale-looking bacteria of (**a**) *Staphylococcus pseudintermedius* and (**b**) *Enterococcus faecium* on the Flexicult Vet agar. For display purposes, the agars were photographed with a dark background.

In comparison with the bacterial identification, antimicrobial susceptibility testing (AST) achieved a slightly better mean accuracy of 79.2% (Table 2). Additionally, AST performance by experts or clinicians was comparable. Flexicult Vet enabled accurate AST results for enrofloxacin (ENR, 88.7%) and bacterial species of *E. coli* and *E. faecalis* (>90.0%). Oppositely, the test performed poorly with the accuracies below 50% for *Proteus* spp. (for all antibiotics) and *S. pseudintermedius* (for penicillin group: ampicillin—AMP; amoxicillin —AMC; oxacillin—OXA). Alarmingly, only 33.3% of methicillin-resistant *S. pseudintermedius* (MRSP) were detected. A very low accuracy (30.0%) was also achieved for *E. faecium* sensitivity to trimethoprim/sulfamethoxazole (STX). A majority (>70%) of AST misestimates happened due to the *Enterococcus* spp. intrinsic resistance to STX, which was either forgotten or discarded since bacteria species were misidentified.

Table 2. Absolute sample counts and AST accuracy (in %, means and 95% confidence intervals, CI, in the squared brackets) for Flexicult Vet, evaluated by experts (E) and clinicians (C). Antibiotic abbreviations are the following: ampicillin (AMP), amoxicillin (AMC), oxacillin (OXA), enrofloxacin (ENR), trimethoprim/sulfamethoxazole (SXT). * denotes a group with one sample less.

| Bacteria | Evaluator | AST | Flexicult Vet | | | | | | | | | |
|---|---|---|---|---|---|---|---|---|---|---|---|---|
| | | | AMP | | AMC | | OXA | | ENR | | SXT | |
| | | | R | S | R | S | R | S | R | S | R | S |
| E. coli, n = 13 | E | R | 9 | 1 | 9 | 1 | | | 6 | 1 | 4 | 1 |
| | | S | – | 3 | – | 3 | | | – | 6 | – | 8 |
| | C | R | 8.83 | 1.17 | 9 | 1 | | | 6 | 1 | 4 | 1 |
| | | S | 0.17 | 2.83 | – | 3 | | | – | 6 | 0.17 | 7.83 |
| | All | | 90.8 [74.1–100] | | 92.3 [75.5–100] | | | | 92.3 [75.5–100] | | 91.5 [74.8–100] | |
| S. pseudintermedius, n = 10 | E | R | 6.75 | 2.25 | 2.50 | 6.50 | 3.13 | 5.88 | 8.75 | 0.25 | 9 | – |
| | | S | – | – | – | – | – | 1 | – | 1 | – | 1 |
| | C | R | 7 | 2 | 2.17 | 6.83 | 3 | 6 | 8.83 | 0.17 | 8.83 | 0.17 |
| | | S | – | – | – | 1 | – | 1 | 0.17 | 0.83 | – | 1 |
| | All | | 76.7 * [53.0–100] | | 33.0 [2.3–63.7] | | 40.5 [11.7–69.3] | | 97.0 [92.2–100] | | 99.0 [96.7–100] | |
| E. faecium, n = 6 | E | R | 2 | – | 2 | – | | | 2 | – | 1.50 | 4.50 |
| | | S | – | 4 | – | 4 | | | – | 4 | – | – |
| | C | R | 1.63 | 0.37 | 1.63 | 0.37 | | | 1.80 | 0.20 | 2 | 4 |
| | | S | 1.27 | 2.73 | – | 4 | | | 0.93 | 3.07 | – | – |
| | All | | 83.7 [77.7–89.7] | | 96.3 [90.3–100] | | | | 88.7 [80.6–96.7] | | 30.0 [7.9–52.1] | |
| E. faecalis, n = 9 | E | R | – | – | – | – | | | 5 | – | 8.50 | 0.50 |
| | | S | – | 8 | – | 8 | | | 1 | 2 | – | – |
| | C | R | – | – | – | – | | | 4.83 | 0.17 | 8.17 | 0.83 |
| | | S | 0.17 | 7.83 | – | 8 | | | 1 | 2 | – | – |
| | All | | 98.7 * [95.8–100] | | 100 * [100–100] | | | | 86.2 * [57.0–100] | | 92.2 [84.4–99.7] | |
| Proteus spp., n = 4 | E | R | 2.25 | 1.75 | – | – | | | – | 2 | – | 2 |
| | | S | – | – | 0.75 | 1.25 | | | – | 2 | 0.75 | 1.25 |
| | C | R | 1.17 | 2.83 | – | 2 | | | – | 2 | – | 2 |
| | | S | – | – | – | 2 | | | – | 2 | 0.33 | 1.67 |
| | All | | 40.0 [0–100] | | 42.5 [0–100] | | | | 50.0 [0–100] | | 37.5 [0–100] | |
| Other, n = 4 | E | R | 2.13 | 0.88 | 1 | 1 | | | 1 | – | – | – |
| | | S | – | – | – | 1 | | | – | 3 | 0.13 | 2.88 |
| | C | R | 2.08 | 0.92 | 1.22 | 0.78 | | | 1 | – | – | – |
| | | S | – | – | 0.33 | 0.67 | | | – | 3 | 0.42 | 2.58 |
| | All | | 70.0 * [5.4–1] | | 64.4 * [0–100] | | | | 100 [100–100] | | 90.0 * [77.6–100] | |
| All samples n = 43 (AMP), 44 (AMC), 10 (OXA), 45 (ENR), 45 (SXT) | All | | 82.1 [73.3–90.9] | | 74.4 [62.1–86.6] | | 40.6 [11.8–69.4] | | 88.7 [80.1–97.3] | | 80.2 [70.4–90.0] | |
| | E | | 86.3 [76.6–96.1] | | 74.4 [62.0–86.9] | | 41.3 [9.7–72.9] | | 90.6 [81.9–99.2] | | 80.3 [70.0–90.6] | |
| | C | | 79.3 [70.5–88.1] | | 74.3 [61.9–86.7] | | 40.2 [12.0–68.4] | | 87.4 [78.8–96.1] | | 80.2 [70.4–89.9] | |
| All together (n = 187) | | | All: 79.2 [74.2–84.2] | | | | E: 80.7 [75.5–85.9] | | | | C: 78.2 [73.2–83.2] | |

## 3. Discussion

Point-of-care (POC) microbiological tests like Flexicult Vet could improve antibiotics use since they offer identification and antimicrobial susceptibility testing (AST) of UTI-causing bacteria. To the best of our knowledge, there are no studies that compared the performance of experts and clinicians in using microbiological POC tests on the controlled monoculture samples. The recent field studies with real urine samples [4,17,18], which included experts and beginners, showed that Flexicult Vet enabled identification of bacteria with an accuracy between 53 and 100%, which is in line with the accuracy of 75.1%, reported in this study. However, evaluator experience plays an important role in the test's performance. Although all evaluators handled Flexicult Vet for the first time, microbiological experts outperformed clinicians in bacteria identification for 15.9 percentage points (accuracies of 84.6% vs. 68.7%). The difference between evaluators was significantly smaller than the one reported by Guardabassi et al. [4], where a beginner recognized only 53% of samples, contrary to the flawless expert (100%). Experts from the other studies [17,18] also achieved an excellent identification accuracy (>97%), which was significantly higher than the one reached by microbiological evaluators in our study (84.6%). However, all other studies included only a single expert evaluator, well familiar with Flexicult Vet, in contrast to the experts in this study, who met Flexicult Vet for the first time.

In general, all evaluators in this study identified colorful bacteria very well (accuracies of >90.0%) (Figure 2). Oppositely, identification of light-colored bacteria was unreliable (Figure 3, *S. pseudintermedius*, accuracy of 57.2%, *E. faecium*, 29.0%). The pale colonies were often recognized as *S. canis*. The mentioned misidentifications could be partially addressed by a prolonged incubation time of 48 h, enabling colonies to develop more characteristic color. Additionally, evaluators should pay more attention to colony size. On Flexicult Vet, *S. pseudintermedius* exhibits moderately sized colonies, but *S. canis* develops only microcolonies.

Recognizing bacteria well is especially important for assuring a high AST accuracy. For example, *E. faecium*, which has an intrinsic resistance to STX, was misidentified in 71% of cases. Since 5 (out of 6) samples did not exhibit any growth in the STX compartment, the clinician could falsely choose STX as an antibiotic of choice. Furthermore, in one *E. faecium* sample, three clinicians and one expert forgot to consider its intrinsic resistance to STX, despite correctly recognizing the strain. As intrinsic resistance also concerns penicillin antibiotics (e.g., *Proteus vulgaris*, *Pseudomonas aeruginosa*), Flexicult Vet could be supplemented with a special AST-deploying protocol, reminding users of a possibility of intrinsic resistance.

Neglecting intrinsic resistance was not the only user error detected. In certain cases (Figure 4), clinical evaluators interpreted growing bacteria as sensitive. Oppositely, the absence of growth led to labeling bacterium as resistant. We speculate that these errors could happen due to mixing up *R* (resistant) and *S* (sensitive) labels when filling the AST results form. We assume that similar administrative mistakes could be even more common when evaluators were in the (often noisy and hectic) clinical environment.

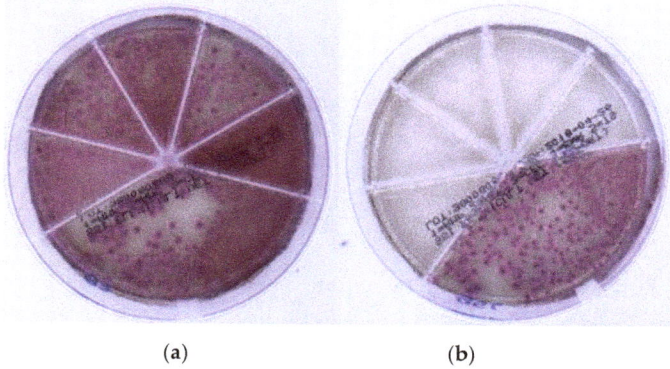

(a)      (b)

**Figure 4.** *Escherichia coli* on Flexicult Vet. The strains were falsely interpreted as (**a**) sensitive (*S*) or (**b**) resistant (*R*) to antibiotics.

In general, Flexicult Vet provided a decent AST for *E. coli* (accuracy of >91.5%) and *E. faecalis* (>86.2%). Despite good identification, poor AST results were achieved for *Proteus* spp. In general, we detected many false sensitive strains (Table 2), which could indicate high antibiotic concentrations. Obviously, appropriate antibiotic concentrations cannot be guaranteed in a single POC test for all bacteria since UTI pathogens (especially *Staphylococcus* spp. versus others) have different AST breakpoints.

The purpose of oxacillin in Flexicult Vet is the detection of methicillin-resistant *S. pseudintermedius* (MRSP). In over a decade, the number of canine MRSP strains in Slovenia has been steadily rising. Moreover, the multidrug-resistant isolates to five or more antimicrobial groups, including oxacillin, penicillin, clindamycin, erythromycin, and trimethoprim, are prevalent [19]. If AST results allow, clinicians often rely on doxycycline for MRSP infection treatment.

Our study included 9 MRSP strains (in addition to one methicillin-sensitive strain). Initially, clinical evaluators had problems recognizing the species since they misidentified 43.8% samples. Additionally, two thirds (6/9) of MRSPs were falsely perceived as sensitive, which led to a conclusion that the OXA concentration is too high. However, this is not in agreement with Guardabassi et al. who showed that 0.125 µg/mL of OXA was the most suitable for cultivating MRSPs and suppressing a methicillin-susceptible *S. pseudintermedius*. The study demonstrated [4] that the larger OXA concentrations, including the CLSI breakpoint (i.e., $R \geq 0.5$ µg/mL [14]), suppressed between 27 and 40% of MRSPs.

## 4. Materials and Methods

We tested a commercially available POC Flexicult Vet Scandinavia (SSI Diagnostica, Hillerød, Denmark) for the identification and AST of UTI-causing bacteria in dogs and cats. Briefly, Flexicult Vet includes the modified chromogenic Müller-Hinton II agar (MH II). The Petri dish was divided into six compartments; one big without antibiotics and five smaller compartments with undisclosed concentrations of ampicillin (AMP), amoxicillin/clavulanate (AMC), oxacillin (OXA), enrofloxacin (ENR), and trimethoprim/sulfamethoxazole (SXT). Bacterial identification is based on the color, shape, and diameter of colonies (CFUs), while the absence or presence of bacterial growth can determine susceptibility to antibiotics (AST). The number of CFUs in the big compartment additionally allows semi-quantitative determination of bacterial concentration in urine, which can reveal clinically relevant bacteriuria due to its correlation with the urine sampling techniques (i.e., free catch, cystocentesis, and catheter specimen thresholds are $\geq 10^5$, $\geq 10^3$, and $\geq 10^4$ CFU/mL, respectively) [4].

The monoculture suspension samples were prepared in a laboratory using 47 common canine and feline UTI strains from the internal bacterial collection at the Institute of Microbiology and Parasitology, Veterinary Faculty, University of Ljubljana. The samples included *E. coli* (13 strains), *S. pseudintermedius* (11, including 9 phenotypically and genetically identified as methicillin-resistant *S. pseudintermedius*, MRSP), *E. faecalis* (9), *E. faecium* (6), *Proteus vulgaris* (2), *Proteus mirabilis* (2), *Klebsiella pneumoniae* (1), *Enterobacter cloacae* (1), *Enterobacter aerogenes* (1), and *P. aeruginosa* (1). At least one reference strain with a known antimicrobial activity was used for each bacterial group, *E. coli* ATCC 25922, *S. aureus* ATCC 29213, *E. faecalis* ATCC 29212, *P. aeruginosa* ATCC 27853, *Klebsiella pneumoniae* ATCC 51503, and *Proteus mirabilis* DSM 788. Other strains were obtained from the different proficiency test trials and clinical isolates. For all strains, we performed AST based on a microdilution method (Sensititre, Thermo Fisher Scientific Inc, Waltham, Massachusetts, USA) or disk diffusion method according to the CLSI standard [14,20]. Bacteria represented by a single sample were joined into a group of *Others*. For a straightforward comparison with Flexicult Vet, intermediate samples were considered as resistant (R).

Monocultures of bacterial suspensions were prepared with various concentrations ($10^4$, $10^5$, and $10^6$ CFU/mL) in sterile saline and inoculated onto Flexicult Vet plates according to the manufacturer's instructions. After the incubation (24 h at 35 °C), 10 participants without any prior Flexicult Vet experience evaluated the plates (Figure 5). There were four *expert* evaluators, microbiologists and microbiology lab assistants in a veterinary microbiological laboratory. Additionally, six veterinary *clinicians* were involved.

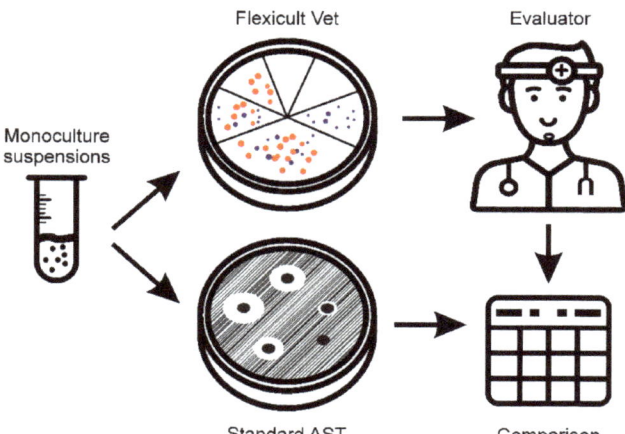

**Figure 5.** Veterinary microbiological experts and veterinary clinicians (Evaluators) performed an identification and antimicrobial susceptibility testing (AST) of UTI bacteria growing on Flexicult Vet plates. The results were compared to the standard AST.

Before the evaluations, we briefly introduced Flexicult Vet to the evaluators. We started with an oral presentation. On a few examples, we additionally demonstrated how to identify bacteria and interpret the plate to obtain AST. First, an evaluator had to provide a bacteria species. In case of doubt, they could list up to three species if selected species were supposedly not crucial for an AST performance. Secondly, the susceptibility (S) or resistance (R) for each antibiotic was retrieved. The final strain score was calculated as a mean of all evaluators' scores. We calculated confidence intervals (CI) as

$$CI = \bar{x} \pm \frac{SD \cdot q}{\sqrt{n}} \quad (1)$$

where $\bar{x}$ and $SD$ are the mean and standard deviation of evaluator scores, $n$ is a number of evaluator scores, and $q$ is a quantile (i.e., the left-tailed inverse of the Student's t-distribution with the probability of 0.975 and the degree of freedom of $n-1$). All calculations were done in the Excel program (Microsoft Excel 2016, 16.0, Microsoft, Redmond, WA, USA). In the end, species and antibiotic score means and confidence intervals were arranged in a tabular form. Plates were photographed by a lightbox (Petriview Box, Vets4science d.o.o., Celje, Slovenia, www.petriview.net, accessed on 1 August 2021).

## 5. Conclusions

Flexicult Vet could be a promising POC test for detecting, identifying, and AST of UTI-causing bacteria. However, to obtain the optimal test performance, which can decrease inappropriate antibiotic use and bacterial resistance, evaluators need to be properly trained; in performing and interpreting Flexicult Vet. Evaluators in this study, regardless of experience, employed the test well for colorful bacteria like *E. coli* and *E. faecalis*. However, experience played an important role in recognizing light-colored bacteria, which can crucially affect the AST accuracy. The study also showed that users could be negligent in considering bacterial intrinsic resistance or selecting R/S labels. Finally, many undiscovered MRSP strains require further studies with *S. pseudintermedius*. Despite the drawbacks mentioned, Flexicult Vet could be useful for veterinary clinicians when dealing with UTI, especially when a pet owner is not willing to cover laboratory AST expenses.

**Author Contributions:** Conceptualization, B.C. and I.Z.; methodology, B.C., M.G. and I.Z.; formal analysis, B.C., M.A., E.Š., T.R. and L.G.; resources, B.C. and I.Z.; data curation, E.Š., L.G.; writing—

original draft preparation, B.C., T.R. and L.G.; writing—review and editing, B.C., M.A., M.G. and I.Z.; visualization, B.C.; supervision, I.Z. All authors have read and agreed to the published version of the manuscript.

**Funding:** This research was funded by the European Society of Veterinary Dermatology (ESVD, Minor grant), the Latvian State Education Development Agency (1.1.1.2/VIAA/3/19/455), and the Slovenian Ministry of Economic Development and Technology under the European Regional Development Fund (Eureka E! 13509).

**Institutional Review Board Statement:** Not applicable.

**Informed Consent Statement:** Not applicable.

**Data Availability Statement:** Data available on request.

**Acknowledgments:** We thank Nina Ružić Gorenjec (Institute for Biostatistics and Medical Informatics, Faculty of Medicine, University of Ljubljana) for her help in analyzing results. We are also very grateful to all evaluators who collaborated in this study.

**Conflicts of Interest:** The authors declare that SSI Diagnostica (Hillerød, Denmark), Flexicult Vet manufacturer, complimentary provided agar samples for this study. However, the company had no role in the design of the study; in the collection, analyses, or interpretation of data; in the writing of the manuscript, or in the decision to publish the results.

## References

1. Dorsch, R.; Teichmann-Knorrn, S.; Sjetne Lund, H. Urinary Tract Infection and Subclinical Bacteriuria in Cats: A Clinical Update. *J. Feline Med. Surg.* **2019**, *21*, 1023–1038. [CrossRef] [PubMed]
2. Smee, N.; Loyd, K.; Grauer, G. UTIs in Small Animal Patients: Part 1: Etiology and Pathogenesis. *J. Am. Anim. Hosp. Assoc.* **2013**, *49*, 83–94. [CrossRef] [PubMed]
3. Weese, J.S.; Blondeau, J.; Boothe, D.; Guardabassi, L.G.; Gumley, N.; Papich, M.; Jessen, L.R.; Lappin, M.; Rankin, S.; Westropp, J.L.; et al. International Society for Companion Animal Infectious Diseases (ISCAID) Guidelines for the Diagnosis and Management of Bacterial Urinary Tract Infections in Dogs and Cats. *Vet. J.* **2019**, *247*, 8–25. [CrossRef] [PubMed]
4. Guardabassi, L.; Hedberg, S.; Jessen, L.R.; Damborg, P. Optimization and Evaluation of Flexicult® Vet for Detection, Identification and Antimicrobial Susceptibility Testing of Bacterial Uropathogens in Small Animal Veterinary Practice. *Acta Vet. Scand.* **2015**, *57*, 72. [CrossRef] [PubMed]
5. Ling, G.V.; Norris, C.R.; Franti, C.E.; Eisele, P.H.; Johnson, D.L.; Ruby, A.L.; Jang, S.S. Interrelations of Organism Prevalence, Specimen Collection Method, and Host Age, Sex, and Breed among 8,354 Canine Urinary Tract Infections (1969–1995). *J. Vet. Intern. Med.* **2001**, *15*, 341–347. [CrossRef] [PubMed]
6. Ball, K.R.; Rubin, J.E.; Chirino-Trejo, M.; Dowling, P.M. Antimicrobial Resistance and Prevalence of Canine Uropathogens at the Western College of Veterinary Medicine Veterinary Teaching Hospital, 2002–2007. *Can. Vet. J. Rev. Vet. Can.* **2008**, *49*, 985–990.
7. Windahl, U.; Holst, B.S.; Nyman, A.; Grönlund, U.; Bengtsson, B. Characterisation of Bacterial Growth and Antimicrobial Susceptibility Patterns in Canine Urinary Tract Infections. *BMC Vet. Res.* **2014**, *10*, 217. [CrossRef] [PubMed]
8. Roberts, M.; White, J.; Lam, A. Prevalence of Bacteria and Changes in Trends in Antimicrobial Resistance of Escherichia Coli Isolated from Positive Canine Urinary Samples from an Australian Referral Hospital over a 5-Year Period (2013–2017). *Vet. Rec. Open* **2019**, *6*, e000345. [CrossRef] [PubMed]
9. De Briyne, N.; Atkinson, J.; Borriello, S.P.; Pokludová, L. Antibiotics Used Most Commonly to Treat Animals in Europe. *Vet. Rec.* **2014**, *175*, 325. [CrossRef] [PubMed]
10. Jessen, L.R.; Sørensen, T.M.; Bjornvad, C.R.; Nielsen, S.S.; Guardabassi, L. Effect of Antibiotic Treatment in Canine and Feline Urinary Tract Infections: A Systematic Review. *Vet. J.* **2015**, *203*, 270–277. [CrossRef] [PubMed]
11. Wong, C.; Epstein, S.E.; Westropp, J.L. Antimicrobial Susceptibility Patterns in Urinary Tract Infections in Dogs (2010–2013). *J. Vet. Intern. Med.* **2015**, *29*, 1045–1052. [CrossRef] [PubMed]
12. Johnson, J.R.; Owens, K.; Gajewski, A.; Clabots, C. Escherichia Coli Colonization Patterns among Human Household Members and Pets, with Attention to Acute Urinary Tract Infection. *J. Infect. Dis.* **2008**, *197*, 218–224. [CrossRef] [PubMed]
13. McEwen, S.A.; Collignon, P.J. Antimicrobial Resistance: A One Health Perspective. *Microbiol. Spectr.* **2018**, *6*, ARBA-0009-2017. [CrossRef] [PubMed]
14. VET01. *Performance Standards for Antimicrobial Disk and Dilution Susceptibility Tests for Bacteria Isolated from Animals*, 4th ed.; CLSI Clinical and Laboratory Standards Institute: Annapolis Junction, MD, USA, 2013.
15. Sørensen, T.M.; Bjørnvad, C.R.; Cordoba, G.; Damborg, P.; Guardabassi, L.; Siersma, V.; Bjerrum, L.; Jessen, L.R. Effects of Diagnostic Work-Up on Medical Decision-Making for Canine Urinary Tract Infection: An Observational Study in Danish Small Animal Practices. *J. Vet. Intern. Med.* **2018**, *32*, 743–751. [CrossRef] [PubMed]

16. Butler, C.C.; Francis, N.A.; Thomas-Jones, E.; Longo, M.; Wootton, M.; Llor, C.; Little, P.; Moore, M.; Bates, J.; Pickles, T.; et al. Point-of-Care Urine Culture for Managing Urinary Tract Infection in Primary Care: A Randomised Controlled Trial of Clinical and Cost-Effectiveness. *Br. J. Gen. Pract.* **2018**, *68*, e268. [CrossRef] [PubMed]
17. Uhl, A.; Hartmann, F.A.; Viviano, K.R. Clinical Performance of a Commercial Point-of-Care Urine Culture System for Identification of Bacteriuria in Dogs. *J. Am. Vet. Med. Assoc.* **2017**, *251*, 922–928. [CrossRef] [PubMed]
18. Olin, S.J.; Bartges, J.W.; Jones, R.D.; Bemis, D.A. Diagnostic Accuracy of a Point-of-Care Urine Bacteriologic Culture Test in Dogs. *J. Am. Vet. Med. Assoc.* **2013**, *243*, 1719–1725. [CrossRef] [PubMed]
19. Papić, B.; Golob, M.; Zdovc, I.; Kušar, D.; Avberšek, J. Genomic Insights into the Emergence and Spread of Methicillin-Resistant Staphylococcus Pseudintermedius in Veterinary Clinics. *Vet. Microbiol.* **2021**, *258*, 109119. [CrossRef]
20. Brložnik, M.; Šterk, K.; Zdovc, I. Prevalence and Resistance Patterns of Canine Uropathogens in Regard to Concurrent Diseases. *Berl. Munch. Tierarztl. Wochenschr.* **2016**, *129*, 340–350. [PubMed]

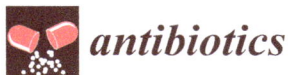 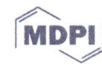

Article

# Antimicrobial Resistance Patterns of *Escherichia coli* Isolated from Sheep and Beef Farms in England and Wales: A Comparison of Disk Diffusion Interpretation Methods

Charlotte Doidge [1], Helen West [2] and Jasmeet Kaler [1,*]

[1] School of Veterinary Medicine and Science, University of Nottingham, Sutton Bonington LE12 5RD, UK; charlotte.doidge@nottingham.ac.uk
[2] School of Biosciences, University of Nottingham, Sutton Bonington LE12 5RD, UK; helen.west@nottingham.ac.uk
\* Correspondence: jasmeet.kaler@nottingham.ac.uk

**Abstract:** Little data exist on the levels of antimicrobial resistance from bacteria isolated from British sheep and beef cattle. The aim of this study was to investigate antimicrobial resistance patterns on sheep and beef farms in England and Wales using multiple interpretation methods. Fecal samples ($n$ = 350) from sheep and beef cattle were collected from 35 farms. Disk diffusion antimicrobial susceptibility testing against ten antimicrobials was carried out for 1115 (699 sheep, 416 beef) β-glucuronidase-positive *Escherichia coli* isolates. Susceptibility was interpreted using clinical breakpoints, which determine clinically resistant bacteria, and epidemiological and livestock-specific cut-off values, which determine microbiological-resistant bacteria (non-wild type). Using livestock-specific cut-off values, a high frequency of wild type for all ten antimicrobials was observed in isolates from sheep (90%) and beef cattle (85%). Cluster analysis was performed to identify patterns in antimicrobial resistance. Interpretation of susceptibility using livestock-specific cut-off values showed a cluster of isolates that were non-wild type to cefotaxime and amoxicillin/clavulanic acid, whereas clinical breakpoints did not. A multilevel logistic regression model determined that tetracycline use on the farm and soil copper concentration were significantly associated with tetracycline non-wild type isolates. The results suggest that using human clinical breakpoints could lead to both the under-reporting and over-reporting of antimicrobial resistance in sheep and beef cattle.

**Keywords:** antibiotic resistance; sheep; beef cattle; *Escherichia coli*; normalised resistance interpretation; antimicrobial susceptibility testing; tetracyclines; farms

**Citation:** Doidge, C.; West, H.; Kaler, J. Antimicrobial Resistance Patterns of *Escherichia coli* Isolated from Sheep and Beef Farms in England and Wales: A Comparison of Disk Diffusion Interpretation Methods. *Antibiotics* **2021**, *10*, 453. https://doi.org/10.3390/antibiotics10040453

Academic Editor: Clair L. Firth

Received: 5 March 2021
Accepted: 14 April 2021
Published: 16 April 2021

**Publisher's Note:** MDPI stays neutral with regard to jurisdictional claims in published maps and institutional affiliations.

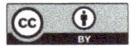

**Copyright:** © 2021 by the authors. Licensee MDPI, Basel, Switzerland. This article is an open access article distributed under the terms and conditions of the Creative Commons Attribution (CC BY) license (https://creativecommons.org/licenses/by/4.0/).

## 1. Introduction

Antimicrobial resistance is a worldwide public health concern. The administration of antimicrobials leads to the selection of antimicrobial-resistant bacteria, and food-producing animals are one of several potential sources of antimicrobial resistance [1]. Although antimicrobial use is thought to be low in sheep and beef cattle [2,3], the large numbers of sheep and cattle in the UK may potentially contribute to the dissemination of antimicrobial-resistant bacteria [4,5]. National surveillance of antimicrobial resistance from bacteria isolated from sheep and beef cattle only uses samples that are submitted for clinical diagnostics [6]. The use of clinical isolates suggests that antimicrobial resistance to commonly used antimicrobials, such as tetracycline and ampicillin, is relatively high in sheep and cattle [7]. However, clinical samples are potentially biased as they usually come from sick animals which may have been treated with antimicrobials. At present in the UK, active national surveillance of healthy sheep or cattle does not exist.

There are few studies investigating antimicrobial susceptibility of organisms isolated from healthy sheep and beef cattle in the UK. These studies suggest that antimicrobial resistance on sheep and beef farms is relatively uncommon [8–10], although extended spectrum beta-lactamase (ESBL)-positive beef farms may be increasing [11,12]. Examining the presence of ESBL *E. coli* has been the focus of more recent studies on beef farms [11,12]. Therefore, other resistance types may have been missed in these studies. Other studies have investigated a larger range of antimicrobial resistances, but only investigated a few farms [8,10]. Hence, variance between farms with respect to antimicrobial resistance patterns was not investigated. More information regarding antimicrobial resistance on sheep and beef farms in the UK is required. Indeed, a systematic review of antimicrobial resistance on British sheep and cattle farms called for additional efforts in collecting farm-level antimicrobial resistance data [7].

Previously identified factors associated with antimicrobial resistance in pigs and veal calves in countries other than the UK include the use of antimicrobials, either as therapeutics to treat sick animals or as growth promoters [13–15]. Antimicrobial growth promoters are not used in the UK. The number of animals on the farm, region of the farm and type of animals sampled have also been reported as factors associated with antimicrobial resistance in bacteria isolated from animals [16,17]. It has been shown that bacterial isolates of animal origin may present with resistance even when the animals have not been exposed to antimicrobials [18,19]. Markland et al. [20] illustrated that when cefotaxime-resistant bacteria were present in samples from beef cattle, resistant bacteria were more abundant in soil samples. This indicated that the environment, such as soils and forage, may be a natural source of antimicrobial-resistant bacteria for food-producing animals [20]. However, the factors that affect the prevalence of antimicrobial-resistant bacteria in soils are unclear [21]. One potential explanation is that heavy metals such as copper and zinc may co-select for antimicrobial resistance in soil. The effect of metal concentrations in soil on the prevalence of antimicrobial resistance in farm animals requires further investigation.

Disk diffusion testing is a commonly used phenotypic method for determining antimicrobial susceptibility. Scientists typically interpret the results of such tests using clinical breakpoints and will mainly adhere to guidelines set by the European Committee on Antimicrobial Susceptibility Testing (EUCAST) or Clinical and Laboratory Standards Institute (CLSI) [22,23]. However, these clinical breakpoints are only relevant for human medicine [24]. CLSI has set very few veterinary clinical breakpoints, and at present, European veterinary breakpoints do not exist. Research suggests that using human clinical breakpoints to interpret veterinary data may lead to calculating a higher antimicrobial resistance prevalence than actually occurs [10].

An alternative method to interpret antimicrobial susceptibility data is to use epidemiological cut-off (ECOFF) values to determine fully susceptible isolates (wild type, WT) from non-fully susceptible isolates (non-wild type, NWT). EUCAST defines a WT organism as one with the absence of acquired and mutational resistance mechanisms to the drug in question [25]. Thus, the ECOFFs determine microbiological resistance, whereas clinical breakpoints determine clinical resistance. The ECOFF values are established by EUCAST through analysis of the distribution of their inhibitory zone diameters [26]. However, the distributions of inhibitory zone diameters for isolates of animal origin may differ from the distributions of inhibitory zone diameters for EUCAST isolates [10,27]. Therefore, ECOFF values may not reflect WT organisms isolated from livestock.

Instead, the normalised resistance interpretation (NRI) method can be used to calculate tailor-made cut-off values. The method was originally developed to calibrate the disk diffusion test to compare results between laboratories [28]. It has also been used to investigate the susceptibility of organisms of animal origin when EUCAST or CLSI breakpoints do not exist [29,30]. Furthermore, the NRI method has been used when clinical breakpoints or ECOFF values do not appear appropriate [10,27]. An inappropriate cut-off value occurs when the cut-off splits the normal distribution of inhibition zone diameters. Therefore, it may be useful to interpret the inhibitory zone diameters of isolates of animal origin using clinical breakpoints, ECOFF values and the NRI method so that comparisons can be made and the appropriate cut-off value can be chosen. A previous study based on isolates from four sheep farms compared these three interpretation methods and suggested that sheep-specific cut-off values were most fitting [10]. There needs to be additional studies with a larger number of participating farms to confirm these results, and similar studies have not been carried out for other livestock species. Additionally, the implications in terms of interpretation of antimicrobial resistance patterns requires further investigation. Therefore, the aim of this study was to investigate and compare antimicrobial resistance patterns on thirty-five sheep and beef farms in England and Wales using multiple interpretation methods, based on bacteria isolated from feces. Further objectives were to identify clusters of antimicrobial resistance and to identify factors that were associated with antimicrobial resistance on sheep and beef farms.

## 2. Results

The total number of isolates tested for each farm is presented in Table 1. A total of 1115 β-glucuronidase-positive *E. coli* isolates underwent antimicrobial susceptibility testing. Of these, 699 isolates were from 203 sheep fecal samples collected from 27 different farms, and 416 isolates were from 134 beef cattle fecal samples from 19 different farms.

**Table 1.** Description of the farms where *E. coli* isolates were obtained including number of animals, region and number of isolates tested.

| Farm No. | Region | n Beef Cattle (All Ages) | n Ewes | n Sheep Isolates | n Beef Isolates |
|---|---|---|---|---|---|
| 1 | West Midlands | 220 | 0 | 0 | 30 |
| 2 | West Midlands | 205 | 370 | 10 | 15 |
| 3 | West Midlands | 281 | 900 | 13 | 16 |
| 4 | Wales | 125 | 750 | 15 | 16 |
| 5 | South West England | 2240 | 0 | 0 | 32 |
| 6 | West Midlands | 172 | 350 | 25 | 15 |
| 7 | West Midlands | 342 | 0 | 0 | 32 |
| 8 | South West England | 500 | 0 | 0 | 36 |
| 9 | South West England | 218 | 1058 | 33 | 0 |
| 10 | Wales | 236 | 840 | 30 | 0 |
| 11 | Wales | 93 | 550 | 26 | 17 |
| 12 | Wales | 0 | 250 | 15 | 0 |
| 13 | Wales | 109 | 584 | 30 | 0 |
| 14 | South East England | 198 | 800 | 10 | 13 |
| 15 | Wales | 39 | 538 | 28 | 0 |
| 16 | Wales | 41 | 500 | 39 | 0 |
| 17 | Wales | 179 | 1850 | 15 | 15 |
| 18 | Wales | 600 | 800 | 15 | 15 |
| 19 | West Midlands | 107 | 0 | 0 | 30 |
| 20 | Wales | 161 | 582 | 30 | 0 |
| 21 | West Midlands | 0 | 300 | 39 | 0 |
| 22 | South West England | 49 | 480 | 29 | 0 |
| 23 | West Midlands | 157 | 520 | 40 | 0 |
| 24 | South West England | 64 | 560 | 30 | 0 |
| 25 | South West England | 209 | 600 | 29 | 0 |
| 26 | North East England | 200 | 500 | 25 | 15 |
| 27 | North West England | 420 | 0 | 0 | 30 |
| 28 | South West England | 241 | 0 | 0 | 30 |
| 29 | Wales | 0 | 300 | 28 | 0 |
| 30 | Wales | 145 | 466 | 27 | 15 |
| 31 | Wales | 23 | 360 | 39 | 0 |
| 32 | Wales | 564 | 1600 | 15 | 15 |
| 33 | West Midlands | 285 | 0 | 0 | 29 |
| 34 | West Midlands | 0 | 600 | 31 | 0 |
| 35 | Wales | 40 | 425 | 33 | 0 |

*n* = number.

## 2.1. Comparison of Methods to Interpret Resistance

The cut-off values determined by the NRI method ($CO_{WT}$) for sheep and beef fecal derived isolates were larger for tetracycline compared with the clinical breakpoints (Table 2). The $CO_{WT}$ values for sheep and beef were larger for ciprofloxacin, sulfamethoxazole-trimethoprim, cefotaxime and imipenem compared with the clinical breakpoints and ECOFF values. However, $CO_{WT}$ values for sheep and beef were smaller for amoxicillin/clavulanic acid and ampicillin compared with the clinical breakpoints and ECOFF values. All $CO_{WT}$ values had a standard deviation < 4.00 mm as recommended by Smith et al. [31]. $CO_{WT}$ values with standard deviation between 3.36–4.00 mm were referred to as tentative $CO_{WT}$ estimates. For beef cattle, four antimicrobials had tentative $CO_{WT}$ estimates, and for sheep, two antimicrobials had tentative $CO_{WT}$ estimates (Table 2).

**Table 2.** Epidemiological cut-off values calculated using the NRI method compared with clinical breakpoints and ECOFF values.

| Antimicrobials | Disk Content | Clinical Breakpoint (S ≥ mm) | ECOFF WT ≥ mm | Sheep $CO_{WT}$ WT ≥ mm | SD | Beef $CO_{WT}$ WT ≥ mm | SD |
|---|---|---|---|---|---|---|---|
| Neomycin | 30 µg | - | - | 13 | 1.46 | 14 | 1.87 |
| Spectinomycin | 100 µg | - | - | 19 | 1.91 | 18 | 2.06 |
| Tetracycline | 30 µg | 15 | - | 25 | 2.25 | 26 | 2.17 |
| Amoxicillin/Clavulanic Acid | 20–10 µg | 19 | 16 | 15 | 3.15 | 15 * | 3.66 |
| Ciprofloxacin | 5 µg | 25 | 25 | 27 * | 3.72 | 32 | 2.42 |
| Ampicillin | 10 µg | 14 | 14 | 12 | 3.26 | 11 * | 3.61 |
| Sulfamethoxazole-Trimethoprim | 23.75–1.25 µg | 14 | 21 | 24 | 2.96 | 24 | 2.72 |
| Chloramphenicol | 30 µg | 17 | 17 | 18 * | 3.50 | 17 * | 3.65 |
| Cefotaxime | 5 µg | 20 | 21 | 26 | 2.26 | 26 | 3.04 |
| Imipenem | 10 µg | 22 | 24 | 27 | 2.82 | 27 * | 3.88 |

* SD > 3.34 mm and therefore $CO_{WT}$ only a tentative estimate. S = susceptible, WT = wild type.

Based on $CO_{WT}$ values, 87.9% (980/1115) of all *E. coli* isolates were defined as WT organisms for all ten antimicrobials. Of the beef fecal isolates, 85.1% (354/416) were defined as WT for all ten antimicrobials. Of the sheep fecal isolates, 89.6% (626/699) were WT for all ten antimicrobials. The *E. coli* isolates had the lowest susceptibility to tetracycline, with 92.1% of sheep isolates being WT (Table 3) and 87.7% of beef isolates being WT (Table 4).

**Table 3.** Prevalence of antimicrobial susceptible (S) and wild type (WT) *E. coli* isolated from sheep using clinical breakpoints, ECOFFs and the NRI method.

| Antimicrobial | n Isolates Sheep | Clinical Breakpoint (% S) | ECOFF (% WT) | Sheep $CO_{WT}$ (% WT) | Kappa |
|---|---|---|---|---|---|
| Neomycin | 699 | - | - | 99.6% | N/A |
| Spectinomycin | 699 | - | - | 95.9% | N/A |
| Tetracycline | 699 | 93.0% | - | 92.1% | 0.938 |
| Amoxicillin/Clavulanic Acid | 699 | 95.4% | 97.4% | 98.1% | 0.689 |
| Ciprofloxacin | 699 | 100% | 100% | 100% | N/A |
| Ampicillin | 699 | 94.7% | 94.7% | 95.1% | 0.971 |
| Sulfamethoxazole-Trimethoprim | 699 | 98.0% | 98.0% | 97.9% | 0.976 |
| Chloramphenicol | 699 | 99.3% | 99.3% | 99.3% | 1.000 |
| Cefotaxime | 699 | 99.7% | 99.1% | 98.7% | 0.585 |
| Imipenem | 699 | 100% | 100% | 100% | N/A |

Table 4. Prevalence of antimicrobial susceptible (S) and wild type (WT) *E. coli* isolated from beef cattle using clinical breakpoints, ECOFFs and the NRI method.

| Antimicrobial | n Isolates Beef | Clinical Breakpoint (% S) | ECOFF (% WT) | Beef CO$_{WT}$ (% WT) | Kappa |
|---|---|---|---|---|---|
| Neomycin | 416 | - | - | 100% | N/A |
| Spectinomycin | 416 | - | - | 99.0% | N/A |
| Tetracycline | 416 | 88.2% | - | 87.7% | 0.977 |
| Amoxicillin/Clavulanic Acid | 416 | 98.3% | 99.5% | 99.8% | 0.395 |
| Ciprofloxacin | 416 | 99.8% | 99.8% | 99.0% | 0.423 |
| Ampicillin | 416 | 97.8% | 97.8% | 97.8% | 1.000 |
| Sulfamethoxazole-Trimethoprim | 416 | 99.5% | 99.5% | 98.1% | 0.495 |
| Chloramphenicol | 416 | 97.6% | 97.6% | 97.6% | 1.000 |
| Cefotaxime | 416 | 99.5% | 99.3% | 99.0% | 0.776 |
| Imipenem | 416 | 100% | 100% | 100% | N/A |

## 2.2. Farm-Level Susceptibility

All *E. coli* isolated from six farms were WT for the ten antimicrobials based on CO$_{WT}$ values (6/35, 17%). Only 26% (9/35) of farms had all isolates WT to tetracycline, whereas all farms (35/35) had all isolates WT to imipenem (Table 5).

Table 5. Farm-level prevalence of antimicrobial susceptibility of all *E. coli* isolated from sheep and beef farms based on the NRI method (CO$_{WT}$) and clinical breakpoints.

| Antimicrobial | Farms Having All Isolates as Wild Type | |
|---|---|---|
| | CO$_{WT}$ | Clinical breakpoint |
| Neomycin | 33/35 (94%) | - |
| Spectinomycin | 21/35 (60%) | - |
| Tetracycline | 9/35 (26%) | 10/35 (29%) |
| Amoxicillin/Clavulanic Acid | 30/35 (86%) | 18/35 (51%) |
| Ciprofloxacin | 32/35 (91%) | 34/35 (97%) |
| Ampicillin | 17/35 (49%) | 16/35 (46%) |
| Sulfamethoxazole-Trimethoprim | 22/35 (63%) | 26/35 (74%) |
| Chloramphenicol | 27/35 (77%) | 27/35 (77%) |
| Cefotaxime | 31/35 (86%) | 32/35 (91%) |
| Imipenem | 35/35 (100%) | 35/35 (100%) |

## 2.3. Cluster Analysis

The dendrograms from the single-linkage cluster analysis of susceptibility to eight antimicrobials in *E. coli* isolates from beef cattle fecal samples and sheep fecal samples are presented in Figure 1.

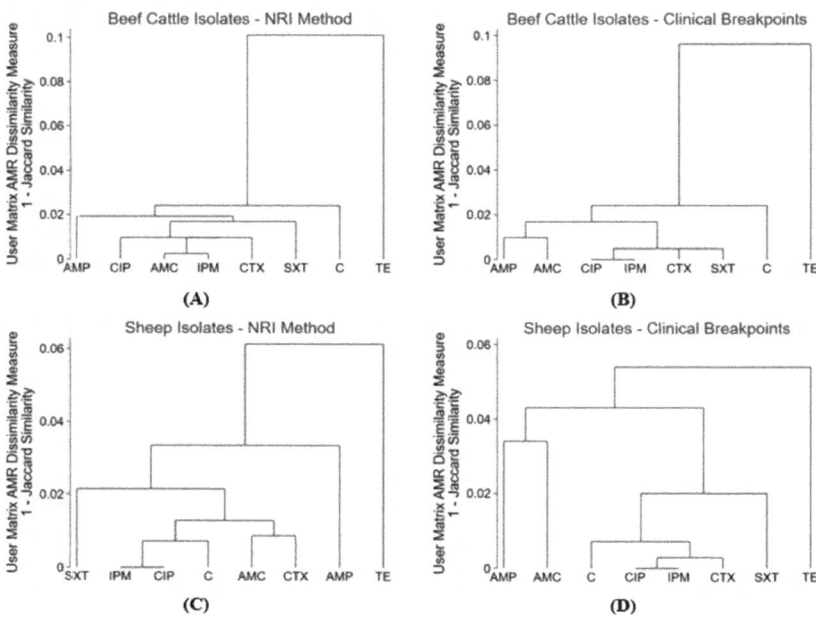

**Figure 1.** Single-linkage clustering dendrograms for non-susceptibility to eight antimicrobials (**A**) based on the NRI $CO_{WT}$ values in *E. coli* isolates from beef cattle fecal samples ($n$ = 416); (**B**) based on clinical breakpoints, in *E. coli* isolates from beef cattle fecal samples ($n$ = 416); (**C**) based on the NRI $CO_{WT}$ values, in *E. coli* isolates from sheep fecal samples ($n$ = 699); and (**D**) based on clinical breakpoints, in *E. coli* isolates from sheep fecal samples ($n$ = 699). AMP = ampicillin, AMC = amoxicillin/clavulanic acid, C = chloramphenicol, CIP = ciprofloxacin, CTX = cefotaxime, IPM = imipenem, SXT = sulfamethoxazole-trimethoprim, TE = tetracycline.

For both the sheep and beef isolates, the cluster analyses using clinical breakpoints identified a cluster of isolates that were non-susceptible to ampicillin and amoxicillin/clavulanic acid. This cluster was not identified when using the NRI $CO_{WT}$ values. In all four cluster analyses, tetracycline was the least related to other antimicrobial susceptibilities. A cluster of sheep isolates non-wild type for cefotaxime and amoxicillin/clavulanic acid was identified using NRI $CO_{WT}$ values, but not using clinical breakpoints.

### 2.4. Multilevel Logistic Regression Model

#### 2.4.1. Base Model

The base multilevel logistic regression model indicated that 16% of the variance of an isolate being defined as non-wild type for tetracycline was due to between-farm differences and 76% of the variance was due to between-sample differences.

#### 2.4.2. Univariable Multilevel Logistic Regression Models

A univariable multilevel logistic regression analysis was carried out to determine potential factors associated with the presence of tetracycline non-wild type isolates. Table 6 presents the associations of potential risk factors.

**Table 6.** Univariable multilevel logistic regression analysis for risk factors associated with *E. coli* defined as non-wild type for tetracycline.

| Factor | Unit | n | Odds Ratio (95% CI) | *p*-Value |
|---|---|---|---|---|
| Flock size | *n* ewes | 1115 | 0.91 (0.46, 1.81) | 0.792 |
| Herd size | *n* cattle > 12 months | 1115 | 0.90 (0.44, 1.82) | 0.761 |
| Region: Wales | No | 737 | | |
| | Yes | 378 | 1.62 (0.37, 7.11) | 0.523 |
| Region: West Midlands (England) | No | 790 | | |
| | Yes | 325 | 1.08 (0.23, 5.13) | 0.924 |
| Region: Southern England | No | 823 | | |
| | Yes | 242 | 0.39 (0.07, 2.25) | 0.292 |
| Indoor samples | No | 568 | | |
| | Yes | 547 | 2.90 (0.77, 10.97) | 0.116 |
| Mixed species farm | No | 362 | | |
| | Yes | 753 | 1.93 (0.41, 9.09) | 0.404 |
| Animal species sample origin | Cattle | 416 | | |
| | Sheep | 699 | 0.38 (0.11, 1.28) | 0.118 |
| Maximum average temperature of sampling month | °C | 1115 | 0.90 (0.45, 1.79) | 0.760 |
| Minimum average temperature of sampling month | °C | 1115 | 0.79 (0.49, 1.95) | 0.939 |
| Average rainfall in sampling month | mm | 1115 | 1.23 (0.62, 2.42) | 0.556 |
| Tetracycline use | No | 159 | | |
| | Yes | 956 | 22.21 (1.46, 337.52) | 0.026 |
| Penicillin use | No | 157 | | |
| | Yes | 958 | 0.62 (0.09, 4.44) | 0.635 |
| Aminoglycoside use | No | 363 | | |
| | Yes | 752 | 0.52 (0.12, 2.19) | 0.376 |
| Macrolide use | No | 634 | | |
| | Yes | 481 | 1.95 (0.48, 7.90) | 0.384 |
| Phenicol use | No | 825 | | |
| | Yes | 290 | 6.98 (1.82, 26.80) | 0.005 |
| Sulphonamide use | No | 993 | | |
| | Yes | 122 | 2.60 (0.32, 21.03) | 0.371 |
| Soil copper concentration | mg/kg | 1115 | 1.72 (0.97–3.05) | 0.062 |
| Soil zinc concentration | mg/kg | 1115 | 0.90 (0.45, 1.78) | 0.755 |
| Soil lead concentration | mg/kg | 1115 | 1.60 (0.85, 3.00) | 0.144 |
| Soil cobalt concentration | mg/kg | 1115 | 0.65 (0.34, 1.26) | 0.206 |

### 2.4.3. Multivariable Multilevel Logistic Regression Model

The odds of isolates being defined as non-wild type for tetracycline were 28 times higher (CrI = 2.50–520.09) when farms used tetracycline antimicrobials in their animals (Table 7). With every standardised unit increase for soil copper concentration, the odds of isolates being defined as non-wild type for tetracycline was 1.78 times higher (CrI = 1.02–3.21).

Table 7. Multivariable multilevel logistic regression analysis for risk factors associated with *E. coli* isolates being defined as non-wild type for tetracycline.

| Variable | Unit | n | Odds Ratio (95% CrI *) | p-Value |
|---|---|---|---|---|
| Tetracycline use | No | 159 | | |
| | Yes | 956 | 28.22 (2.50, 520.09) | 0.014 |
| Soil copper concentration | mg/kg | 1115 | 1.78 (1.02, 3.21) | 0.046 |
| **Random Effects** | | | **Variance Estimate (95% CrI *)** | |
| Farm | | | 1.24 (0.003, 4.47) | |
| Sample | | | 9.36 (4.86, 16.38) | |

* CrI = credible interval.

The multivariable multilevel logistic regression model indicated that 9% of the residual variance of an isolate being defined as non-wild type for tetracycline was due to between-farm differences and 76% of the residual variance was due to between-sample differences.

## 3. Discussion

In this study, antimicrobial resistance patterns in *E. coli* isolated from sheep and beef farms were assessed using different interpretation methods. The results show that antimicrobial resistance in feces on sheep and beef farms in England and Wales is generally low regardless of interpretation method, compared with samples from other livestock species in the UK [6]. However, interpretation method can have important implications on the understanding of resistance patterns. Different clusters of resistance patterns were determined when using clinical breakpoints compared with bespoke cut-off values using the NRI method.

The comparison of susceptibility interpretation methods showed that differences in the proportion of susceptible isolates may occur depending on the method used. There was little correlation between interpretations of susceptibility using clinical breakpoints, ECOFFs and $CO_{WT}$ values for amoxicillin/clavulanic acid in particular. For the beef isolates, there was also little correlation between the interpretations for ciprofloxacin and sulfamethoxazole-trimethoprim. This is possibly because clinical breakpoints detect human clinical resistance, whereas ECOFFs and $CO_{WT}$ values detect microbiological resistance. The results suggest that clinical breakpoints and ECOFFs are not appropriate for interpreting antimicrobial resistance in bacteria isolated from sheep or cattle feces as they do not fit the wild type distribution of isolates. Silva et al. [10] also showed that clinical breakpoints and ECOFFs may be inappropriate for the classification of ovine isolates as resistant and that these interpretation methods may over-report antimicrobial resistance in sheep populations [10]. Our results also indicate that clinical breakpoints and/or ECOFFs may slightly under-report, as well as over-report, antimicrobial resistance in sheep and beef isolates, particularly for sulfamethoxazole-trimethoprim, tetracycline and cefotaxime.

Silva et al. [10] further suggest that the sheep industry could establish sheep-specific cut-offs to avoid over-interpretation of resistance in ovine isolates. It is important to highlight that some of the sheep-specific cut-offs determined in the study by Silva et al. [10] were vastly different to those determined in our study. For example, Silva et al. [10] calculated the sheep $CO_{WT}$ for tetracycline to be 14 mm, whereas we calculated a sheep $CO_{WT}$ of 25 mm. The difference could be because of differences in the study population. The present study investigated sheep samples from 27 farms in England and Wales, whereas Silva et al. [10] used samples from just three farms in Scotland and one farm in Norway. Additionally, some isolates collected by Silva et al. [10] were from diseased animals and not from fecal samples. Nevertheless, this demonstrates the need for large-scale data collection from a variety of different farms before industry-wide cut-off values can be developed. These results also demonstrate the need to use the NRI method to calibrate the disk diffusion test to compare results between laboratories.

The differences in interpretation methods led to disparities in the groupings of antimicrobial resistances through cluster analysis. There was a cluster of isolates that were non-susceptible to ampicillin and amoxicillin/clavulanic acid for both the sheep and beef samples when the clinical breakpoints were used, but were not clustered as non-wild type when $CO_{WT}$ values were used. A cluster of sheep isolates that were non-wild type for cefotaxime and amoxicillin/clavulanic acid was only determined with the $CO_{WT}$ values. This may have implications for elucidating resistance mechanisms. Non-susceptibility to amoxicillin/clavulanic acid and ampicillin or cefotaxime suggests mechanisms of beta-lactam resistance, which requires further investigation through genotypic analysis [32]. These non-susceptibility and non-wild type patterns may have been missed if only one interpretation method was used.

A few cases of cefotaxime non-susceptibility in sheep and beef fecal isolates were reported in this study. Reduced susceptibility to cefotaxime has been reported in British beef cattle [12]. Although cefotaxime resistance in isolates from sheep has previously been reported in England and Wales, this was from clinical diagnostic samples [11], and to the authors' knowledge, it has not been reported for apparently healthy sheep in England and Wales before. This may be because third-generation cephalosporins are very rarely used on sheep farms. The use of highest-priority critically important antimicrobials should only be used as a last resort, when susceptibility testing has been conducted and no other antimicrobial would be effective. As resistance to other lower priority antimicrobials is uncommon in sheep and beef cattle, the use of third-generation cephalosporins is usually not required. It has previously been shown that cefotaxime-resistant bacteria may be present on beef farms without any antimicrobial use and that the environment may be a source of cefotaxime resistance [19,20]. The presence of cefotaxime non-susceptibility raises concerns around the existence of extended spectrum beta-lactamases (ESBLs) in healthy sheep and beef cattle [32], especially as a group of sheep isolates resistant to both cefotaxime and amoxicillin/clavulanic acid was identified from the cluster analysis. Further screening of the cefotaxime non-susceptible isolates is required to determine the presence of ESBL resistance mechanisms [33].

The results suggest that antimicrobial resistance to commonly used antimicrobials (such as tetracycline and penicillin) in apparently healthy sheep and beef cattle in England and Wales is much lower than that reported from national clinical surveillance [6,34]. This is probably because clinical samples are more likely to come from sick animals that have already been treated with antimicrobials before submission. Additionally, beef and dairy cattle samples are often not separated when reporting antimicrobial resistance [6]. In apparently healthy dairy cattle, the proportion of resistant isolates is much higher than the beef cattle reported here [35]. Although antimicrobial resistance appears to be low on sheep and beef farms in England and Wales, these figures were higher than what was reported historically. In 1999, 3% of isolates from sheep, and 6% of isolates from cattle were resistant to one or more antimicrobials [9]. In contrast, in our study, 10% of isolates from sheep, and 15% of isolates from cattle were non-wild type for one or more antimicrobials. Similarly, less than 4% of *E. coli* isolates from Scottish beef farms between 2001 and 2004 were resistant to tetracycline [8], compared with 12% of beef isolates in our study. This difference in susceptibility may be due to differences in study design, for example, differences in the antimicrobials studied or sampling technique. Additionally, the use of different interpretation methods may play a role in the varying antimicrobial susceptibilities as an organism that is classed as non-wild type does not necessarily display clinical resistance. Alternatively, differences in susceptibilities between the studies may be due to changes in farm practices over the last twenty years. This highlights the need for regular and consistent surveillance of antimicrobial resistance on sheep and beef farms in the UK so that longitudinal comparisons can be made.

The majority of the variance in antimicrobial susceptibility between isolates was due to between-sample differences, whereas only a small proportion of variance was due to between-farm differences. Around half of the between-farm variance could be explained by the use of tetracycline on the farm and the concentration of copper in the soils; however, there was still a large proportion of between-sample variation that was unexplained. This suggests that differences in antimicrobial resistance patterns are due to the variability in management of individual animals rather than any whole flock or herd management practices. The results probably reflect that antimicrobials are not usually used as routine prophylactic (preventative) treatments on sheep and beef farms in the UK, and in most cases farmers only use antimicrobials for the treatment of sick individual animals [3,36]. This is encouraging as there has been a large push in the UK agriculture industry to voluntarily reduce antimicrobial use over the last five years, particularly targeted at whole flock and herd treatments [36,37]. The large sample-level variance may also be due to the individual characteristics of the animals. For example, cattle over the age of 25 months have been shown to carry significantly less antimicrobial-resistant *E. coli* compared with younger cattle [17]. It was not possible to gather much sample-level information in this study as fecal samples were collected from the ground rather than directly from the animals. To understand the sources of variance at the sample level, further investigation using samples obtained directly from individual animals is recommended. The high variability between samples suggests that future studies that aim to understand the drivers of antimicrobial resistance on farms should consider taking individual animal samples rather than pooled samples.

The use of phenicols and tetracyclines was significantly associated with tetracycline non-wild type isolates in the univariable analysis. The association between tetracycline use and tetracycline non-wild type isolates is not surprising and has previously been reported for other livestock species [13,15]. The use of a particular antimicrobial will result in the direct selection of the corresponding resistance [38]. Phenicol use might indirectly select for tetracycline resistance via cross-resistance mechanisms. Alternatively, phenicol use may be associated with tetracycline non-wild type isolates if farmers change their antimicrobial drug of choice from tetracycline to phenicol when they find tetracyclines are no longer as effective for them. Tetracyclines are used as first-line treatments for livestock in the UK, whereas phenicols are in a higher category of antimicrobial which should only be used when first-line treatments are unavailable, for example, in cases of clinical tetracycline resistance [39]. Other factors that were identified as significant influences on antimicrobial resistance in previous studies, such as weather [35] and farm size [17], were not significant in our study. One possible reason for this is that for the dependent variable, there was only a small proportion of non-wild type isolates for tetracycline.

The concentration of copper in the soils in the farm area and the use of tetracyclines were significantly associated with tetracycline non-wild type isolates in the multivariable analysis. Previous research indicates that the geochemical conditions of soils, particularly copper concentrations, are correlated with the abundance of antimicrobial resistance genes [40,41]. Furthermore, copper has been shown to co-select for tetracycline resistance in experimental conditions [42], and mathematical models suggest that this co-selection may occur at copper concentrations as low as 5.5 mg/mL [43]. Our results suggest that tetracycline non-susceptibility may be more prevalent on some farms due to the environmental exposure to copper in soils. There needs to be further investigation into the presence of copper resistance genes in the tetracycline non-wild type isolates obtained in this study.

*Limitations*

The study sample was small; however, the number of farms was comparable to that of similar studies investigating antimicrobial resistance at the farm level and the farms represented a range of farm types and sizes [44,45]. Additionally, the farms were mainly located in Wales and the West of England, where sheep and cattle are more densely populated [46,47]. This was a cross-sectional study and so changes in antimicrobial resistance over time could not be measured. Additionally, information was mainly only collected at the farm level, but analysis indicated that most of the variation in resistance was at the sample level. Further investigation using a longitudinal study design and collecting sample-level information from individual animals is required to understand additional variation in resistance levels on farms. The β-glucuronidase-positive *E. coli* isolates were the focus here, although other species not studied are likely to also be environmentally important.

## 4. Materials and Methods

### 4.1. Participant Recruitment

Farmers identified for participation in the study were those that had previously completed a sheep flock health survey, beef herd health survey or both. The survey was distributed by a British retailer; therefore, all farms participating in this study supply to the retailer. Those that indicated that they would be interested in sharing their antimicrobial use data in the survey were contacted by their preferred form of contact, either telephone or email. Farmers were contacted in order of preference until thirty-five farms were recruited. Preference was farms that had sheep and/or cattle numbers that were representative of the producer average based on previous survey data [3].

The study was approved by the University of Nottingham School of Veterinary Medicine and Science Ethics Committee (No. 1850 160916).

### 4.2. Sample Collection

Each farm was visited between February and October 2019. Ten fecal samples from either sheep or beef cattle were taken at each farm. Random samples of fresh feces were taken from the field or pen floor and each placed into a sterile bag. Previous research shows that taking samples from the floor provides similar antimicrobial resistance profiles to taking samples directly from the rectum of the animals [48,49]. Therefore, samples from the floor were taken to reduce stress on the animals. Location of sample collection was not the same for each farm due to the different production systems. Therefore, sample collection location was recorded (e.g., indoor pen or outdoor pasture). Farmers were asked if they thought any of the animals in the field/pen had been given antimicrobials in the past two weeks. If so, the fecal samples were excluded from further analysis. The samples were kept cool and were processed within 24 h at laboratories at the University of Nottingham.

### 4.3. Isolation of Escherichia coli

For each sample, 2 g of feces was weighed and suspended in 18 mL of Maximum Recovery Diluent (MRD) (Oxoid). Samples were serially diluted, and 200 µL aliquots were plated onto Tryptone Bile X-glucuronide (TBX) agar (Oxoid) for the detection of β-glucuronidase-positive *E. coli*. *E. coli* form blue colonies on these plates while other Enterobacteriaceae form white colonies. TBX plates were incubated at 35 °C for 24 h. For each sample, the number of colonies with a typical *E. coli* phenotype were counted. The plate with between 30 and 300 colonies was chosen, and six blue colonies from each plate were picked for streak plating. Single colonies were streaked onto Luria-Bertani (LB) agar (Lennox) and incubated at 35 °C for 24 h. From each plate, a single colony was put into a Microbank (Pro-Lab Diagnotics UK) and placed in a −80 °C freezer.

### 4.4. Antimicrobial Susceptibility Testing

At least three isolates from each sample were chosen for antimicrobial susceptibility testing. Antimicrobial susceptibility testing was undertaken following the EUCAST guidelines [22]. Antimicrobial resistance testing was carried out for ten antimicrobials using the disk diffusion method. Colonies were suspended in MRD until it reached 0.5 McFarland standard. The dilution was then streaked across a Mueller-Hinton Agar plate (Oxoid), and the 10 antimicrobial disks were placed onto the surface of the agar. The plates were incubated for 24 h at 35 °C. The zone diameters were then recorded using the EUCAST guidelines where possible [24]. For antimicrobials that do not have EUCAST breakpoints available, CLSI guidelines were followed [23]. All antimicrobials used are shown in Table 8 and were supplied by Oxoid (Basingstoke, UK).

Table 8. Disk contents used to determine antimicrobial susceptibility of *E. coli* isolates and source of clinical breakpoints.

| Antimicrobials | Disk Content | Source |
| --- | --- | --- |
| Neomycin | 30 µg | N/A |
| Spectinomycin | 100 µg | N/A |
| Tetracycline | 30 µg | CLSI |
| Amoxicillin/Clavulanic Acid | 20–10 µg | EUCAST |
| Ciprofloxacin | 5 µg | EUCAST |
| Ampicillin | 10 µg | EUCAST |
| Sulfamethoxazole-Trimethoprim | 23.75–1.25 µg | EUCAST |
| Chloramphenicol | 30 µg | EUCAST |
| Cefotaxime | 5 µg | EUCAST |
| Imipenem | 10 µg | EUCAST |

### 4.5. Terminology

Epidemiological cut-off values determined by EUCAST are referred to by the acronym ECOFF. For differentiation from the ECOFF values, the sheep-specific and beef-specific cut-off values determined by the NRI method in this study are referred to by the acronym sheep $CO_{WT}$ and beef $CO_{WT}$, respectively.

$CO_{WT}$ and ECOFF values determine WT and NWT organisms, where WT organisms are characterised as devoid of phenotypically detectable acquired resistance mechanisms. The term "resistant" is reserved for clinically resistant organisms. Clinical breakpoints determine susceptible (S) and resistant (R) organisms, where S organisms are characterised by a level of antimicrobial activity associated with a high likelihood of therapeutic success [25].

### 4.6. Data Analysis

Data cleaning, descriptive analysis, cluster analyses and univariable multilevel logistic regression modelling were carried out in Stata software (Stata SE/16.1, Stata Corp., College Station, TX, USA). The isolates obtained from three samples from Farm 2 were excluded from analysis as the sampled sheep were recently administered antimicrobials. The data used for this study are available in the Supplementary Material.

#### 4.6.1. Determining Cut-Off Values

Clinical breakpoints, ECOFFs and $CO_{WT}$ values were used to determine the proportion of fully susceptible/wild type organisms. The normalised resistance interpretation (NRI) method was used to calculate sheep $CO_{WT}$ and beef $CO_{WT}$. NRI is based on the assumption that the wild type distribution is normal. The mean and the standard deviation are calculated from a plot of probit values of their cumulative frequencies of observations against their respective susceptibility measures [28]. The $CO_{WT}$ was determined as 2.5 standard deviations from the mean. The automatic and manual Excel programs used to calculate the $CO_{WT}$ were made available through courtesy by P. Smith, W. Finnegan and G. Kronvall [50].

Upon inspection of the disk plots produced using the NRI automatic cut-off calculator, the calculated cut-offs for ciprofloxacin and chloramphenicol for sheep and imipenem and chloramphenicol for beef were deemed inappropriate. This was because of an outlying peak in the high-zone part. For these four NRI calculations, the manual NRI calculator was used instead. Usually, the first drop in the rolling means determines the putative peak used for the NRI calculations, whereas if there was an outlying peak in the high-zone part, the second drop in the rolling means was used to determine the putative peak [28].

The NRI method was used with permission from the patent holder, Bioscand AB, TÄBY, Sweden (European patent No 1383913, US Patent No. 7,465,559).

### 4.6.2. Descriptive Statistics

The proportion of susceptible/wild type *E. coli* isolates was calculated for each antimicrobial used for the susceptibility testing. The kappa-statistic was used to measure the level of agreement between the interpretations of clinical breakpoints, ECOFFs and CO$_{WT}$ values. A score of 1 indicates perfect agreement, and a score of 0 indicates the amount of agreement that would be expected to be observed by chance [51]. The proportion of farms that had full susceptibility/wild type to each antimicrobial was also calculated.

### 4.6.3. Cluster Analysis

To determine potential groupings in antimicrobial resistances, single-linkage hierarchical agglomerative clustering was implemented [52]. The Jaccard similarity measure was used to compare antimicrobial susceptibility for ten antimicrobials, saving one minus the Jaccard measure as a dissimilarity matrix. Cluster analysis was performed four times to produce dendrograms for antimicrobial susceptibility for (1) sheep isolates using the CO$_{WT}$ values, (2) sheep isolates using clinical breakpoints, (3) beef isolates using CO$_{WT}$ values and (4) beef isolates using clinical breakpoints. A low dissimilarity measure indicated that two antimicrobial susceptibilities were related. A dissimilarity measure of zero indicated that all isolates were susceptible to both antimicrobials.

### 4.6.4. Multilevel Logistic Regression Base Model

A binary variable for tetracycline non-wild type (based on CO$_{WT}$ values) was chosen as the dependent variable as this antimicrobial had the lowest proportion of antimicrobial susceptibility for both sheep and beef isolates. Multilevel logistic regression was not performed for the other antimicrobials because there were very few isolates that were non-susceptible to the other antimicrobial families. A base model with no predictor variables and three levels was run. If $y_{ijk} = 1$ if the ith isolate from sample j from farm k is non-wild type for tetracycline and $y_{ijk} = 0$ if it is wild type for tetracycline, then we model:

$$y_{ijk} \sim \text{Bernouilli}\left(\pi_{ijk}\right) \quad (1)$$

$$\text{logit}\left(\pi_{ijk}\right) = \beta + v_k + u_{jk} \quad (2)$$

$$v_k = N\left(0, \sigma_v^2\right), \ u_{jk} \sim N(0, \sigma_u^2) \quad (3)$$

where $\beta$ is the probability of the isolate being non-wild type, $u_{jk}$ is the sample effects (with variance $\sigma_u^2$) and $v_k$ is the farm effects (with variance $\sigma_v^2$).

The intraclass correlation coefficients were determined to understand the underlying variation in susceptibility at the sample and farm level.

### 4.6.5. Multivariable Multilevel Random-Intercept Logistic Regression

Additional data were collected to investigate risk factors that might be associated with tetracycline non-susceptibility, based on the findings of previous research [13,14,16,20]. Meteorological data were extracted from UK Meteorological Office data [53]. The average maximum and minimum temperature (°C), and rainfall (mm) from the closest weather station for the month of sample collection were recorded for each farm. Soil data were extracted from the UK Soil Observatory based on the postcode of each farm [54]. Antimicrobial use data were collected using the bin method [55]. In a visit prior to the sample collection, farms were instructed to place any empty antimicrobial packaging used in sheep/beef cattle into a bin. The contents of the bin were collected during the sampling visit. From this, a binary variable for the presence/absence of each antimicrobial class was produced.

A univariable three-level logistic regression analysis was carried out to determine associations with isolates being tetracycline non-wild type. Variables with $p \leq 0.2$ were considered for the multivariable three-level random-intercept logistic regression model.

The multivariable multilevel logistic regression model was fitted in MLwiN 3.02 [56]. Initially, model exploration was conducted using first-order marginal quasi-likelihood. Then, Markov-chain Monte Carlo (MCMC) simulations using Metropolis–Hastings sampling with diffuse priors, a burn-in length of 5000 and a run of 50,000 iterations were used to fit the multivariable model. The Raftery–Lewis diagnostic suggested that a Markov chain of at least 435,000 was needed to estimate the 2.5% quantile for the intercept coefficient. Therefore, MCMC simulations with a burn-in length of 10,000 and a run of 500,000 iterations were used to fit the final multivariable multilevel logistic regression model. A forward and backward selection stepwise model-building approach was used, where only variables with $p \leq 0.05$ were selected to remain in the model. If $y_{ijk} = 1$ if the ith isolate from sample j from farm k is non-wild type to tetracycline and $y_{ijk} = 0$ if it is wild type to tetracycline, then we model:

$$y_{ijk} \sim \text{Bernouilli}\left(\pi_{ijk}\right) \tag{4}$$

$$\text{logit}\left(\pi_{ijk}\right) = \beta_0 + \beta_1 \text{TetracyclineUse}_{ijk} + \beta_2 \text{CuConc}_{ijk} + v_k + u_{jk} \tag{5}$$

$$v_k = N\left(0, \sigma_v^2\right),\ u_{jk} \sim N(0, \sigma_u^2) \tag{6}$$

where $\beta_0$ is the intercept; $\beta_1$ is the coefficient for the effect of a unit increase of the predictor TetracyclineUse$_{ijk}$ on the outcome; $\beta_2$ is the coefficient for the effect of a unit increase of the predictor CuConc$_{ijk}$ on the outcome; and $v_k$ and $u_{jk}$ are the random effects at the farm and sample level, respectively.

The variance partitioning coefficients were calculated under the latent variable method, which assumes the binary outcome arises from an underlying continuous distribution and that the level 1 variance on the logit scale is $\pi^2/3$ [57].

$$\text{VPC}_k = \sigma_v^2 / (\sigma_v^2 + \sigma_u^2 + \pi^2/3) \tag{7}$$

$$\text{VPC}_j = (\sigma_v^2 + \sigma_u^2) / (\sigma_v^2 + \sigma_u^2 + \pi^2/3) \tag{8}$$

where VPC$_k$ is the VPC at the farm level, VPC$_j$ is the VPC at the sample level, $\sigma_v^2$ is the variance at the farm level, and $\sigma_u^2$ is the variance at the sample level.

Selection of the best fitting model was based on the value of Bayesian Deviance Information Criterion (DIC). The model with the lowest DIC value was considered the best fitting model.

## 5. Conclusions

Antimicrobial non-susceptibility of *E. coli* isolated from healthy sheep and beef cattle in England and Wales appears to be low compared with reports from clinical diagnostic isolates. However, antimicrobial non-susceptibility from healthy animals may have increased in the past twenty years. The use of tetracyclines on farms and environmental copper exposure in soils may contribute to tetracycline resistance. Uniform methods of antimicrobial susceptibility testing are required to make longitudinal comparisons and monitor long-term changes in resistance patterns. Using human clinical breakpoints could lead to the under-reporting and over-reporting of antimicrobial resistance in sheep and beef cattle. The use of livestock-specific cut-off values for interpreting antimicrobial susceptibility can provide more appropriate estimates of susceptibility for sheep and beef cattle.

**Supplementary Materials:** The data used for this study are available in the Supplementary Material available online at https://www.mdpi.com/article/10.3390/antibiotics10040453/s1.

**Author Contributions:** Conceptualisation, C.D., H.W. and J.K.; methodology, C.D., H.W. and J.K.; formal analysis, C.D.; investigation, C.D.; resources, H.W. and J.K.; data curation, C.D.; writing—original draft preparation, C.D.; writing—review and editing, H.W. and J.K.; visualisation, C.D.; supervision, H.W. and J.K.; project administration, C.D., H.W. and J.K.; funding acquisition, J.K. All authors have read and agreed to the published version of the manuscript.

**Funding:** C.D. was funded by the Agricultural and Horticultural Development Board, ref. 61110063.

**Institutional Review Board Statement:** The study was approved by the University of Nottingham School of Veterinary Medicine and Science Ethics Committee (No. 1850 160916).

**Informed Consent Statement:** Informed consent was obtained from all farmers involved in the study.

**Data Availability Statement:** The data presented in this study are available in the Supplementary Material.

**Acknowledgments:** We would like to thank the farmers who took part in the study, Nikki Bollard for her technical help, and Lis King for her useful comments on the manuscript.

**Conflicts of Interest:** The authors declare no conflict of interest. The funders had no role in the design of the study; in the collection, analyses, or interpretation of data; in the writing of the manuscript, or in the decision to publish the results.

## References

1. Marshall, B.M.; Levy, S.B. Food Animals and Antimicrobials: Impacts on Human Health. *Clin. Microbiol. Rev.* **2011**, *24*, 718–733. [CrossRef] [PubMed]
2. Davies, P.; Remnant, J.G.; Green, M.J.; Gascoigne, E.; Gibbon, N.; Hyde, R.; Porteous, J.R.; Schubert, K.; Lovatt, F.; Corbishley, A. Quantitative analysis of antibiotic usage in British sheep flocks. *Vet. Rec.* **2017**, *181*, 511. [CrossRef] [PubMed]
3. Doidge, C.; Hudson, C.D.; Burgess, R.; Lovatt, F.; Kaler, J. Antimicrobial use practices and opinions of beef farmers in England and Wales. *Vet. Rec.* **2020**, *187*, e119. [CrossRef]
4. DEFRA. Farming Statistics Final Land Use, Livestock Populations and Agricultural Workforce at 1 June 2018—England. Available online: https://assets.publishing.service.gov.uk/government/uploads/system/uploads/attachment_data/file/869064/structure-jun2018final-eng-28feb20.pdf (accessed on 4 November 2020).
5. Welsh Government. Farming Facts and Figure, Wales. 2019. Available online: https://gov.wales/sites/default/files/statistics-and-research/2019-07/farming-facts-and-figures-2019-492.pdf (accessed on 12 December 2020).
6. VMD. UK Veterinary Antibiotic Resistance and Sales Surveillance Report. 2019. Available online: https://assets.publishing.service.gov.uk/government/uploads/system/uploads/attachment_data/file/936107/UK-VARSS_2019_Report__2020_.pdf (accessed on 19 November 2020).
7. Hennessey, M.; Whatford, L.; Payne-Gifford, S.; Johnson, K.F.; Van Winden, S.; Barling, D.; Häsler, B. Antimicrobial & antiparasitic use and resistance in British sheep and cattle: A systematic review. *Prev. Vet. Med.* **2020**, *185*, 105174. [CrossRef] [PubMed]
8. Vali, L.; Hamouda, A.; Hoyle, D.V.; Pearce, M.C.; Whitaker, L.H.R.; Jenkins, C.; Knight, H.I.; Smith, A.W.; Amyes, S.G.B. Antibiotic resistance and molecular epidemiology of *Escherichia coli* O26, O103 and O145 shed by two cohorts of Scottish beef cattle. *J. Antimicrob. Chemother.* **2007**, *59*, 403–410. [CrossRef] [PubMed]
9. Enne, V.I.; Cassar, C.; Sprigings, K.; Woodward, M.J.; Bennett, P.M. A high prevalence of antimicrobial resistant *Escherichia coli* isolated from pigs and a low prevalence of antimicrobial resistant *E. coli* from cattle and sheep in Great Britain at slaughter. *FEMS Microbiol. Lett.* **2008**, *278*, 193–199. [CrossRef]
10. Silva, N.; Phythian, C.J.; Currie, C.; Tassi, R.; Ballingall, K.T.; Magro, G.; McNeilly, T.N.; Zadoks, R.N. Antimicrobial resistance in ovine bacteria: A sheep in wolf's clothing? *PLoS ONE* **2020**, *15*, e0238708. [CrossRef]
11. Snow, L.C.; Wearing, H.; Stephenson, B.; Teale, C.J.; Coldham, N.G. Investigation of the presence of ESBL-producing *Escherichia coli* in the North Wales and West Midlands areas of the UK in 2007 to 2008 using scanning surveillance. *Vet. Rec.* **2011**, *169*, 656. [CrossRef] [PubMed]
12. Velasova, M.; Smith, R.P.; Lemma, F.; Horton, R.A.; Duggett, N.; Evans, J.; Tongue, S.C.; Anjum, M.F.; Randall, L. Detection of extended-spectrum β-lactam, AmpC and carbapenem resistance in Enterobacteriaceae in beef cattle in Great Britain in 2015. *J. Appl. Microbiol.* **2019**, *126*, 1081–1095. [CrossRef] [PubMed]
13. Varga, C.; Rajić, A.; McFall, M.E.; Reid-Smith, R.J.; Deckert, A.E.; Checkley, S.L.; McEwen, S.A. Associations between reported on-farm antimicrobial use practices and observed antimicrobial resistance in generic fecal *Escherichia coli* isolated from Alberta finishing swine farms. *Prev. Vet. Med.* **2009**, *88*, 185–192. [CrossRef]
14. Bosman, A.; Wagenaar, J.; Stegeman, J.; Vernooij, J.; Mevius, D. Antimicrobial resistance in commensal *Escherichia coli* in veal calves is associated with antimicrobial drug use. *Epidemiol. Infect.* **2014**, *142*, 1893–1904. [CrossRef]
15. Gibbons, J.F.; Boland, F.M.; Egan, J.B.; Fanning, S.W.; Markey, B.K.; Leonard, F.C. Antimicrobial Resistance of Faecal *Escherichia coli* Isolates from Pig Farms with Different Durations of In-feed Antimicrobial Use. *Zoonoses Public Health* **2016**, *63*, 241–250. [CrossRef]
16. Berge, A.C.; Hancock, D.D.; Sischo, W.M.; Besser, T.E. Geographic, farm, and animal factors associated with multiple antimicrobial resistance in fecal Escherichia coli isolates from cattle in the western United States. *J. Am. Vet. Med. Assoc.* **2010**, *236*, 1338–1344. [CrossRef]

17. Mainda, G.; Bessell, P.R.; Muma, J.B.; McAteer, S.P.; Chase-Topping, M.E.; Gibbons, J.; Stevens, M.P.; Gally, D.L.; Bronsvoort, B.M.D. Prevalence and patterns of antimicrobial resistance among *Escherichia coli* isolated from Zambian dairy cattle across different production systems. *Sci. Rep.* **2015**, *5*, srep12439. [CrossRef] [PubMed]
18. Mir, R.A.; Weppelmann, T.A.; Johnson, J.A.; Archer, D.; Morris, J.G., Jr.; Jeong, K.C. Identification and Characterization of Cefotaxime Resistant Bacteria in Beef Cattle. *PLoS ONE* **2016**, *11*, e0163279. [CrossRef]
19. Mir, R.A.; Weppelmann, T.A.; Teng, L.; Kirpich, A.; Elzo, M.A.; Driver, J.D.; Jeong, K.C. Colonization Dynamics of Cefotaxime Resistant Bacteria in Beef Cattle Raised Without Cephalosporin Antibiotics. *Front. Microbiol.* **2018**, *9*, 500. [CrossRef] [PubMed]
20. Markland, S.; Weppelmann, T.A.; Ma, Z.; Lee, S.; Mir, R.A.; Teng, L.; Ginn, A.; Lee, C.; Ukhanova, M.; Galindo, S.; et al. High Prevalence of Cefotaxime Resistant Bacteria in Grazing Beef Cattle: A Cross Sectional Study. *Front. Microbiol.* **2019**, *10*, 176. [CrossRef]
21. Lee, S.; Mir, R.A.; Park, S.H.; Kim, D.; Kim, H.-Y.; Boughton, R.K.; Morris, J.G., Jr.; Jeong, K.C. Prevalence of extended-spectrum β-lactamases in the local farm environment and livestock: Challenges to mitigate antimicrobial resistance. *Crit. Rev. Microbiol.* **2020**, *46*, 1–14. [CrossRef] [PubMed]
22. EUCAST. EUCAST Disk Diffusion Method for Antimicrobial Susceptibility Testing. Available online: https://www.eucast.org/fileadmin/src/media/PDFs/EUCAST_files/Disk_test_documents/2020_manuals/Manual_v_8.0_EUCAST_Disk_Test_2020.pdf (accessed on 24 November 2020).
23. CLSI. *Performance Standards for Antimicrobial Susceptibility Testing*, 30th ed.; Clinical and Laboratory Standards Institute: Pittsburgh, PA, USA, 2020.
24. EUCAST. *Breakpoint Tables for Interpretation of MICs and Zone Diameters*; Version 8.1; EUCAST: Växjö, Sweden, 2018; Available online: http://www.eucast.org (accessed on 24 November 2020).
25. EUCAST. EUCAST Definitions of Clinical Breakpoints and Epidemiological Cutoff Values. Available online: https://www.eucast.org/fileadmin/src/media/PDFs/EUCAST_files/EUCAST_SOPs/EUCAST_definitions_of_clinical_breakpoints_and_ECOFFs.pdf (accessed on 24 November 2020).
26. Kahlmeter, G. Defining antibiotic resistance-towards international harmonization. *Upsala J. Med Sci.* **2014**, *119*, 78–86. [CrossRef]
27. Dias, D.; Torres, R.T.; Kronvall, G.; Fonseca, C.; Mendo, S.; Caetano, T. Assessment of antibiotic resistance of *Escherichia coli* isolates and screening of *Salmonella* spp. in wild ungulates from Portugal. *Res. Microbiol.* **2015**, *166*, 584–593. [CrossRef]
28. Kronvall, G.; Smith, P. Normalized resistance interpretation, the NRI method. *APMIS* **2016**, *124*, 1023–1030. [CrossRef] [PubMed]
29. Pereira, R.V.; Siler, J.D.; Ng, J.C.; Davis, M.A.; Grohn, Y.T.; Warnick, L.D. Effect of on-farm use of antimicrobial drugs on resistance in fecal *Escherichia coli* of preweaned dairy calves. *J. Dairy Sci.* **2014**, *97*, 7644–7654. [CrossRef] [PubMed]
30. Lim, Y.-J.; Kim, D.-H.; Roh, H.J.; Park, M.-A.; Park, C.-I.; Smith, P. Epidemiological cut-off values for disc diffusion data generated by standard test protocols from *Edwardsiella tarda* and *Vibrio harveyi*. *Aquac. Int.* **2016**, *24*, 1153–1161. [CrossRef]
31. Smith, P.; Schwarz, T.; Verner-Jeffreys, D.W. Use of normalised resistance analyses to set interpretive criteria for antibiotic disc diffusion data produce by *Aeromonas* spp. *Aquaculture* **2012**, *326–329*, 27–35. [CrossRef]
32. Li, X.-Z.; Mehrotra, M.; Ghimire, S.; Adewoye, L. β-Lactam resistance and β-lactamases in bacteria of animal origin. *Vet. Microbiol.* **2007**, *121*, 197–214. [CrossRef]
33. EUCAST. Subcommittee for Detection of Resistance Mechanisms and Specific Resistances of Clinical and/or Epidemiological Importance. EUCAST Guidelines for Detection of Resistance Mechanisms and Specific Resistances of Clinical and/or Epidemiological Importance, Version 2.0. Available online: http://www.eucast.org/fileadmin/src/media/PDFs/EUCAST_files/Resistance_mechanisms/EUCAST_detection_of_resistance_mechanisms_170711.pdf (accessed on 24 November 2020).
34. Cheney, T.E.A.; Smith, R.P.; Hutchinson, J.P.; Brunton, L.A.; Pritchard, G.; Teale, C.J. Cross-sectional survey of antibiotic resistance in *Escherichia coli* isolated from diseased farm livestock in England and Wales. *Epidemiol. Infect.* **2015**, *143*, 2653–2659. [CrossRef]
35. Schubert, H.; Morley, K.; Puddy, E.F.; Arbon, R.; Findlay, J.; Mounsey, O.; Gould, V.C.; Vass, L.; Evans, M.; Rees, G.M.; et al. Reduced Antibacterial Drug Resistance and blaCTX-M β-Lactamase Gene Carriage in Cattle-Associated *Escherichia coli* at Low Temperatures, at Sites Dominated by Older Animals, and on Pastureland: Implications for Surveillance. *Appl. Environ. Microbiol.* **2021**, *87*, e01468-20. [CrossRef]
36. Doidge, C.; Ruston, A.; Lovatt, F.; Hudson, C.; King, L.; Kaler, J. Farmers' Perceptions of Preventing Antibiotic Resistance on Sheep and Beef Farms: Risk, Responsibility, and Action. *Front. Vet. Sci.* **2020**, *7*, 524. [CrossRef]
37. RUMA. Targets Task Force Report. Available online: https://www.ruma.org.uk/wp-content/uploads/2020/11/Targets-Task-Force-Report-2020-FINAL-181120-download.pdf (accessed on 30 November 2020).
38. Harada, K.; Asai, T. Role of antimicrobial selective pressure and secondary factors on antimicrobial resistance prevalence in *Escherichia coli* from food-producing animals in Japan. *J. Biomed. Biotechnol.* **2010**, *2010*, 180682. [CrossRef]
39. EMA. Categorisation of Antibiotics in the European Union. Available online: https://www.ema.europa.eu/en/documents/report/categorisation-antibiotics-european-union-answer-request-european-commission-updating-scientific_en.pdf (accessed on 30 November 2020).
40. Knapp, C.W.; McCluskey, S.M.; Singh, B.K.; Campbell, C.D.; Hudson, G.; Graham, D.W. Antibiotic Resistance Gene Abundances Correlate with Metal and Geochemical Conditions in Archived Scottish Soils. *PLoS ONE* **2011**, *6*, e27300. [CrossRef]
41. Knapp, C.W.; Callan, A.C.; Aitken, B.; Shearn, R.; Koenders, A.; Hinwood, A. Relationship between antibiotic resistance genes and metals in residential soil samples from Western Australia. *Environ. Sci. Pollut. Res.* **2017**, *24*, 2484–2494. [CrossRef]

Dust samples from only one farm were found to be positive for MRSA, this isolate was found to contain the *mecC* gene.

### 2.3. Antimicrobial Use Data

The total Defined Daily Doses per cow and year (DDDvet/cow/year) for all disease indications on each farm was calculated according to the standardised Defined Daily Dose (DDDvet) values published by the European Medicines Agency [21]. Total antimicrobial use (AMU) for all disease indications ranged from 2.47 to 8.04 DDDvet/cow/year in the high use group (mean 4.35; median 3.82 DDDvet/cow/year), compared to 0.01 to 0.63 DDDvet/cow/year in the low use group (mean 0.29; median 0.31 DDDvet/cow/year). As would be expected, the two groups ("high" and "low" AMU in DDDvet/cow/year) of antimicrobial use showed a highly statistically significant difference in the Mann–Whitney U-test (U score 0, Z score 4.88, $p < 0.00001$).

Among high antimicrobial users on ESBL-producing *E. coli* positive farms, the median AMU was 3.38 DDDvet/cow/year (mean 3.77, $n = 5$); compared to the negative farms where the median AMU was 4.14 DDDvet/cow/year (mean 4.50, $n = 20$). On farms classed as low users, the median AMU was 0.40 DDDvet/cow/year (mean 0.31, $n = 8$) on farms where at least one sample tested positive, compared to a median of 0.29 DDDvet/cow/year (mean 0.28, $n = 17$) on negative farms.

The comparison of antimicrobial classes used on both ESBL-producing *E. coli* positive and negative farms is shown in Figure 1. On ESBL-producing *E. coli* positive farms, beta-lactamase sensitive penicillins (such as benzylpenicillin) had the highest DDDvet/cow/year (mean 0.49, median 0.12, maximum 1.95 DDD/cow/year); while the DDDvet/cow/year for third/fourth-generation cephalosporins was higher on the ESBL-producing *E. coli*-negative farms (mean 1.13, median 0.19, maximum 6.39 DDD/cow/year) (for details, see Figure 1). As would be expected on dairy farms, the majority of antimicrobial treatment on all farms was for udder diseases (53.8% as calculated as a total of the DDDvet/cow/year), followed by a much lower proportion of treatments for reproductive disorders (17.8% of the total DDDvet/cow/year) (for details, see Table 2 and Figure 2).

**Table 2.** Antimicrobial treatments by disease indication, according to DDDvet/cow/year, and whether farms tested positive or negative for ESBL-producing *E. coli*.

|  | Proportion of Overall Antimicrobial Treatments (%) Based on Total DDDvet/Cow/Year | Proportion of Antimicrobial Treatments by Disease Indication | |
|---|---|---|---|
|  |  | Non-HPCIA * | HPCIA * |
| **ESBL-POSITIVE FARMS (N = 13)** |  |  |  |
| Respiratory disease | 13.2% | 54.8% | 45.2% |
| Musculoskeletal/Locomotory disease | 5.2% | 32.5% | 67.5% |
| Udder disease (excluding DCT #) | 52.2% | 79.0% | 21.0% |
| Reproductive disorders | 20.4% | 99.4% | 0.6% |
| Other diseases | 9.0% | 47.8% | 52.2% |
| **ESBL-NEGATIVE FARMS (N = 37)** |  |  |  |
| Respiratory disease | 12.4% | 78.1% | 21.9% |
| Musculoskeletal/Locomotory disease | 8.4% | 10.6% | 89.4% |
| Udder disease (excluding DCT #) | 54.1% | 37.4% | 62.6% |
| Reproductive disorders | 16.4% | 95.2% | 4.8% |
| Other diseases | 8.6% | 45.4% | 54.6% |

* HPCIA—highest priority critically important antimicrobials as defined by the World Health Organization [22]. For this study, HPCIA included third and fourth generation cephalosporins, macrolides, and fluoroquinolones.
# DCT—dry cow therapy.

group, the mean herd size was 57.1 head of cattle (median 52; range 11–157), including 29.6 dairy cows (median 24; range 5–77). In the high use group, 17/25 (68.0%) farms were run conventionally, while just 2/25 (8.0%) farms were organic producers. No production type was reported for the remaining six farms (24.0%) as the farmers did not complete the farm management survey (as previously described elsewhere [20]). In the low use group, 7/25 (28.0%) farms were run organically, 14/25 (56.0%) conventionally, and production type was not known for the remaining 4 farms. Of the 40 farmers in the overall study group who completed the farm management survey, 27 (67.5%) reported that they routinely fed waste/discard milk containing antimicrobial residues (from the treatment of cows) to calves on their farms. For further details, see Table 1.

**Table 1.** Demographics of study farms, total AMU in DDDvet/cow/year, and results of ESBL-producing *E. coli* screening.

| DDDvet/Cow/Year | HIGH (N = 25) | | LOW (N = 25) | |
|---|---|---|---|---|
| Range | 2.47–8.04 | | 0.01–0.63 | |
| Median | 3.82 | | 0.31 | |
| Mean | 4.35 | | 0.29 | |
| | Freestall ($n = 17$) | Tie-stall ($n = 8$) | Freestall ($n = 16$) | Tie-stall ($n = 9$) |
| **Production system** | | | | |
| Conventional | 12 | 5 | 11 | 3 |
| Organic | 2 | 0 | 5 | 2 |
| No answer given [#] | 3 | 3 | 0 | 4 |
| **Waste milk * routinely fed to calves** | | | | |
| Yes | 12 | 3 | 9 | 3 |
| No | 2 | 2 | 7 | 2 |
| No answer given [#] | 3 | 3 | 0 | 4 |
| **ESBL-producing *E. coli* present on farm** | | | | |
| Cowshed boot swabs | 2 | 1 | 3 | 1 |
| Calf samples | 3 | 1 | 5 | 2 |
| Youngstock samples | 2 | 2 | 0 | 0 |
| Total number of farms with at least one positive ESBL-producing *E. coli* sample | 3 | 2 | 6 | 2 |
| Total number of farms where all three samples were ESBL-producing *E. coli* positive | 2 | 1 | 0 | 0 |

* Waste milk is defined here as non-saleable milk, usually containing antimicrobial residues, or within the milk withholding period. [#] Farmer did not complete farm management survey; therefore this information is not available for this farm.

### 2.2. Bacteriology of Farm Samples

ESBL-producing *E. coli* were isolated in faecal samples from 13 (26%) of the 50 participating farms. Of these 11 pooled calf samples, seven pooled cowshed boot swab samples and four pooled youngstock samples were positive (for details, see Table 1). Three "high use" farms were found to be positive in all types of bovine faecal samples (i.e., cows, calves, and youngstock); while two of the "low use" farms were positive in both the cow and calf sample types and no youngstock were present at the time of sampling. One "high use" farm kept enough calves and youngstock (>5 head in each group) to require two pooled samples to be taken; however, these additional samples were negative, as were the other samples from this farm. In total, additional pooled samples were taken from three "low use" farms with sufficient animals. On two of these farms, all samples were negative and on one farm, the samples from cows and calves were positive for ESBL-producing *E. coli* in both the standard and additional samples.

production, while 19.7% are for use in cattle (of which, around 7% are for dairy cows and 9% for beef cattle) and the remaining 6.7% for use in poultry [6].

Whilst a proven relationship between antimicrobial use (AMU) and the selection for antimicrobial-resistant (AMR) bacteria remains a contentious issue, a number of studies have assessed the possibility of such a correlation. In 2014, a report on seven European countries (including Austria) determined a strong association between total antimicrobial use in livestock in each country and the reported prevalence of AMR in *E. coli* in those countries [7]. Similarly, a study of outpatient antimicrobial consumption and AMR in human patients determined a strong linear relationship between macrolide use and resistant *S. pneumoniae* (MRSP) in 16 countries (including Austria) [8]. Meanwhile, a study from the Netherlands determined no association between total AMU on farms and the presence of ESBL/AmpC-producing *E. coli*, although a correlation between increasing third- and fourth-generation cephalosporin use and increasing levels of these cephalosporin-resistant bacteria was detected [9]. More recently, a Swedish study of antimicrobial use on dairy farms analysed the presence of resistant phenotypes among *E. coli* and found no link between overall AMU and *E. coli* resistance [10]. However, the study's authors noted that AMU in Sweden is generally much lower than in other EU countries [10].

With respect to the risk to humans from antimicrobial-resistant bacteria in food, a number of studies have found evidence of AMR bacteria [11–13], including an Austrian study in 2014 which reported the presence of ESBL-producing *E. coli* in 20% of minced pork/beef samples tested, as well as MRSA in 9% of these samples [14]. As part of the EU AMR monitoring system, the European Food Standards Agency (EFSA) and the European Centre for Disease Control and Prevention (ECDC) publish joint annual summary reports on AMR in zoonotic and indicator bacteria from humans, animals, and food. The Austrian health authorities provide data for these reports and the most recent national monitoring results in 2019 reported the isolation of ESBL/AmpC-producing *E. coli* in 4 of 340 (1.2%) beef samples, as well as MRSA in 6 of 228 (2.8%) beef samples [15–17]. A recent pan-European study of 11 countries, including Austria, failed to detect a statistically significant association between ESBL and/or AmpC-producing *E. coli* (i.e., those resistant to third-generation cephalosporins) in humans and calves under one year of age [18]. Nevertheless, a source attribution model of ESBL-producing *E. coli* in the Netherlands highlighted that transmission to and from non-human sources (including cattle) is necessary to continue the intra-community spread of ESBL-producing *E. coli* and plasmid-mediated AmpC-producing *E. coli* [19].

The study presented here represents initial data from a pilot study of a small group of dairy farms, where extensive data on antimicrobial use over a one-year period, as well as farm management practices, were available. These data, as well as whether farms were considered "high" or "low" users of antimicrobials relative to the study population, were compared with the prevalence of ESBL-producing *E. coli* and MRSA obtained from samples collected on farms.

## 2. Results

In total, 138 voided faecal samples were collected from 50 farms (25 classified as "high" antimicrobial users and 25 as "low" users). Samples from the areas of the barn where cows were kept were available from all 50 farms. Calves were present on 46/50 farms (92.0%) and pooled samples (1–5 animals per pool) were taken from calf holding areas/hutches. Youngstock (>six months of age) were present on 32/50 farms (64.0%) and pooled samples (1–5 animals per pool) were taken from their pens. An additional ten pooled samples were taken from calves and youngstock on four farms, which reared more than 50 head of cattle. Dust samples were taken from all 50 farms.

### 2.1. Farm Population

In the "high" AMU group, the mean herd size was 47.3 head of cattle (median 38; range 14–128), including 22.6 dairy cows (median 17; range 8–56); whereas in the "low" AMU

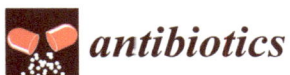

Article

# Analysis of Antimicrobial Use and the Presence of Antimicrobial-Resistant Bacteria on Austrian Dairy Farms—A Pilot Study

Clair L. Firth [1,*], Annemarie Käsbohrer [1], Peter Pless [2], Sandra Koeberl-Jelovcan [3] and Walter Obritzhauser [1,4]

1. Unit of Veterinary Public Health and Epidemiology, Institute of Food Safety, Food Technology & Veterinary Public Health, University of Veterinary Medicine, 1210 Vienna, Austria
2. Veterinary Directorate and Administration, Styrian Provincial Government, 8010 Graz, Austria
3. Institute for Medical Microbiology and Hygiene, Centre for Foodborne Infectious Diseases, Division for Public Health, Austrian Agency for Health and Food Safety (AGES GmbH), 8010 Graz, Austria
4. Veterinary Practice, 8605 Parschlug, Austria
* Correspondence: clair.firth@vetmeduni.ac.at

**Abstract:** The assumed link between high levels of antimicrobial use on farms and selection for antimicrobial-resistant (AMR) bacteria on that farm remains difficult to prove. In the pilot study presented here, we analysed total antimicrobial use on 50 dairy farms in Austria and also collected environmental samples to ascertain whether specific AMR bacteria were present. Antimicrobial use (AMU) analysis was based on electronic veterinary treatment records over a one-year period. Faecal samples for the assessment of extended-spectrum beta-lactamase (ESBL)-producing *E. coli* were collected from cowsheds, calf pens, and youngstock housing areas, as well as dust samples from barns, to isolate methicillin-resistant *Staphylococcus aureus* (MRSA). Bacteriological cultures were carried out on selective agar. Farms were split into groups of 25 of the highest antimicrobial users and 25 of the lowest users. Overall, samples from 13/50 (26.0%) farms were found to be positive for the presence of ESBL-producing *E. coli*. Of these, eight farms were in the low user group and five were in the high user group. Only one farm was confirmed to harbour MRSA. Statistical analyses demonstrated that there was no significant difference in this study population between high or low antimicrobial use with respect to the presence of ESBL-producing *E. coli* on farms ($p = 0.33$). In conclusion, the presence of specific AMR bacteria on farms in this study population was not found to have a statistically proven relationship with their level of antimicrobial use.

**Keywords:** antimicrobial resistance; antibiotics; dairy; ESBL; MRSA; farms; veterinary

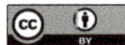

## 1. Introduction

Globally, the excessive use of antimicrobials and the increasing level of antimicrobial-resistant bacterial infections in both humans and animals are continuing to cause concern among veterinarians, medics, and the general public [1]. Veterinary antimicrobial use worldwide is expected to increase by an estimated 11.5% by 2030 (based on 2017 figures), and so the problem will persist [2]. While many countries (such as China, Brazil, the USA, and Australia) continue to misuse antimicrobials for non-therapeutic growth promotion, such use has been banned in the European Union (EU) since 2006 [3,4]. In Austria, antimicrobials for use in animals are only available from veterinarians and never over the counter. Injectable antimicrobials are further restricted and can only be dispensed to farmers who are members of the Animal Health Service (*Tiergesundheitsdienst*) and have completed a specific training course in medication administration and documentation. Since 2015, all antimicrobials dispensed for use in food-producing animals by veterinarians must also be reported to the relevant authorities [5]. Based on the latest national reports (for 2020), the vast majority of dispensed antimicrobials (73.4%) are provided for use in Austrian pig

42. Song, J.; Eensing, C.; Holm, P.E.; Virta, M.; Brandt, K.K. Comparison of Metals and Tetracycline as Selective Agents for Development of Tetracycline Resistant Bacterial Communities in Agricultural Soil. *Environ. Sci. Technol.* **2017**, *51*, 3040–3047. [CrossRef] [PubMed]
43. Arya, S.; Williams, A.; Reina, S.V.; Knapp, C.W.; Kreft, J.-U.; Hobman, J.L.; Stekel, D.J. Towards a general model for predicting minimal metal concentrations co-selecting for antibiotic resistance plasmids. *Environ. Pollut.* **2021**, *275*, 116602. [CrossRef] [PubMed]
44. Carson, C.A.; Reid-Smith, R.; Irwin, R.J.; Martin, W.S.; McEwen, S.A. Antimicrobial resistance in generic fecal *Escherichia coli* from 29 beef farms in Ontario. *Can. J. Vet. Res.* **2008**, *72*, 119–128.
45. Schmid, A.; Hörmansdorfer, S.; Messelhäusser, U.; Käsbohrer, A.; Sauter-Louis, C.; Mansfeld, R. Prevalence of Extended-Spectrum β-Lactamase-Producing *Escherichia coli* on Bavarian Dairy and Beef Cattle Farms. *Appl. Environ. Microbiol.* **2013**, *79*, 3027–3032. [CrossRef]
46. APHA. Livestock Demographic Data Group: Cattle Population Report. Available online: http://apha.defra.gov.uk/documents/surveillance/diseases/lddg-pop-report-cattle-1118.pdf (accessed on 2 February 2021).
47. APHA. Livestock Demographic Data Group: Sheep Population Report. Available online: http://apha.defra.gov.uk/documents/surveillance/diseases/lddg-pop-report-sheep-1118.pdf (accessed on 2 February 2021).
48. Benedict, K.M.; Gow, S.P.; Checkley, S.; Booker, C.W.; McAllister, T.A.; Morley, P.S. Methodological comparisons for antimicrobial resistance surveillance in feedlot cattle. *BMC Vet. Res.* **2013**, *9*, 216. [CrossRef] [PubMed]
49. Rosager, W.N.; Peter, N.J.; Lind, J.S.E.; Svend, H.; Matthew, D.; Steen, P.K. Comparison of antimicrobial resistance in *E. coli* isolated from rectal and floor samples in pens with diarrhoeic nursery pigs in Denmark. *Prev. Vet. Med.* **2017**, *147*, 42–49. [CrossRef]
50. Smith, P.; Finnegan, W.; Ngo, T.; Kronvall, G. Influence of incubation temperature and time on the precision of MIC and disc diffusion antimicrobial susceptibility test data. *Aquaculture* **2018**, *490*, 19–24. [CrossRef]
51. Fleiss, J.L.; Levin, B.; Paik, M.C. *Statistical Methods for Rates and Proportions*, 3rd ed.; John Wiley & Sons: Hoboken, NJ, USA, 2003.
52. Romesburg, C. *Cluster Analysis for Researchers*; Lulu Press: Morrisville, NC, USA, 2004.
53. Met Office. Historic Station Data. Available online: https://www.metoffice.gov.uk/research/climate/maps-and-data/historic-station-data (accessed on 24 November 2020).
54. UK Soil Observatory. Advanced Soil Geochemical Atlas of England and Wales. Available online: http://ukso.org/static-maps/advanced-soil-geochemical-atlas-of-england-and-wales.html (accessed on 5 December 2020).
55. Saini, V.; McClure, J.; Léger, D.; Dufour, S.; Sheldon, A.; Scholl, D.; Barkema, H. Antimicrobial use on Canadian dairy farms. *J. Dairy Sci.* **2012**, *95*, 1209–1221. [CrossRef]
56. Charlton, C.; Rabash, J.; Browne, W.; Healy, M.; Cameron, B. *MLwiN*; 3.02; Centre for Multilevel Modelling, University of Bristol: Brisotl, UK, 2017.
57. Leyland, A.H.; Groenewegen, P.P. Apportioning Variation in Multilevel Models. In *Multilevel Modelling for Public Health and Health Services Research*; Leyland, A.H., Groenewegen, P.P., Eds.; Springer: Cham, Switzerland, 2020; pp. 89–104. [CrossRef]

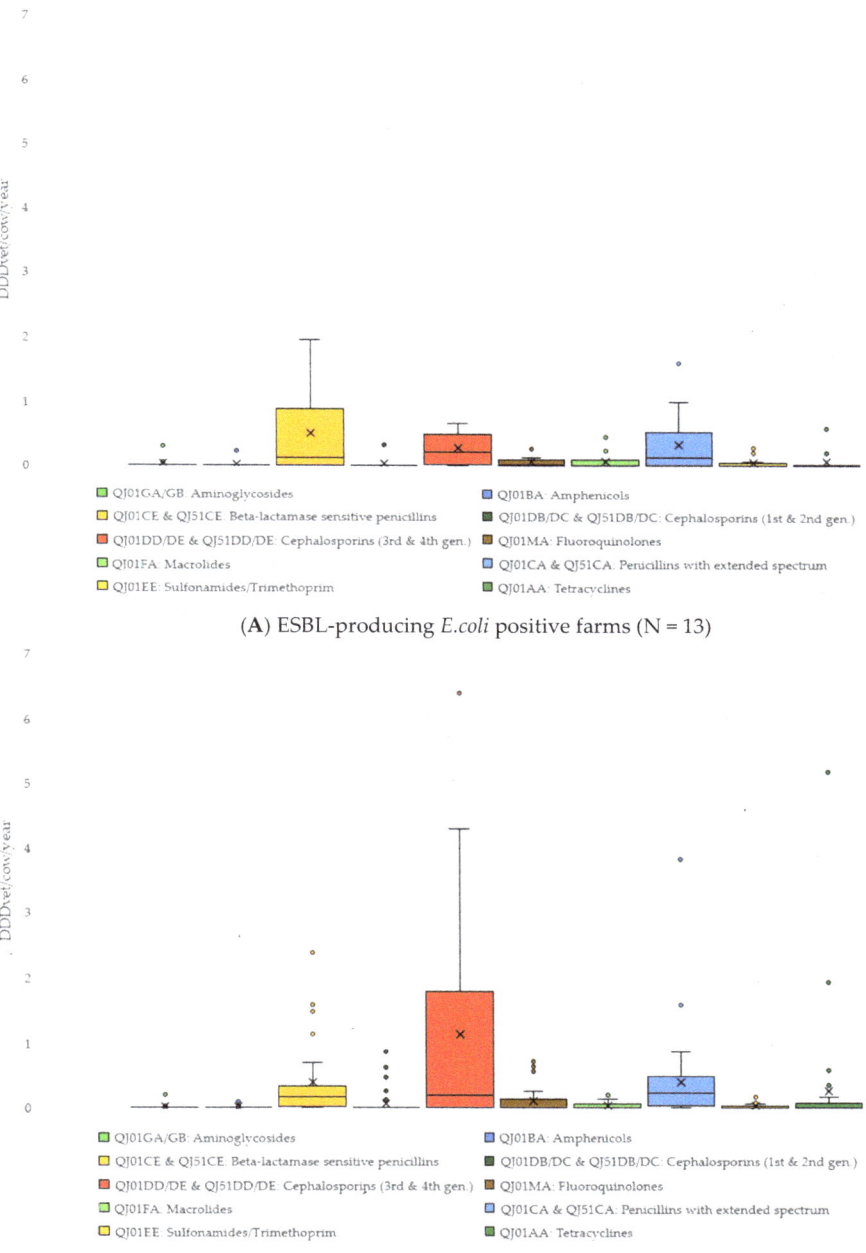

**Figure 1.** Antimicrobial treatments by antimicrobial class (and ATCVet code), divided into those farms where faecal samples tested positive for ESBL-producing *E. coli* (**A**) and those where samples tested negative for ESBL-producing *E. coli* (**B**).

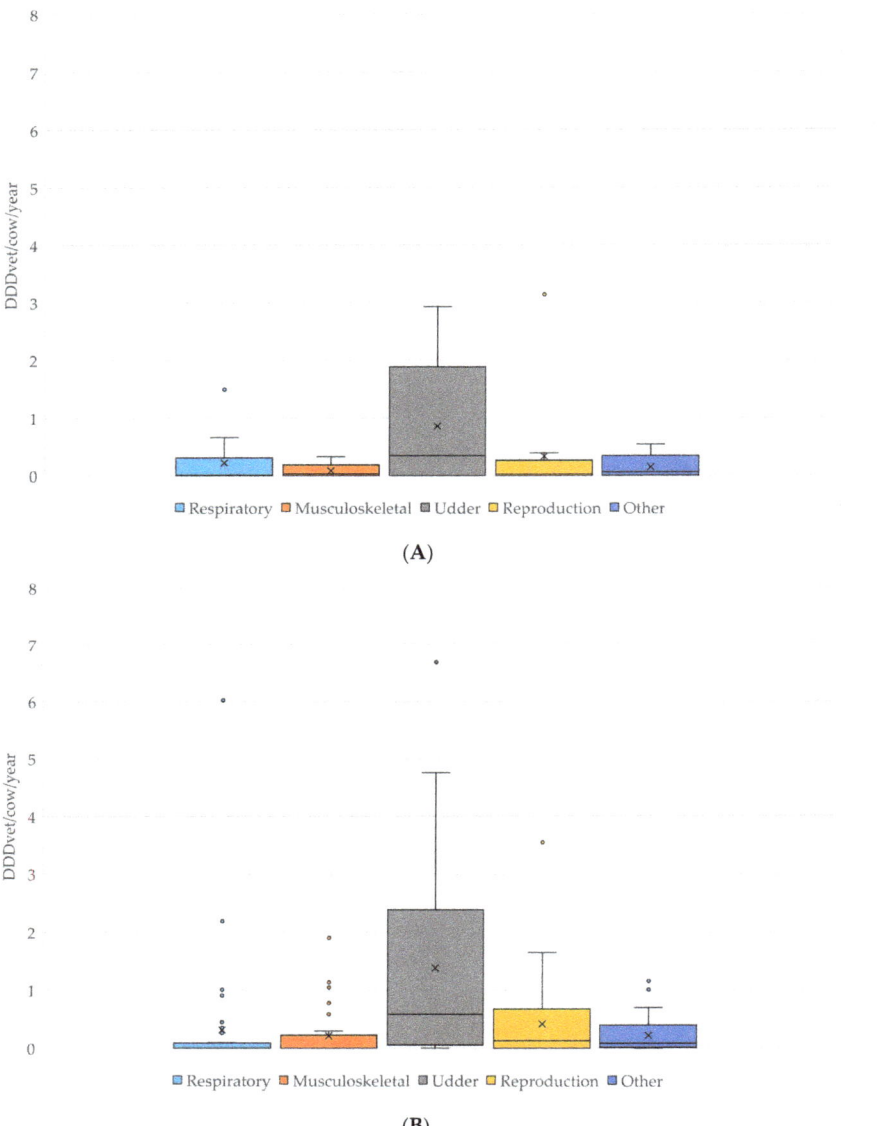

**Figure 2.** (**A**): Comparison of antimicrobial use in DDDvet/cow/year by disease indication on farms which tested POSITIVE for the presence of ESBL-producing *E. coli* (N = 13). (**B**): Comparison of antimicrobial use in DDDvet/cow/year by disease indication on farms which tested NEGATIVE for the presence of ESBL-producing *E. coli* (N = 37). X—mean; horizontal line—median; box—range between 1st and 3rd quartile; dots—outliers.

Dry cow therapy was analysed by Defined Course Dose (DCDvet) per cow and year and is shown in Figure 3. Among farms where at least one sample tested positive for the presence of ESBL-producing *E. coli*, the median was 0.53 DCDvet/cow/year (mean 0.71), whereas on negative farms the median was 0.50 DCDvet/cow/year (mean 0.77).

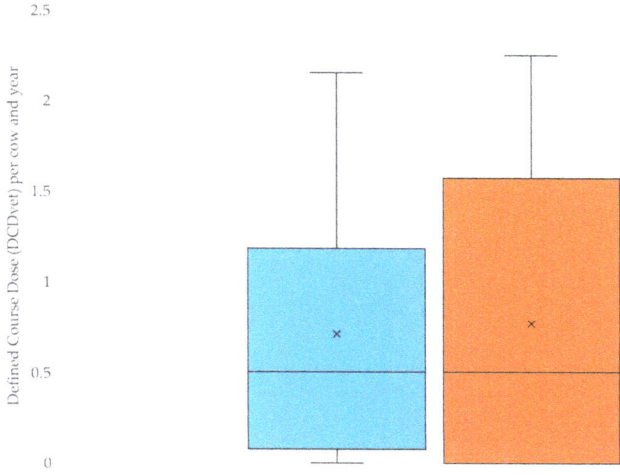

**Figure 3.** Comparison of antimicrobial dry cow therapy in Defined Course Dose per cow and year (DCDvet/cow/year).

### 2.4. Statistical Analysis

Using the Mann–Whitney U-test for independent samples, no statistically significant difference was determined between AMU in DDDvet/cow/year on each of the farms which were classified as ESBL-producing *E. coli* positive or negative (Mann–Whitney U score 187.0, Z score 1.17, $p = 0.24$). With respect to the use of third and fourth generation cephalosporins, the Mann–Whitney U-test similarly showed no statistically significant difference between the levels of use of this antimicrobial group regardless of whether ESBL-producing *E. coli* were isolated on the farm or not (Mann–Whitney U score 206.5, Z score 0.74, $p = 0.46$).

Using the Chi-squared test, no statistical significance was found at the 5% level between ESBL-positive *E. coli* or negative farms with respect to either "high" ($\geq 2.47$ DDDvet/cow/year) or "low" ($\leq 0.63$ DDDvet/cow/year) use groups ($p = 0.33$), or the number of dairy cows ($p = 0.42$) (Tables 3 and 4).

**Table 3.** 2 × 2 contingency table with respect to high and low AMU. Observed frequencies of ESBL-producing *E. coli* positive or negative farms (expected frequencies in brackets).

|  | High AMU Group $\geq 2.47$ DDDvet/Cow/Year | Low AMU Group $\leq 0.63$ DDDvet/Cow/Year | Total |
|---|---|---|---|
| ESBL-producing *E. coli*—positive | 5 (6.5) | 8 (6.5) | 13 |
| ESBL-producing *E. coli*—negative | 20 (18.5) | 17 (18.5) | 37 |
| Total | 25 | 25 | 50 |

Chi-squared test statistic 0.93, $p = 0.33$.

**Table 4.** 2 × 2 contingency table with respect to numbers of dairy cows. Observed frequencies of ESBL-producing *E. coli* positive or negative farms (expected frequencies in brackets).

|  | $\leq 20$ Dairy Cows | >20 Dairy Cows | Total |
|---|---|---|---|
| ESBL-producing *E. coli*—positive | 5 (6.2) | 8 (6.8) | 13 |
| ESBL-producing *E. coli*—negative | 19 (17.8) | 18 (19.2) | 37 |
| Total | 24 | 26 | 50 |

Chi-squared test statistic 0.64, $p = 0.42$.

With respect to feeding calves waste milk, no statistically significant difference was determined for the presence of ESBL-producing *E. coli* between those farms routinely feeding calves waste milk containing antimicrobial residues and those which did not (Fisher's exact test, $p$ = 0.44) (Table 5).

**Table 5.** 2 × 2 contingency table with respect to whether calves were fed waste milk containing antimicrobial residues on the farm. Observed frequencies of ESBL-producing *E. coli* positive (at least one positive sample) or negative farms.

|  | Waste Milk Fed to Calves | Waste Milk NOT Fed to Calves | Total |
|---|---|---|---|
| ESBL-producing *E. coli*—positive | 5 | 4 | 9 |
| ESBL-producing *E. coli*—negative | 22 | 9 | 31 |
| Total | 27 | 13 | 40 * |

Fisher's exact test, $p$ = 0.44. * Details on which farms fed waste milk were obtained via a questionnaire, which was completed by 40/50 of the farmers included in this study.

### 3. Discussion

To the authors' knowledge, this is the first study to analyse the presence of antimicrobial-resistant bacteria in relation to antimicrobial use on Austrian dairy farms. The current study represents the first steps in data collection on 50 dairy farms participating in a larger study of 250 farms. Analyses of faecal samples from the farm environment (boot swabs from alleyways of the cowshed, pooled faecal samples from calves and youngstock) determined a low prevalence of ESBL-producing *E. coli*, with approximately one quarter (26.0%) of the 50 farms testing positive in at least one sample. This is relatively low in comparison to neighbouring Bavaria (Germany) where a previous study of dairy and beef farms reported at least one positive ESBL-producing *E. coli* sample was found on 86.7% of the 45 farms tested [23]. Similarly, a study in the Netherlands collected ESBL/AmpC-positive samples on 41% of 100 conventionally run dairy farms [9]. A follow-up to this Dutch study carried out two years later after a change in local legislation to restrict the use of third- and fourth-generation cephalosporins demonstrated that the herd prevalence between matching herds fell from 32.7% ESBL/AmpC *E. coli*-positive in 2011 to 18.0% in 2013 [24]. However, the results determined here in Austria are not surprising as they correspond to the most recent official statistics published by the European Food Safety Authority and the European Centre for Disease Prevention and Control in 2020, where 20.5% of slaughtered calves (<1 year of age) in Austria were found to have presumptive ESBL-producing *E. coli* in their caeca, compared to a similar prevalence in Switzerland (19.1%), slightly higher in the Netherlands (36.4%), and much higher prevalences in Germany (66.8%), Belgium (64.8%), and Italy (86.8%) [25].

The statistical analysis presented here demonstrated that there was no statistically significant correlation between farms classified as "high" ($\geq$2.47 DDDvet/cow/year) antimicrobial users or "low" ($\leq$0.63 DDDvet/cow/year) antimicrobial users in this study population and the presence of ESBL-producing *E. coli* on these farms. This trend has also been reported in the Netherlands, where researchers found that the total annual animal-defined daily dose (DDDA) did not significantly differ between ESBL/AmpC-positive and negative farms [9,26]. Furthermore, the results presented here did not show a relationship between the presence of ESBL-producing *E. coli* and the use of third and fourth generation cephalosporins, contrasting with a Dutch study which found the use of these highest priority critically important antimicrobials (HPCIAs) led to an 8.05-fold increase in the odds of testing positive for ESBL/AmpC-producing *E. coli* [9]. A German study comparing dairy farms, which either did or did not use antimicrobials for a one-year period prior to sampling, found that 30% of the 10 control farms (no antimicrobial use) were ESBL-producing *E. coli* positive, while 39/45 (86.7%) of the dairy farms using antimicrobials tested positive [23]. A recent pan-European analysis on the prevalence of ESBL and/or AmpC-producing *E. coli* in slaughtered veal calves aged under one year (as well as broilers, turkeys, and fattening pigs) has also shown a statistically significant association between the national consumption of third and fourth generation cephalosporins in food-producing animals and the presence of these AMR bacteria (logistic regression based on national data from 31 countries, including Austria, in 2017–2018, odds ratio 1.29 (95% CI: 1.14; 1.46), $p < 0.001$) [18].

A study in France demonstrated that young calves (<7 weeks of age) on dairy farms were harbouring a variety of AMR bacteria in their intestinal microbiome [27]. In particular, this study demonstrated that the proportion of ESBL-producing *E. coli* as determined by selective media, fell slightly from 22% at 15 days of age to 19% at 7 weeks [27]; a trend which has been observed in many other studies of the intestinal flora of dairy calves [28–31]. While the feeding of waste milk containing antimicrobial residues to calves did not appear to have a statistically significant effect on the farms sampled in the current study, a number of other studies have shown that feeding such milk to calves leads to a transient increase in the presence of AMR bacteria in their faeces [31–34]. It is important to note that, similar to a Canadian study investigating extended-spectrum cephalosporin-resistant *E. coli* in calf faeces [34], the survey of farm management practices in the current study only provided "herd level" information and did not confirm that the calves sampled here had actually received waste milk containing antimicrobial residues, only that it was a routine practice on that farm. Furthermore, we did not investigate the impact of the prevalence of AMR bacteria on this practice.

Although data on MRSA on dairy farms are limited, other European studies in dairy cattle have reported a much higher prevalence of MRSA than that determined in the present study, where only one farm tested positive. A German study of three dairy herds more than a decade ago found that 46.7% (7/15) of cows tested were MRSA-positive and at a similar time, a Belgian study reported 9.3% of the 118 dairy farms tested were MRSA-positive [35,36]. The results determined for MRSA on these 50 Austrian farms are, however, comparable to the extremely low proportion of cattle testing positive for MRSA in a study of patients at the University of Veterinary Medicine in Vienna's ruminant clinic, where only 0.45% (95% CI: 0.01; 2.90%) of 221 cattle were MRSA-positive [37].

A previous study of human patients in the federal state of Upper Austria reported that 16/21 (76.2%) patients testing positive for MRSA CC398 were either pig or poultry farmers or had relatives with direct animal contact [38]. The Austrian researchers authoring that study suggested that the high level of doxycycline resistance (19/21, 90.5%) of MRSA isolates determined among these MRSA-positive patients could be connected to the relatively high proportion of tetracycline use on pig and poultry farms in Austria at this time [38]. However, a more recent Austrian study reported that human patients were much more likely to become infected with resistant *S. aureus* just through living in rural areas rather than working directly in animal production (OR 1.53 (95% CI: 1.02; 2.30) vs. OR 0.54 (95% CI: 0.19; 1.55)), although this may have been due to the relatively small number of livestock farmers (96/3309; 2.9%) included in that study population [39].

A study from the United States reported that, of 18 dairy farms sampled, 50% were positive for antimicrobial-resistant *Enterobacteriaceae* in environmental sampling and that on three (17%) of these farms such strains were isolated from 75.1 to 100% of all tested surfaces [40]. This study found that over 60% of "shared human and animal contact surfaces" were positive for AmpC and over 20% were positive for ESBL-producing *Enterobacteriaceae*, a finding which is extremely relevant for the possible transfer of antimicrobial resistance from animals to humans [40].

A meta-analysis of 181 studies to assess possible associations between antimicrobial use in food-producing animals and antimicrobial resistance in such animals and humans was published in 2017 [41]. A total of 81 studies on animals and 13 studies on humans were included in the final meta-analysis. In this study, the pooled absolute risk differences when interventions were introduced into livestock farming systems to reduce antimicrobial use led to a 10 to 15% (range 1–39%) lower proportion of resistant isolates in these systems compared to the control group, where no interventions were implemented [41]. The authors of this meta-analysis reported that there is sufficient evidence to demonstrate that a transfer of AMR bacteria can occur between livestock and farm workers and that this appears to occur less frequently when AMU in animal populations is reduced. However, they also pointed out that farmworkers are also the most commonly investigated group and that the evidence is, therefore, weaker for the general human population [41].

While the milk produced in this study population was not specifically tested for ESBL-producing *E. coli*, other European studies have investigated the presence of these AMR bacteria in the milk. A German study of bulk tank milk detected ESBL-producing *Enterobacteriaceae* in 9.5% of the 866 dairy farms tested [42], while a Swiss study of 100 dairy farms did not determine any ESBL-producing *E. coli* [43] in saleable milk.

In the present study, no statistically significant relationship could be proven between AMU and AMR on farms. It is important to note, however, that AMU on these Austrian dairy farms was relatively low compared to the dairy industry in other European countries [44–47], as well as the pig and poultry sector as a whole, and it is also unlikely that definitive conclusions can be made based on the small number of samples isolated which tested positive for ESBL-producing *E. coli*.

The main limitation of the current study was that the study population was not randomised and the data on antimicrobial use in this population of dairy cows cannot, therefore, be extrapolated to the rest of the Austrian dairy cow population. However, given the potentially sensitive nature of collecting diagnosis and antimicrobial treatment data directly from herd veterinarians, as well as the high level of commitment required by both veterinarian and farmer to complete all required study tasks, the decision was made to invite veterinarians to participate (convenience sampling) and that they should, in turn, suggest farmers from their client base to join the study (respondent-driven sampling). The subpopulation of 50 farms included here to investigate AMR bacteria was actually part of a much larger study containing around 250 dairy farms. Over a one-year period, the following data were collated from the 250 farms: AMU, bacteriological milk culturing results, veterinary diagnoses, milk recording results, animal movement data, and many other farm management factors [20,44]. While it is true that the enrolment of the 50 farms in the current study does indeed introduce a certain level of bias into the study population, we are of the opinion that this bias was limited as neither the farmers nor their herd vets knew which farms would be sampled for AMR bacteria at enrolment. The larger observational study commenced in October 2015, the faecal/dust samples included here were taken in July 2017, and the farms included in the current study were based on their AMU in 2015–2016. We do not believe that the herd veterinarians were able to influence the inclusion or exclusion of specific farms with antimicrobial resistance problems as the initial enrolment of farmers took place in winter 2014/2015, i.e., more than two years prior to AMR samples being collected.

A further limitation may have been the decision to include only the highest and lowest AMU farms in one geographical region in the subpopulation. In theory, the low use farms would have had either no or a low level of selection pressure on the bacteria present leading to a lower probability of resistant bacteria being favoured in the farm environment. In contrast, the high use farms could have had such a broad use of antimicrobials such that even ESBL-producing *E. coli* were not able to thrive. Nevertheless, we do not believe either of these cases to be true, as we determined no statistically significant difference between the prevalence of ESBL-producing *E. coli* on high or low AMU farms in this study, and the overall AMU on Austrian dairy farms is known to be relatively low (even the maximum use of antimicrobials on the highest using farm was <8.10 DDD/cow/year (median 3.82 DDD/cow/year), compared to other countries [44,45,47–49]).

## 4. Materials and Methods

### 4.1. Study Population

The sample of farms included in this pilot study was taken from a larger nationwide study of 248 Austrian dairy farms, as described elsewhere [20,44]. Overall antimicrobial use (AMU) was analysed as part of the previous study [44] and a subset of 50 farms in the federal state of Styria were chosen to participate in this pilot study based on their total AMU over a one-year period. These farms were selected to include the 25 highest users of all AMU and the 25 lowest users in the federal state who were participating in the larger study. The analysis of AMU was based on the Defined Daily Dose metric (DDDvet) as assigned for each antimicrobial active ingredient by the European Medicines Agency [21].

Farms were selected solely on their AMU calculated in DDDvet per cow per year in the previous year, no adjustments were made for housing system, production system (organic or conventional), herd size, or any other farm-related factors.

Bacteriological culture results from milk samples taken from these farms over the one-year study period were available, as described in detail for all 248 farms elsewhere [50]. The most common mastitis pathogens in the larger study population were *Staphylococcus* spp. (40.1%), *Streptococcus* spp. (24.1%), and *Enterobacteriaceae* (13.3%) [50]. A total of 3020 quarter samples from 647 cows on 166 farms were analysed as part of the wider study and it was determined that multiresistant (MDR, i.e., resistant to at least 3 antimicrobials from different classes [51]) strains were most common among *Enterobacteriaceae* spp., with 14.3% (19/133) of isolates, followed by *Staphylococcus* spp. with 5.5% (22/402) MDR isolates [50].

### 4.2. Background Information on Udder Health and Herd Management

Detailed information on the farms included in this pilot study is available in the form of questionnaire responses (see Supplementary Materials), as previously described with respect to mastitis risk factors and overall farm management [20].

### 4.3. Total Antimicrobial Use in Defined Daily Dose (DDDvet/Cow/Year)

Total AMU was calculated from veterinary treatment records covering 1 October 2015 to 30 September 2016, as detailed elsewhere [44,52]. A total of 11 veterinary practices provided data for this pilot study of 50 farms. Briefly, the number of DDDvet were calculated for each antimicrobial substance by dividing the total amount of active substance in milligrams by the European Medicines Agency's predefined DDDvet values [21].

Intramammary treatments were calculated slightly differently, as the European Medicines Agency classes each udder tube as 1 DDDvet, regardless of milligrams of active substance or standardised cow live weight (for details, see [21,44]).

DDDvet values have not been assigned by the EMA for dry cow therapy (DCT) intramammary tubes, only Defined Course Doses (DCDvet). For this reason, DCT was excluded from the majority of the AMU analyses included here. However, as dry cow therapy is an important part of the antimicrobial use statistics of dairy farms, a comparison of the corrected DCDvet/cow/year was carried out between those farms testing positive for the presence of ESBL-producing *E. coli* and those testing negative. The DCD/cow/year value was corrected by the replacement rate and calving interval for each of the farms included here, as described elsewhere [53].

No antimicrobial treatments were excluded in the present study (with the exception of unquantifiable sprays), regardless of diagnosis.

### 4.4. Farm Sampling and Bacteriological Culture

Each farm was sampled by one of two authors (CLF and WO). Personal protective equipment (PPE) in the form of disposable overalls, gloves, and boot covers were used to ensure that each site was not contaminated. As many Austrian dairy farms keep dual-purpose Simmental cows (Austrian *Fleckvieh*) for milk production, they frequently rear a number of female replacement heifers, as well as some male animals for beef production. For this reason, cows, calves, and youngstock are often found in the same building or on the same farm.

Each farm was visited in July 2017 and the following samples were collected:

- 2 pairs of boot swabs either from the alleyways of freestalls where lactating cows were housed or the slurry passage immediately behind cows in tie-stalls
- 1–2 pooled faecal samples from calf pens or freshly voided faeces if calves defaecated while researchers were present (1–5 calves per sample; 2 pooled samples were taken from farms with >50 head of cattle)
- 1–2 pooled faecal samples from youngstock (>6 months) pens (if youngstock were present on the farm, 1–5 head per sample; 2 pooled samples were taken from farms with >50 head of cattle)

Additionally, one dust sample was collected on dry gauze from 3 to 5 faeces-free areas of the main cowshed (for the isolation of MRSA).

Samples were immediately stored in an insulated cool box until they could be refrigerated. Faecal samples were transported to the laboratory of the Styrian Provincial Government Veterinary Authorities in Graz. Approximately 2 g faeces from each sample were pre-enriched in 200 mL buffered peptone water (BPW) at 37 °C for 18–24 h and then subsequent selective plated on ChromID-ESBL agar (bioMerieux, Marcy-L'Etoile, France). Plates were incubated at 37 °C for 24–28 h. Broth microdilution of the presumptive ESBL-producing *E. coli* was performed using the Sensititre™ EU Surveillance ESBL (EUVSEC2) plate (Thermo Fisher Scientific, Waltham, MA, USA) according to the manufacturer's instructions (briefly, each well was filled with 50 µL inoculum, the plate was then sealed and incubated at 34–36 °C for 18 h in a non-CO2 incubator). The Sensititre™ EU Surveillance ESBL (EUVSEC2) plate includes wells containing cefotaxime and ceftazidime with or without clavulanic acid, as well as cefoxitin, ertapenem, imipenem, meropenem, cefipime, temocillin, and positive control wells. An ESBL phenotype was categorised according to the EFSA/ECDC standard EU surveillance method, namely a minimal inhibitory concentration (MIC) >1 mg/L for cefotaxime and/or ceftazidime, a positive synergy test for these antimicrobials with clavulanic acid, an MIC $\leq 8$ mg/L for cefoxitin, and an MIC $\leq 0.12$ mg/L for meropenem [54].

Dust samples for MRSA isolation were transported to the National Reference Laboratory for Antimicrobial Resistance at the Institute for Medical Microbiology & Hygiene, Graz (part of the Austrian Agency for Health and Food Safety (AGES)). Swabs were inoculated in 100 mL Mueller–Hinton broth supplemented with 6.5% sodium chloride (NaCl) and incubated for 16–20 h at 37 °C. A 10 µL loopful of pre-enrichment broth was spread on chromID MRSA agar (bioMerieux, Marcy-L'Etoile, France) and incubated for 24–48 h at 37 °C. In addition, 1 mL of pre-enrichment broth was added to 9 mL tryptone soya broth (TSB) containing 3.5 mg/L cefoxitin and 75 mg/L aztreonam and incubated for another 16–20 h at 37 °C. A total of 10 µL of the selective enrichment broth were spread on chromID MRSA agar (bioMerieux) and incubated for 24–48 h at 37 °C. Presumptive MRSA colonies were confirmed by Time of Flight Mass Spectrometry (MALDI-TOF MS) and subsequent PCR targeting mecA and mecC according to methods described elsewhere [55,56], with minor deviations (for details, see the Supplementary Materials).

*4.5. Statistical Analysis*

Statistical analyses were carried out using the SPSS (IBM, Armonk, NY, USA) statistical software and Microsoft Excel (Microsoft Corporation, WA, USA). A non-parametric test of independent samples, the Mann–Whitney U-test, was done using the total DDDvet/cow/year for each of the 50 farms and whether at least one sample from the farm tested positive for the presence of ESBL-producing *E. coli*. This test was then repeated using the DDDvet/cow/year for third and fourth generation cephalosporins for each farm. Furthermore, using $2 \times 2$ contingency tables, the Chi-squared test was carried out on group sizes larger than five, while contingency tables where one or more category was smaller than five were assessed using Fisher's *t*-test. Statistical significance was set at $p < 0.05$ in all cases.

## 5. Conclusions

The level of antimicrobial resistance on the study farms was assessed by means of environmental samples collected from 50 dairy farms in the Austrian federal state of Styria chosen for either their high or low levels of overall AMU over a one-year period. The most frequent indication for antimicrobial use was the treatment of udder disease. No statistically significant relationships between high AMU in DDDvet/cow/year and the presence of these AMR bacteria were determined. While the low prevalence of ESBL-producing *E. coli* in cattle determined here correspond with national AMR monitoring of young calves, our findings may also have been due to the generally low level of antimicrobial use and subsequent lack of selection pressure for resistance genes on the study farms and, therefore, further investigation is needed with a larger sample size.

**Supplementary Materials:** The following supporting information can be downloaded at: https://www.mdpi.com/article/10.3390/antibiotics11020124/s1, S1: English summary of the farm management questionnaire; S2: Description of PCR methods.

**Author Contributions:** Conceptualisation, C.L.F. and W.O.; methodology, C.L.F., A.K., P.P., S.K.-J. and W.O.; formal analysis, C.L.F. and W.O.; investigation, C.L.F., P.P., S.K.-J. and W.O.; resources, A.K.; data curation, C.L.F. and W.O.; writing—original draft preparation, C.L.F.; writing—review and editing, C.L.F., A.K., P.P., S.K.-J. and W.O.; supervision, W.O. and A.K.; project administration, W.O. and A.K.; funding acquisition, W.O. All authors have read and agreed to the published version of the manuscript.

**Funding:** The K-Projekt ADDA—Advancement of Dairying in Austria was supported by the Austrian Ministry for Transport, Innovation and Technology (BMVIT), the Federal Ministry of Science, Research and Economy (BMWFJ), the province of Lower Austria and the city of Vienna within the framework of COMET—Competence Centers for Excellent Technologies. The COMET program is handled by the Austrian Research Promotion Agency (FFG). C.L.F. is partly funded by the K-Project "D4Dairy" which is supported by BMVIT, BMDW, the province of Lower Austria and the city of Vienna.

**Institutional Review Board Statement:** In accordance with national legislation and good scientific practice (GSP) guidelines, the study was registered with the institutional ethics and animal welfare committee of the University of Veterinary Medicine, Vienna (Ref No. ETK-13/11/2015). No invasive procedures were performed as part of this study.

**Informed Consent Statement:** Written informed consent was obtained from all farmers and veterinarians involved in the study.

**Data Availability Statement:** The authors do not own the antimicrobial use data analysed here. These data were collected from the veterinarians who were treating the animals included in the study. Under the data privacy agreement signed by the farmers and veterinarians, these data are not available to be published.

**Acknowledgments:** The authors would like to thank all the veterinarians and farmers who participated in this study, and Stefanie Klatovsky for help with PCR amplification of mecA/mecC.

**Conflicts of Interest:** The authors declare no conflict of interest. The funders had no role in the design of the study; in the collection, analyses, or interpretation of data; in the writing of the manuscript, or in the decision to publish the results.

## References

1. O'Neill, J. *Antimicrobials in Agriculture and the Environment: Reducing Unnecessary Use and Waste*; HM Government: London, UK, 2015.
2. Tiseo, K.; Huber, L.; Gilbert, M.; Robinson, T.P.; Boeckel, T.P. Van Global Trends in Antimicrobial Use in Food Animals from 2017 to 2030. *Antibiotics* **2020**, *9*, 918. [CrossRef]
3. Maron, D.F.; Smith, T.J.S.; Nachman, K.E. Restrictions on antimicrobial use in food animal production: An international regulatory and economic survey. *Global. Health* **2013**, *9*, 1–11. [CrossRef]
4. European Medicines Agency. Sales of Veterinary Antimicrobial agents in 31 European Countries in 2019 and 2020 (11th ESVAC Report); 2021. Available online: https://www.ema.europa.eu/en/documents/report/sales-veterinary-antimicrobial-agents-31-european-countries-2019-2020-trends-2010-2020-eleventh_en.pdf (accessed on 23 December 2021).

5. BMG Verordnung des Bundesministers für Gesundheit, mit der ein System zur Überwachung des Vetriebs und Verbrauchs von Antibiotika im Veterinärbereich eingereicht wird (Veterinär-Antibiotika-Mengenströme-VO) sowie die Verordnung über die Einrichtung und Führung der Tierärzteliste. Available online: https://www.ris.bka.gv.at/Dokumente/BgblAuth/BGBLA_2014_II_83/BGBLA_2014_II_83.pdf (accessed on 1 June 2017).
6. Fuchs, R.; Fuchs, K. Bericht über den Vertrieb von Antibiotika in der Veterinärmedizin in Österreich 2016–2020 (Report on Veterinary Antimicrobial Sales/Dispensing in Austria 2016–2020); Graz, Austria, 2021. Available online: https://www.ages.at/download/0/0/f290c2127644b5369881327c484607518e526e66/fileadmin/AGES2015/Themen/AGES_Schwerpunktthemen/Antibiotika/AB_Mengen_AUT_Bericht_2020.pdf (accessed on 22 December 2021).
7. Chantziaras, I.; Boyen, F.; Callens, B.; Dewulf, J. Correlation between veterinary antimicrobial use and antimicrobial resistance in food-producing animals: A report on seven countries. *J. Antimicrob. Chemother.* **2014**, *69*, 827–834. [CrossRef]
8. Albrich, W.C.; Monnet, D.L.; Harbarth, S. Antibiotic Selection Pressure and Resistance in Streptococcus pneumoniae and Streptococcus pyogenes—Volume 10, Number 3—March 2004—Emerging Infectious Diseases journal—CDC. *Emerg. Infect. Dis.* **2004**, *10*, 514–517. [CrossRef]
9. Gonggrijp, M.A.; Santman-Berends, I.M.G.A.; Heuvelink, A.E.; Buter, G.J.; van Schaik, G.; Hage, J.J.; Lam, T.J.G.M. Prevalence and risk factors for extended-spectrum β-lactamase- and AmpC-producing Escherichia coli in dairy farms. *J. Dairy Sci.* **2016**, *99*, 9001–9013. [CrossRef] [PubMed]
10. Sjöström, K.; Hickman, R.A.; Tepper, V.; Antillón, G.O.; Järhult, J.D.; Emanuelson, U.; Fall, N.; Lewerin, S.S. Antimicrobial Resistance Patterns in Organic and Conventional Dairy Herds in Sweden. *Antibiotics* **2020**, *9*, 834. [CrossRef] [PubMed]
11. Irrgang, A.; Roschanski, N.; Tenhagen, B.-A.; Grobbel, M.; Skladnikiewicz-Ziemer, T.; Thomas, K.; Roesler, U.; Käsbohrer, A. Prevalence of mcr-1 in E. coli from Livestock and Food in Germany, 2010–2015. *PLoS ONE* **2016**, *11*, e0159863. [CrossRef]
12. Roschanski, N.; Guenther, S.; Vu, T.T.T.; Fischer, J.; Semmler, T.; Huehn, S.; Alter, T.; Roesler, U. VIM-1 carbapenemase-producing Escherichia coli isolated from retail seafood, Germany 2016. *Eurosurveillance* **2017**, *22*, 17-00032. [CrossRef]
13. George, A. Antimicrobial resistance, trade, food safety and security (Editorial Commentary). *One Health* **2018**, *5*, 6–8. [CrossRef] [PubMed]
14. Petternel, C.; Galler, H.; Zarfel, G.; Luxner, J.; Haas, D.; Grisold, A.J.; Reinthaler, F.F.; Feierl, G. Isolation and characterization of multidrug-resistant bacteria from minced meat in Austria. *Food Microbiol.* **2014**, *44*, 41–46. [CrossRef]
15. Much, P.; Sun, H. Bericht zur AntibiotikaresistenzÜberwachung gemäß Durchführungsbeschluss der Kommission 2013/652/EU in Österreich, 2019. In *Resistenzbericht Österreich AURES 2019*; Bundesministerium für Soziales, Gesundheit, Pflege und Konsumentenschutz (BMSGPK): Vienna, Austria, 2021; pp. 357–394.
16. EFSA/ECDC. Annex E—Data on presumptive ESBL-, AmpC- and/or carbapenemase- producing microorganisms and their resistance occurrence (routine and specific monitoring). *EFSA J.* **2021**, *19*, 2015–2019. [CrossRef]
17. EFSA/ECDC. Annex F—Data reported on antimicrobial resistance in MRSA from food- producing animals and derived meat. *EFSA J.* **2021**, *19*, 1–17. [CrossRef]
18. ECDC; EFSA; EMA. Antimicrobial Consumption and Resistance in Bacteria from Humans and Animals Third Joint Inter-Agency Report on Integrated Analysis of Antimicrobial agent Consumption and Occurrence of Antimicrobial Resistance in Bacteria from Humans and Food-Producing an. Available online: https://www.ecdc.europa.eu/sites/default/files/documents/JIACRA-III-Antimicrobial-Consumption-and-Resistance-in-Bacteria-from-Humans-and-Animals.pdf (accessed on 24 November 2021).
19. Mughini-Gras, L.; Dorado-García, A.; van Duijkeren, E.; van den Bunt, G.; Dierikx, C.M.; Bonten, M.J.M.; Bootsma, M.C.J.; Schmitt, H.; Hald, T.; Evers, E.G.; et al. Attributable sources of community-acquired carriage of Escherichia coli containing β-lactam antibiotic resistance genes: A population-based modelling study. *Lancet Planet. Heal.* **2019**, *3*, e357–e369. [CrossRef]
20. Firth, C.L.; Laubichler, C.; Schleicher, C.; Fuchs, K.; Käsbohrer, A.; Egger-Danner, C.; Köfer, J.; Obritzhauser, W. Relationship between the probability of veterinary-diagnosed bovine mastitis occurring and farm management risk factors on small dairy farms in Austria. *J. Dairy Sci.* **2019**, *102*, 4452–4463. [CrossRef]
21. EMA Defined Daily Doses for Animals (DDDvet) and Defined Course Doses for Animals (DCDvet): European Surveillance of Veterinary Antimicrobial Consumption (ESVAC). Available online: http://www.ema.europa.eu/docs/en_GB/document_library/Other/2016/04/WC500205410.pdf (accessed on 1 July 2021).
22. WHO. *Critically Important Antimicrobials for Human Medicine— 5th Revision 2016*; Cambridge University Press: Geneva, Switzerland, 2017.
23. Schmid, A.; Hörmansdorfer, S.; Messelhäusser, U.; Käsbohrer, A.; Sauter-Louis, C.; Mansfeld, R. Prevalence of extended-spectrum beta-lactamase-producing Escherichia coli on Bavarian dairy and beef cattle farms. *Appl. Environ. Microbiol.* **2013**, *79*, 3027–3032. [CrossRef]
24. Heuvelink, A.E.; Gonggrijp, M.A.; Buter, R.G.J.; ter Bogt-Kappert, C.C.; van Schaik, G.; Velthuis, A.G.J.; Lam, T.J.G.M. Prevalence of extended-spectrum and AmpC β-lactamase-producing Escherichia coli in Dutch dairy herds. *Vet. Microbiol.* **2019**, *232*, 58–64. [CrossRef]
25. EFSA/ECDC. The European Union Summary Report on Antimicrobial Resistance in zoonotic and indicator bacteria from humans, animals and food in 2017/2018. *EFSA J.* **2020**, *18*, e06007. [CrossRef]
26. Santman-Berends, I.M.G.A.; Gonggrijp, M.A.; Hage, J.J.; Heuvelink, A.E.; Velthuis, A.; Lam, T.J.G.M.; van Schaik, G. Prevalence and risk factors for extended-spectrum β-lactamase or AmpC-producing Escherichia coli in organic dairy herds in the Netherlands. *J. Dairy Sci.* **2017**, *100*, 562–571. [CrossRef] [PubMed]

27. Jarrige, N.; Cazeau, G.; Bosquet, G.; Bastien, J.; Benoit, F.; Gay, E. Effects of antimicrobial exposure on the antimicrobial resistance of Escherichia coli in the digestive flora of dairy calves. *Prev. Vet. Med.* **2020**, *185*, 105177. [CrossRef] [PubMed]
28. Pereira, R.V.V.; Siler, J.D.; Bicalho, R.C.; Warnick, L.D. In Vivo Selection of Resistant E. coli after Ingestion of Milk with Added Drug Residues. *PLoS ONE* **2014**, *9*, e115223. [CrossRef]
29. Pereira, R.V.V.; Carroll, L.M.; Lima, S.; Foditsch, C.; Siler, J.D.; Bicalho, R.C.; Warnick, L.D. Impacts of feeding preweaned calves milk containing drug residues on the functional profile of the fecal microbiota. *Sci. Rep.* **2018**, *8*, 554. [CrossRef]
30. EFSA Panel on Biological Hazards; Ricci, A.; Allende, A.; Bolton, D.; Chemaly, M.; Davies, R.; Fernández Escámez, P.S.; Girones, R.; Koutsoumanis, K.; Lindqvist, R.; et al. Risk for the development of Antimicrobial Resistance (AMR) due to feeding of calves with milk containing residues of antibiotics. *EFSA J.* **2017**, *15*, e04665. [CrossRef]
31. Firth, C.L.; Kremer, K.; Werner, T.; Käsbohrer, A. The Effects of Feeding Waste Milk Containing Antimicrobial Residues on Dairy Calf Health. *Pathogens* **2021**, *10*, 112. [CrossRef] [PubMed]
32. Horton, R.A.; Duncan, D.; Randall, L.P.; Chappell, S.; Brunton, L.A.; Warner, R.; Coldham, N.G.; Teale, C.J. Longitudinal study of CTX-M ESBL-producing E. coli strains on a UK dairy farm. *Res. Vet. Sci.* **2016**, *109*, 107–113. [CrossRef] [PubMed]
33. Maynou, G.; Terré, M.; Bach, A.; Chester-Jones, H.; Migura-Garcia, L.; Ziegler, D. Effects of feeding pasteurized waste milk to dairy calves on phenotypes and genotypes of antimicrobial resistance in fecal Escherichia coli isolates before and after weaning. *J. Dairy Sci.* **2017**, *100*, 7967–7979. [CrossRef] [PubMed]
34. Awosile, B.; McClure, J.; Sanchez, J.; Rodriguez-Lecompte, J.C.; Keefe, G.; Heider, L.C. Salmonella enterica and extended-spectrum cephalosporin-resistant Escherichia coli recovered from Holstein dairy calves from 8 farms in New Brunswick, Canada. *J. Dairy Sci.* **2018**, *101*, 3271–3284. [CrossRef] [PubMed]
35. Vanderhaeghen, W.; Cerpentier, T.; Adriaensen, C.; Vicca, J.; Hermans, K.; Butaye, P. Methicillin-resistant Staphylococcus aureus (MRSA) ST398 associated with clinical and subclinical mastitis in Belgian cows. *Vet. Microbiol.* **2010**, *144*, 166–171. [CrossRef]
36. Spohr, M.; Rau, J.; Friedrich, A.; Klittich, G.; Fetsch, A.; Guerra, B.; Hammerl, J.A.; Tenhagen, B.A. Methicillin-resistant Staphylococcus aureus (MRSA) in three dairy herds in southwest Germany. *Zoonoses Public Health* **2011**, *58*, 252–261. [CrossRef]
37. Schauer, B.; Krametter-Frötscher, R.; Knauer, F.; Ehricht, R.; Monecke, S.; Feßler, A.T.; Schwarz, S.; Grunert, T.; Spergser, J.; Loncaric, I. Diversity of methicillin-resistant Staphylococcus aureus (MRSA) isolated from Austrian ruminants and New World camelids. *Vet. Microbiol.* **2018**, *215*, 77–82. [CrossRef]
38. Krziwanek, K.; Metz-Gercek, S.; Mittermayer, H. Methicillin-resistant staphylococcus aureus ST398 from human patients, Upper Austria. *Emerg. Infect. Dis.* **2009**, *15*, 766–769. [CrossRef] [PubMed]
39. Hoffmann, K.; den Heijer, C.D.J.; George, A.; Apfalter, P.; Maier, M. Prevalence and resistance patterns of commensal S. aureus in community-dwelling GP patients and socio-demographic associations: A cross-sectional study in the framework of the APRES-project in Austria. *BMC Infect. Dis.* **2015**, *15*, 1–9. [CrossRef]
40. Adams, R.J.; Kim, S.S.; Mollenkopf, D.F.; Mathys, D.A.; Schuenemann, G.M.; Daniels, J.B.; Wittum, T.E. Antimicrobial-resistant Enterobacteriaceae recovered from companion animal and livestock environments. *Zoonoses Public Health* **2018**, *65*, 519–527. [CrossRef] [PubMed]
41. Tang, K.L.; Caffrey, N.P.; Nóbrega, D.B.; Cork, S.C.; Ronksley, P.E.; Barkema, H.W.; Polachek, A.J.; Ganshorn, H.; Sharma, N.; Kellner, J.D.; et al. Restricting the use of antibiotics in food-producing animals and its associations with antibiotic resistance in food-producing animals and human beings: A systematic review and meta-analysis. *Lancet Planet. Health* **2017**, *1*, e316–e327. [CrossRef]
42. Odenthal, S.; Akineden, Ö.; Usleber, E. Extended-spectrum β-lactamase producing Enterobacteriaceae in bulk tank milk from German dairy farms. *Int. J. Food Microbiol.* **2016**, *238*, 72–78. [CrossRef] [PubMed]
43. Geser, N.; Stephan, R.; Hächler, H. Occurrence and characteristics of extended-spectrum β-lactamase (ESBL) producing Enterobacteriaceae in food producing animals, minced meat and raw milk. *BMC Vet. Res.* **2012**, *8*, 1–9. [CrossRef] [PubMed]
44. Firth, C.L.; Käsbohrer, A.; Schleicher, C.; Fuchs, K.; Egger-Danner, C.; Mayerhofer, M.; Schobesberger, H.; Köfer, J.; Obritzhauser, W. Antimicrobial consumption on Austrian dairy farms: An observational study of udder disease treatments based on veterinary medication records. *PeerJ* **2017**, *5*, e4072. [CrossRef] [PubMed]
45. Stevens, M.; Piepers, S.; Supré, K.; Dewulf, J.; De Vliegher, S. Quantification of antimicrobial consumption in adult cattle on dairy herds in Flanders, Belgium, and associations with udder health, milk quality, and production performance. *J. Dairy Sci.* **2016**, *99*, 2118–2130. [CrossRef] [PubMed]
46. Kuipers, A.; Koops, W.J.; Wemmenhove, H. Antibiotic use in dairy herds in the Netherlands from 2005 to 2012. *J. Dairy Sci.* **2016**, *99*, 1632–1648. [CrossRef]
47. More, S.J.; Clegg, T.A.; McCoy, F. The use of national-level data to describe trends in intramammary antimicrobial usage on Irish dairy farms from 2003 to 2015. *J. Dairy Sci.* **2017**, *100*, 1–14. [CrossRef] [PubMed]
48. Pol, M.; Ruegg, P.L. Treatment practices and quantification of antimicrobial drug usage in conventional and organic dairy farms in Wisconsin. *J. Dairy Sci.* **2007**, *90*, 249–261. [CrossRef]
49. Saini, V.; McClure, J.T.; Scholl, D.T.; DeVries, T.J.; Barkema, H.W. Herd-level association between antimicrobial use and antimicrobial resistance in bovine mastitis Staphylococcus aureus isolates on Canadian dairy farms. *J. Dairy Sci.* **2012**, *95*, 1921–1929. [CrossRef] [PubMed]

50. Schabauer, A.; Pinior, B.; Gruber, C.-M.; Firth, C.L.; Käsbohrer, A.; Wagner, M.; Rychli, K.; Obritzhauser, W. The relationship between clinical signs and microbiological species, spa type, and antimicrobial resistance in bovine mastitis cases in Austria. *Vet. Microbiol.* **2018**, *227*, 52–60. [CrossRef]
51. Magiorakos, A.-P.; Srinivasan, A.; Carey, R.B.; Carmeli, Y.; Falagas, M.E.; Giske, C.G.; Harbarth, S.; Hindler, J.F. Multidrug-resistant, Extensively Drug-resistant and Pandrug-resistant Bacteria: An International Expert Proposal for Interim Standard Definitions for Acquired Resistance. *Clin. Microbiol. Infect.* **2012**, *18*, 268–281. [CrossRef]
52. Firth, C.L. Analysis of antimicrobial use for the treatment of mastitis and antimicrobial resistance of clinically-relevant and commensal bacterial isolates on dairy farms in Austria, University of Veterinary Medicine Vienna, 2018. Available online: https://permalink.obvsg.at/UVW/AC15385467 (accessed on 22 December 2021).
53. Firth, C.L.; Käsbohrer, A.; Egger-Danner, C.; Fuchs, K.; Pinior, B.; Roch, F.F.; Obritzhauser, W. Comparison of defined course doses (DCDvet) for blanket and selective antimicrobial dry cow therapy on conventional and organic farms. *Animals* **2019**, *9*, 707. [CrossRef] [PubMed]
54. EFSA/ECDC Annex A—Materials and methods: The European Union Summary Report on Antimicrobial Resistance in zoonotic and indicator bacteria from humans, animals and food in 2018/2019. *EFSA J.* **2021**, *19*, 6490. [CrossRef]
55. Murakami, K.; Minamide, W.; Wada, K.; Nakamura, E.; Teraoka, H.; Watanabe, S. Identification of methicillin-resistant strains of staphylococci by polymerase chain reaction. *J. Clin. Microbiol.* **1991**, *29*, 2240–2244. [CrossRef]
56. Cuny, C.; Layer, F.; Strommenger, B.; Witte, W. Rare occurrence of methicillin-resistant Staphylococcus aureus CC130 with a novel mecA homologue in humans in Germany. *PLoS ONE* **2011**, *6*, e24360. [CrossRef]

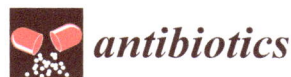 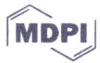

Article

# Antimicrobial Resistance Profiles of *Escherichia coli* from Diarrheic Weaned Piglets after the Ban on Antibiotic Growth Promoters in Feed

**Do Kyung-Hyo [1], Byun Jae-Won [2] and Lee Wan-Kyu [1],***

[1] Department of Veterinary Bacteriology and Infectious Diseases, College of Veterinary Medicine, Chungbuk National University, Cheongju 28544, Korea; pollic@chungbuk.ac.kr
[2] Animal Disease Diagnostic Division, Animal and Plant Quarantine Agency, Gimcheon 39660, Korea; jaewon8911@korea.kr
* Correspondence: wklee@cbu.ac.kr

Received: 3 October 2020; Accepted: 27 October 2020; Published: 29 October 2020

**Abstract:** This study aimed to survey the antimicrobial resistance profiles of 690 pathogenic *Escherichia coli* isolates obtained from Korean pigs with symptoms of enteric colibacillosis between 2007 and 2017, while assessing the change in antimicrobial resistance profiles before and after the ban on antibiotic growth promoters (AGPs). Following the Clinical and Laboratory Standards Institute guidelines, the antimicrobial resistance phenotype was analyzed through the disk diffusion method, and the genotype was analyzed by the polymerase chain reaction. After the ban on AGPs, resistance to gentamicin (from 68.8% to 39.0%), neomycin (from 84.9% to 57.8%), ciprofloxacin (from 49.5% to 39.6%), norfloxacin (from 46.8% to 37.3%), and amoxicillin/clavulanic acid (from 40.8% to 23.5%) decreased compared to before the ban. However, resistance to cephalothin (from 51.4% to 66.5%), cefepime (from 0.0% to 2.4%), and colistin (from 7.3% to 11.0%) had increased. We confirmed a high percentage of multidrug resistance before (95.0%) and after (96.6%) the ban on AGPs. The *AmpC* gene was the most prevalent from 2007 to 2017 (60.0%), followed by the *blaTEM* gene (55.5%). The *blaTEM* was prevalent before (2007–2011, 69.3%) and after (2012–2017, 49.2%) the ban on AGPs. These results provide data that can be used for the prevention and treatment of enteric colibacillosis.

**Keywords:** *Escherichia coli*; antimicrobial resistance; swine; weaned piglet; antibiotic growth promoters

## 1. Introduction

Weaned piglets are vulnerable to disease for many reasons such as changes in environmental conditions, a decline in maternal antibody titers, and various stresses. Presently, enteric colibacillosis, such as postweaning diarrhea and/or edema disease, is frequent in swine farms [1]. *Escherichia coli* (*E. coli*) in weaned piglets can result in serious economic losses due to diarrhea, growth retardation, and increased mortality [2].

Antimicrobials are used to treat colibacillosis in diarrheic weaned piglets. They play a significant role in the prevention and treatment of diseases and have also been used as a feed additive to promote swine growth [3]. However, the widespread and indiscriminate use of antimicrobials has resulted in the emergence of antimicrobial-resistant bacteria and the appearance of antibiotic residues in meat products [4]. Antimicrobial-resistant bacteria represent a threat to the successful treatment of disease in swine farms. As such, antibiotic growth promoters (AGPs) in feeds were banned in Korea in July 2011 [5].

Due to the emergence of antimicrobial resistance as a global problem, Denmark [6], Japan [7], and Canada [8] have started to formally monitor the state of antibiotic resistance. The antimicrobial-resistant profiles of pathogenic *E. coli* are changing based on geographical and temporal variations and previous exposures to antimicrobial agents [9]. Thus, devising control measures for colibacillosis in piggeries requires data regarding the prevalence of antimicrobial susceptibility [9].

Information on the antimicrobial resistance of pathogenic *E. coli* will be useful in establishing treatment and prevention strategies for colibacillosis in the swine industry. Although there have been many studies on the antimicrobial resistance of *E. coli* [10–12], few studies have examined annual trends in antimicrobial resistance profiles of *E. coli* over a decade. Additionally, there was little data comparing the changes in antimicrobial resistance profiles before and after the ban on AGPs. This study aimed to survey the antimicrobial resistance profiles of 690 pathogenic *E. coli* isolates obtained from Korean pigs with symptoms of enteric colibacillosis between 2007 and 2017, while assessing the change in antimicrobial resistance profiles before and after the ban on AGPs.

## 2. Results

### 2.1. Antimicrobial Susceptibility Test

The results of the antimicrobial susceptibility tests are shown in Table 1. We confirmed high resistance rates to tetracycline (598 isolates, 86.7%), ampicillin (586 isolates, 84.9%), streptomycin (589 isolates, 85.4%). On the other hand, the strains showed low resistance to cefepime (10 isolates, 1.4%) and colistin (68 isolates, 9.9%).

After the ban on AGPs, resistance to gentamicin (68.8% to 39.0%), neomycin (84.9% to 57.8%), ciprofloxacin (49.5% to 39.6%), norfloxacin (46.8% to 37.3%), and amoxicillin/clavulanic acid (40.8% to 23.5%) decreased with respect to that before the ban. There was a rapid decline in the resistance rates of those antimicrobials between 2012 to 2013 and 2014 to 2015. The resistance rates of gentamicin, ciprofloxacin, and norfloxacin in 2012–2013 were 62.4%, 59.6%, and 58.2%, respectively. However, those were decreased to 35.3%, 29.4%, and 27.1% in 2016–2017, respectively. On the other hand, the resistance rate of cephalothin (51.4% to 69.5%) increased, with an emergence of resistance to cefepime (0.0% to 2.1%) after the ban on AGPs. When we compared the resistance to colistin between 2012 to 2013 and 2014 to 2015 using a Chi-square test, there was a significant increase in resistance to colistin (7.1% to 19.9%, $p < 0.01$).

### 2.2. Multidrug Resistance

The results of the analysis of multidrug resistance rates are shown in Table 2. Before and after the ban on AGPs, the percentage of isolates resistant to seven subclasses were 22.9% and 21.0%, respectively, which were the most prevalent. Before the ban on AGPs, 1.4%, 6.4%, and 10.6% of isolates showed patterns of resistance to three, four, and eight antimicrobial subclasses, respectively. These rates increased to 4.0%, 9.3%, and 16.1% after the ban. However, rates of resistance to 6 and 10 subclasses decreased from 18.3% to 14.8% and from 11.9% to 7.4%, respectively. In terms of multidrug resistance for those with resistance to 3 or more subclasses of drugs among the 12 subclasses of drugs tested, 207 (95.0%) strains before the ban on AGPs, and 456 (96.6%) strains after the ban on AGPs, respectively, showed multidrug resistance.

### 2.3. Antimicrobial Resistance Genes

Table 3 shows the prevalence of antimicrobial resistance genes of *E. coli* isolated from diarrheic weaned piglets before and after the ban on AGPs. The *AmpC* gene was the most prevalent from 2007 to 2017 (414 isolates, 60.0%), followed by the *blaTEM* gene (383 isolates, 55.5%). Although the percentage decreased after the ban on AGPs, the *blaTEM* gene was still prevalent in 2007–2011 (69.3%) and 2012–2017 (49.2%). Before the ban on AGPs, only five isolates (2.3%) encoded the *blaSHV* gene. However, after the ban on AGPs, 29 isolates (6.1%) tested *blaSHV* positive. Additionally, there was the emergence of *blaCTX-M* group 2 after the ban on AGPs (0.0% to 1.7%). There was no isolate encoding the *mcr-2* gene in this study. Rates of the *tetA* gene increased annually. From 2007 to 2011, there were 46 (21.1%) *tetA*-gene-encoding isolates. However, it increased to 32.4% (153 isolates) in 2012–2017.

Table 1. Antimicrobial-resistant pathogenic *Escherichia coli* isolates (%) from weaned piglets with diarrhea in Korea from 2007 to 2017.

| Antimicrobial Subclasses | Agents [1] | Before the Ban on AGPs | | | | After the Ban on AGPs | | | | Total (2007–2017) (n = 690) | Differences in before and after Ban on AGPs [2] |
|---|---|---|---|---|---|---|---|---|---|---|---|
| | | 2007–2009 (n = 118) | 2010–2011 (n = 100) | Subtotal (2007–2011) (n = 218) | 2012–2013 (n = 141) | 2014–2015 (n = 161) | 2016–2017 (n = 170) | Subtotal (2012–2017) (n = 472) | | | |
| Aminoglycosides | GM ** | 84 (71.2) | 66 (66.0) | 150 (68.8) | 88 (62.4) | 36 (22.4) | 60 (35.3) | 184 (39.0) | 334 (48.4) | (29.8) |
| | S | 99 (83.9) | 85 (85.0) | 184 (84.4) | 122 (86.5) | 131 (81.4) | 152 (89.4) | 405 (85.8) | 589 (85.4) | (−1.4) |
| | N ** | 100 (84.7) | 85 (85.0) | 185 (84.9) | 95 (67.4) | 89 (55.3) | 89 (52.4) | 273 (57.8) | 458 (66.4) | (27.1) |
| Cephalosporin I | CF ** | 66 (55.9) | 46 (46.0) | 112 (51.4) | 95 (67.4) | 120 (74.5) | 113 (66.5) | 328 (69.5) | 440 (63.8) | (−18.1) |
| | CZ | 23 (19.5) | 18 (18.0) | 41 (18.8) | 30 (21.3) | 55 (34.2) | 22 (12.9) | 107 (22.7) | 148 (21.4) | (−3.9) |
| Cephalosporin IV | FEP * | 0 (0.0) | 0 (0.0) | 0 (0.0) | 1 (0.7) | 5 (3.1) | 4 (2.4) | 10 (2.1) | 10 (1.4) | (−2.1) |
| Cephamycin | FOX | 20 (16.9) | 13 (13.0) | 33 (15.1) | 24 (17.0) | 31 (19.3) | 6 (3.5) | 61 (12.9) | 94 (13.6) | (2.2) |
| Quinolones | NA | 97 (82.2) | 66 (66.0) | 163 (74.8) | 108 (76.6) | 109 (67.7) | 105 (61.8) | 322 (68.2) | 485 (70.3) | (6.6) |
| Fluoroquinolone | CIP * | 67 (56.8) | 41 (41.0) | 108 (49.5) | 84 (59.6) | 53 (32.9) | 50 (29.4) | 187 (39.6) | 295 (42.8) | (9.9) |
| | NOR * | 63 (53.4) | 39 (39.0) | 102 (46.8) | 82 (58.2) | 48 (29.8) | 46 (27.1) | 176 (37.3) | 278 (40.3) | (9.5) |
| Aminopenicillin | AM | 103 (87.3) | 86 (86.0) | 189 (86.7) | 116 (82.3) | 131 (81.4) | 150 (88.2) | 397 (84.1) | 586 (84.9) | (2.6) |
| BL/BLI [3] | AMC ** | 36 (30.5) | 53 (53.0) | 89 (40.8) | 54 (38.3) | 43 (26.7) | 14 (8.2) | 111 (23.5) | 200 (29.0) | (17.3) |
| FPI [4] | SXT | 92 (78.0) | 41 (41.0) | 133 (61.0) | 94 (66.7) | 97 (60.2) | 96 (56.5) | 287 (60.8) | 420 (60.9) | (0.2) |
| Phenicols | C | 104 (88.1) | 90 (90.0) | 194 (89.0) | 125 (88.7) | 130 (80.7) | 154 (90.6) | 409 (86.7) | 603 (87.4) | (2.3) |
| Polymyxins | CL | 9 (7.6) | 7 (7.0) | 16 (7.3) | 10 (7.1) | 32 (19.9) | 10 (5.9) | 52 (11.0) | 68 (9.9) | (−3.7) |
| Tetracyclines | TE ** | 111 (94.1) | 90 (90.0) | 201 (92.2) | 119 (84.4) | 127 (78.9) | 151 (88.8) | 397 (84.1) | 598 (86.7) | (8.1) |

[1] Significant differences between before (2007–2011) and after (2012–2017) the ban on antibiotic growth promoters in feed were expressed as * ($p < 0.05$) and ** ($p < 0.01$); GM: gentamicin, S: streptomycin, N: neomycin, CF: cephalothin, CZ: cefazolin, FEP: cefepime, FOX: cefoxitin, NA: nalidixic acid, CIP: ciprofloxacin, NOR: norfloxacin, AM: ampicillin, AMC: amoxicillin/clavulanic acid, SXT: trimethoprim/sulfamethoxazole, C: chloramphenicol, CL: colistin, TE: tetracycline. [2] Difference of the subtotals before (2007–2011) minus after (2012–2017) the ban on antibiotic growth promoters in feed. [3] BL/BLI: β-lactam/β-lactamase inhibitor combination. [4] FPI: Folate pathway inhibitors.

Table 2. Multidrug-resistant pathogenic *Escherichia coli* isolates (%) from weaned piglets with diarrhea in Korea from 2007 to 2017.

| Antimicrobial Subclass [1] | Before the Ban on AGPs | | | After the Ban on AGPs | | | | Total (2007–2017) (n = 690) | Differences in before and after Ban on AGPs [2] |
|---|---|---|---|---|---|---|---|---|---|
| | 2007–2009 (n = 118) | 2010–2011 (n = 100) | Subtotal (2007–2011) (n = 218) | 2012–2013 (n = 141) | 2014–2015 (n = 161) | 2016–2017 (n = 170) | Subtotal (2012–2017) (n = 472) | | |
| 0 subclass ** | 4 (3.4) | 0 (0.0) | 4 (1.8) | 0 (0.0) | 0 (0.0) | 0 (0.0) | 0 (0.0) | 4 (0.6) | (1.8) |
| 1 subclass | 2 (1.7) | 0 (0.0) | 2 (0.9) | 3 (2.1) | 1 (0.6) | 2 (1.2) | 6 (1.3) | 8 (1.2) | (−0.4) |
| 2 subclasses | 0 (0.0) | 5 (5.0) | 5 (2.3) | 4 (2.8) | 4 (2.5) | 2 (1.2) | 10 (2.1) | 15 (2.2) | (0.2) |
| 3 subclasses | 1 (0.8) | 2 (2.0) | 3 (1.4) | 3 (2.1) | 10 (6.2) | 6 (3.5) | 19 (4.0) | 22 (3.2) | (−2.6) |
| 4 subclasses | 2 (1.7) | 12 (12.0) | 14 (6.4) | 7 (5.0) | 14 (8.7) | 23 (13.5) | 44 (9.3) | 58 (8.4) | (−2.9) |
| 5 subclasses | 10 (8.5) | 21 (21.0) | 31 (14.2) | 21 (14.9) | 17 (10.6) | 34 (20.0) | 72 (15.3) | 103 (14.9) | (−1.1) |
| 6 subclasses | 27 (22.9) | 13 (13.0) | 40 (18.3) | 17 (12.1) | 19 (11.8) | 34 (20.0) | 70 (14.8) | 110 (15.9) | (3.5) |
| 7 subclasses | 28 (23.7) | 22 (22.0) | 50 (22.9) | 32 (22.7) | 26 (16.1) | 41 (24.1) | 99 (21.0) | 149 (21.6) | (1.9) |
| 8 subclasses | 17 (14.4) | 6 (6.0) | 23 (10.6) | 23 (16.3) | 36 (22.4) | 17 (10.0) | 76 (16.1) | 99 (14.3) | (−5.5) |
| 9 subclasses | 11 (9.3) | 8 (8.0) | 19 (8.7) | 11 (7.8) | 19 (11.8) | 7 (4.1) | 37 (7.8) | 56 (8.1) | (7.9) |
| 10 subclasses | 16 (13.6) | 10 (10.0) | 26 (11.9) | 18 (12.8) | 13 (8.1) | 4 (2.4) | 35 (7.4) | 61 (8.8) | (4.5) |
| 11 subclasses | 0 (0.0) | 1 (1.0) | 1 (0.5) | 2 (1.4) | 2 (1.2) | 0 (0.0) | 4 (0.8) | 5 (0.7) | (−0.3) |
| Multi-resistant (≥3 Subclasses) | 112 (94.9) | 95 (95.0) | 207 (95.0) | 134 (95.0) | 156 (96.9) | 166 (97.6) | 456 (96.6) | 663 (96.1) | (−2.6) |

[1] Significant differences between before (2007–2011) and after (2012–2017) the ban on antibiotic growth promoters in feed were expressed as ** ($p < 0.01$) Antimicrobial subclass are defined by the Clinical and Laboratory Standards Institute. [2] Difference of the subtotals before (2007–2011) minus after (2012–2017) the ban on antibiotic growth promoters in feed.

Table 3. Antimicrobial resistance genes (%) of pathogenic *Escherichia coli* from weaned piglets with diarrhea in Korea from 2007 to 2017.

| Antimicrobial Resistance GENES [1] | Before the Ban on AGPs | | | After the Ban on AGPs | | | | | Total (2007–2017) ($n = 690$) | Differences in before and after Ban on AGPs [2] |
|---|---|---|---|---|---|---|---|---|---|---|
| | 2007–2009 ($n = 118$) | 2010–2011 ($n = 100$) | Subtotal (2007–2011) ($n = 218$) | 2012–2013 ($n = 141$) | 2014–2015 ($n = 161$) | 2016–2017 ($n = 170$) | | Subtotal (2012–2017) ($n = 472$) | | |
| *bla*TEM ** | 79 (66.9) | 72 (72.0) | 151 (69.3) | 62 (44.0) | 65 (40.4) | 105 (61.8) | | 232 (49.2) | 383 (55.5) | (20.1) |
| *bla*SHV * | 2 (1.7) | 3 (3.0) | 5 (2.3) | 11 (7.8) | 16 (9.9) | 2 (1.2) | | 29 (6.1) | 34 (4.9) | (−3.8) |
| *bla*OXA | 10 (8.5) | 14 (14.0) | 24 (11.0) | 19 (13.5) | 18 (11.2) | 9 (5.3) | | 46 (9.7) | 70 (10.1) | (1.3) |
| *bla*CTX-M group 1 | 0 (0.0) | 4 (4.0) | 4 (1.8) | 2 (1.4) | 5 (3.1) | 2 (1.2) | | 9 (1.9) | 13 (1.9) | (−0.1) |
| *bla*CTX-M group 2 | 0 (0.0) | 0 (0.0) | 0 (0.0) | 0 (0.0) | 8 (5.0) | 0 (0.0) | | 8 (1.7) | 8 (1.2) | (−1.7) |
| *bla*CTX-M group 9 | 0 (0.0) | 4 (4.0) | 4 (1.8) | 3 (2.1) | 9 (5.6) | 2 (1.2) | | 14 (3.0) | 18 (2.6) | (−1.2) |
| *mcr*-1 | 0 (0.0) | 1 (1.0) | 1 (0.5) | 3 (2.1) | 3 (1.9) | 1 (0.6) | | 7 (1.5) | 8 (1.2) | (−1.0) |
| *mcr*-2 | 0 (0.0) | 0 (0.0) | 0 (0.0) | 0 (0.0) | 0 (0.0) | 0 (0.0) | | 0 (0.0) | 0 (0.0) | (0.0) |
| *mcr*-3 | 1 (0.8) | 2 (2.0) | 3 (1.4) | 5 (3.5) | 0 (0.0) | 0 (0.0) | | 5 (1.1) | 8 (1.2) | (0.3) |
| *AmpC* ** | 54 (45.8) | 43 (43.0) | 97 (44.5) | 88 (62.4) | 105 (65.2) | 124 (72.9) | | 317 (67.2) | 414 (60.0) | (−22.7) |
| *tetA* ** | 20 (16.9) | 26 (26.0) | 46 (21.1) | 38 (27.0) | 60 (37.3) | 55 (32.4) | | 153 (32.4) | 199 (28.8) | (−11.3) |

[1] Significant differences between before (2007–2011) and after (2012–2017) the ban on antibiotic growth promoters in feed were expressed as * ($p < 0.05$) and ** ($p < 0.01$). [2] Difference of the subtotals before (2007–2011) minus after (2012–2017) the ban on antibiotic growth promoters in feed.

## 3. Discussion

Antibiotics are used in intensive pig production systems to control infectious diseases. This widespread use is suspected to be a major cause of antimicrobial resistance [13]. To treat colibacillosis, antimicrobial agents including broad-spectrum-activity drugs, such as β-lactams and fluoroquinolones, are frequently used in veterinary medicine [14]. Usage of antimicrobial agents could be a cause for increasing antimicrobial resistance [15]. Thus, diseased animals might constitute an important reservoir of antimicrobial resistance [14].

In the previous study, we isolated 690 pathogenic *E. coli* strains from weaned piglets showing signs of enteric colibacillosis from 2007 to 2017, and investigated these isolates for adherence (F4, F5, F6, F18, F41, eae, paa, AIDA-I) and toxin (LT, STa, STb, Stx2e, EAST-I) genes [4]. Further, in this study, we tested antimicrobial resistance phenotypes and genotypes. We sought to provide data on the annual antimicrobial resistance profiles in Korean pig farms.

The frequencies of resistance to antimicrobials (gentamicin: 48.4%, neomycin: 66.4%, nalidixic acid 70.3%, ampicillin 84.9%, trimethoprim/sulfamethoxazole 60.9%, and tetracycline 86.7%) observed in this study are clearly higher than the EU average resistance figures (nalidixic acid 59.8%, ampicillin 58.0%, and tetracycline 47.1%), and the USA average resistance figures (gentamicin: 23.9%, neomycin 33.8%, ampicillin 68.1%, and trimethoprim/sulfamethoxazole 22.0%) [16,17].

Caution must be exercised when comparing such data because of the differences in methodologies used, particularly with the use of Clinical and Laboratory Standards Institute (CLSI) clinical breakpoints in this study compared with the use of epidemiological cut-off values (ECOFF's) in the EFSA (European Food Safety Authority) report. The results of this study are based on multiple isolates from diseased piglets. In contrast, the EFSA data were gathered mainly from the national monitoring program based on the sampling of healthy porcine carcasses at slaughter with all samples derived from distinct epidemiological units. The differences in resistance data across countries are not completely unexpected, as intensive pig production throughout Europe operates to different standards and utilizes distinct management practices.

Additionally, the pathogenic *E. coli* strains isolated in this study exhibited high resistance to ampicillin (84.9%), tetracycline (86.7%), and streptomycin (85.4%). This result is similar to the results of studies published in Denmark [6], Japan [7], and Canada [8]. The comparisons of resistance rates to the antimicrobials tested revealed that the isolates were more frequently resistant to ampicillin, tetracycline, and streptomycin—drugs that have been extensively used in large quantities in Korea [18]. Similar results have been described in other Korean reports. Cho et al. reported that the rate of resistance to tetracycline was the highest (97.8%), followed by ampicillin (89.1%) [19]. Lim et al. also reported a high resistance rate of *E. coli* to tetracycline (76.1%), ampicillin (64.6%), and streptomycin (58.4%) [10]. However, the resistance rates reported in this study were higher than those reported by Lim et al. [10]. This might be due to the differences in the origins of the isolates. We isolated from weaned piglets showing symptoms of colibacillosis, however, Lim et al. isolated from healthy pigs. According to the Korean national antimicrobial resistance monitoring systems, pathogenic bacteria tend to be more resistant to antimicrobials than bacteria isolated from normal livestock [20]. Lim et al. [10] assessed the resistance rates of *E. coli* from normal livestock; whereas in this study, we tested the antimicrobial resistance of pathogenic *E. coli* encoding at least one or more virulence factors isolated from pigs with diarrhea.

After the ban on AGPs, resistance rates to gentamicin had dramatically decreased (68.8% to 39.0%). Additionally, there was the emergence of resistance to cefepime (0.0% to 2.1%) and an increase in resistance rates to cephalothin (51.4% to 69.5%) and colistin (7.3% to 11.0%). Antimicrobial resistance is dependent on the level of antimicrobial usage [4]. The sales for antimicrobial agents that are usually used for growth promotion in Korea decreased from 2010 to 2017. Antimicrobial classes, tetracyclines and aminoglycosides, sold as much as 283,865 kg and 58,975 kg in 2010, respectively. However, this decreased to 254,541 kg and 50,503 kg in 2017, respectively. On the other hand, the sales for cephalosporins and phenicols, which are frequently used to treat enteric diseases in swine, increased from 2010 (4980 kg, and 63,882 kg, respectively) to 2017 (11,312 kg, and 114,716 kg, respectively) [21]. These changes in sales for antimicrobial agents could affect the resistance of isolates. Due to the rare occurrence of bacteria with resistance to it, as well as a paucity of horizontal transmission of resistance mechanisms, colistin has been regularly used for the treatment of enteric colibacillosis [22]. Additionally, the World Health Organization (WHO) has classified colistin as one of the "Highest Priority Critically Important Antimicrobials" in humans [23]. Recently, the plasmid-mediated colistin resistance gene, *mcr* was reported in Korea [24,25]. The observed increase in resistance rates could be attributed to this *mcr* gene. Increased resistance to colistin could pose serious problems not only in veterinary medicine but also in public health. Restrictions on the use of colistin are required to reduce resistance rates.

We confirmed a high frequency of multidrug resistance before (207 isolates, 95.0%) and after (456 isolates, 96.6%) the ban on AGPs. Due to the different types of antimicrobial tested, it is hard to directly compare multidrug resistance rates in comparison to the multidrug resistance rates (30.9%) of pigs with *E. coli* of US origin [26], the multidrug resistance rates of Korean piglets were very high. Since the regulation of the use of antimicrobials is not as strict in Korea as it is in other developed countries, it is considered that the use of antimicrobials by nonspecialists such as livestock workers and not veterinarians might be the cause of this phenomenon [18].

*E. coli* develop resistance mechanisms by using instructions provided by their DNA. Often, antimicrobial resistance genes are found within plasmids. This means that some bacteria can share their antimicrobial resistance genes and make other bacteria become resistant [3]. Extended spectrum β-lactamases (ESBLs) have been reported worldwide, most frequently in Enterobacteriaceae. ESBLs and *AmpC* are plasmid-encode, which are capable of inactivating a large number of beta-lactam antibiotics [15]. Additionally, colistin has been regularly used for the treatment of enteric colibacillosis such as postweaning diarrhea and edema disease due to the rare existence of resistant bacteria and lacking horizontal transmission mechanisms. However, very recently, the plasmid-mediated colistin resistance gene, *mcr* was found in Korea [5].

The *AmpC* gene encodes cephalosporinases and gives rise to serious therapeutic challenges in veterinary medicine. In this study, 414 isolates (60.0%) were positive for *AmpC* gene. β-lactam resistance in *E. coli* generally occurs as a result of the deregulation of the putative *AmpC* gene or the acquisition of a mobile genetic element containing an *AmpC* gene [15]. Consequently, high rates of ampicillin-resistant isolates are to be expected. In this study, we found that there was a high rate of resistance to ampicillin (84.9%).

Both TEM and SHV enzymes belong to the class A family of β-lactamases and are widely disseminated among the *Enterobacteriaceae* from veterinary sources [27] In this study, *blaTEM* was identified in over half the porcine *E. coli* isolates. However, *blaSHV* was detected in only 4.9% of isolates. There was also a decrease in the frequency of *blaTEM* after the ban on AGPs. TEM enzymes often co-exist with CTX-M enzymes in bacteria of animal origin [28]. However, the number of *blaCTX-M* group-positive isolates in this study was low (group 1: 13 isolates, group 2: 8 isolates, group 9: 18 isolates, total: 39 isolates). These results are of interest considering the current epidemiology of these genes.

We also confirmed that the antimicrobial resistance varied according to regions (Tables S1–S3). Resistance to chloramphenicol, gentamicin, neomycin, nalidixic acid, ciprofloxacin, and trimethoprim/sulfamethoxazole was higher in the northern farms than middle and southern farms after the ban on AGPs. The antimicrobial resistance phenotypes, and the multidrug resistance rates and prevalence of the *tetA* gene increased after the ban on AGPs in the northern farms, unlike in the middle and southern farms. This result is probably due to the fact that more antimicrobials were used in the northern farms than in the middle and southern farms. From 2001 in Korea, sales of antimicrobials for domestic livestock products and fisheries by use, breed, and antimicrobials were analyzed by a comprehensive management system created by the Korean Animal Health Products Association [20]. However, the analyses were not carried out by region [10]. The WHO/FAO/OIE stresses that overall sales, livestock, annual, periodic, and regional sales data for the use of antimicrobials that can be compared internationally and shared together should be investigated in a standardized way and the results should be expressed in standardized units [29]. Proper risk assessment, guidelines, and policy decisions for antimicrobial resistance management require data on the use of antimicrobials in each region. Therefore, in order to obtain a more accurate use of antimicrobials, it will be necessary to classify antimicrobials used in livestock production in accordance with the International Standards Classification Act and to develop a surveillance system that can further refine the methods of investigation (such as route of administration, breeding, breeding stage, and disease), to enter all prescribed antimicrobial agents, and to train clinical veterinarians.

In this study, we analyzed and compared the antimicrobial resistance phenotypes and genotypes of *E. coli* isolated from Korean diarrheic weaned piglets before and after the ban on AGPs. The trend in our findings suggests a decrease in resistance to gentamicin, neomycin, ciprofloxacin, norfloxacin, and amoxicillin/clavulanic acid after the ban on AGPs. However, resistance to cephalothin, cefepime, and colistin increased. Additionally, there was still a high frequency of multidrug-resistant isolates. Among the tested antimicrobial resistance genes, *AmpC* and *blaTEM* genes were the most prevalent. After the ban on AGPs, the frequency of the *AmpC* gene increased. On the other hand, the frequency of the *blaTEM* gene decreased. These results provide data that can be used for the prevention and treatment of enteric colibacillosis, as well as important data for assessing the impact of banning AGPs on the antimicrobial resistance profiles of *E. coli* isolates. Further studies are needed to determine the specific association of exposures to antimicrobial agents with antimicrobial resistance profiles.

## 4. Materials and Methods

### 4.1. Escherichia coli Isolates

Between 2007 and 2017, 690 *E. coli* isolates were obtained from weaned piglets showing symptoms of enteric colibacillosis and/or edema disease. The sampled farms consisted of 150 different pig herds (50 to 100 sows per herd) located in 3 areas: the northern (35 farms encompassing the Gangwon, Gyeonggi, and Incheon provinces), middle (46 farms, Chungbuk and Chungnam provinces), and southern (69 farms, Chonbuk, Chonnam, Gyeongbuk, and Gyeongnam provinces) areas of South Korea. The strains were not collected repeatedly from the same farm. The aseptically collected intestinal contents and feces were inoculated on a MacConkey agar (Becton Dickinson, Sparks, MD, USA) and blood agar (Asan Pharmaceutical, Seoul, Korea). After overnight incubation at 37 °C, only pure or nearly pure cultured colonies were selected and transferred to blood agar. Suspected colonies were identified as *E. coli* using the VITEK 2 GN ID card via VITEK II system (bioMéreiux, Marcy l'Etoile, France). The isolates were stored in 20% glycerol at −70 °C for further experimentation.

### 4.2. Antimicrobial Susceptibility Test

The following 16 antimicrobials were selected following the marketing amounts for animal use in Korea: gentamicin (10 µg), streptomycin (10 µg), neomycin (30 µg), ampicillin (10 µg), amoxicillin/clavulanic acid (20/10 µg), cephalothin (30 µg), cefoxitin (30 µg), cefazolin (30 µg), cefepime (30 µg), nalidixic acid (30 µg), ciprofloxacin (5 µg), norfloxacin (10 µg), sulfamethoxazole/trimethoprim (23.75/1.25 µg), chloramphenicol (30 µg), colistin (10 µg), and tetracycline (30 µg). Each antimicrobial disc was purchased from Becton-Dickinson (Sparks, MD, USA). Antimicrobial susceptibility testing was carried out using the Kirby Bauer disk diffusion method [30]. The isolates were inoculated on Mueller-Hinton agar (Becton-Dickinson). The antimicrobial discs were dropped on the agar and incubated at 37 °C for 18 h. *Escherichia coli* ATCC 25922 was used for quality control of the experiment. The interpretation of zone of inhibition was determined according to the CLSI standards *Enterobacteriaceae* breakpoints [31]. Intermediate isolates were grouped with resistant isolates. CLSI classified antimicrobial agents by class including several subclasses [31]. We categorized antimicrobial agents according to CLSI antimicrobial subclasses. Strains resistant to 3 or more CLSI subclasses of drugs were considered as multidrug-resistant strains.

*4.3. Antimicrobial Resistance Genes*

The *E. coli* genes for antimicrobial resistance were amplified by polymerase chain reaction (PCR) analysis. Bacterial colonies were suspended in 200 µL of distilled water and boiled for 10 min. After centrifugation at 8000× $g$, the supernatant was used as a template for PCR. We tested colistin-resistant *mcr* genes [5], tetracycline-resistant *tetA* genes [32], ampicillin-resistant *AmpC* genes [33], and extended-spectrum β-lactamase: *blaTEM*, *blaSHV*, *blaOXA*, *blaCTX-M* group 1, group 2, and group 9 [34], according to previously-described protocols (Supplementary Table S4). Bacterial colonies were suspended in 200 µL of distilled water and boiled for 10 min. After centrifugation at 8000× $g$, the supernatant was used as a template. The reaction volume, 20 µL, was composed of 2× EmeraldAmp Master Mix (Takara, Otsu, Japan), 2 µM of each primer, and 2 µL of template DNA. PCR product was electrophoresed on 2% agarose gel using Mupid-exU AD140 (Takara), stained with Ethidium bromide, and visualized on a UV trans-illuminator.

*4.4. Statistical Analysis*

All statistical analyses were performed using SPSS version 12.0 program (SPSS inc., Chicago, IL, USA). To compare antimicrobial resistance before and after the ban on AGPs, chi-square test was performed.

**Supplementary Materials:** The following are available online at http://www.mdpi.com/2079-6382/9/11/755/s1, Table S1. Antimicrobial-resistant pathogenic Escherichia coli isolates (%) from weaned piglets with diarrhea in northern, middle, and southern Korean farms before and after the ban on AGPs in feed, Table S2. Multidrug-resistant pathogenic Escherichia coli isolates (%) from weaned piglets with diarrhea in northern, middle, and southern Korean farms before and after the ban on AGPs in feed, Table S3. Antimicrobial resistance genes (%) of pathogenic Escherichia coli from weaned piglets with diarrhea in northern, middle, and southern Korean farms before and after the ban on AGPs in feed, Table S4. Primers for detection of antimicrobial resistance genes.

**Author Contributions:** Conceptualization: D.K.-H., B.J.-W., and L.W.-K.; methodology: B.J.-W.; validation: D.K.-H.; formal analysis: D.K.-H. and B.J.-W.; investigation: D.K.-H.; resources: B.J.-W. and L.W.-K.; data curation: D.K.-H.; writing/original draft preparation: D.K.-H.; writing, reviewing and editing: D.K.-H., B.J.-W., and L.W.-K; visualization: D.K.-H.; supervision: L.W.-K; project administration: L.W.-K; funding acquisition: L.W.-K. All authors have read and agreed to the published version of the manuscript.

**Funding:** This work was supported by "Korea Institute of Planning and Evaluation for Technology in Food, Agriculture, Forestry and Fisheries (IPET) through Agriculture, Food and Rural Affairs Convergence Technologies Program for Educating Creative Global Leader, funded by Ministry of Agriculture, Food and Rural Affairs (MAFRA) (grant number: 320005-4)".

**Conflicts of Interest:** The authors declare no conflict of interest.

# References

1. Straw, B.E.; Zimmerman, J.J.; D'Allaire, S.; Taylorm, D.J. *Escherichia coli*. In *Diseases of Swine*, 9th ed.; Wiley-Blackwell: Hoboken, NJ, USA, 2006; pp. 387–395.
2. Fairbrother, J.M.; Nadeau, E.; Gyles, C.L. *Escherichia coli* in postweaning diarrhea in pigs: An update on bacterial types, pathogenesis, and prevention strategies. *Anim. Health Res. Rev.* **2005**, *6*, 17–39. [CrossRef] [PubMed]
3. Wegener, H.C. Antibiotics in animal feed and their role in resistance development. *Curr. Opin. Microbiol.* **2003**, *6*, 439–445. [CrossRef] [PubMed]
4. Lim, S.-K.; Lee, J.-E.; Lee, H.-S.; Nam, H.-M.; Moon, D.-C.; Jang, G.-C.; Park, Y.-J.; Jung, Y.-G.; Jung, S.-C.; Wee, S.-H. Trends in antimicrobial sales for livestock and fisheries in Korea during 2003–2012. *Korean J. Vet. Res.* **2014**, *54*, 81–86. [CrossRef]
5. Do, K.-H.; Park, H.-E.; Byun, J.-W.; Lee, W.-K. Virulence and antimicrobial resistance profiles of *Escherichia coli* encoding mcr gene from diarrhoeic weaned piglets in Korea during 2007–2016. *J. Glob. Antimicrob. Resist.* **2020**, *20*, 324–327. [CrossRef]

6. DANMAP 2013: Use of Antimicrobial Agents and Occurrence of Antimicrobial Resistance in Bacteria from Food Animals, Food and Humans in Denmark. Available online: https://www.danmap.org/-/media/arkiv/projekt-sites/danmap/danmap-reports/danmap-2013/danmap-2013.pdf?la=en%20 (accessed on 27 October 2020).
7. Tamura, Y. The Japanese veterinary antimicrobial resistance monitoring system (JVARM). In *OIE International Standards on Antimicrobial Resistance*; OIE (World organization for animal health): Paris, France, 2003; pp. 206–210.
8. Deckert, A.; Gow, S.; Rosengren, L.; Léger, D.; Avery, B.; Daignault, D.; Dutil, L.; Reid-Smith, R.; Irwin, R. Canadian Integrated Program for Antimicrobial Resistance Surveillance (CIPARS) Farm Program: Results from Finisher Pig Surveillance. *Zoonoses Public Health* **2010**, *57*, 71–84. [CrossRef]
9. Alonso, C.A.; Mora, A.; Díaz, D.; Blanco, M.; González-Barrio, D.; Ruiz-Fons, J.F.; Simón, C.; Blanco, J.; Torres, C. Occurrence and characterization of stx and/or eae-positive *Escherichia coli* isolated from wildlife, including a typical EPEC strain from a wild boar. *Vet. Microbiol.* **2017**, *207*, 69–73. [CrossRef]
10. Lim, S.-K.; Nam, H.-M.; Moon, D.-C.; Jang, G.-C.; Jung, S.-C.; Korean Veterinary Antimicrobial Resistance Monitoring group. Antimicrobial resistance of *Escherichia coli* isolated from healthy animals during 2010–2012. *Korean J. Vet. Res.* **2014**, *54*, 131–137. [CrossRef]
11. Gibbons, J.; Boland, F.; Egan, J.; Fanning, S.; Markey, B.K.; Leonard, F.C. Antimicrobial Resistance of Faecal *Escherichia coli* Isolates from Pig Farms with Different Durations of In-feed Antimicrobial Use. *Zoonoses Public Health* **2015**, *63*, 241–250. [CrossRef]
12. Kusumoto, M.; Ogura, Y.; Gotoh, Y.; Iwata, T.; Hayashi, T.; Akiba, M. Colistin-Resistant *mcr-1*–Positive Pathogenic *Escherichia coli* in Swine, Japan, 2007–2014. *Emerg. Infect. Dis.* **2016**, *22*, 1315–1317. [CrossRef]
13. Diana, A.; Manzanilla, E.G.; Díaz, J.A.C.; Leonard, F.C.; Boyle, L.A. Correction: Do weaner pigs need in-feed antibiotics to ensure good health and welfare? *PLoS ONE* **2017**, *12*, e0189434. [CrossRef]
14. Luppi, A. Swine enteric colibacillosis: Diagnosis, therapy and antimicrobial resistance. *Porc. Health Manag.* **2017**, *3*, 16. [CrossRef]
15. Lalak, A.; Wasyl, D.; Zając, M.; Skarżyńska, M.; Hoszowski, A.; Samcik, I.; Woźniakowski, G.; Szulowski, K. Mechanisms of cephalosporin resistance in indicator *Escherichia coli* isolated from food animals. *Vet. Microbiol.* **2016**, *194*, 69–73. [CrossRef] [PubMed]
16. The European Union Summary Report on Antimicrobial Resistance in Zoonotic and Indicator Bacteria from Humans, Animals and Food in 2016. Available online: https://www.ecdc.europa.eu/sites/default/files/documents/AMR-zoonotic-bacteria-humans-animals-food-2016_Rev3.pdf (accessed on 27 October 2020).
17. Hayer, S.S.; Rovira, A.; Olsen, K.; Johnson, T.J.; Vannucci, F.; Rendahl, A.; Perez, A.; Alvarez, J. Prevalence and trend analysis of antimicrobial resistance in clinical *Escherichia coli* isolates collected from diseased pigs in the USA between 2006 and 2016. *Transbound. Emerg. Dis.* **2020**. [CrossRef] [PubMed]
18. Do, K.-H.; Byun, J.-W.; Lee, W.-K. Serogroups, Virulence Genes and Antimicrobial Resistance of F4+ and F18+ *Escherichia coli* Isolated from Weaned Piglets. *Pak. Vet. J.* **2019**, *39*, 266–270. [CrossRef]
19. Cho, J.K.; Ha, J.S.; Kim, K.S. Antimicrobial drug resistance of *Escherichia coli* isolated from cattle, swine and chicken. *Korean J. Vet. Public Health* **2006**, *30*, 9–18.
20. Lim, S.-K. *Establishment of Antimicrobial Resistance Surveillance System for Livestock 2012*; Animal and Plant Quarantine Agency: Seoul, Korea, 2015.
21. Animal and Plant Quarantine Agency (APQA). *Antimicrobial Use and Antimicrobial Resistance Monitoring in Animals and Animal Products*; APQA: Gimcheon, Korea, 2019.
22. Rhouma, M.; Fairbrother, J.M.; Beaudry, F.; Letellier, A. Post weaning diarrhea in pigs: Risk factors and non-colistin-based control strategies. *Acta Vet. Scand.* **2017**, *59*, 31. [CrossRef] [PubMed]
23. Arcilla, M.S.; Van Hattem, J.M.; Matamoros, S.; Melles, D.C.; Penders, J.; De Jong, M.D.; Schultsz, C. Dissemination of the *mcr-1* colistin resistance gene. *Lancet Infect. Dis.* **2016**, *16*, 147–149. [CrossRef]
24. Lim, S.-K.; Kang, H.Y.; Lee, K.; Moon, D.-C.; Lee, H.-S.; Jung, S.-C. First Detection of the *mcr-1* Gene in *Escherichia coli* Isolated from Livestock between 2013 and 2015 in South Korea. *Antimicrob. Agents Chemother.* **2016**, *60*, 6991–6993. [CrossRef]
25. Belaynehe, K.M.; Shin, S.W.; Park, K.Y.; Jang, J.Y.; Won, H.G.; Yoon, I.J.; Yoo, H.S. Emergence of *mcr-1* and *mcr-3* variants coding for plasmid-mediated colistin resistance in *Escherichia coli* isolates from food- producing animals in South Korea. *Int. J. Infect. Dis.* **2018**, *72*, 22–24. [CrossRef]

26. Sayah, R.S.; Kaneene, J.B.; Johnson, Y.; Miller, R. Patterns of Antimicrobial Resistance Observed in *Escherichia coli* Isolates Obtained from Domestic- and Wild-Animal Fecal Samples, Human Septage, and Surface Water. *Appl. Environ. Microbiol.* **2005**, *71*, 1394–1404. [CrossRef]
27. Yang, F.; Zhang, K.; Zhi, S.; Li, J.; Tian, X.; Gu, Y.; Zhou, J. High prevalence and dissemination of β-lactamase genes in swine farms in northern China. *Sci. Total Environ.* **2019**, *651*, 2507–2513. [CrossRef]
28. Cantón, R.; Novais, A.; Valverde, A.; Machado, E.; Peixe, L.; Baquero, F.; Coque, T. Prevalence and spread of extended-spectrum β-lactamase-producing Enterobacteriaceae in Europe. *Clin. Microbiol. Infect.* **2008**, *14*, 144–153. [CrossRef]
29. Silley, P.; Simjee, S.; Schwarz, S. Surveillance and monitoring of antimicrobial resistance and antibiotic consumption in humans and animals. *Rev. Sci. Tech.* **2012**, *31*, 105–120. [CrossRef]
30. Bauer, M.A.W.; Kirby, M.W.M.M.; Sherris, M.J.C.; Turck, M.M. Antibiotic Susceptibility Testing by a Standardized Single Disk Method. *Am. J. Clin. Pathol.* **1966**, *45*, 493–496. [CrossRef] [PubMed]
31. CLSI. *Performance Standards for Antimicrobial Susceptibility Testing*, 28th ed.; CLSI Supplement M100; Clinical and Laboratory Standards Institute: Wayne, PA, USA, 2018.
32. Pakpour, S.; Jabaji, S.; Chénier, M.R. Frequency of Antibiotic Resistance in a Swine Facility 2.5 Years after a Ban on Antibiotics. *Microb. Ecol.* **2012**, *63*, 41–50. [CrossRef] [PubMed]
33. Gonggrijp, M.; Santman-Berends, I.; Heuvelink, A.; Buter, G.; Van Schaik, G.; Hage, J.; Lam, T. Prevalence and risk factors for extended-spectrum β-lactamase- and AmpC-producing *Escherichia coli* in dairy farms. *J. Dairy Sci.* **2016**, *99*, 9001–9013. [CrossRef] [PubMed]
34. Dallenne, C.; Da Costa, A.; Decré, D.; Favier, C.; Arlet, G. Development of a set of multiplex PCR assays for the detection of genes encoding important β-lactamases in Enterobacteriaceae. *J. Antimicrob. Chemother.* **2010**, *65*, 490–495. [CrossRef]

**Publisher's Note:** MDPI stays neutral with regard to jurisdictional claims in published maps and institutional affiliations.

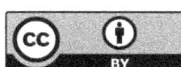

© 2020 by the authors. Licensee MDPI, Basel, Switzerland. This article is an open access article distributed under the terms and conditions of the Creative Commons Attribution (CC BY) license (http://creativecommons.org/licenses/by/4.0/).

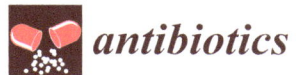

Article

# Risk Factors for Antimicrobial Resistance in Turkey Farms: A Cross-Sectional Study in Three European Countries

Mayu Horie [1,*], Dongsheng Yang [1], Philip Joosten [2], Patrick Munk [3], Katharina Wadepohl [4], Claire Chauvin [5], Gabriel Moyano [6], Magdalena Skarżyńska [7], Jeroen Dewulf [2], Frank M. Aarestrup [3], Thomas Blaha [4], Pascal Sanders [5], Bruno Gonzalez-Zorn [6], Dariusz Wasyl [7], Jaap A. Wagenaar [8,9], Dick Heederik [1], Dik Mevius [8,9], Heike Schmitt [1,10], Lidwien A. M. Smit [1] and Liese Van Gompel [1] on behalf of the EFFORT-Group [†]

[1] Institute for Risk Assessment Sciences, Utrecht University, Yalelaan 3, 3584 CM Utrecht, The Netherlands; d.yang@uu.nl (D.Y.); d.heederik@uu.nl (D.H.); h.schmitt@uu.nl (H.S.); l.a.smit@uu.nl (L.A.M.S.); l.vangompel@uu.nl (L.V.G.)

[2] Veterinary Epidemiology Unit, Department of Obstetrics, Reproduction and Herd Health, Faculty of Veterinary Medicine, Ghent University, Salisburylaan 133, 9820 Merelbeke, Belgium; philip.joosten@ugent.be (P.J.); jeroen.dewulf@ugent.be (J.D.)

[3] Research Group for Genomic Epidemiology, The National Food Institute, Technical University of Denmark, Kemitorvet, 2800 Kgs. Lyngby, Denmark; pmun@food.dtu.dk (P.M.); fmaa@food.dtu.dk (F.M.A.)

[4] Field Station for Epidemiology, University of Veterinary Medicine Hannover, Büscheler Straße 9, 49456 Bakum, Germany; katharina.wadepohl@tiho-hannover.de (K.W.); thomas.blaha@tiho-hannover.de (T.B.)

[5] Epidemiology, Health and Welfare Unit, The French Agency for Food, Environmental and Occupational Health & Safety (ANSES), 22440 Ploufragan, France; claire.chauvin@anses.fr (C.C.); pascal.sanders@anses.fr (P.S.)

[6] Antimicrobial Resistance Unit (ARU), Animal Health Departement, Faculty of Veterinary Medicine and VISAVET Health Surveillance Centre, Complutense University of Madrid, 28040 Madrid, Spain; gmoyano@ucm.es (G.M.); bgzorn@ucm.es (B.G.-Z.)

[7] Department of Microbiology, National Veterinary Research Institute (PIWet), Partyzantów Avenue 57, 24-100 Puławy, Poland; magdalena.skarzynska@piwet.pulawy.pl (M.S.); wasyl@piwet.pulawy.pl (D.W.)

[8] Department of Infectious Diseases and Immunology, Faculty of Veterinary Medicine, Utrecht University, Yalelaan 1, 3584 CL Utrecht, The Netherlands; j.wagenaar@uu.nl (J.A.W.); d.j.mevius@uu.nl (D.M.)

[9] Department of Bacteriology and Epidemiology, Wageningen Bioveterinary Research, Houtribweg 39, 8221 RA Lelystad, The Netherlands

[10] National Institute for Public Health and the Environment, P.O. Box 1, 3720 BA Bilthoven, The Netherlands

* Correspondence: m.horie@uu.nl

[†] EFFORT-Group: see acknowledgments.

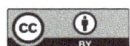

**Abstract:** Food-producing animals are an important reservoir and potential source of transmission of antimicrobial resistance (AMR) to humans. However, research on AMR in turkey farms is limited. This study aimed to identify risk factors for AMR in turkey farms in three European countries (Germany, France, and Spain). Between 2014 and 2016, faecal samples, antimicrobial usage (AMU), and biosecurity information were collected from 60 farms. The level of AMR in faecal samples was quantified in three ways: By measuring the abundance of AMR genes through (i) shotgun metagenomics sequencing ($n$ = 60), (ii) quantitative real-time polymerase chain reaction (qPCR) targeting *ermB*, *tetW*, *sul2*, and *aph3'-III*; ($n$ = 304), and (iii) by identifying the phenotypic prevalence of AMR in *Escherichia coli* isolates by minimum inhibitory concentrations (MIC) ($n$ = 600). The association between AMU or biosecurity and AMR was explored. Significant positive associations were detected between AMU and both genotypic and phenotypic AMR for specific antimicrobial classes. Beta-lactam and colistin resistance (metagenomics sequencing); ampicillin and ciprofloxacin resistance (MIC) were associated with AMU. However, no robust AMU-AMR association was detected by analyzing qPCR targets. In addition, no evidence was found that lower biosecurity increases AMR abundance. Using multiple complementary AMR detection methods added insights into AMU-AMR associations at turkey farms.

**Keywords:** antimicrobial use; antimicrobial resistance; turkeys; poultry; farm; antimicrobial resistance genes; biosecurity; risk factor; metagenomics; qPCR; isolates

## 1. Introduction

Antimicrobial resistance (AMR) is a global public health concern causing a substantial health and economic burden [1]. The types of antimicrobials used in food-producing animals are often the same or closely related to those used in human medicine [2]. Besides, resistance can spread rapidly and unpredictably through various environments. Therefore, AMR developed in animals can also be transferred to humans. To combat this, AMR is being addressed as part of a One Health approach [3,4].

Turkeys and turkey meat are possible sources for the transmission of AMR [5]. Within the European poultry sector, turkey fattening is the second biggest meat production sector after broiler production, accounting for around 14% of overall poultry meat production [6]. Recently, monitoring data in European countries has shown that a substantial proportion of isolates from turkeys are resistant to several classes of antimicrobials [7].

Farm-level risk factors for AMR in turkeys, such as antimicrobial usage (AMU) and biosecurity measures, have been examined in specific countries [8–13]. For example, AMU in the flock and evidence of mice were reported as risk factors for ciprofloxacin resistance in *Escherichia coli* (*E. coli*) in Great Britain [8]. In Germany, the floor design of turkey houses did not affect the development of resistance to enrofloxacin and ampicillin in *E. coli* isolates from turkeys [12,13]. However, it is unclear if these risk factors are country specific or not, because large variation exists between countries and farms in terms of the amount and type of antimicrobials used [14]. Furthermore, farming practices, including biosecurity measures, vary between countries and farms. Therefore, risk factors for AMR at a regional level may not be predictive for other regions or countries.

So far, all studies in turkeys have focused on the prevalence and characteristics of phenotypic resistance. Bacterial species such as *E. coli*, *Salmonella enterica*, and *Campylobactor* spp. were isolated from faeces and minimum inhibitory concentrations (MIC) were determined for fixed panels of antimicrobials [8–15]. There are many mechanisms by which these specific bacteria acquire resistance to antimicrobials. For example, there are multiple gene families encoding extended spectrum beta-lactamases (ESBL) or plasmid-mediated AmpC beta-lactamases. The enterobacteriaceae producing these enzymes are resistant to antibiotics such as penicillins and 3rd and 4th generation cephalosporins. These isolates can then transfer ESBL or AmpC genes to other bacteria in the gut environment or through the food chain. In poultry production pyramids, ESBLs are frequently found [16]. Therefore, culture-dependent methods may underestimate AMR in unculturable gut microbiota. Genotypic methods enable faecal AMR gene detection. When using metagenomics or quantitative real-time polymerase chain reaction (qPCR), the abundance and diversity of AMR genes present in samples can be measured without culturing bacteria. Combining this kind of AMR data with data on AMU and other potential on-farm risk factors, allows for exposure-response relationships to be explored [17–19]. Comparing AMR detection methods provides a better understanding of the complex mechanisms behind AMR occurrence in food-producing animals.

As part of the Ecology from Farm to Fork of Microbial Drug Resistance and Transmission (EFFORT) project (http://www.effort-against-amr.eu/, accessed on 28 March 2021), the present study aimed to explore AMR in turkeys from 60 farms in three European countries. The objectives of this paper were to (i) quantify the abundance and diversity of AMR genes in turkey faeces by applying metagenomics and qPCR, and to (ii) determine risk factors for AMR such as AMU as well as other potential farm-level risk factors. In addition, the used AMR quantification methods were compared.

## 2. Results

### 2.1. Overview of the Sampled Farms and Flocks

General characteristics of the sampled farms ($n = 60$) are shown in Table 1. The total number of turkeys per farm varied considerably (median 10,000 turkeys per farm, range: 2950–56,850). We carried out sampling across all seasons: Spring ($n = 21$), summer ($n = 8$), autumn ($n = 16$), and winter ($n = 15$). All farms in country H were sampled in spring and summer. The weight of turkeys at the set up differed substantially between the three countries, and within country B. In country H, all the farms followed an integrated fattening process where the turkeys were introduced to the fattening farms after 28 days of life in breeding, resulting in a small variation in set up weights.

**Table 1.** Characteristics of the sampled turkey farms and flocks by country and overall countries.

| Characteristics | Country | | | Overall |
|---|---|---|---|---|
| | B | E | H | |
| **Farm Information** | | | | |
| Included farms, n | 20 | 20 | 20 | 60 |
| No. of turkeys present on the farm, median (Min-Max) | 12,683 (5000–46,500) | 7275 (2950–38,000) | 12,609 (4404–56,850) | 10,055 (2950–56,850) |
| Farms where other livestock is present, n (%) | 4 (20) | 11 (55) | 4 (20) | 19 (32) |
| No. of people working at the farm, median (Min-Max) | 2 (1–28) | 1.5 (1–3) | 1 (1–4) | 1.5 (1–28) |
| Farms sampled in spring and summer, n (%) | 4 (20) | 5 (25) | 20 (100) | 29 (48) |
| **Flock Information** | | | | |
| No. of turkeys at sampling, median (Min-Max) [a] | 4213 (2050–11,660) | 4140 (450–9155) | 6422 (302–21,356) | 4710 (450–21,356) |
| No. of turkeys at set-up in the current round in the sampled house, median (Min-Max) [b] | 5040 (2997–13,000) | 9180 (4240–22,000) | 7020 (3000–21,794) | 7850 (2997–22,000) |
| Weight of turkeys at set-up, kg, median (Min-Max) [c] | 1.5 (0.1–6.4) | 0.1 (0.1–0.5) | 1.1 (0.9–1.3) | 1.1 (0.1–6.4) |
| Age of turkeys at sampling, days, median (Min-Max) [b] | 134 (96–147) | 116 (74–140) | 101 (86–118) | 115 (74–147) |
| Average expected age at delivery to slaughter, days, median (Min-Max) [b] | 146 (106–154) | 109 (79–138) | 117 (95–127) | 118 (79–154) |
| **Biosecurity at the Farm** | | | | |
| Visitor access more than once a month (family members, technicians, etc), n (%) | 8 (40) | 20 (100) | 16 (80) | 44 (73) |
| Outdoor access possible for turkeys, n (%) | 14 (70) | 0 (0) | 0 (0) | 14 (23) |
| Different age categories of turkeys present, n (%) | 10 (50) | 5 (25) | 0 (0) | 15 (25) |
| Bird- and vermin-proof grids placed on the air inlets, n (%) | 20 (100) | 15 (75) | 18 (90) | 53 (88) |
| Staff keeps turkeys or birds at home, n (%) | 2 (10) | 7 (35) | 1 (5) | 10 (17) |
| Disinfecting footbaths present on the farm, n (%) | 14 (70) | 10 (50) | 10 (50) | 34 (57) |
| The nearest turkey farm within 500 m, n (%) | 4 (20) | 5 (25) | 4 (20) | 13 (22) |
| Other livestock farm present within 500 m, n (%) | 12 (60) | 18 (90) | 7 (35) | 37 (62) |
| Wild birds can enter the stables, n (%) | 1 (5) | 6 (30) | 8 (40) | 15 (25) |

Missing observations were excluded to calculate the average. [a,b,c] The number of farms with missing observations: [a] 2, [b] 1, [c] 10. Biosecurity status displayed in the table are those significantly associated with the AMR in the applied models.

The median age of turkeys at sampling was 115 days. Flocks were separated by sex in country B and H, with the exception of country E where both cocks and hens were usually housed together with a mobile fence. Therefore, some of the hens within those flocks had been removed from the house prior to sampling of the cocks. The overall expected slaughter age was 118 days. For some flocks we could not exactly determine how many days before slaughter sampling was performed, since these included several groups with a different expected slaughter date. Consequently, we calculated the average expected slaughter age per flock.

The biosecurity status at the farm was reduced to two levels. Due to a large number of questions, the questions that were significantly related with AMR in the applied models were shown in Table 1 with the number of farms that answered yes. The proportion of farms that answered yes differed between countries for several biosecurity statuses. For instance, farms where turkeys had outdoor access were only included in country B (70% of the farms in country B).

### 2.2. Antimicrobial Usage

Antimicrobial group treatments applied during the entire rearing period of the sampled flock were quantified using treatment incidence (TI) as a unit of measurement.

There were differences in amounts and types of antimicrobials used between countries (Figure 1). The mean TI per farm was 8.03, 9.95, and 18.4, in country B, E, and H, respectively. Aminoglycosides and spectinomycins, and macrolides and lincomycins were grouped together because they have a common resistance mechanism. The most frequently used antimicrobial groups across all the farms were beta-lactams, polymyxins, and quinolones.

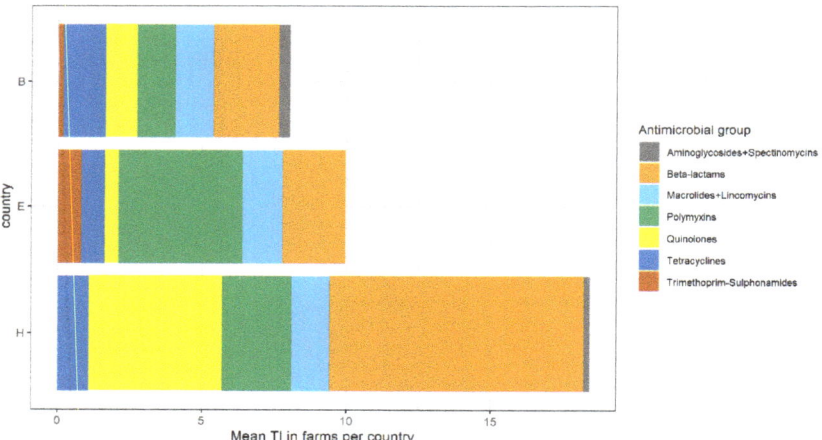

**Figure 1.** Average antimicrobial usage on farm level in 60 turkey farms in three countries. Mean treatment incidence (TI) shows the average number of treatment days per 100 days. Antimicrobials were grouped after TI was calculated for lincomycin-spectinomycin combination product and subsequently divided and added to macrolides and aminoglycosides, respectively. Beta-lactams included aminopenicillins and penicillins. Quinolones included fluoroquinolones and other quinolones (flumequine). Countries were anonymized as B, E, and H.

The sum of TI at 60 farms is shown in Figure S2. Across all farms, 7 (11.7%) did not use any antimicrobials (country B:3, E:3, and H:1).

### 2.3. AMR Genes Identified by Metagenomics
#### 2.3.1. The Abundance and Composition of AMR Genes

In total, 573 different AMR genes were identified in samples from 60 turkey farms using ResFinder as a reference database [20]. The abundance of AMR genes were quantified using normalized fragments per kilobase reference per million bacterial fragments (FPKM) values. The FPKM values for the different AMR genes were summed for each antimicrobial class. In general, the composition of AMR genes appeared rather homogenous across farms despite the difference in AMU, and even when comparing farms that did or did not use antimicrobials (Figure 2). The clusters of AMR genes encoding for resistance to tetracyclines, macrolides, and aminoglycosides were most abundant. Moreover, AMR gene clusters encoding for resistance to aminoglycosides, beta-lactams, macrolides, phenicols, sulphonamides, tetracyclines, and trimethoprim classes were detected on all farms. A stacked bar chart showing FPKM values (i.e., not proportional) is shown in Figure S3.

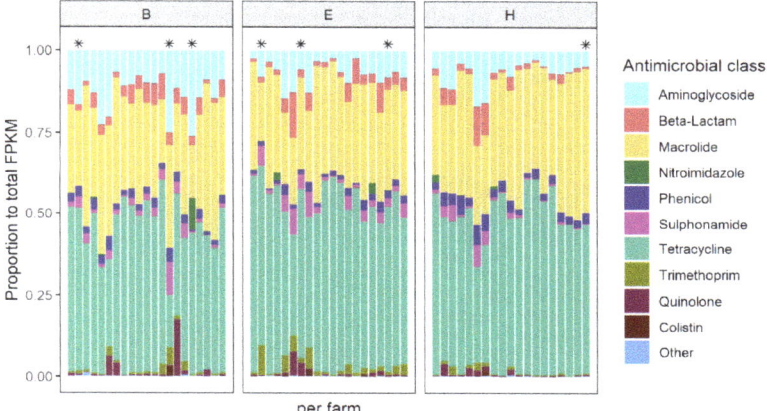

**Figure 2.** Relative abundance of antimicrobial (AMR) genes expressed as a proportion of total fragments per kilobase reference per million bacterial fragments (FPKM). Columns represent 60 samples from 60 farms from three countries (B: $n$ = 21, E: $n$ = 20, and H: $n$ = 19). One additional farm was visited in country B due to incomplete questionnaire data in one of the farms, resulting in 21 samples in total. One sample in country H was removed due to errors during processing. The AMR genes were aggregated to antimicrobial classes. Seven farms where no antimicrobial use was reported in the sampled flock are indicated with an asterisk above the columns.

The total abundance of AMR genes, expressed as the summed FPKM values differed between the three countries. The mean total abundance on the farms in country E was significantly lower than that of country H (One-way ANOVA, Tukey HSD, $p < 0.01$) (Figure S4).

2.3.2. Factors Associated with the Abundance of AMR Gene Clusters

Factors associated with the abundance of AMR gene clusters of eight antimicrobial classes were investigated for 57 farms with complete data (country B: $n$ = 18, E: $n$ = 20, and H: $n$ = 19). Using a random-effects meta-analysis by country, Table 2 presents the associations between AMU and the abundance of AMR gene cluster of the corresponding antimicrobial class. Three significant associations between AMU and the corresponding AMR gene cluster were detected: Beta-lactam use (penicillin and aminopenicillins) and beta-lactam resistance, polymyxin use, and colistin resistance, and aminoglycosides or spectinomycin use (binary variable), and aminoglycoside resistance ($p$ value < 0.1 adjusted for multiple testing). At farms that reported a higher TI of beta-lactam and polymyxins, a higher faecal abundance of the corresponding AMR gene clusters was observed. Farms with reported aminoglycosides or spectinomycin use had a higher faecal abundance of aminoglycoside resistance genes compared to the farms that did not use these antimicrobial classes. However, only one and five farms reported usage of aminoglycoside and lincomycin-spectinomycin, respectively.

Table 2. Associations between antimicrobial usage (AMU) and relative abundance of the corresponding antimicrobial resistance (AMR) genes detected by metagenomics, obtained from a random-effects meta-analysis by country.

| AMU | AMR Gene Cluster [a] | Estimate | Adjusted $p$ Value [b] | 95% CI | Country and Number of Farms with Reported AMU |
|---|---|---|---|---|---|
| $Log_{10}$ TI beta-lactam | Beta-lactam | **1.06** | **0.033** | **[0.29–1.84]** | B-15, E-14, H-18 |
| $Log_{10}$ TI polymixin | Colistin | **0.99** | **0.033** | **[0.29–1.69]** | B-4, E-11, H-5 |
| Aminoglycosides or spectinomycin used (ref:no) | Aminoglycoside | 0.92 | 0.097 | [0.08–1.76] | B-3, H-3 |
| Trimethoprim-sulphonamides used (ref:no) | Trimethoprim | 0.78 | 0.221 | [−0.15–1.71] | B-2, E-3 |
| Trimethoprim-sulphonamides used (ref:no) | Sulphonamide | 0.68 | 0.282 | [−0.26–1.61] | B-2, E-3 |
| $Log_{10}$ TI quinolone | Quinolone | 0.69 | 0.338 | [−0.43–1.81] | B-5, E-4, H-12 |
| $Log_{10}$ TI tetracyclines | Tetracycline | 0.09 | 0.948 | [−0.82–1.00] | B-6, E-6, H-9 |
| $Log_{10}$ TI macrolides + lincomycin | Macrolide | −0.17 | 0.948 | [−1.35–1.01] | B-6, E-12, H-7 |
| $Log_{10}$ TI total AMU | Total FPKM | −0.02 | 0.948 | [−0.62–0.58] | B-15, E-17, H-18 |

Associations in bold have an adjusted $p$ value < 0.1. In the models, 57 farms with complete data were included (country B: $n = 18$, E: $n = 20$, and H: $n = 19$). AMU = Antimicrobial usage; AMR = Antimicrobial resistance; 95% CI = 95% Confidence interval; TI = Treatment incidence. [a]: Relative abundance of AMR genes were clustered per antimicrobial class and calculated as a sum of fragments per kilobase reference per million bacterial fragments. [b]: $p$ values were adjusted with Benjamini–Hochberg correction with a false discovery rate set to 10%.

None of the other farm characteristics than AMU were significantly associated with the abundance of AMR gene clusters after Benjamini–Hochberg multiple testing correction (adjusted $p$ value $\geq 0.1$).

### 2.4. ermB, tetW, sul2, and aph3′-III Identified by qPCR

#### 2.4.1. Abundance of ermB, tetW, sul2, and aph3′-III

In total, 304 samples were analyzed by qPCR. Across all samples, the number of 16S rRNA gene copies varied ($log_{10}$ copies median = 10.8, min = 7.73, and max = 12.8). The number of 16S rRNA copies were used subsequently to calculate relative concentrations of the AMR gene copies. After the qPCR quality check, in order to include samples with a low concentration of *sul2* (11 samples) and *aph3′-III* (20 samples) that were below the limit of detection or limit of quantification, the following values were assigned: *sul2*: 5.10; *aph3′-III*: 3.62. The unit was the number of gene copies ($log_{10}$ copies) before normalization with 16S rRNA. Of those, two *aph3′-III* samples were removed due to a low abundance of 16S rRNA ($log_{10}$ 16S rRNA copies < 8.51). As a result, 283 (93.1%), 287 (94.4%), 262 (86.1%), and 269 (88.5%) samples for *ermB*, *tetW*, *sul2*, and *aph3′-III*, respectively, were available for analysis. The abundance of the four genes relative to bacterial DNA (16S rRNA), stratified per country and gene is shown in Figure 3.

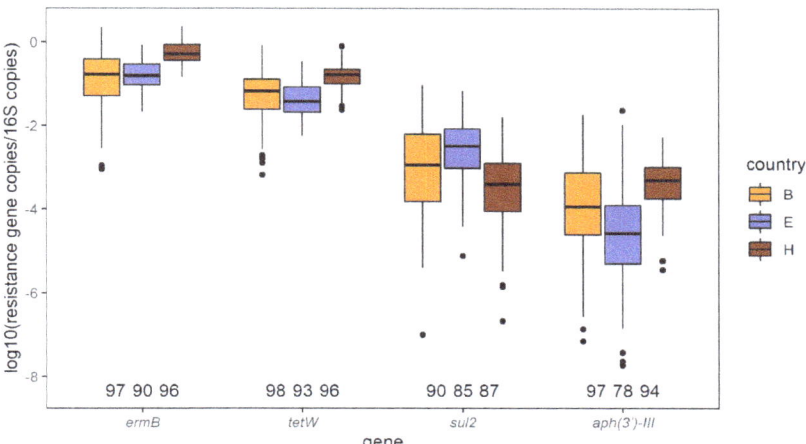

**Figure 3.** Relative abundance of *ermB*, *tetW*, *sul2*, *and aph3′-III* in turkey faeces sampled in three countries, detected by qPCR. Resistance gene $\log_{10}$ copies were normalized using 16S rRNA abundances. The numbers displayed above the horizontal axis are the number of the samples eligible for analysis.

2.4.2. Factors Associated with the Abundance of *ermB*, *tetW*, *sul2*, and *aph3′-III*

In the univariate analysis, total AMU (summed TI of all the antimicrobial classes at farm level) was positively associated with the abundance of *ermB* (Geometric Mean Ratio, GMR = 1.86) and *tetW* (GMR = 1.81). No significant association between AMU and the corresponding resistance gene abundances were detected (Table S1).

Table 3 presents GMR estimates and 95% confidence intervals of the final multivariable models mutually adjusted for technical farm characteristics and biosecurity. None of the biosecurity variables were associated with the abundance of *sul2*. Linear mixed models with random effect for country were fitted for all the genes, however, there was no variance between countries in the final *sul2* model.

Trimethoprim-sulphonamide treatment in flocks was positively associated with the abundance of *sul2* in turkey faeces, when adjusted for sampling season and the presence of other livestock at the farm (GMR = 7.38). No association was detected between the abundance of *ermB*, *tetW*, and *aph3′-III* and the use of corresponding AMU in multivariable models. Three biosecurity variables remained in the final *ermB* model, and two in the final *tetW* and *aph3′-III* models. The abundance of *ermB* and *tetW* in faeces was significantly lower at farms where visitor access was granted more than once a month, and at farms where turkeys had outdoor access. The concentration of *ermB* in faeces was lower if there were different age categories of turkeys present on the farm. For the abundance of *aph3′-III*, having wild bird- and vermin-proof grids placed on the air inlets was positively associated while having a permanent staff that keeps turkeys or birds at home was negatively associated.

*2.5. Phenotypic Resistance Identified by Minimum Inhibitory Concentrations*
2.5.1. *E. coli* Resistance to Antimicrobials

Ceccarelli et al., previously described the MIC values derived from the turkey faeces collected in this study [21]. *E. coli* was successfully isolated from 596 out of 600 samples, and MIC values were determined by broth microdilution for a fixed panel of 14 antimicrobials for those isolates. Epidemiological cut-off values were used to determine non-wild type susceptible (i.e.microbiological resistant) isolates. However, misinterpretation of sulphamethoxazole MIC-endpoints (overestimation of resistance) for country B led to the exclusion of these data from the analysis.

Table 3. Multivariable model associations between antimicrobial usage (AMU), characteristics, biosecurity measures of the turkey farms, and the median relative faecal abundance of *ermB*, *tetW*, *sul2*, and *aph3'-III* per farm.

| Model Variables | ermB GMR | [95% CI] | tetW GMR | [95% CI] | sul2 GMR | [95% CI] | aph3'-III GMR | [95% CI] |
|---|---|---|---|---|---|---|---|---|
| **AMU** | | | | | | | | |
| $Log_{10}$ TI macrolides + lincomycin | 1.57 | [0.77, 3.23] | | | | | | |
| $Log_{10}$ TI tetracyclines | | | 1.54 | [0.80, 2.97] | | | | |
| Trimethoprim-sulphonamides used (ref:no) | | | | | **7.38** | **[1.61, 33.8]** | | |
| Aminoglycosides or spectinomycin used (ref:no) | | | | | | | 1.47 | [0.42, 5.14] |
| **Technical farm characteristics** | | | | | | | | |
| Age of turkeys at sampling (standardized) | **0.73** | **[0.54, 0.98]** | | | | | | |
| Other livestock present (ref:no) | | | | | **2.89** | **[1.17, 7.14]** | **0.38** | **[0.15, 0.95]** |
| Sampling season (ref: autumn, winter) | | | | | **0.21** | **[0.09, 0.48]** | | |
| **Biosecurity** | | | | | | | | |
| Visitor access more than once a month (ref:no) | **0.41** | **[0.22, 0.75]** | **0.36** | **[0.21, 0.60]** | | | | |
| Outdoor access possible for turkeys (ref:no) | **0.35** | **[0.17, 0.75]** | **0.37** | **[0.19, 0.74]** | | | | |
| Different age categories of turkeys present (ref:no) | **0.45** | **[0.25, 0.83]** | | | | | | |
| Bird- and vermin-proof grids placed on the air inlets (ref:no) | | | | | | | **6.32** | **[1.76, 22.73]** |
| Staff keeps turkeys or birds at home (ref:no) | | | | | | | **0.27** | **[0.09, 0.83]** |

Associations in bold have a *p* value < 0.05. Technical farm characteristics and biosecurity variables displayed in the table are those significantly associated with the abundance of each gene in the final models. AMU = Antimicrobial usage; GMR = Geometric mean ratio; 95% CI = 95% Confidence Interval; TI = Treatment incidence.

The proportions of resistant *E. coli* isolates differed between countries and between antimicrobials [21]. The proportion of isolates resistant to ampicillin and tetracycline was higher than 70% in all three countries. The proportion of isolates resistant to ciprofloxacin, nalidixic acid and chloramphenicol was higher than 55% in country H, whereas those in both country B and E were less than 35%. Less than 10% of all the isolates were resistant to cefotaxime, ceftazidime, meropenem, azithromycin, gentamicin, and tigecycline. All meropenem-resistant isolates were confirmed to be negative for known carbapenemases by PCR.

2.5.2. Factors Associated with *E. coli* Resistance

The univariate association between potential risk factors and the occurrence of *E. coli* resistant to ampicillin, tetracycline, and ciprofloxacin from the mixed effect logistic models are presented in Table S2. These three antimicrobials were selected for this analysis because both (i) the number of farms on which corresponding antimicrobial classes were used and (ii) the prevalence of isolates resistant to the antimicrobials were higher than 10%. Significant positive associations were detected between AMU and the occurrence of *E. coli* resistant to ampicillin, tetracycline, and ciprofloxacin. The total amount of AMU was also positively related to resistance to all three antimicrobials. In addition to these three antimicrobials, a univariate association between polymyxin use and resistance to colistin was detected ($p = 0.001$). However, because of model convergence failure, the multivariable model for colistin resistance could not be investigated. A random intercept for farms was included in all the models and country intercept was also added to the ciprofloxacin model because it significantly improved the model fit.

Table 4 shows that there was a significant positive association between AMU at the farm and resistance of *E. coli* isolates for ampicillin and ciprofloxacin when mutually adjusted for other farm characteristics. The presence of a turkey farm within 500 m was negatively associated with ciprofloxacin resistance of *E. coli* isolates. Other associations between biosecurity and resistance of *E. coli* isolates were not statistically significant after mutual adjustment for potential other determinants identified in the univariate analysis.

**Table 4.** Multivariable associations between antimicrobial usage (AMU) and characteristics and biosecurity measures of the turkey farms and the occurrence of *E. coli* isolates from turkey faeces resistant to ampicillin, tetracycline, and ciprofloxacin.

| Model Variables | AMP | | TET | | CIP | |
|---|---|---|---|---|---|---|
| | OR | [95% CI] | OR | [95% CI] | OR | [95% CI] |
| **AMU** | | | | | | |
| $Log_{10}$ TI aminopenicillins | **4.10** | **[1.37, 12.30]** | | | | |
| $Log_{10}$ TI tetracyclines | | | 3.32 | [0.75, 14.7] | | |
| $Log_{10}$ TI quinolones | | | | | **12.85** | **[4.00, 41.2]** |
| **Technical farm characteristics** | | | | | | |
| Age of turkeys at sampling (standardized) | 0.83 | [0.53, 1.31] | 0.74 | [0.48, 1.13] | | |
| Sampling season (ref: autumn, winter) | | | 2.13 | [0.85, 5.31] | | |
| **Biosecurity** | | | | | | |
| Other livestock farms present within 500 m (ref: no) | 0.48 | [0.19, 1.18] | | | | |
| Wild birds can enter the stables (ref: no) | | | 2.67 | [0.90, 7.87] | | |
| Different age categories of turkeys present (ref: no) | | | 0.48 | [0.19, 1.20] | | |
| The nearest turkey farm within 500 m (ref: no) | | | | | **0.28** | **[0.11, 0.69]** |

Associations in bold have a $p < 0.05$. All OR shown in the table are mutually adjusted for class specific AMU and farm characteristics/biosecurity variables for the specific column. AMU = Antimicrobial usage; OR = Odds ratio; 95% CI = 95% Confidence interval; AMP = Ampicillin; TET = Tetracycline; CIP = ciprofloxacin; TI = Treatment incidence.

*2.6. Correlations between AMR Genes Abundances Detected by Metagenomics and qPCR*

The correlation between an abundance of *ermB*, *tetW*, *sul2*, and *aph3′-III* detected by metagenomics and qPCR is shown in Figure S5. Metagenomics samples were pooled at a farm level and the median of the qPCR samples per farm were used. A significant but modest correlation was observed for all four genes ($p < 0.001$, Spearman rho = 0.47–0.74). The highest correlation was observed for *ermB* (rho = 0.74).

The abundance of metagenomically-derived AMR genes clustered at the 90% identity level and present within the macrolide, tetracycline, sulphonamide, and aminoglycoside class clusters were shown in Table S3. The abundance of *ermB*, *tetW*, *sul2*, and *aph3′-III* accounted for 69.0%, 42.3%, 42.6%, and 25.3% of the macrolide, tetracycline, sulphonamide, and aminoglycoside resistance class clusters, respectively.

## 3. Discussion

In this multi-country risk factor study on 60 turkey farms, we investigated risk factors for the faecal abundance of AMR genes in turkeys detected by both metagenomics and qPCR, as well as the prevalence of resistance in *E. coli* isolates in turkey faeces collected in Germany, France, and Spain. We detected positive associations between AMU and both genotypic and phenotypic AMR, specifically for beta-lactam and colistin resistance (metagenomics) as well as ampicillin and ciprofloxacin resistance (MIC).

Substantial differences in AMU were observed between farms and countries. The most frequently used antimicrobial groups were beta-lactams (aminopenicillins and penicillins), followed by polymyxins, and quinolones (fluoroquinolones and other quinolones). A previous study on Italian turkey farms reported that polymyxins, penicillins (including aminopenicillins), and sulphonamides were widely used [22]. A substantial variation in the use of antimicrobial classes within and between countries is expected since there are many possible explanations such as differences in antimicrobial stewardship of veterinarians, differences in availability of pharmaceutical products, and national legislations [23]. A similar high variation in AMU was observed on broiler farms from nine European countries [24].

The relative AMR gene composition detected by metagenomics was similar across the 60 included farms, including flocks that did not receive any antimicrobial treatment. This was in accordance with European broiler studies, where the faecal AMR genes composition appeared to be roughly similar between farms, despite the absence of AMU in many flocks [18,25]. Genes encoding for resistance to tetracyclines were the most dominant cluster, followed by macrolides and aminoglycosides, when clustered at the antimicrobial class level. This is consistent with previously published gut microbiome data in Polish turkeys [26]. These classes, however, did not correspond with the most frequently used antimicrobials in our study. The presence of these AMR gene classes in the faeces of other animal species is reported in multiple countries, regardless of AMU [25–27]. These AMR genes may be present in various bacterial species in the gut of turkeys. It suggests that there are other factors that affect the composition of AMR genes in the gut environment, in addition to direct AMU. This could include the co-selection of resistance by AMU in the production round or in previous rounds at the farm, through which antimicrobial residues and resistant bacteria remained in the environment. The physical transfer of bacteria via the movement of animals may have contributed as well [28].

Significant positive associations were detected between AMU and the abundance of corresponding AMR genes for some antimicrobial classes. The result of the random effects meta-analyses using metagenomics data showed that flocks that received more beta-lactam and colistin antimicrobials had a higher abundance of the corresponding AMR genes. Horizontal gene transfer plays a role in the acquisition of beta-lactam and colistin resistance in addition to chromosomal mutations [29,30]. Therefore, AMU may select for and thus accelerate such transmission.

Fluoroquinolone use has previously been identified as a risk factor for increased fluoroquinolone resistance in *E. coli* [9,12,13]. These studies also reported an increased prevalence of ampicillin resistant isolates in trials in the absence of ampicillin use [12,13].

In line with these studies, we also observed that increased fluoroquinolone use was related to higher proportions of *E. coli* isolates being resistant to ciprofloxacin. In addition, we observed an AMU-AMR association for ampicillin in *E. coli* isolates. Boulianne et al. reported associations between tetracycline use and the occurrence of tetracycline resistance in *E. coli* isolates in Canadian turkey flocks [11]. We also observed positive phenotypic AMU-AMR associations on tetracycline in our study, which were statistically significant in the univariate analysis, but with a wide confidence interval. To study more phenotypic AMU-AMR associations, susceptibility testing in gram positive bacteria such as *Enterococcus* spp. could be considered [11].

We found no evidence that good biosecurity measures were related to lower faecal AMR abundance in turkeys. Our results differ from earlier findings on the association between biosecurity measures and fluoroquinolone resistance in *E. coli* in turkey faeces in Great Britain [8]. They reported that the on-farm presence of mice was a risk factor, while disinfection of floors and walls at depopulation appeared protective. However, information on the quantity of AMU in the sampled flock was not included in their study, so it may be possible that AMU was correlated with the biosecurity factors. In our study, we could not verify if the presence of mice increases the risk, but we observed that bird- and vermin-proof grids placed on the air inlets were associated with a higher risk for *aph3'-III* detected by qPCR. Additionally, the fact that all the farms provided the same answer for "there is a preventive vermin control program" and "stables are disinfected after every round" in our study may suggest that these measures are not associated with variations of AMR on turkey farms. Chuppava et al. reported that the floor design of the turkey house did not correlate with the development of ampicillin- and enrofloxacin-resistant *E. coli* isolates [12,13]. Furthermore, there was little evidence for associations between farm biosecurity and the abundance of AMR genes in European broilers [18]. Interestingly, poor biosecurity such as staff having contact with other birds among others, were in fact related to a lower faecal abundance of *aph3'-III* detected by qPCR. In addition, the presence of a turkey farm within 500 m was negatively associated with *E. coli* resistance to ciprofloxacin. However, we cannot explain this phenomenon biologically. Therefore, the relationship between biosecurity and AMR on turkey farms remains uncertain.

Three different AMR detection methods were used in this study. We observed modest correlations between the abundance of AMR genes quantified by metagenomics and qPCR. A possible reason may be the difference in sample selection. For metagenomic sequencing, the samples were pooled per farm before DNA extraction to represent the farm, whereas DNA was extracted from five to six samples individually for qPCR analysis to detect variations within farms. Pooled samples provide a composition representative of the common AMR genes at the farm [31], whereas the abundance of particular genes may vary between individual samples. Additionally, a low correlation could be due to the low concentration of the target genes or inhibition of gene expression [32]. We chose multiple genes in metagenomic sequencing based on 90% identity level and summed to compare with qPCR, but we can also speculate that there might have been more genes that qPCR detects. On the other hand, the agreement between the abundance of genotypic resistance and phenotypic resistance was not tested. This is because genotypic resistance in this study represents the abundance in the total faecal bacterial community whereas phenotypic resistance is specific to *E. coli*. To compare and predict phenotypic resistance in specific isolates, whole genome sequencing studies could be performed [33].

Detecting total genotypic resistance in samples, rather than isolating specific bacteria, is a good choice to find risk factors for AMR genes associated with horizontal gene transfer. Genotypic detection methods in our study enabled to confirm that AMR genes were widely present in turkey faeces for some antimicrobial classes such as macrolides and aminoglycosides, despite low phenotypic resistance to specific antimicrobials expressed in *E. coli*. The strength of metagenomic sequencing was that it showed the composition of AMR genes in the resistome (the collection of all resistance genes in a sample). Moreover, AMR genes could be analyzed at several grouping levels, such as at a gene and antimicrobial class level. On the other hand, qPCR may be a better choice for detecting specific genes of interest because of lower costs and simple procedures over metagenomic sequencing. However, the selection of the most appropriate target gene may be difficult. Our qPCR target genes were the most abundant gene clusters within the respective antimicrobial classes. However, such information may not always be available beforehand. Limitations for both metagenomic sequencing and qPCR lie in the difficulty to compare the results with other studies since genotypic AMR data in turkeys is still scarce and methods can vary between studies. In contrast, phenotypic AMR in specific bacteria has been studied in a standardized manner for monitoring purposes, making it easier to compare results between studies or to monitor trends over time. However, using dichotomized outcomes by epidemiological cut-off in our study hampered data analysis for antimicrobial classes in which the resistant proportion of isolates were low. In summary, we showed that these methods are complementary and the choice depends on the research question.

Our study is unique considering that farms were included from three European countries using standardized sampling, which enabled the identification of risk factors that are not country-specific. We also related AMU and multiple farm-level factors to both genotypic and phenotypic AMR. However, information on purchased AMU at a farm level was not available in all countries and could therefore not be studied as an alternative to group treatments. This could explain the on-farm background levels of AMR in the absence of reported usage. Moreover, although we included group treatments data at breeding farms, farm characteristics of those farms were not collected. Both AMU and biosecurity information of the sampled farms were from farmers' reports rather than registered data. Therefore, underreporting of AMU and misclassification or missing biosecurity answers could have led to social desirability bias. We quantified the 16S rRNA gene to normalize AMR gene results detected by qPCR, but many bacterial species have more than one copy of the 16S rRNA gene. There is no suitable approach to correct for copy numbers in microbiome data [34,35]. Although gut bacterial composition between turkeys may differ, we expect that this taxonomic difference will not have a large effect on the between group comparisons. Error in quantification of the 16S rRNA gene that we used to normalize the AMR genes would lead to a less precise estimate of AMR, resulting in the attenuation of risk estimates (e.g., AMU-AMR associations). Despite these limitations, our study shows an association between AMU and AMR on turkey farms, which is a potential exposure route to humans.

## 4. Materials and Methods

### 4.1. Selection of Farms

Between October 2014 and October 2016, 60 conventional fattening turkey farms were visited in 3 countries (Germany, France, and Spain, 20 farms per country). German farms were geographically spread over the country, while all French and Spanish farms were concentrated in Brittany and Andalusia, respectively, both being the major turkey production sites of these countries (Figure S1). The preferable selection of farms was based on the following criteria: Conventional farms with an all-in-all-out system and containing 3000–15,000 birds per farm. However, the size criteria were not always met. Farms included in the study were unrelated. Both farms and countries were anonymized (country B, E, and H) to ensure that the results cannot be traced back, consistent with previous EFFORT publications in which data from 9 countries (A to I) was analyzed. The selected farms cannot be considered representative for the respective countries.

Each farm was visited once to collect faecal samples. On each farm, the unit for sampling was a turkey house with a flock that had not been moved or mixed with other flocks except the removal of individual birds before the sampling time. In the flocks, all animals had received the same group treatments by water, medicated feed, or injection during their lifetime. The sampling was intended at maximally one week before the final slaughter date of the hens, but samples were collected randomly regardless of sex. Farms were visited across all seasons.

## 4.2. Questionnaire Data: Antimicrobial Usage, Farm Characteristics, and Biosecurity

Information on all antimicrobials administered as group treatments to the sampled flock during their whole lifetime were documented by the farmers with the supervision of the researchers or veterinarians. Before introducing the sampled flock, researchers informed the farmers on how to document the antimicrobial treatments. Group treatment data included not only those administered in the sampled farms but also in previous breeding farms if applicable. Technical farm characteristics and biosecurity status were obtained by a questionnaire filled out by the participating farmers. Answers in the questionnaire were entered into EpiData version 3.1 Software (EpiData Association, Odense, Denmark).

## 4.3. Quantification of AMU

To quantify AMU, TI was calculated based on antimicrobials administered to the sampled flock, as previously described [21,24]. Defined Daily Dose for turkeys ($DDD_{turkey}$) were assigned for all the antimicrobials used on the included farms. Therefore, TI is expressed as the number of $DDD_{turkey}$ administered per 100 turkey days at risk or the number of days per 100 turkey days that the flock received a standardized dose of antimicrobials (1). The latter can also be interpreted as the percentage of time that a turkey is treated with antimicrobials in its life:

$$TI = \frac{Total\ amount\ of\ active\ substance\ administered\ (mg)}{DDD\ turkey\ (mg/kg/day) \times number\ of\ days\ at\ risk \times kg\ turkey\ at\ risk} \times 100\ turkeys\ at\ risk \quad (1)$$

For determining "kg turkey at risk", a standard weight of 6 kg was used according to the European Surveillance of Veterinary Antimicrobial Consumption (ESVAC) guidelines [36]. Then, the standard weight was multiplied by the number of turkeys at setup. "Number of days at risk" was equal to the expected age of slaughter at each farm. When there were a few different age groups of slaughter batches within the sampled flock, the average age within the sampled flock was used. From this formula, TI was calculated for each antimicrobial class per farm. Total TI per farm was also calculated.

For the risk factor analyses, the sum of TI at farm level for each antimicrobial class was used. Furthermore, we grouped antimicrobials (TIs) that possessed similar mechanisms of resistance, i.e., macrolides and lincomycin, aminoglycosides and spectinomycin. Since lincomycin and spectinomycin were administered as combination products with a fixed ratio (lincomycin:spectinomycin, 1:2) [37], TI was first calculated using $DDD_{turkey}$ for lincomycin-spectinomycin and subsequently divided for each active substance. Aminopenicillin and penicillin were grouped as beta-lactam, fluoroquinolones, and other quinolones (flumequine) were grouped together as quinolones.

## 4.4. Sampling and Processing of Faecal Samples

Per farm, 25 fresh faecal droppings were collected from the floor of one turkey house. After collection, each sample was refrigerated at 4 °C and transported to the laboratories within 24 h.

On arrival at the laboratory of each sampling country, samples for *E. coli* isolation were processed. Simultaneously, samples for metagenomics and qPCR were prepared and stored at −80 °C until shipment. Frozen samples were shipped on dry ice to the Institute for Risk Assessment Sciences (IRAS, Utrecht, the Netherlands).

## 4.5. Metagenomic Sequencing and Processing Data

Metagenomic sequencing and processing was performed as described previously, with modifications [25,38]. The reads are available in the European Nucleotide Archive, under project accession number PRJEB39685.

At the laboratory, the individual faecal samples were homogenized by stirring thoroughly with a tongue depressor or a spoon for a few minutes. Twenty-five individual samples from the same farm were pooled with 0.5 g of faeces from each sample and stirred for a few minutes. DNA extraction was centrally performed at the Technical University of Denmark (The National Food institute, Kgs. Lyngby, Denmark). From a 0.2-g sample,

DNA was extracted using a modified QIAmp Fast DNA Stool Mini Kit (QIAGEN, Hilden, Germany) [39]. The samples were sequenced on the NovaSeq 6000 platform (Illumina Inc, CA, USA) by Admera Health (South Plainfield, NJ, USA), using a $2 \times 150$-bp paired-end (PE) read approach, aiming for 35 M PE reads per sample.

After removing low-quality nucleotides as well as adaptor sequences, trimmed read pairs corresponding to each farm-level sample were aligned to the ResFinder database and, separately, to a merged database of genomic sequences using the k-mer alignment software KMA (v1.2.8). The ResFinder database repository was accessed on 13 February 2019, and contained 3081 AMR genes. Read was aligned to the ResFinder database using the KMA parameters '-mem_mode -ef -1t1 -cge -nf -nc'. In order to filter out low-coverage alignments, alignments that were lower than a 20% consensus of the corresponding reference were removed. The genomic sequence database was described previously [40]. Reads were assigned to the the genomic database using KMA parameters '-mem_mode -ef -1t1 -apm f -nf -nc'. The sum of sequencing fragments mapped to the bacteria, archaea, plasmid, bacteria_draft, HumanMicrobiome, and MetaHitAssembly sub-databases was used as the sample size factor for the FPKM calculation.

As the unit of outcome, FPKM values were computed as previously described [25]. The values were aggregated at the antimicrobial class cluster level for risk factor analysis. Distribution was checked and a pseudocount of one and $\log_{10}$ transformation was applied to FPKM values. Furthermore, the values were aggregated at the 90% identity clustering [41], to analyze the abundance of the specific AMR genes.

*4.6. qPCR Analysis*

For qPCR analysis, 5 to 6 samples per farm were randomly selected, resulting in 304 samples. Five samples per farm were incldued to depict between-animal variation which is assumed to be small within one turkey house. From each sample, 0.5 g of faeces were transferred to a 2-mL cryotube. From a 0.2-g sample, DNA was extracted using a modified QIAmp Fast DNA Stool Mini Kit (QIAGEN, Hilden, Germany) [39]. For all the samples, DNA extraction was performed centrally at IRAS, in the Netherlands.

Four AMR genes, *ermB*, *tetW*, *sul2*, and *aph3'-III*, were selected as qPCR targets. These genes encode resistance against macrolides, tetracyclines, sulphonamides, and aminoglycosides, respectively. These antibiotic classes of public health relevance were chosen based on their abundance in metagenomic data of pooled pig and broiler faeces samples collected within the EFFORT project [25]. In addition, 16S rRNA was targeted for normalization of the AMR genes to bacterial DNA in each sample. Three gene targets of qPCR assay (16S rRNA, *sul2*, and *aph3'-III*) were performed at the National Veterinary Institute (PIWet, Puławy, Poland), while the other two (*ermB* and *tetW*) were at IRAS. Overall results were centrally analyzed at IRAS.

A qPCR assay was performed as previously described [*ermB*, *tetW*, 16S rRNA [42]; *sul2* and *aph3'-III* [19]]. Briefly, all samples were run in two technical PCR duplicates with a non-competitive internal amplification control (IAC) to control quality. From raw amplification data, Ct values were derived by the R project package "chipPCR" [43]. For each gene, the number of copies derived from the Ct values were normalized to bacterial load ($\log_{10}$ (copies of AMR gene/copies 16S rRNA)).

Among the samples passing the qPCR quality criteria (IAC and replicate consistency), those without a quantifiable 16S rRNA concentration were excluded from further analysis (14 samples). Additionally, *sul2* (11 samples) and *aph3'-III* (20 samples) were below the limit of detection or limit of quantification. Those samples were assigned a value (in $\log_{10}$ copies) corresponding to the 1st percentile of the distribution when considering all values of all samples together per gene (*sul2*: 5.10; *aph3'-III*: 3.62). Of those, the samples with a low abundance of 16S rRNA (lower than the 1st percentile of the copy unit of all 16S rRNA concentrations) were excluded from data analyses because these present very high normalized values.

*4.7. E. coli Isolation and MIC Determination*

Isolation of *E. coli* and MIC determination was performed as previously described [21]. The individual samples were suspended in buffered peptone water 1/10 ($w/v$) with 20% glycerol in a 2-mL cryotube and thoroughly mixed. Ten samples from each farm were selected (no. 2, 4, 6, 8, 10, 12, 14, 16, 18, and 20), resulting in 600 samples for *E. coli* isolation. Briefly, all samples were inoculated on MacConkey agar and after incubating 24 h overnight, suspected colonies were isolated and confirmed as *E. coli*. Isolated samples were stored individually in buffered peptone water with 20% glycerol at −80 °C. Next, MIC values by broth microdilution were determined for a fixed panel of antimicrobials by commercially-available microtitre plates (Sensititre, EUVSEC, Themo Fisher Scientific UK Ltd., Loughborough, UK). The European Committee on Antimicrobial Susceptibility Testing (EUCAST) epidemiological cut-off values were used to differentiate between wild type and non-wild-type susceptibility.

*4.8. Variable Selection and Statistical Analysis*

First, to examine the association between AMR and farm level factors, univariate models with AMR, and the corresponding AMU were applied, as well as with other farm-level variables selected from the questionnaires. Next, according to the association observed in univariate models, multivariable models were built.

All statistical analyses were performed in R version 3.6.1 (https://www.R-project.org, accessed on 28 March 2021).

4.8.1. Explanatory Variables

The distributions of continuous variables (i.e., AMU, "total number of turkeys at the farm", "age of turkeys at sampling") were explored and $\log_{10}$ transformed in case of skewness. Age of turkeys was standardized by subtracting the mean and dividing it by the standard deviation to avoid modeling errors due to scale differences between variables. As only a limited number of farms (<10) used trimethoprim-sulphonamide, aminoglycosides, or spectinomycin, we dichotomized these variables. From the questionnaires, the most important farm characteristics variables were selected based on expert knowledge and prior studies [8,17,19,44,45].

In the case of a high correlation between technical farm characteristics and biosecurity variables (Spearman $\rho > 0.7$), technical farm characteristics variables were selected. Variables without contrast and those with missing values were excluded. One missing value of age of turkeys in country B was replaced with the median age of the sampled birds in country B (134 days). All categorical variables were reduced to two levels to avoid convergence errors in modeling.

Four technical farm characteristics variables, namely, "total number of turkeys at the farm", "age of turkeys at sampling", "other livestock is present at the farm", and "season of the sampling", as well as 19 biosecurity variables fulfilling the above criteria were considered in the following models (Supplementary Material Part B).

4.8.2. Factors Associated with AMR Gene Clusters Identified by Metagenomics Sequencing

Three samples from farms for which the metagenomic data could not be matched with the questionnaire data were excluded in the risk factor analysis, resulting in 57 farms to be analyzed (country B: $n = 18$, E: $n = 20$, and H: $n = 19$). The abundance of AMR genes clustered at the antimicrobial class level were used as the outcome variable. Eight clusters with the reported corresponding AMU were chosen for the models. Random effects meta-analyses by country were performed as previously described [17,18]. First, linear regressions were calculated per country, after which the overall associations were calculated using a random effect for country to take the between country variance into account. To prevent certain countries from largely influencing the estimates, the outcome variable were standardized (mean 0, SD 1) by country. R package Metafor was used [46].

Briefly, univariate associations between AMR gene clusters and corresponding AMU, technical farm characteristics, and biosecurity variables were examined. Additionally, the association between the summed FPKM of all the clusters (total FPKM) and total AMU at the farm was analyzed. $p$-values were adjusted for multiple testing by the Benjamini–Hochberg procedure with the false discovery rate set to 10% [47].

4.8.3. Factors Associated with *ermB*, *tetW*, *sul2*, and *aph3′-III* Identified by qPCR

The abundances of the four genes were averaged at the farm level using the median value of the five to six samples within each farm to remove correlation in the farms (i.e., 60 samples in total), instead of adding a random effect for the farms. Random effect for both the farm and country resulted in convergence errors when modeling. Linear mixed models with random intercept for each country were applied for both univariate and multivariable analyses.

First, univariate models were built for each gene to look for factors significantly influencing the AMR gene concentrations. Subsequently, we applied the step function of the R lmerTest package, which performs a backward elimination of non-significant effects in multivariable models [48]. We applied this to the fixed effects while keeping the random effect for country. The variables included in the full models were: (i) The corresponding AMU variable, (ii) the variables significantly related with AMR in the univariate analysis (Satterthwaite's degrees of freedom method, $p$ value < 0.05), and (iii) four technical farm characteristics variables because these may be related with AMU and biosecurity variables. Fixed effect variables were eliminated backward from the full models according to the $p$ value (alpha = 0.05), while keeping the corresponding AMU variable. To make the model coefficients more interpretable, all estimates and their 95% CIs were expressed as GMR values by exponentiating with base 10 coefficients (Table 3, Table S1).

4.8.4. Factors Associated with *E. coli* Resistance

The occurrence of *E. coli* isolates resistant to ampicillin, tetracycline, and ciprofloxacin were used as the outcome variables. These three antimicrobials were selected because there were more than six farms (i.e., 10% of all the farms) with the reported corresponding AMU and there were more than 60 resistant isolates (i.e., 10% of all the isolates). Nalidixic acid was not selected but ciprofloxacin was selected for quinolone resistance. This is because when using the epidemiological cut-off to define non-wild type susceptible isolates, nalidixic acid and the fluoroquinolone ciprofloxacin show the same results in proportions of non-wild type strains. Corresponding AMU variables were aminopenicillin, tetracycline, and quinolone use (fluoroquinolone and other quinolones). Penicillins were not included since *E. coli* is intrinsically resistant to penicillin. At first, it was intended to investigate the association between polymyxin use and colistin-resistant *E. coli*, but many models failed to converge in univariate analysis, which made it impossible to further investigate risk factors. Mixed effects logistic models with random intercept for farm were applied. A country random intercept was added when it improved the fit in null models.

Following univariate analysis, the variables significantly related in univariate analysis ($p$ value < 0.05) were added in the multivariable models. All ORs and their 95% CIs are shown in the results (Table 4, Table S2).

4.8.5. Comparisons between Metagenomics and qPCR

First, two genotypic resistance methods, namely metagenomics and qPCR samples were compared. Metagenomics samples were pooled at the farm level while for qPCR samples, the median value of the five to six samples within each farm were used. Associations between the abundance of *ermB*, *tetW*, *sul2*, and *aph3′-III* clusters as identified by metagenomics and the abundance of these genes by qPCR were examined by calculating the Spearman correlation coefficient (Figure S5). In addition, total abundance (i.e., summed FPKM of all the farms) per gene level cluster was calculated and the proportion of the respective gene within the according macrolide, tetracycline, sulphonamide, and aminoglycoside class level cluster was calculated (Table S3).

## 5. Conclusions

We investigated risk factors for AMR in European turkey farms using three different AMR detection methods. Positive AMU-AMR associations were detected for both genotypic and phenotypic AMR: Beta-lactam and colistin (metagenomic sequencing) and aminopenicillin and fluoroquinolone (MIC). No robust AMU-AMR association was detected by analyzing qPCR targets. No evidence was found that lower biosecurity increases AMR abundance. We showed AMR genes encoding for some antimicrobial classes were abundant in faeces despite the low prevalence of phenotypic resistance in *E. coli* isolates. Since different AMR detection methods provide information on different aspects of AMR, the choice depends on the availability of resources and research questions. We have shown that using multiple complementary AMR detection methods adds insights into AMU-AMR associations in turkey farms.

**Supplementary Materials:** The following are available online at https://www.mdpi.com/article/10.3390/antibiotics10070820/s1, Part A: Figure S1: Distribution of the 60 turkey farms across three countries; Figure S2: Antimicrobial usage in 60 farms in three countries, expressed as the sum of treatment incidence (TI); Figure S3: Abundance of antimicrobial resistance (AMR) genes detected by metagenomics per farm, expressed as fragments per kilobase reference per million bacterial fragments (FPKM); Figure S4: Total abundance of antimicrobial resistance (AMR) genes detected by metagenomics per country, expressed as the sum of fragments per kilobase reference per million bacterial fragments (FPKM); Figure S5: Correlations between the abundance of *ermB*, *tetW*, *sul2*, and *aph3'-III* genes detected by metagenomics and those genes detected by qPCR; Table S1: Univariate associations between antimicrobial usage (AMU), technical farm characteristics, biosecurity measures of turkey farms, and the median relative faecal abundance of *ermB*, *tetW*, *sul2*, and *aph3'-III* per farm; Table S2. Univariate associations between antimicrobial usage (AMU), characteristics, biosecurity measures of the turkey farms, and the occurrence of *E. coli* isolates from turkey faeces resistant to ampicillin, tetracycline, and ciprofloxacin; Table S3: Ten most abundant antimicrobial resistance (AMR) genes in turkey faeces quantified by metagenomics and their proportion within the macrolide, tetracycline, sulphonamide, and aminoglycoside class clusters; Part B: Selected biosecurity check questions from the questionnaire used in risk factor analyses.

**Author Contributions:** All authors have read and agreed to the published version of the manuscript. Conceptualization, J.A.W., D.H., D.M., H.S., L.A.M.S. and L.V.G.; methodology, P.J., P.M., D.M., H.S., L.A.M.S. and L.V.G.; software, D.Y., L.V.G.; formal analysis, M.H., D.Y.; investigation, P.M., K.W., C.C., G.M. and M.S.; resources, P.M., K.W., C.C. and G.M.; data curation, D.Y., P.J., P.M. and H.S.; writing—original draft preparation, M.H.; writing—review and editing, all authors; visualization, M.H.; supervision, D.M., L.A.M.S. and L.V.G.; project administration, J.A.W.; funding acquisition, J.D., F.M.A., T.B., P.S., B.G.-Z., D.W., J.A.W, D.H. and D.M.

**Funding:** This work was part of the Ecology from Farm to Fork of Microbial drug Resistance and Transmission (EFFORT) project (http://www.effort-against-amr.eu, accessed on 28 March 2021), co-funded by the European Commission, 7th Framework Programme for Research and Innovation (FP7-KBBE-2013–7, grant agreement: 613754). Research at the National Veterinary Research Institute (PIWet), Poland, was also supported by the donation of the Polish Ministry of Science, no. 3173/7PR/2014/2.

**Institutional Review Board Statement:** No ethical approval was obtained because this study did not involve invasive animal sampling.

**Informed Consent Statement:** The participation of this study was voluntary and consent was obtained from all farmers involved in the study.

**Data Availability Statement:** The data presented in this study are available upon request from the corresponding author.

**Acknowledgments:** The authors would like to thank all participating farmers. We would also like to thank all researchers of the EFFORT consortium, especially those involved in sampling: Rodolphe

Thomas (ANSES), Jenna Coton (ANSES), Denis Leon (ANSES), and Julie David (ANSES); laboratory analysis and data analysis: Roosmarijn E.C. Luiken (IRAS), Eri van Heijnsbergen (IRAS), Inge M. Wouters (IRAS), Peter Scherpenisse (IRAS), Gerdit D Greve (IRAS), Monique HG Tersteeg-Zijderveld (IRAS), Katharina Juraschek (BfR), and Jennie Fisher (BfR).

**EFFORT-Group:** Haitske Graveland (UUVM), Steven Sarrazin (UGENT), Alieda van Essen (WBVR), Julie David (ANSES), Antonio Battisti (IZSLT), Andrea Caprioli (IZSLT), Maximiliane Brandt (TIHO), Tine Hald (DTU), Ana Sofia Ribeiro Duarte (DTU), Magdalena Zając (PIWet), Andrzej Hoszowski (deceased) (PIWet), Hristo Daskalov (NDRVI), Helmut W. Saatkamp (BEC), and Katharina D.C. Stärk (SAFOSO).

**Conflicts of Interest:** The authors declare no conflict of interest. Author M.H. was also employed by the Ministry of Health, Labour, and Welfare, Japan during the time of the analyses and has no conflicts of interest to declare.

## References

1. O'Neill, J. Antimicrobial Resistance: Tackling a Crisis for the Health and Wealth of Nations the Review on Antimicrobial Resistance Chaired. Available online: http://www.jpiamr.eu/wp-content/uploads/2014/12/AMR-Review-Paper-Tackling-a-crisis-for-the-health-and-wealth-of-nations_1-2.pdf (accessed on 1 May 2021).
2. World Health Organization. Critically Important Antimicrobials for Human Medicine. Available online: https://apps.who.int/iris/bitstream/handle/10665/312266/9789241515528-eng.pdf (accessed on 1 May 2021).
3. World Health Organization. Global Action Plan on Antimicrobial Resistance. Available online: https://apps.who.int/iris/bitstream/handle/10665/193736/9789241509763_eng.pdf?sequence=1 (accessed on 30 January 2021).
4. European Comission. A European One Health Action Plan against Antimicrobial Resistance (AMR). Available online: https://ec.europa.eu/health/sites/health/files/antimicrobial_resistance/docs/amr_2017_action-plan.pdf (accessed on 30 March 2021).
5. Mughini-Gras, L.; Dorado-García, A.; van Duijkeren, E.; van den Bunt, G.; Dierikx, C.M.; Bonten, M.J.M.; Bootsma, M.C.J.; Schmitt, H.; Hald, T.; Evers, E.G.; et al. Articles Attributable Sources of Community-Acquired Carriage of *Echerichia coli* Containing β-Lactam Antibiotic Resistance Genes: A Population-Based Modelling Study. *Lancet* **2019**, *8*, 357–369. [CrossRef]
6. DG AGRI DASHBOARD: POULTRY MEAT. Available online: https://ec.europa.eu/info/sites/info/files/food-farming-fisheries/farming/documents/poultry-meat-dashboard_en.pdf (accessed on 29 March 2021).
7. European Food Safety Authority and European Centre for Disease Prevention and Control. The European Union Summary Report on Antimicrobial Resistance in Zoonotic and Indicator Bacteria from Humans, Animals and Food in 2018/2019. *EFSA J.* **2021**, *19*, e06007. [CrossRef]
8. Jones, E.M.; Snow, L.C.; Carrique-Mas, J.J.; Gosling, R.J.; Clouting, C.; Davies, R.H. Risk Factors for Antimicrobial Resistance in *Escherichia coli* Found in GB Turkey Flocks. *Vet. Rec.* **2013**, *173*, 422. [CrossRef] [PubMed]
9. Taylor, N.M.; Wales, A.D.; Ridley, A.M.; Davies, R.H. Farm Level Risk Factors for Fluoroquinolone Resistance in *E. coli* and Thermophilic *Campylobacter* spp. on Poultry Farms. *Avian Pathol.* **2016**, *45*, 559–568. [CrossRef]
10. Agunos, A.; Gow, S.P.; Leger, D.F.; Carson, C.A.; Deckert, A.E.; Bosman, A.L.; Loest, D.; Irwin, R.J.; Reid-Smith, R.J. Antimicrobial Use and Antimicrobial Resistance Indicators—Integration of Farm-Level Surveillance Data from Broiler Chickens and Turkeys in British Columbia, Canada. *Front. Vet. Sci.* **2019**, *6*, 131. [CrossRef] [PubMed]
11. Boulianne, M.; Arsenault, J.; Daignault, D.; Archambault, M.; Letellier, A.; Dutil, L. Drug Use and Antimicrobial Resistance among *Escherichia coli* and *Enterococcus* spp. Isolates from Chicken and Turkey Flocks Slaughtered in Quebec, Canada. *Can. J. Vet. Res.* **2016**, *80*, 49–59. [PubMed]
12. Chuppava, B.; Keller, B.; Meißner, J.; Kietzmann, M.; Visscher, C. Effects of Different Types of Flooring Design on the Development of Antimicrobial Resistance in Commensal *Escherichia coli* in Fattening Turkeys. *Vet. Microbiol.* **2018**, *217*, 18–24. [CrossRef]
13. Chuppava, B.; Keller, B.; El-Wahab, A.; Meißner, J.; Kietzmann, M.; Visscher, C. Resistance of *Escherichia coli* in Turkeys after Therapeutic or Environmental Exposition with Enrofloxacin Depending on Flooring. *Int. J. Environ. Res. Public Health* **2018**, *15*, 1993. [CrossRef] [PubMed]
14. European Centre for Disease Prevention and Control, European Food Safety Authority and European Medicines Agency. ECDC/EFSA/EMA Second Joint Report on the Integrated Analysis of the Consumption of Antimicrobial Agents and Occurrence of Antimicrobial Resistance in Bacteria from Humans and Food-Producing Animals: Joint Interagency Antimicrobial Consumption and Resistan. *EFSA J.* **2017**, *15*, e05017. [CrossRef]
15. European Food Safety Authority and European Centre for Disease Prevention and Control. The European Union Summary Report on Antimicrobial Resistance in Zoonotic and Indicator Bacteria from Humans, Animals and Food in 2017/2018. *EFSA J.* **2020**, *18*, e06007. [CrossRef]
16. Dierikx, C.M.; van der Goot, J.A.; Smith, H.E.; Kant, A.; Mevius, D.J. Presence of ESBL/AmpC -Producing *Escherichia coli* in the Broiler Production Pyramid: A Descriptive Study. *PLoS ONE* **2013**, *8*, e79005. [CrossRef]

17. Van Gompel, L.; Luiken, R.E.C.; Sarrazin, S.; Munk, P.; Knudsen, B.E.; Hansen, R.B.; Bossers, A.; Aarestrup, F.M.; Dewulf, J.; Wagenaar, J.A.; et al. The Antimicrobial Resistome in Relation to Antimicrobial Use and Biosecurity in Pig Farming, a Metagenome-Wide Association Study in Nine European Countries. *J. Antimicrob. Chemother.* **2019**, *74*, 865–876. [CrossRef] [PubMed]
18. Luiken, R.E.C.; Van Gompel, L.; Munk, P.; Sarrazin, S.; Joosten, P.; Dorado-García, A.; Borup Hansen, R.; Knudsen, B.E.; Bossers, A.; Wagenaar, J.A.; et al. Associations between Antimicrobial Use and the Faecal Resistome on Broiler Farms from Nine European Countries. *J. Antimicrob. Chemother.* **2019**, *74*, 2596–2604. [CrossRef]
19. Yang, D.; Van Gompel, L.; Luiken, R.E.C.; Sanders, P.; Joosten, P.; van Heijnsbergen, E.; Wouters, I.M.; Scherpenisse, P.; Chauvin, C.; Wadepohl, K.; et al. Association of Antimicrobial Usage with Faecal Abundance of *aph(3')-III*, *ermB*, *sul2* and *tetW* Resistance Genes in Veal Calves in Three European Countries. *Int. J. Antimicrob. Agents* **2020**, *56*, 106131. [CrossRef] [PubMed]
20. Zankari, E.; Hasman, H.; Cosentino, S.; Vestergaard, M.; Rasmussen, S.; Lund, O.; Aarestrup, F.M.; Larsen, M.V. Identification of Acquired Antimicrobial Resistance Genes. *J. Antimicrob. Chemother.* **2012**, *67*, 2640–2644. [CrossRef] [PubMed]
21. Ceccarelli, D.; Hesp, A.; van der Goot, J.; Joosten, P.; Sarrazin, S.; Wagenaar, J.A.; Dewulf, J.; Mevius, D.J. Antimicrobial Resistance Prevalence in Commensal *Escherichia coli* from Broilers, Fattening Turkeys, Fattening Pigs and Veal Calves in European Countries and Association with Antimicrobial Usage at Country Level. *J. Med. Microbiol.* **2020**, *69*, 537–547. [CrossRef] [PubMed]
22. Caucci, C.; Di Martino, G.; Dalla Costa, A.; Santagiuliana, M.; Lorenzetto, M.; Capello, K.; Mughini-Gras, L.; Gavazzi, L.; Bonfanti, L. Trends and Correlates of Antimicrobial Use in Broiler and Turkey Farms: A Poultry Company Registry-Based Study in Italy. *J. Antimicrob. Chemother.* **2019**, *74*, 2784–2787. [CrossRef] [PubMed]
23. Sanders, P.; Vanderhaeghen, W.; Fertner, M.; Fuchs, K.; Obritzhauser, W.; Agunos, A.; Carson, C.; Borck Høg, B.; Dalhoff Andersen, V.; Chauvin, C.; et al. Monitoring of Farm-Level Antimicrobial Use to Guide Stewardship: Overview of Existing Systems and Analysis of Key Components and Processes. *Front. Vet. Sci.* **2020**, *7*, 540. [CrossRef]
24. Joosten, P.; Sarrazin, S.; Van Gompel, L.; Luiken, R.E.C.; Mevius, D.J.; Wagenaar, J.A.; Heederik, D.J.J.; Dewulf, J.; Graveland, H.; Schmitt, H.; et al. Quantitative and Qualitative Analysis of Antimicrobial Usage at Farm and Flock Level on 181 Broiler Farms in Nine European Countries. *J. Antimicrob. Chemother.* **2019**, *74*, 798–806. [CrossRef]
25. Munk, P.; Knudsen, B.E.; Lukjacenko, O.; Duarte, A.S.R.; Van Gompel, L.; Luiken, R.E.C.; Smit, L.A.M.; Schmitt, H.; Garcia, A.D.; Hansen, R.B.; et al. Abundance and Diversity of the Faecal Resistome in Slaughter Pigs and Broilers in Nine European Countries. *Nat. Microbiol.* **2018**, *3*, 898–908. [CrossRef]
26. Skarżyńska, M.; Leekitcharoenphon, P.; Hendriksen, R.S.; Aarestrup, F.M.; Wasyl, D. A Metagenomic Glimpse into the Gut of Wild and Domestic Animals: Quantification of Antimicrobial Resistance and More. *PLoS ONE* **2020**, *15*, e0242987. [CrossRef] [PubMed]
27. Joyce, A.; McCarthy, C.G.P.; Murphy, S.; Walsh, F. Antibiotic Resistomes of Healthy Pig Faecal Metagenomes. *Microb. Genom.* **2019**, *5*, e000272. [CrossRef]
28. Davies, R.; Wales, A. Antimicrobial Resistance on Farms: A Review Including Biosecurity and the Potential Role of Disinfectants in Resistance Selection. *Compr. Rev. Food Sci. Food Saf.* **2019**, *18*, 753–774. [CrossRef] [PubMed]
29. Alba, P.; Leekitcharoenphon, P.; Franco, A.; Feltrin, F.; Ianzano, A.; Caprioli, A.; Stravino, F.; Hendriksen, R.S.; Bortolaia, V.; Battisti, A. Molecular Epidemiology of *mcr*-Encoded Colistin Resistance in *Enterobacteriaceae* from Food-Producing Animals in Italy Revealed through the EU Harmonized Antimicrobial Resistance Monitoring. *Front. Microbiol.* **2018**, *9*, 1217. [CrossRef] [PubMed]
30. Saliu, E.M.; Vahjen, W.; Zentek, J. Types and Prevalence of Extended-Spectrum Beta-Lactamase Producing *Enterobacteriaceae* in Poultry. *Anim. Health Res. Rev.* **2017**, *18*, 46–57. [CrossRef] [PubMed]
31. Andersen, V.D.; Jensen, M.S.; Munk, P.; Vigre, H. Robustness in Quantifying the Abundance of Antimicrobial Resistance Genes in Pooled Faeces Samples from Batches of Slaughter Pigs Using Metagenomics Analysis. *J. Glob. Antimicrob. Resist.* **2021**, *24*, 398–402. [CrossRef] [PubMed]
32. Andersen, S.C.; Fachmann, M.S.R.; Kiil, K.; Nielsen, E.M.; Hoorfar, J. Gene-Based Pathogen Detection: Can We Use qPCR to Predict the Outcome of Diagnostic Metagenomics? *Genes* **2017**, *8*, 332. [CrossRef] [PubMed]
33. Bortolaia, V.; Kaas, R.S.; Ruppe, E.; Roberts, M.C.; Schwarz, S.; Cattoir, V.; Philippon, A.; Allesoe, R.L.; Rebelo, A.R.; Florensa, A.F.; et al. ResFinder 4.0 for Predictions of Phenotypes from Genotypes. *J. Antimicrob. Chemother.* **2020**, *75*, 3491–3500. [CrossRef] [PubMed]
34. Starke, R.; Pylro, V.S.; Morais, D.K. 16S rRNA Gene Copy Number Normalization Does Not Provide More Reliable Conclusions in Metataxonomic Surveys. *Microb. Ecol.* **2021**, *81*, 535–539. [CrossRef] [PubMed]
35. Louca, S.; Doebeli, M.; Parfrey, L.W. Correcting for 16S rRNA Gene Copy Numbers in Microbiome Surveys Remains an Unsolved Problem. *Microbiome* **2018**, *6*, 41. [CrossRef]
36. European Medicines Agency. Revised ESVAC Reflection Paper on Collecting Data on Consumption of Antimicrobial Agents per Animal Species, on Technical Units of Measurement and Indicators for Reporting Consumption of Antimicrobial Agents in Animals. Available online: https://www.ema.europa.eu/en/documents/scientific-guideline/revised-european-surveillance-veterinary-antimicrobial-consumption-esvac-reflection-paper-collecting_en.pdf (accessed on 30 March 2021).
37. European Medicines Agency. Questions and Answers on Veterinary Medicinal Products Containing a Combination of Lincomycin and Spectinomycin to Be Administered Orally to Pigs and/or Poultry. Lincomycin and Spectinomycin Article 35 Referral—Annex

I, II, III. Available online: https://www.ema.europa.eu/en/documents/referral/lincomycin-spectinomycin-article-35-referral-annex-i-ii-iii_en.pdf (accessed on 15 June 2021).
38. Duarte, A.S.R.; Röder, T.; Van Gompel, L.; Petersen, T.N.; Hansen, R.B.; Hansen, I.M.; Bossers, A.; Aarestrup, F.M.; Wagenaar, J.A.; Hald, T. Metagenomics-Based Approach to Source-Attribution of Antimicrobial Resistance Determinants—Identification of Reservoir Resistome Signatures. *Front. Microbiol.* **2021**, *11*, 601407. [CrossRef] [PubMed]
39. Knudsen, B.E.; Bergmark, L.; Munk, P.; Lukjancenko, O.; Priemé, A.; Aarestrup, F.M.; Pamp, S.J. Impact of Sample Type and DNA Isolation Procedure on Genomic Inference of Microbiome Composition. *mSystems* **2016**, *1*, e00095-16. [CrossRef] [PubMed]
40. Osakunor, D.N.M.; Munk, P.; Mduluza, T.; Petersen, T.N.; Brinch, C.; Ivens, A.; Chimponda, T.; Amanfo, S.A.; Murray, J.; Woolhouse, M.E.J.; et al. The Gut Microbiome but Not the Resistome Is Associated with Urogenital Schistosomiasis in Preschool-Aged Children. *Commun. Biol.* **2020**, *3*, 155. [CrossRef]
41. Macedo, G.; van Veelen, H.P.J.; Hernandez-Leal, L.; van der Maas, P.; Heederik, D.; Mevius, D.; Bossers, A.; Schmitt, H. Science of the Total Environment Targeted Metagenomics Reveals Inferior Resilience of Farm Soil Resistome Compared to Soil Microbiome after Manure Application. *Sci. Total Environ.* **2021**, *770*, 145399. [CrossRef]
42. Van Gompel, L.; Dohmen, W.; Luiken, R.E.C.; Bouwknegt, M.; Heres, L.; van Heijnsbergen, E.; Jongerius-Gortemaker, B.G.M.; Scherpenisse, P.; Greve, G.D.; Tersteeg-Zijderveld, M.H.G.; et al. Occupational Exposure and Carriage of Antimicrobial Resistance Genes (*tetW*, *ermB*) in Pig Slaughterhouse Workers. *Ann. Work Expo. Health* **2020**, *64*, 125–137. [CrossRef] [PubMed]
43. Rödiger, S.; Burdukiewicz, M.; Schierack, P. ChipPCR: An R Package to Pre-Process Raw Data of Amplification Curves. *Bioinformatics* **2015**, *31*, 2900–2902. [CrossRef]
44. Hille, K.; Felski, M.; Ruddat, I.; Woydt, J.; Schmid, A.; Friese, A.; Fischer, J.; Sharp, H.; Valentin, L.; Michael, G.B.; et al. Association of Farm-Related Factors with Characteristics Profiles of Extended-Spectrum β-Lactamase- / Plasmid-Mediated AmpC β-Lactamase-Producing *Echerichia coli* Isolates from German Livestock Farms. *Vet. Microbiol.* **2018**, *223*, 93–99. [CrossRef]
45. Birkegård, A.C.; Halasa, T.; Græsbøll, K.; Clasen, J.; Folkesson, A.; Toft, N. Association between Selected Antimicrobial Resistance Genes and Antimicrobial Exposure in Danish Pig Farms. *Sci. Rep.* **2017**, *7*, 9683. [CrossRef]
46. Viechtbauer, W. Conducting Meta-Analyses in {R} with the {metafor} Package. *J. Stat. Softw.* **2010**, *36*, 1–48. [CrossRef]
47. Yoav Benjamini, Y.H. Controlling the False Discovery Rate: A Practical and Powerful Approach to Multiple Testing. *J. R. Stat. Soc. Ser. B* **1995**, *57*, 289–300. [CrossRef]
48. Kuznetsova, A.; Brockhoff, P.B.; Christensen, R.H.B. {lmerTest} Package: Tests in Linear Mixed Effects Models. *J. Stat. Softw.* **2017**, *82*, 1–26. [CrossRef]

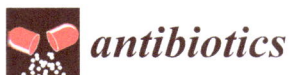 

Article

# Quantitative Risk Assessment for the Introduction of Carbapenem-Resistant Enterobacteriaceae (CPE) into Dutch Livestock Farms

Natcha Dankittipong [1,*], Egil A. J. Fischer [1], Manon Swanenburg [2], Jaap A. Wagenaar [3], Arjan J. Stegeman [1] and Clazien J. de Vos [2]

1. Department Population Health Sciences, Farm Animal Health, Utrecht University, Martinus G. de Bruingebouw, Yalelaan 7, 3584 CL Utrecht, The Netherlands; e.a.j.fischer@uu.nl (E.A.J.F.); j.a.stegeman@uu.nl (A.J.S.)
2. Wageningen Bioveterinary Research, Wageningen University & Research, Houtribweg 39, 8221 RA Lelystad, The Netherlands; manon.swanenburg@wur.nl (M.S.); clazien.devos@wur.nl (C.J.d.V.)
3. Department Biomolecular Health Science, Infectious Diseases & Immunology, Utrecht University, Androclusgebouw, Yalelaan 1, 3584 CL Utrecht, The Netherlands; j.wagenaar@uu.nl
* Correspondence: n.dankittipong@uu.nl

**Abstract:** Early detection of emerging carbapenem-resistant Enterobacteriaceae (CPE) in food-producing animals is essential to control the spread of CPE. We assessed the risk of CPE introduction from imported livestock, livestock feed, companion animals, hospital patients, and returning travelers into livestock farms in The Netherlands, including (1) broiler, (2) broiler breeder, (3) fattening pig, (4) breeding pig, (5) farrow-to-finish pig, and (6) veal calf farms. The expected annual number of introductions was calculated from the number of farms exposed to each CPE source and the probability that at least one animal in an exposed farm is colonized. The total number of farms with CPE colonization was estimated to be the highest for fattening pig farms, whereas the probability of introduction for an individual farm was the highest for broiler farms. Livestock feed and imported livestock are the most likely sources of CPE introduction into Dutch livestock farms. Sensitivity analysis indicated that the number of fattening pig farms determined the number of high introductions in fattening pigs from feed, and that uncertainty on CPE prevalence impacted the absolute risk estimate for all farm types. The results of this study can be used to inform risk-based surveillance for CPE in livestock farms.

**Keywords:** carbapenems; CPE; meat-producing animal; companion animal; travelers; feed; risk assessment; introduction risk; stochastic risk model

Citation: Dankittipong, N.; Fischer, E.A.J.; Swanenburg, M.; Wagenaar, J.A.; Stegeman, A.J.; de Vos, C.J. Quantitative Risk Assessment for the Introduction of Carbapenem-Resistant Enterobacteriaceae (CPE) into Dutch Livestock Farms. *Antibiotics* **2022**, *11*, 281. https://doi.org/10.3390/antibiotics11020281

Academic Editor: Clair L. Firth

Received: 13 January 2022
Accepted: 15 February 2022
Published: 21 February 2022

**Publisher's Note:** MDPI stays neutral with regard to jurisdictional claims in published maps and institutional affiliations.

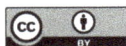

**Copyright:** © 2022 by the authors. Licensee MDPI, Basel, Switzerland. This article is an open access article distributed under the terms and conditions of the Creative Commons Attribution (CC BY) license (https://creativecommons.org/licenses/by/4.0/).

## 1. Introduction

Antimicrobial-resistant (AMR) bacteria have been one of the greatest public health challenges since the 1950s [1]. Increased use of broad-spectrum antibiotics has resulted in a race between resistant bacteria and treatments. The lagging development of new antibiotics and the speed at which resistance emerges are propelling the healthcare sector toward using "drugs of last resort", administered only after other antibiotics have failed. One antimicrobial class of last resort, carbapenems, represents extremely potent, broad-spectrum drugs for treating serious infections, primarily from multidrug-resistant Enterobacteriaceae [2]. Enterobacteriaceae with carbapenem-resistant genes have a 50% mortality rate in humans due to the absence of alternative antibiotic treatments [3]. Carbapenemase-producing Enterobacteriaceae (CPE) have spread globally since early 2010 in hospital facilities and have risen at an alarming rate in the human community [4,5].

CPE quickly disseminate resistant genes between bacteria through horizontal transfer, specifically plasmid-mediated gene transfer [6]. A plasmid is a mobile circular DNA carrying useful genes for adaptation and moving within and between species of bacteria.

Inter-host transmission of resistant genes via plasmids enables the development of CPE cases in humans, not from using antibiotics directly, but from interacting with environments and hosts colonized with CPE [7]. As an illustration, plasmid-mediated, extended-spectrum β-lactamase-producing *Escherichia coli* (ESBL-EC) in the Dutch community is partly attributable to ESBL-EC in food, the environment, and animals [8].

AMR has rapidly disseminated worldwide in the community and hospitals due to excessive antibiotic usage, international travel, and global trade networks. The multiple sources of the AMR pandemic have prompted the European Union (EU), since 2010, to extend its surveillance of AMR to include food-producing animals. Cecal samples from live fattening pigs, veal calves, and broilers are collected at slaughterhouses and tested for resistant genes. Since 2016, this surveillance also includes CPE [9,10]. The current compulsory and harmonized AMR surveillance carried out by all EU member states is adequate to detect widespread AMR but will not quickly detect a newly emerging resistant bacterium due to the limited sample sizes and sampling frequency. In the current EU surveillance protocol, EU member states must annually collect a total of 170–300 samples, depending on the states' production volume, from each species of food-producing animal. This sample size was set to detect CPE with 95% confidence, provided the prevalence is at least 2%. However, because the sampling is conducted only once a year, CPE could be widespread before they are detected. Enhancing EU surveillance to detect emerging CPE is possible through an increased sampling frequency, increased sample sizes, and risk-based surveillance.

This study aimed to inform risk-based surveillance for CPE *E. coli* (referred to as CPE in the remainder of the text of this paper) by ranking the farm types according to the likelihood of CPE introduction using a quantitative risk assessment model. We based our study on The Netherlands, but it is scalable to the European Union. We included six farm types at risk of CPE introduction: broiler farm, broiler breeder farm, fattening pig farm, breeding pig farm, farrow-to-finish pig farm, and veal calf farm. The reason for this selection was that these farm types are the ones most associated with AMR in The Netherlands [11]. Seven potential sources of CPE relevant to the Dutch livestock sector were identified in the literature review [7,12,13] Figure S1. These potential sources are hospital patients, returning travelers from abroad, companion animals, wild animals, wastewater from hospitals, imported livestock, and animal feed (Supplementary File S1). The results from expert elicitation highlight returning travelers, wastewater from hospitals, and imported veal calves as the most important sources of CPE introduction (Supplementary File S2).

## 2. Results

To estimate the risk of introduction, first, the number of farms exposed to CPE sources (Section 2.1) and the probability of colonization after exposure (Section 2.2) were estimated. These were combined into the risk of introduction by calculating the number of expected introductions (Section 2.3). The sensitivity of model output to model input parameters was determined by two methods of sensitivity analysis (Section 2.4). First, Spearman correlation coefficients were used to identify important uncertain parameters. Second, one-at-a-time sensitivity analysis was used to investigate the robustness of the ranking of risks to changes in each of the input parameters. Finally, different scenarios with respect to contamination of feed, restrictions on imports, and biosecurity were studied (Section 2.5).

### 2.1. Number of Farms Exposed to CPE

Based on our model calculations, fattening pig farms have the highest risk of CPE exposure, with over 600 farms in The Netherlands being exposed to at least one CPE source annually (Figure 1). The results indicate that 22% of the 2652 fattening pig farms and 12% of the 4513 pig farms (all farm types) in The Netherlands would be exposed to CPE. The numbers of broiler, breeding pig, and veal calf farms exposed to CPE is lower, though still considerable, with more than 100 farms exposed annually. The risk of CPE exposure is the lowest for broiler breeder farms with only 18 CPE expected exposures annually (Figure 1).

The main sources of exposure are livestock feed, imported livestock, and returning travelers, while the small number of farms exposed to companion animals (four) and hospitalized patients is negligible (one).

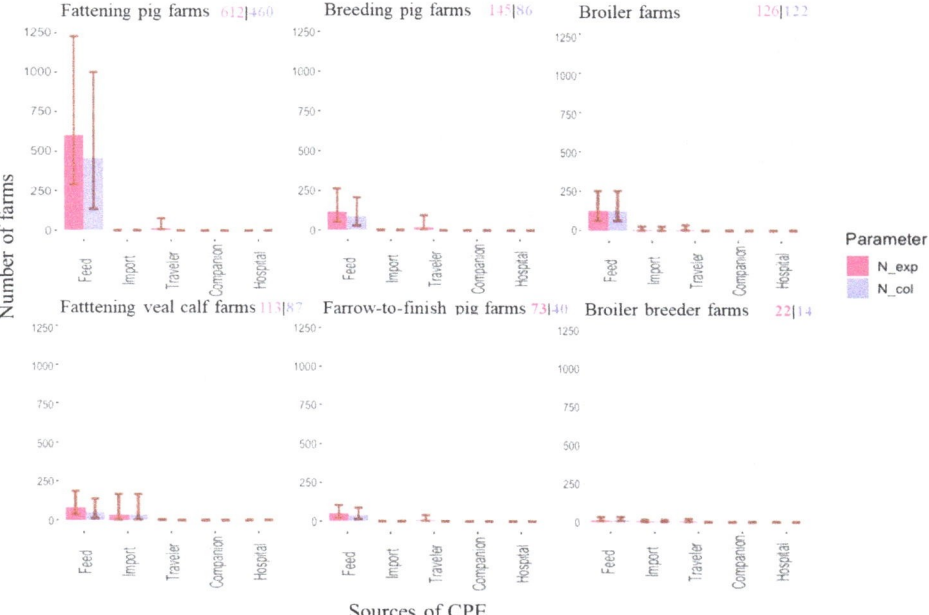

**Figure 1.** Baseline result: median (whisker: 5th and 95th percentiles) annual number of farms exposed to (red) and colonized by (blue) *CPE* in each farm type from five sources (feed, imported livestock, returning travelers, companion animals, and hospital patients). The color-coded numbers in the right upper corner of each plot are the total number of farms exposed to *CPE* and the total number of farms in which CPE has been introduced.

## 2.2. Probability of Colonization Given Exposure to CPE

This probability was not calculated for imported livestock, since introduction of a colonized animal on the farm immediately results in colonization of the farm (where colonization of a farm was defined as the presence of at least one colonized animal on the farm). Livestock feed had the highest probability of colonization in the exposed farms (Table 1). Farm workers and veterinarians posed a very low probability of colonization to the exposed farms. The probability of colonization by exposure to companion animals was not calculated for the baseline scenario because we assumed that companion animals would not enter the barns, resulting in zero introduction to the small number of exposed farms. In the farm type comparison, exposed broiler and broiler breeder farms had the highest probability of colonization if exposed. The probability of colonization on a veal calf farm exposed to contaminated feed was the lowest of all farm types. The probabilities of colonization in veal calf and all three pig farm types exposed to CPE-colonized humans were equivalent. The probability of colonization was the lowest in all three pig farm types and veal calf fattening farms exposed to colonized returning veterinarians from overseas travel and hospital.

**Table 1.** Probability of at least one animal colonized on a farm given exposure of the farm to CPE. The companion animal source resulted in zero probability, and there was no calculation for imported livestock.

| Farms at Risk | Median Probability of at Least One Animal Being Colonized Given Exposure by a Specific CPE Source (5th and 95th Percentiles) | | |
| --- | --- | --- | --- |
| Farm Types | Feed | Farm Workers Returning from Travel and Hospital | |
| | | Farm Workers | Veterinarians |
| Broiler | 1.00 (1.00, 1.00) | $1 \times 10^{-4}$ ($1 \times 10^{-5}$, $8 \times 10^{-4}$) | $2 \times 10^{-6}$ ($2 \times 10^{-7}$, $2 \times 10^{-5}$) |
| Broiler breeder | 1.00 (1.00, 1.00) | $1 \times 10^{-4}$ ($1 \times 10^{-5}$, $8 \times 10^{-4}$) | $2 \times 10^{-6}$ ($2 \times 10^{-7}$, $2 \times 10^{-5}$) |
| Fattening pig | 0.88 (0.22, 1.00) | $2 \times 10^{-7}$ ($1 \times 10^{-8}$, $5 \times 10^{-6}$) | $4 \times 10^{-9}$ ($2 \times 10^{-10}$, $9 \times 10^{-8}$) |
| Breeding pig | 0.92 (0.26, 1.00) | $2 \times 10^{-7}$ ($1 \times 10^{-8}$, $5 \times 10^{-6}$) | $4 \times 10^{-9}$ ($2 \times 10^{-10}$, $9 \times 10^{-8}$) |
| Farrow-to-finish | 0.92 (0.26, 1.00) | $2 \times 10^{-7}$ ($1 \times 10^{-8}$, $5 \times 10^{-6}$) | $4 \times 10^{-9}$ ($2 \times 10^{-10}$, $9 \times 10^{-8}$) |
| Veal calf | 0.73 (0.15, 1.00) | $2 \times 10^{-7}$ ($1 \times 10^{-8}$, $5 \times 10^{-6}$) | $4 \times 10^{-9}$ ($2 \times 10^{-10}$, $9 \times 10^{-8}$) |

### 2.3. Ranking the Risk of Introduction: Combining Exposure and Colonization

The estimated number of fattening pig farms with CPE introduction was the highest, followed by broiler, fattening veal calf, and breeding pig farms (Figure 1). Farrow-to-finish farms and broiler breeder farms ranked lowest in terms of numbers of introductions. Exposure to contaminated feed was most likely to result in CPE introduction, with probabilities of colonization varying between 73% and 100% (Table 1). Exposure to hospitalized farm workers and returning travelers, on the contrary, was estimated to hardly ever result in CPE introduction to the farm due to a very low probability of colonization in exposed farms (Table 1). The expected annual number of CPE introductions to livestock farms in The Netherlands due to returning travelers was $5 \times 10^{-5}$, which equals an introduction once every 20,000 years. For an individual farm, the estimated probability of colonization was highest on broiler farms (0.23, Table 2). Probabilities of colonization in fattening pig and farrow-to-finish farms were slightly lower (between 0.16 and 0.17). The probabilities of colonization in other farm types were lower than 0.1.

**Table 2.** Expected number of farms exposed and colonized combined with the total number of farms to calculate the probability of exposure and colonization for an individual farm of a specific type.

| | | | Broiler | Fattening Pig | Farrow-to-Finish | Veal Calf | Broiler Breeder | Breeding Pig | Total |
| --- | --- | --- | --- | --- | --- | --- | --- | --- | --- |
| | | Total number of farms in The Netherlands | 524 | 2652 | 260 | 1298 | 255 | 1601 | 6590 |
| Expected number | | Farms exposed | 126 | 612 | 73 | 113 | 22 | 145 | 1091 |
| | | Farms colonized | 122 | 460 | 40 | 87 | 14 | 86 | 810 |
| Probability per individual farm | | Exposure | 0.24 | 0.23 | 0.28 | 0.09 | 0.09 | 0.09 | 0.17 |
| | | Colonization | 0.23 | 0.17 | 0.16 | 0.07 | 0.05 | 0.05 | 0.13 |
| | Probability of exposure due to | Feed | 0.229 | 0.228 | 0.196 | 0.059 | 0.051 | 0.067 | 0.148 |
| | | Imported livestock | 0.004 | $3 \times 10^{-4}$ | 0.002 | 0.025 | 0.004 | 0.001 | 0.007 |
| | | Returning traveler | 0.008 | 0.006 | 0.040 | 0.006 | 0.015 | 0.069 | 0.143 |
| | | Companion animal | 0.001 | 0.004 | $3 \times 10^{-4}$ | 0.002 | $3 \times 10^{-4}$ | 0.002 | 0.009 |
| | | Hospital patient | $1.8 \times 10^{-4}$ | 0.001 | $2 \times 10^{-4}$ | $4 \times 10^{-4}$ | $8 \times 10^{-5}$ | $5 \times 10^{-4}$ | 0.003 |

## 2.4. Result from Sensitivity Analysis

First, the Spearman rank correlation, a non-parametric metric between $-1$ and 1, was calculated for all input parameters with an uncertainty distribution to estimate the extent to which these input parameters determined the model results for each source (Section 2.4.1). Secondly, one-at-a-time (OAT) sensitivity analysis was performed (Section 2.4.2). In this additional sensitivity analysis, the value of a single input parameter was either increased or decreased. The outcome of each adjustment was compared to the baseline scenario to investigate the impact of all input parameters on the estimated number of introductions. OAT sensitivity analysis was performed separately for each source. Then, to evaluate if changes in input parameters would affect the ranking of sources, we compared the results of the OAT sensitivity analysis across sources (Section 2.4.3).

### 2.4.1. Result from Spearman Rank Correlation

Based on the model results, feed is indicated as the main contributor of CPE introduction for all livestock farm types (Table 2). The Spearman rank correlation for this source revealed that the prevalence of CPE-colonized patients in Dutch hospitals ($P_{CPE_{NL}}$), which was combined with *E. coli* prevalence to infer the prevalence of CPE in feed ($P_{CPE_{feed}}$), 50% infectious dose (*ID*50), and the average batch size of feed ($V_{batch}$) are inputs that are strongly correlated with the expected number of introductions from feed (Figure 2). However, these parameters are not expected to affect the ranking of farm types for their introduction risk because these inputs are identical for all farm types apart from 50% infectious dose (*ID*50), which differs between farm types (Figure S3). CPE prevalence in livestock i in country j ($P_{CPE_A}$) is highly correlated with the expected number of CPE introductions from imported animals to all farm types. Though CPE prevalence in humans ($P_{CPE_{NL}}$ and $P_{CPE}$) is correlated with the number of introductions from both hospitalized patients and returning travelers, the average number of farmers per farm ($AVG_{farmers}$) and the probability of admission to hospital during travel ($P_{admit}$) were more correlated with pig and veal calf farm introductions than CPE prevalence in the returning traveler source. Introductions from returning travelers and hospitalized patients were also correlated with input parameters for probability of colonization given exposure such as infectious dose at 50% colonization (*ID*50) and proportion of CPE transferred from fomite to finger and vice versa ($C_{tran_E}$ and $C_{tran_A}$).

### 2.4.2. One-at-a-Time Sensitivity Analysis per Source

One-at-a-time sensitivity analysis of the input parameters for introduction by feed unveiled two parameters that had a huge impact on the estimated number of introductions in different farm types: the total number of animals in The Netherlands ($N_{animal}$) and the amount of feed consumed per animal per day ($C_a$) (Figure 3). The total number of farms ($N_{farm}$) was used twice in the model, i.e., to obtain the number of animals per farm and the number of farms exposed, which compiled into a lower effect toward introductions than the total number of animals in The Netherlands ($N_{animal}$) and the amount of feed consumed per animal per day ($C_a$). Parameters with the least impact on introduction in all farm types were the number of bacteria in contaminated feed ($Ecoli_{concF}$) and the median infectious dose (*ID*50). These two parameters were involved in calculating the probability of colonization in an exposed farm ($P_{col_s}$), while other parameters were involved in calculating the number of exposed farms ($N_{col_s}$).

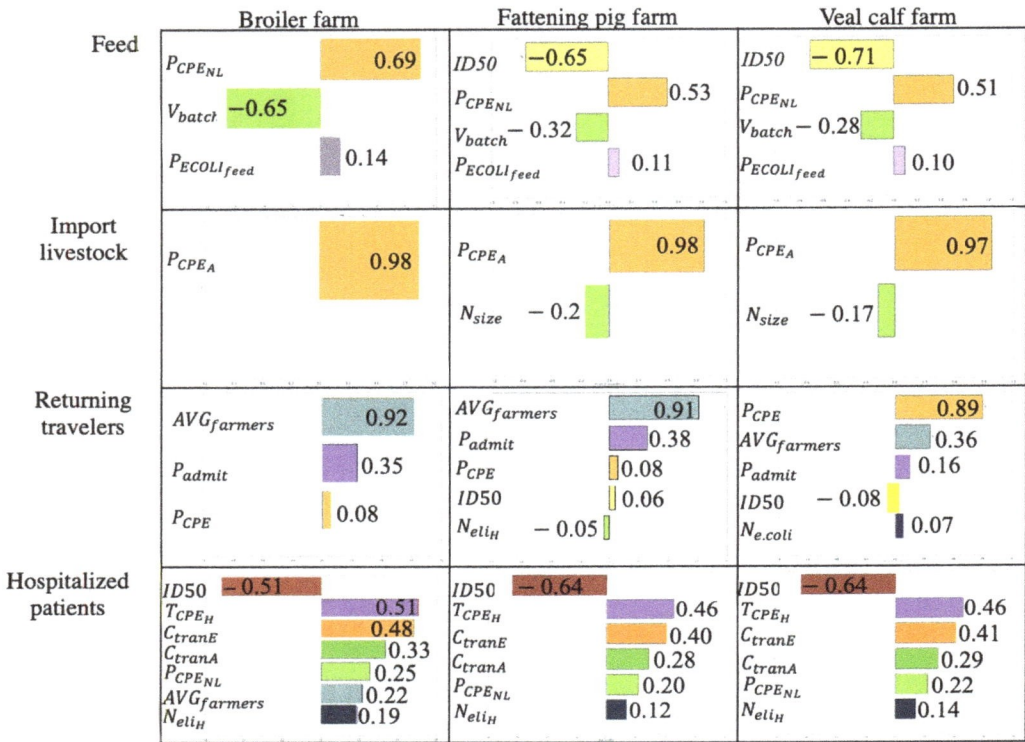

**Figure 2.** Results of Spearman rank correlation for broiler farm, fattening pig farm, and veal calf farm. Each row shows rank correlation of input parameters with the expected number of CPE colonizations from feed, imported livestock, returning travelers, and hospitalized patients. Only input parameters with a Spearman rank correlation coefficient >|0.1| are included in the plots. Spearman rank correlation of companion animals is excluded from the figure because the introduction is zero.

Input values of three impactful parameters, namely, the total number of animals ($N_{animal}$), total number of local farms ($N_{farm}$), and grams of feed ingested per livestock per day ($C_a$), in the baseline model were compared across all farm types (Supplementary File S6). Fattening pig farms had the highest total number of farms ($N_{farm}$) but a moderate total number of fattening pigs ($N_{animal}$) and grams of feed ingested per fattening pig per day ($C_a$) compared to other farm types. The high number of introductions to veal calf farms arose from imported livestock. Two essential parameters that directly facilitate introduction to fattening veal calf farms are CPE prevalence in the source country ($P_{CPE_A}$) and the number of livestock i per shipment ($N_{size}$) (Figure S2). When the number of livestock i per shipment was enhanced two-fold, the number of farms exposed was also enhanced two-fold (Supplementary File S8). It should be noted that the number of livestock per shipment is directly correlated with the annual number of animals imported ($N_{imp}$). However, a two-fold increase in the CPE prevalence in livestock in source countries ($P_{CPE_A}$) increases the number of introductions only slightly because of the very low prevalence estimates based on the zero CPE cases in livestock (as reported by most source countries).

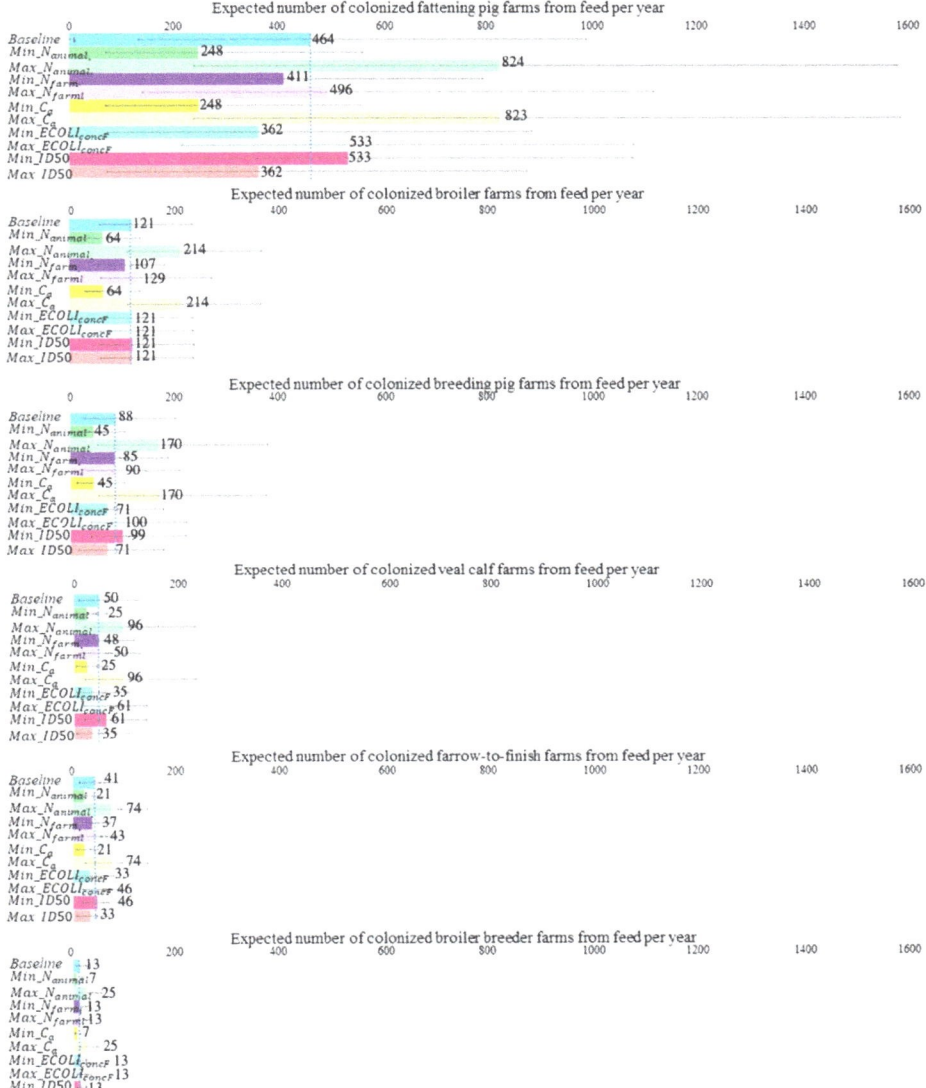

**Figure 3.** One-at-a-time sensitivity analysis of the number of introductions from feed to six farm types calculated in which one parameter either increases or decreases two-fold. Farm types are ordered according to the highest to lowest number of introductions in the baseline model. Dotted blue line indicates the estimated number of introductions in the baseline model. Only parameters that differed between farm types are included in this figure.

Fattening pig farms and veal calf farms remained the highest in farm types with introductions from livestock feed and imported livestock in the OAT sensitivity analysis. None of the OAT analysis resulted in increased introduction from human sources. However, one scenario of the OAT analysis indicated introduction to fattening pig farms from the companion animal source.

### 2.4.3. One-at-a-Time Sensitivity Analysis between Sources

To evaluate if changes in input parameters would affect the ranking of sources, we performed a pairwise comparison of the results of the OAT sensitivity analysis of individual sources (Table S6). For example, for the comparison of feed and imported livestock, we compared 15 outcomes (7 parameters that were both increased and decreased, and the baseline) of the feed source to 7 outcomes of the imported livestock source (3 parameters that were both increased and decreased, and the baseline). This resulted in a total of 105 combinations of outcomes including 1 combination of baseline parameters for both sources (Table S7). Of all the other 104 outcome combinations, we recorded if the ranking of the sources was different from the comparison of the baseline parameters in both sources. Feed consistently ranked as the source with the highest expected number of CPE introductions in all farm types, except for veal calf farms, when comparing sensitivity tests across all sources (Supplementary File S9). Forty-four percent of the adjusted input parameters resulted in a higher introduction from imported livestock to veal calf farms than feed. In the baseline model, the colonization risk of imported livestock and feed for veal calf farms was on the same order of magnitude, with the risk of feed being slightly higher, whereas for all other farm types, the risk of imported livestock was very low compared to feed (Figure 1). On the other hand, all sensitivity tests produced non-zero introduction from feed, while a small proportion of sensitivity tests (19%) resulted in negligible introduction from imported livestock to most farm types except fattening pig and veal calf farms. Imported livestock always had a higher introduction risk than returning travelers, hospitalized patients, and companion animals (Supplementary File S9: Tables S8 and S9).

### 2.5. Result from What-If Analysis

The effects of higher contamination levels in feed, less strict biosecurity at the farm level, and a ban on livestock imports from countries sampling less than 100 animals for CPE surveillance were explored by adjusting input parameters and evaluating the model outcome (number of introductions) in what-if scenario analysis.

CPE was introduced into eight (one breeding, five fattening pig, and two veal calf) additional farms when the number of *E. coli* contaminations increased to the maximum limit for rejecting feed as given by GMP+. This addition is small compared to the 767 expected introductions in the baseline model (Table 3). Interestingly, banning imports from countries with a low surveillance level (less than 100 animals sampled) reduced the risk of introduction from imported livestock by 71%. Following a minor increase in introduction from companion animals in a flexible biosecurity scenario, companion animals would be reclassified from no risk to a low-risk source. Conversely, introduction from returning travelers and hospitalized patients remained negligible when the number of bacteria on a person's palms increased four times due to non-compliance with hand hygiene protocols.

**Table 3.** What-if analysis related to probability of colonization in feed, restriction on import of animals from countries with weak surveillance for *CPE*, and less strict biosecurity practice in local farms.

| Scenario | CPE Source Affected | Parameter Changed | Baseline Number of Introductions from Affected Source (95% Range) | Changed Number of Introductions from Affected Source (95% Range) |
|---|---|---|---|---|
| Contamination of *E. coli* in feed reaches concentration of maximum rejection limit according to GMP+ | Feed | $Ecoli_{concF}$ | 767 (244, 1679) | 775 (246, 1668) |

Table 3. Cont.

| Scenario | CPE Source Affected | Parameter Changed | Baseline Number of Introductions from Affected Source (95% Range) | Changed Number of Introductions from Affected Source (95% Range) |
|---|---|---|---|---|
| The Netherlands only allows import of livestock from EU member states that sample ≥100 animals in CPE surveillance | Imported livestock | $P_{CPE_A}$ | 48 (4, 214) | 14 (0, 58) |
| Lower biosecurity: companion animals have full access to livestock areas in broiler, pig, and veal calf farms | Companion animals | $P_{barnC}$ | 0 (0, 0) | 2 (1, 7) |
| Lower biosecurity: non-compliance with hand hygiene | Travelers and hospitalized patients | $Ecoli_{hand}$ | $1 \times 10^{-4}$ ($9 \times 10^{-6}, 8 \times 10^{-4}$) | $4 \times 10^{-3}$ ($3 \times 10^{-4}, 3 \times 10^{-2}$) |

## 3. Discussion

This is the first risk assessment that quantifies the risk of CPE introduction into livestock farms in The Netherlands. The results indicate that fattening pig farms ranked the highest with respect to the expected annual number of CPE-colonized farms. However, when considering the probability of CPE introduction per individual farm, broiler farms have the highest introduction risk. Our model indicates that feed is a major potential source of CPE introduction, but this risk estimate has a high uncertainty. Imported livestock is indicated as an important CPE source specifically for veal calf farms. Other sources (companion animals, hospital patients, and returning travelers) were assessed to be of minor or negligible importance.

The number of exposed farms was most important in determining the introduction risk expressed as the expected number of colonized farms for high-rank sources (feed and imported livestock), due to the high probability of colonization upon exposure ($P_{col_s}$) in both sources (probability varying between 0.73 and 1 for feed (Table 1), probability of 1 for livestock imports). The probability of an individual farm exposed to CPE due to feed was similar in broiler, fattening pig, and farrow-to-finish farms (Table 2). This probability equaled the probability of receiving at least one CPE-contaminated batch of feed ($P_{CPE_{batch}}$). Although broilers require much less feed per animal than pigs due to their relatively small size, the number of broilers kept per farm is higher, resulting in a similar amount of feed delivered to all farm types.

The overall probability of introduction for an individual farm resulting from all sources was the highest in the broiler sector. If exposed to CPE, broilers have a higher probability of colonization than pigs and veal calves due to the very low median infectious dose ($ID50$) in broilers. This parameter mainly affected the colonization probabilities of farms exposed to CPE-colonized humans because, for this source, the dose to which the animals are exposed is low. With high exposure doses, as was the case with feed, the probabilities of colonization are high, even when the $ID50$ is high. The total number of CPE introductions is thus mainly determined by the total number of farms exposed to CPE given the high probability of colonization upon exposure by the two major sources (0.73–1 probability). Consequently, the effect of changing the probability of colonization is much smaller than that of changing the number of exposed farms.

According to our model, thirteen percent of Dutch farms are estimated to be colonized by CPE each year, mainly via feed, which is clearly an overestimation as such a percentage of farms being colonized would be detectable under the current national surveillance protocol [14,15]. Still, an undetected CPE presence in Dutch livestock is possible, as the current national surveillance protocol was designed to detect at least one colonized animal with 95% certainty, provided the prevalence is 1% [14]. However, this surveillance protocol does not take into account clustering of colonization at the farm level, which decreases the sensitivity of the surveillance. Furthermore, introductions could have escaped detection because most farms for meat production (broiler, fattening pig, and veal calf) apply an all-in-all-out system that produces more than one batch of livestock annually, while the national surveillance collects samples only once a year from a single animal per batch at slaughter from part of the farms. Thus, for each farm unit, multiple samples distributed over time are necessary to calculate an accurate prevalence [16].

In our calculation, a major source of CPE introduction is feed, although no carbapenemase-producing bacteria have been found thus far in feed. The probability that batches are CPE-contaminated and the concentration of CPE in contaminated batches were both inferred from the CPE prevalence among humans, *E. coli* prevalence in feed, and the ratios of CPE, ESBL, and other *E. coli* in water sources. Using these proxy measures introduces uncertainty in the calculations. Multiple studies, however, indicated the presence of *E. coli* in feed to be as prominent as Salmonella, which is a major hazard in animal feed [1,17–21]. Despite no CPE detection in livestock feed, a small percentage of *E. coli* from feed collected in Portugal and the United States carried resistant genes against ampicillin and cefotaxime [19,22,23]. It is, therefore, reasonable to assume that CPE contamination of feed is possible. Although halving the CPE prevalence in feed lowered the risk of feed considerably (Supplementary File S8; Figure S3), feed still remained an important source of CPE introduction, still being higher than the risk of imported animals. It is therefore recommended to investigate this source of CPE in more detail to either discard this source as a risk or to enable mitigation strategies.

The probability of batches of feed contaminated with CPE ($P_{CPE\,feed}$), the number of batches delivered to a farm each year ($N_{batch}$), the median infectious dose ($ID50$), and the concentration of CPE *E. coli* (cfu/g) in contaminated animal feed ($CPE_{concF}$) are four parameters worth further examination because they had a large impact on the introduction risk and are surrounded by considerable uncertainty. Uncertainty in the probability of batches of feed contaminated with CPE ($P_{CPE\,feed}$), and the concentration of CPE *E. coli* (cfu/g) in contaminated animal feed were due to lack of data for CPE, and these parameters were therefore inferred from the prevalence and concentration of *E. coli* in feed and other sources. Equally, no data were available on the median infectious dose ($ID50$) for CPE in livestock, and therefore estimates from studies on ESBL in broilers and pigs were used. Uncertainty in the number of batches delivered to a farm each year ($N_{batch}$) stems from generalizing highly variable parameters into an average value. The impact of overestimating these parameters was assessed in a sensitivity analysis, where the number of introductions from feed was reduced by, at most, 47% (Tables S7–S9). Still, the 47% reduction in the number of introductions from feed remains higher than other sources (Supplementary File S9).

Whereas most farm types have a low risk of introduction via routes other than feed, veal calf farms have a high risk of introduction by imported animals. Farms received a higher number of batches of imported veal calves than other animal types due to a high number of imported animals and small batch sizes. Furthermore, the inferred CPE prevalence in veal calves in source countries ($P_{CPE_A}$) is higher than the estimated CPE prevalence in pigs and broilers [9,24]. Eighteen EU member states did not collect any samples from veal calves for CPE surveillance (Supplementary File S10; Figure S4). Therefore, the CPE prevalence in veal calves in these member states was inferred from ESBL surveillance in bovine meat (Supplementary File S3 & Table S2), resulting in a higher CPE prevalence in our calculations for veal calves. Both countries from which a high number of veal calves are imported ($N_A$) and countries with a high inferred probability that imported veal calf batches are colonized with CPE ($P_{CPE_A}$) (Supplementary File S9: Table S10) have a high risk of CPE introduction. This outcome resembles a risk assessment by EFSA, which concluded that EU member states with higher volumes of livestock trading have a higher risk of disseminating AMR-ESBL bacteria [2,25]. We believe that the high risk level expected for veal calves from the model could be an overestimation given the lack of CPE detection in veal calves in EU surveillance (EARS-net). The high prevalence estimates for source countries were thus not based on reported detections but resulted from uncertainty due to low sample sizes. However, CPE cases in cows were detected in European countries [26], and imported veal calves were ranked first for risk of CPE in our expert elicitation (Supplementary File S2). The scenario of reducing risk by only allowing countries that sample more than 100 animals annually to export to The Netherlands was shown to be an effective mitigation strategy in the what-if analysis. The expected number of introductions was reduced by 71%. It should, however, be kept in mind that this strategy reduces the potential CPE introductions resulting from uncertainty in CPE prevalence in veal calves in source countries. Countries with an effective surveillance program in calves that do find CPE in calves might, in reality, pose a higher risk to the Dutch veal calf sector. A more reliable estimate of the CPE introduction risk via imported livestock can be obtained via enacting EU-wide mandatory surveillance with enough samples in all countries exporting veal calves to EU member states.

Humans were initially thought to be a high-risk source because of high numbers of overseas travel and CPE presence in hospitals [4], but the risk of these sources was found to be very low. In spite of a non-zero number of farms exposed to returning travelers and hospitalized patients (the probability of exposure of an individual farm is as high as for imported livestock (Table 2)), the extremely small calculated dose of CPE ingested by livestock leads to a very low number of expected colonizations in the exposed farms (Table 1). The prevalence of the clinically relevant CPE Klebsiella pneumoniae in humans is slightly higher than CPE *E. coli* [10]. Only the latter was considered in this risk assessment. Including CPE Klebsiella pneumoniae is, however, not expected to result in a change in the ranking of sources given the huge difference in the estimated risk between feed and imported livestock, on the one hand, and travelers and hospitalized patients, on the other. Likewise, CPE introduction from the companion animal source was assessed to be negligible because there is no exposure of farm animals to colonized companion animals if strict biosecurity is applied. What-if analysis evaluated the effect of reduced biosecurity in farms, where hand hygiene and exclusion of companion animals from the barns were not complied with [27–31]. This scenario still resulted in a very low number of expected introductions from human and companion animal sources. This is explained by the low number of humans and companion animals attributed per farm and the very low probability of colonization of the farm if exposed to CPE-colonized humans or companion animals.

The outcome of this introduction risk assessment was used to rank farm types and sources of their CPE introduction risk. The results for the absolute numbers of exposures and introductions have a large uncertainty and cannot be viewed as accurate quantitative risk estimates. The results of the sensitivity analysis provide good indications of the uncertain input parameters that have the largest impact on the model results. Parameters with both a large uncertainty and a large impact are important knowledge gaps that can be targeted in future studies. Despite these uncertainties, the ranking of farm types and sources was robust and the outcome of this risk assessment can thus be used for targeted CPE surveillance [32–34].

## 4. Materials and Methods

We quantitatively assessed the risk of CPE introduction to broiler, pig, and veal calf farms from five potential CPE sources, i.e., imported livestock, livestock feed, companion animals, hospital patients, and returning travelers, and ranked farm types by the expected number of farms with CPE introduction and the probability of CPE introduction for an individual farm. This quantitative risk assessment followed the guidelines for import risk assessment provided by the World Organisation for Animal Health (OIE) [32,33] to assess the risk of exposure of farms, and the guidelines for microbial risk assessment provided by the Codex Alimentarius to assess the risk of infection upon exposure [35,36].

We conducted sensitivity analysis to assess the effect of uncertainty surrounding important input parameters toward the output and evaluated alternative biosecurity practices and trade restrictions via scenarios analysis.

Despite being highlighted as an important potential CPE source, wastewater from hospitals was excluded from the model because CPE will be effectively removed in the wastewater treatment facilities. Additionally, although small traces of CPE could be present in surface water due to overflow from rainfall, the vast majority of the meat-producing animals of our concern (veal calf, fattening pig, breeding pig, broiler, and broiler breeder) were raised in a closed system where they drink tap water. This water source undergoes extensive purification, ensuring no traces of resistant bacteria such as CPE [37–39]. Wild mammals and birds were also excluded from the model. Small mammals such as rodents move locally and thus would not be exposed to CPE from outside The Netherlands. Interactions between local target farms and wild birds are mostly prevented as livestock live in closed barns.

### 4.1. Risk Model

#### 4.1.1. Model Outline

CPE introduction was defined as the colonization of at least one animal with CPE upon exposure of a farm to any of the sources included in the model. The risk of CPE introduction was modeled with two submodels (Figure 4). The first submodel used scenario tree modeling to estimate the number of farms exposed to CPE-colonized sources ($N_{col}$). The second submodel was a microbial risk assessment model to estimate the probability that at least one animal will be colonized on an exposed farm ($P_{col}$) given the dose to which the animals on the farm are exposed ($CPE_{ing}$), using an exponential dose–response model. The outputs of both submodels were combined to calculate the expected annual numbers of farms on which CPE is introduced ($N_{intro}$). Parameters and values used in the model are presented in Table 1.

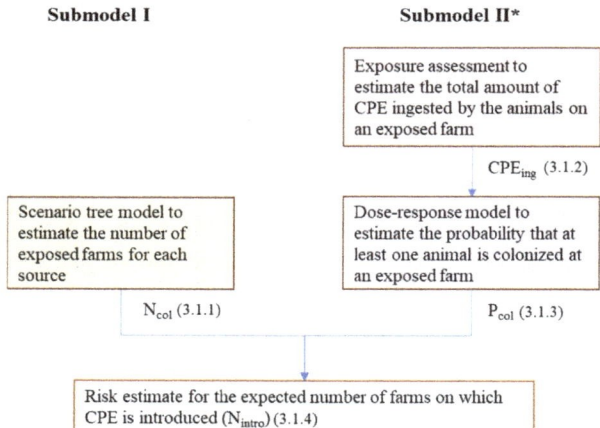

**Figure 4.** Outline of the risk model to estimate the introduction risk of CPE into Dutch livestock farms from five sources: imported livestock, livestock feed, companion animals (cats and dogs), hospital patients, and returning travelers. * Submodel II is not used for imported livestock because the introduction of a colonized animal into a livestock farm automatically results in colonization of the farm.

The annual expected number of CPE introductions via each source was calculated using multiple input parameters, some of which are uncertain. Parameters on CPE prevalence, CPE concentration, number of animals in transport, and colonization duration were chosen to be included with a distribution to account for uncertainty and variability. Less variable data, such as total numbers of farms and livestock in The Netherlands, were entered as point estimates. The impact of these parameters on the model results was studied by a sensitivity analysis where the input values were increased and decreased two-fold. We ran 10,000 iterations using Monte Carlo sampling in ModelRisk, an add-on for Microsoft Excel version 1908® [40].

4.1.2. Submodel I: Scenario Tree Model

The exposure of the following six farm types: broilers, broiler breeders, fattening pigs, breeding pigs, farrow-to-finish, and veal calves, to CPE from sources s (imported livestock (A), livestock feed (F), companion animals (C), farm workers being hospitalized (H), and farm workers traveling abroad (T)) was calculated by multiplying the number of farms in contact with people or animals or receiving feed, $N_s$, or by the probability that these persons or animals are colonized with CPE, or that the feed is contaminated with CPE, $P_{CPE_s}$. Mixed species livestock farms were not considered in the risk assessment because they represented a small proportion of local farms [41].

$$N_{col_s} = N_s \cdot P_{CPE_s} \tag{1}$$

Imported Livestock

The number of farms exposed to CPE from imported animals, $N_{col_A}$, was calculated by multiplying the annual number of batches of animals imported from the source country—among all EU member states in 2017—to six farm types ($N_A$) by the probability that an imported batch from the source country which is delivered to an individual farm type is colonized with CPE ($P_{CPE_A}$).

We assumed that CPE colonization is maintained during transport and will reach local farms without detection. Sustained CPE colonization in animals during transportation between EU member states is likely within the maximum 24 h transport time [42], because in livestock, ESBL colonization can be maintained for 30 to 180 days [43–46]. Within the EU, antimicrobial testing in imported animals is not obligatory and not conducted [2]. The probability of detecting a CPE-colonized animal is thus negligible and was not accounted for in the calculations.

Livestock Feed

The number of farms exposed to CPE-colonized feed, $N_{col_F}$, was calculated as the product of the total number of six farm types in The Netherlands ($N_{farm}$) and the probability that an individual farm would receive at least one batch of feed contaminated with CPE ($P_{CPE_{batch}}$). $P_{CPE_{batch}}$ was calculated from the probability that a batch of feed is contaminated with CPE ($P_{CPE_{feed}}$) and the annual number of feed batches received by a farm ($N_{batch}$). The estimated value for $P_{CPE_{feed}}$ was used for all farm types because no data were available to estimate $P_{CPE_{feed}}$ separately for each farm type.

$$P_{CPE_{batch}} = 1 - \left(1 - P_{CPE_{feed}}\right)^{N_{batch}} \tag{2}$$

Companion Animals

The number of farms exposed to CPE-colonized companion animals ($N_{col_C}$) was derived by multiplying the number of farms with companion animals ($N_C$) by the probability that companion animals in The Netherlands are colonized with CPE ($P_{cCPE_{NL}}$). The number of farms having companion animals ($N_C$) was calculated from the total number of farms ($N_{farm}$) multiplied by the probability of farms having a companion animal ($P_{farmC}$).

Farm Workers

CPE introduction from humans is possible when farm-related workers k (farmers, veterinarians) acquire CPE during holidays outside The Netherlands or in local hospitals

(Figure 5). Here, the number of farm workers acquiring CPE in hospital ($N_{colH_k}$) was calculated by multiplying the number of farm workers hospitalized ($N_H$) by the probability that patients acquire CPE in Dutch hospitals ($P_{CPENL}$). The number of farm workers hospitalized ($N_H$) was estimated by multiplying the number of farm workers and veterinarians in The Netherlands ($N_k$) by the annual probability of hospital admission in the general population ($P_{admit_{NL}}$).

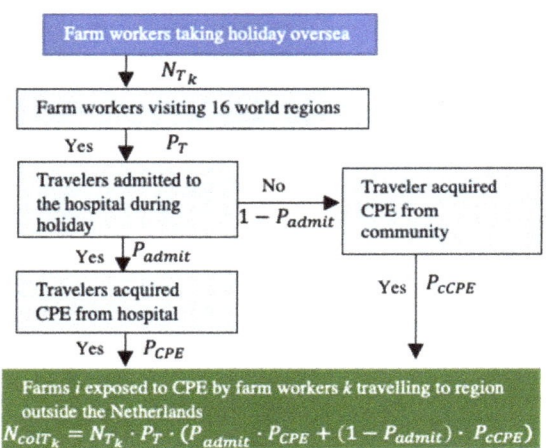

**Figure 5.** Scenario tree to calculate the number of farms exposed to CPE by farm workers returning from travel abroad.

The number of farms exposed to CPE through infected farm workers returning from travel abroad ($N_{colT_k}$) was calculated by multiplying the number of farm workers returning from abroad ($N_{T_k}$) by the probability of travelers acquiring CPE during travel. The probability of traveler-acquired CPE differed according to the 16 regions of destination based on the United Nations geoscheme excluding The Netherlands [47] (Supplementary File S6), and therefore calculations were performed for each region individually. The number of farmers returning from each of these regions was estimated based on the probability of Dutch travelers visiting each region ($P_T$). Both the probability of acquiring CPE in the hospital ($P_{CPE}$) and the probability of acquiring CPE from the community ($P_{cCPE}$) during travel were considered in the model. The probability of hospital-acquired CPE during holidays ($P_{CPE}$) was multiplied by the probability of travelers being hospitalized ($P_{admit}$). The probability of community-acquired CPE ($P_{cCPE}$) was multiplied by the probability of non-hospitalized travelers ($1 - P_{admit}$) (Figure 2). The estimated value for was used for all regions because no data were available to estimate $P_{admit}$ separately for each region.

### 4.1.3. Submodel II: Exposure Assessment

We estimated the numbers of farms where CPE was introduced by multiplying the number of exposed farms ($N_{col_s}$) by the probability that at least one animal on an exposed farm would become colonized ($P_{col_s}$). The probability that at least one animal on an exposed farm would become colonized was calculated with an exponential dose–response model using the total number of CPE *E. coli* bacteria ingested by the animals on the farm ($CPE_{ings}$) as the dose. The ingested dose ($CPE_{ings}$) was calculated separately for each farm type and CPE source s, as described in Equations (3)–(5). These calculations were not performed for the source imported livestock, since the introduction of a colonized animal into a livestock farm directly results in a colonized farm.

Animal Feed

The ingested dose of CPE from contaminated feed on a single farm ($CPE_{ing_F}$) was estimated as the product of the concentration of CPE *E. coli* (cfu/g) in contaminated animal feed delivered to a farm ($CPE_{concF}$) and the average weight of one batch of feed in grams ($V_{batch}$).

$$CPE_{ing_F} = CPE_{concF} \cdot V_{batch} \quad (3)$$

Companion Animals

To estimate the total CPE deposited by companion animals in the farm environment, we multiplied the concentration of CPE in companion animal feces ($CPE_{gramC}$) (cfu/g) by the average weight (grams) of feces defecated by a companion animal in each defecation ($W_{fec}$), the daily defecation frequency of companion animals ($N_{eli_C}$), the length of the colonization period in companion animals in days ($T_{CPE_C}$), and the proportion of time that a companion animal is present in the barn ($P_{barnCi}$). The total CPE ingested by the farm animals ($CPE_{ing_C}$) was subsequently calculated by multiplying the deposited CPE in the farm environment by the proportion of excreted bacteria taken up by the livestock animals from the farm environment ($C_{tranA}$) (Table 1).

$$CPE_{ing_C} = W_{fec} \cdot N_{eli_C} \cdot T_{CPE_C} \cdot CPE_{gramC} \cdot P_{barnC} \cdot C_{tranA} \quad (4)$$

Farm Workers

The number of CPE bacteria ingested by colonized farm workers ($CPE_{ing_H}$) was calculated in a similar manner to the ingested dose from companion animals ($CPE_{ing_C}$), albeit with different inputs. The transmission event started after the colonized farm worker (farmer or veterinarian) used the toilet for defecation. We assumed CPE contaminated their hands after toilet usage and that not all would be removed by hand washing. Thus, $CPE_{hand}$ was the number of CPE (cfu) remaining on a farm worker's hands after hand washing. The number of CPE deposited in the farm environment was then calculated by multiplying this number by the daily defecating frequency of humans ($N_{eli_H}$), the length of the colonization period of CPE in humans in days ($T_{CPE_H}$), the proportion of bacteria transferred from the farm worker's hand to the farm environment ($C_{tran_E}$), and the proportion of the day that a worker is in the barn ($P_{barnH}$). The last parameter is different between farm workers and veterinarians, assuming that a farmer spends much more time in the barn of a single farm than a vet. The total CPE ingested by the farm animals ($CPE_{ing_H}$) was subsequently calculated by multiplying the deposited CPE in the farm environment by the proportion of bacteria taken up by the livestock animals from the farm environment ($C_{tranA}$).

$$CPE_{ing_H} = CPE_{hand} \cdot N_{eli_H} \cdot T_{CPE_H} \cdot C_{tran_E} \cdot P_{barnH} \cdot C_{tran_A} \quad (5)$$

4.1.4. Submodel II: Dose–Response Model

The probability that at least one animal at farm type i is colonized with CPE ($P_{col_s}$) is a function of the CPE ingested dose from a source s ($CPE_{ing_s}$) and the dose–response parameter. The dose–response parameter gives the probability of a single CPE bacterium colonizing an animal's gut ($P$) and is calculated from the $ID50$ (the dose at which 50% of the animals are expected to be colonized). An exponential dose–response model was used, and P was calculated as $\frac{ln2}{ID50}$. The probability that at least one animal is colonized with CPE was then calculated as

$$P_{col_s} = 1 - e^{-(P \cdot CPE_{ing_s})} \quad (6)$$

4.1.5. Risk Estimate Combining Submodel I and Submodel II

The expected number of introductions to each farm type from each source s ($N_{intro_s}$) was calculated by multiplying the number of farms exposed to each source s ($N_{col_s}$) by the probability that at least one animal on an exposed farm is colonized ($P_{col_s}$).

$$N_{intro_s} = N_{col_s} \cdot P_{col_s} \quad (7)$$

The absolute risk of CPE introduction into local Dutch farms was given as the expected annual number of introductions per farm type ($N_{intro}$) from all CPE sources considered in the model. The probability of CPE introduction for an individual farm was estimated by dividing the number of expected introductions per farm type by the total number of farms of this type in The Netherlands.

4.2. Input Parameters

4.2.1. Imported Livestock

Data on the number of livestock imported into The Netherlands from EU member states ($N_{imp}$) were available for the period 2016 to 2020 and fluctuated slightly. Import data for the year 2017 were used in the baseline model to be consistent with the data used for the number of farms and veterinarians. The livestock import records were derived from two publicly available sources, namely, Statistics Netherlands (CBS) and The Netherlands Enterprise Agency (RVO) (Supplementary File S6 and Table 4) [48]. To estimate the number of imported batches ($N_A$), the annual number of imported animals was divided by the average number of livestock per shipment ($N_{size}$). In estimating the number of animal batches delivered to each farm type annually ($N_{batch}$), we assumed that all imported one-day-old broilers would go to broiler farms, all imported parent broilers would go to broiler breeder farms, all imported veal calves would go to veal calf farms, all imported piglets would go to fattening pig farms, and all imported breeding pigs would go to breeding pig farms and farrow-to-finish pig farms in a ratio of 2:1, representing the ratio of these farms in The Netherlands.

The probability that imported animals from EU member states are colonized with CPE ($P_{CPE_A}$) was directly inferred from national surveillance data provided by the European Antimicrobial Resistance Surveillance Network [9,24]. CPE surveillance in livestock consisted of random sampling of fecal samples from live animals at slaughter, the results of which were used as a proxy for herd prevalence in the risk model. Data on surveillance in pigs and broilers were available for all EU member states, EFTA countries, and the UK, whereas only 9 EU member states and 2 EFTA countries (Norway and Switzerland) reported on CPE surveillance in calves. For countries that had no data on surveillance in calves, the probability of CPE colonization was inferred from the surveillance in bovine meat (Supplementary File S3, Supplementary Tables S1 and S2). The probability that imported animals are colonized with CPE ($P_{CPE_A}$) was estimated using a beta distribution based on the number of animals sampled (n), the number of animals that tested positive (s), and test sensitivity (se) (Table 4).

4.2.2. Animal Feed

The average number of batches of feed received by individual farms ($N_{batch}$) was calculated as

$$N_{batch} = \frac{n_a \cdot c_a \cdot 365}{V_{batch}} \quad (8)$$

where $n_a$ is the average number of animals on a farm of type $i$, $c_a$ is the average consumption of feed per day per animal on each farm type (in grams), and $V_{batch}$ is the average size of a batch of feed delivered to a farm (in grams). The average number of animals on farm type $i$ ($n_a$) was calculated by dividing the total number of animals in The Netherlands present at each farm type ($N_{animal}$) by the total number of farms at each farm type in The Netherlands ($N_{farm}$). The number of Dutch farms ($N_{farm}$) and livestock heads ($N_{animal}$) was based on

2017 data provided by Statistics Netherlands. Due to a lack of farm-specific data, $V_{batch}$ was set equal for all farm types.

Since feed ingredients are heat-treated, CPE contamination was expected to result from cross-contamination during processing and storage in a local feed mill. The probability of feed colonized with CPE was therefore based on Dutch data. As there is no CPE surveillance conducted on animal feed at all, the probability of batches of feed contaminated with CPE ($P_{CPE_{feed}}$) was inferred from the ratio between E. coli prevalence in feed ($P_{ec_{feed}}$) and in humans ($P_{ec_{NL}}$) under the presumption that the ratio of E. coli in the two aforementioned sources is the same as the CPE ratio (Equation (9)). $P_{ec_{feed}}$ was based on the prevalence of compound feed for cattle contaminated with E. coli in the EU [23], and $P_{ec_{NL}}$ was based on the prevalence of E. coli in Dutch residents reported in the national surveillance of antimicrobial resistance [11]. No data were available for the CPE prevalence in the Dutch community ($P_{cCPE_{NL}}$). However, we had data on CPE prevalence in Dutch hospitals ($P_{CPE_{NL}}$). Therefore, $P_{cCPE_{NL}}$ was inferred from the ratio between ESBL E. coli in the community and in clinical settings ($C_{com: cli}$), under the presumption that the CPE correlation between the community and the clinical setting is similar to the ESBL E. coli correlation in European countries. The CPE prevalence in Dutch hospitals ($P_{CPE_{NL}}$) was therefore multiplied by the ratio of ESBL E. coli in the community versus ESBL in a clinical setting, $C_{com: cli}$. This ratio was estimated to be 0.79 based on the Pearson correlation between ESBL prevalence in the community and in the clinical setting in the EU, as observed in five studies [49–53]. The derived value of $P_{CPE_{feed}}$ was used for all farm types owing to the lack of data on E. coli in feed for other animal species.

$$P_{CPE_{feed}} = \frac{P_{cCPE_{NL}}}{P_{ec_{NL}}} \cdot P_{ec_{feed}} \tag{9}$$

No data were available on the concentration of CPE in feed if it was contaminated. The concentration of CPE in feed ($CPE_{concF}$) was estimated by multiplying the strict concentrations of E. coli allowed (minimum rejection limit) in feed components ($Ecoli_{concF}$) as given by GMP+ [54] by the ratio of E. coli carrying CPE genes to non-resistant E. coli ($P_{CPE:EC}$), as observed in samples from 100 Dutch wastewater treatment facilities [37].

4.2.3. Companion Animals

The number of farms with a companion animal ($N_C$) was calculated by multiplying the total number of farms in The Netherlands ($N_{farm}$) by the proportion of farms with companion animals ($P_{farmC}$). No data were available on the proportion of farms with companion animals in The Netherlands. Assuming that farmers' behavior in The Netherlands does not greatly deviate from other Western regions, we used surveillance data of farmers' behavior in the United States of America to estimate $P_{farmC}$.

The probability of companion animals colonized with CPE in The Netherlands was set equal to the CPE prevalence in the Dutch community ($P_{cCPE_{NL}}$). Although some information on numbers of colonized companion animals in The Netherlands was available from the Monitoring of Antimicrobial Resistance and Antibiotic Usage in Animals in The Netherlands report [55], these numbers were not considered representative as these were cases from animals visiting a veterinary clinic only (Supplementary file S5). The concentration of CPE (cfu/g) in feces ($CPE_{gramC}$) was estimated from the concentration of ESBL E. coli (cfu/g) in animal feces ($ESBL_{gramFec}$) measured in an observational study of healthy dogs in the United States [56] and the proportion of ESBL E. coli carrying CPE genes ($P_{CPE:ESBL}$) [37].

The frequency of defecating ($N_{eliC}$) was based on a report from a commercial feed company in the United Kingdom [57]. The weight (grams) of feces defecated by a companion animal was based on a study in healthy medium-sized dogs in the United States ($W_{fec}$) [58]. Time spent in the livestock area ($P_{barnC}$) was set to zero for all farm types in the default calculations, assuming compliance with biosecurity protocols in The Netherlands.

However, we explored non-zero $P_{barnC}$ reflecting farms with a lower biosecurity standard in a what-if analysis (Section 2.5 & Table 3). The proportions of CPE transfer from the environment to animal ($C_{tranA}$) were based on a study that measured the proportion of *Acinobacter* transferred from fomite to finger [59]. The CPE colonization period in companion animals ($T_{CPE_C}$) was set equal to the ESBL *E. coli* colonization period in healthy dogs in The Netherlands [60].

#### 4.2.4. Farm Workers

The total number of farms in The Netherlands ($N_{farm}$) was multiplied by the average number of employees per farm ($Avg_{farmer}$) to parameterize the number of farmers ($N_{farmers}$). Each farm is typically visited by a single veterinarian, and therefore the number of veterinarians ($N_{vet}$) in the model was set equal to the total number of farms in The Netherlands ($N_{farm}$). The number of farm-related workers spending their holiday abroad ($N_{T_k}$) was calculated by multiplying the number of farm workers ($N_{farmer}$) and veterinarians ($N_{vet}$) by the probability of farm workers and veterinarians traveling abroad for their holidays ($P_{holiday}$). The probability of farmers taking a holiday abroad was derived from an online survey among 300 Dutch farmers conducted by a farm-oriented magazine, Boerderij (Farm) [61]. The probability of veterinarians taking a holiday abroad was based on data from Statistics Netherlands [41] for the general Dutch population. The proportion of Dutch travelers visiting each UN region ($P_T$) was based on Statistics Netherlands data from 2013, where the number of holidays to each region was divided by the total number of holidays taken by Dutch citizens (Supplementary File S6). To estimate the probability of hospital admission for farm workers ($P_{admit_{NL}}$), the number of Dutch inpatients in 2017 was divided by the total population of The Netherlands in 2017. The prevalence of CPE in hospital ($P_{CPE_{NL}}$) was based on data provided by EARS-Net [10]. The probability of hospital admission during holidays outside of The Netherlands ($P_{admit}$) was derived from a study among 2000 Dutch travelers. The probability of acquiring CPE during hospitalization ($P_{CPE}$) in non-European countries was parameterized from national surveillance on CPE prevalence from multiple countries around the world reported in the WHO's global report of surveillance [62] and independent academic publications [63,64]. The probability of non-hospitalized travelers acquiring CPE from the community in a foreign country ($P_{cCPE}$) was inferred by multiplying the hospital CPE prevalence ($P_{CPE}$) by the ratio of ESBL in the community versus ESBL in the clinical setting ($C_{com:\ cli}$) (Supplementary File S4). The number of CPE (cfu) remaining on a farm worker's hands after hand washing ($CPE_{hand}$) was estimated from an observational study in Mexico among tomato farmers, in which the number of *E. coli* on hands after toilet use followed by hand washing ($Ecoli_{hand}$) was measured. $Ecoli_{hand}$ was multiplied by the probability of *E. coli* carrying CPE genes ($P_{CPE:EC}$) to calculate CPE (cfu) on farm workers' hands. The number of defecations per day ($N_{eli_H}$) was retrieved from an observational study of 2000 returning Dutch travelers (Arcilla et al., 2016). Proportion of time spent in the livestock area ($P_{barnH}$) was estimated at eight hours a day for farmers and one hour per week for veterinarians. The proportions of CPE transfer from the hands to the environment ($C_{tranE}$) were based on the same study used to estimate the proportions of CPE transfer from the environment to the animal ($C_{tranA}$) [59].

#### 4.2.5. Dose–Response Parameter

The median infectious dose ($ID50$) was used to calculate the dose–response parameter (P). The median infectious dose ($ID50$) was based on experimental studies for ESBL in broilers and pigs. No data were available to estimate the $ID50$ for veal calves, and, therefore, it was set equal to the median infectious dose of pigs.

Table 4. Input parameters for the model to assess the risk of CPE introduction into Dutch livestock farms.

| Input * | Description | Value Distribution ** | Value in Sensitivity Analysis | References |
|---|---|---|---|---|
| $N_{intro}$ | Expected annual number of farms on which CPE is introduced | | | |
| $N_{col_s}$ | Number of farms exposed to CPE-colonized sources s (imported livestock (A), livestock feed (F), companion animals (C), farm workers being hospitalized (H), and farm workers traveling abroad (T)) | | | |
| $N_s$ | Number of farms in contact with people, import animals, companion animals, and livestock feed | | | |
| $P_{CPE_s}$ | Probability of sources exposed to farm are colonized/contaminated with CPE | | | |
| $P_{CPE batch}$ | Probability that an individual farm receives at least one batch of feed contaminated with CPE | | | |
| $N_{batch}$ | Annual number of feed batches received by a farm | | | |
| $P_{CPE_{feed}}$ | Probability that a batch of feed is contaminated with CPE | | | |
| $N_C$ | Number of farms with companion animals | | | |
| $N_H$ | Number of farm workers/vets hospitalized | | | |
| $N_{T_k}$ | Number of farm workers/vets returning from abroad | | | |
| $CPE_{ing_s}$ | Total number of CPE E. coli bacteria ingested by the animals on an exposed farm | | | |
| $CPE_{concF}$ | Total number of CPE E. coli (cfu/g) in contaminated animal feed | | | |
| $CPE_{gramC}$ | Total number of CPE E. coli (cfu/g) in companion animal feces | | | |
| $CPE_{hand}$ | Total number of CPE E. coli (cfu) remaining on a farm worker's hands after hand washing | | | |
| $p$ | Probability of a single CPE bacterium colonizing an animal's gut | | | |
| $N_{imp}$ | Annual number of imported broilers, parent broilers, piglets, breeding pigs, and veal calves from EU member states j to farm type i in The Netherlands | Supplementary File S7 | Yes | [41,48] |
| $se$ | CPE surveillance sensitivity | 0.85 | Yes | [14] |
| $P_{CPE_A}$ $P_{CPE_{NL}}$ | CPE prevalence in livestock i in country j CPE prevalence in hospitalized patients in The Netherlands | Beta ($\alpha$/se, $\beta$) (values of beta distribution in EFSA reference) Beta (8/se, 6676) | Yes | [9,10,24] |
| $P_{CPE}$ | CPE prevalence in hospital patients in region m | Beta ($\alpha$/se, $\beta$) (values of beta distribution are in Table S5) | Yes | [63–83] |
| $C_{com: cli}$ | Ratio of ESBL in the community versus ESBL in a clinical setting | 0.79 | N | Table S3 |
| $P_{ec_{feed}}$ | Prevalence of E. coli-contaminated feed in compound cattle feed | Beta (59, 46) | Yes | [23] |

**Table 4.** *Cont.*

| Input * | Description | Value Distribution ** | Value in Sensitivity Analysis | References |
|---|---|---|---|---|
| $P_{ec_{NL}}$ | Prevalence of *E. coli* in Dutch residents | Beta (159,620, 280,677) | Yes | [55] |
| $N_{size}$: broiler<br>$N_{size}$: piglet<br>$N_{size}$: breeding pig<br>$N_{size}$: veal calf | Number of livestock *i* per shipment | Pert (45,00, 47,000, 55,000)<br>Pert (100, 260, 300)<br>Pert (65, 80, 95)<br>Pert (30, 150, 200) | Yes | [29] |
| $N_{farm}$ and $N_{animal}$ | Total number of farm types *i* and total number of animals *i* in The Netherlands | Table S5 | Yes | [41] |
| $N_K$ | Total number of farm workers and veterinarians in The Netherlands | Table S5 | Yes | [41] |
| $c_a$ | The average grams of feed consumed by livestock *i* per day | Table S5 | Yes | [84–86] |
| $V_{batch}$ | The average grams of feed delivered to a farm derived from the volume of a standard transport truck | Pert ($3 \times 10^6$, $16 \times 10^6$, $3 \times 10^7$) | Yes | [29] |
| $Ecoli_{concF}$: broiler<br>$Ecoli_{concF}$: fattening pig<br>$Ecoli_{concF}$: breeding pig<br>$Ecoli_{concF}$: veal calf | Concentrations of *E. coli* in feed components following minimum rejection limit by GMP+ (cfu/g) | 11.8<br>11.8<br>14.3<br>7.3 | Yes | [54] |
| $Ecoli_{hand}$ | The amount of *E. coli* remaining on a farm worker's hands after toilet use and subsequent hand washing (cfu) | Log-normal (63, 5.02) | Yes | [28] |
| $ESBL_{gramFec}$ (cfu/g) | Number of *E. coli* (cfu) in a gram of healthy companion animal's feces | Normal (70, 35) | Yes | [87] |
| $P_{CPE:EC}$<br>$P_{CPE:ESBL}$ | Proportion of *E. coli* carrying CPE genes and proportion of ESBL *E. coli* carrying CPE genes | 0.00004<br>0.00424 | N | [37] |
| $ID50$: broiler<br>$ID50$: pig and veal calf | Infectious dose of ESBL *E. coli* at which, on average, 50% of livestock species *i* are colonized (cfu) | Log-normal (5, 5)<br>Log-normal (4695, 9187) | Yes | [56,88,89] |
| $P_{farm_C}$ | Proportion of farms that have companion animals | Beta (298, 148) | Yes | [56] |
| $W_{fec}$ (grams) | Grams of feces defecated by a companion animal in one defecation | Normal (70, 35) | Yes | [58] |
| $N_{eli_C}$<br>$N_{eli_H}$ | The average number of defecations by companion animals and humans per day | Pert (1, 2, 5)<br>Uniform (1, 3) | Yes | [57] Assumption |
| $T_{CPE_C}$<br>$T_{CPE_H}$ | Colonization duration of CPE in companion animals and humans (days) | Pert (0, 120, 180)<br>Pert (1, 30, 365) | Yes | [60,90] |
| $P_{barnC}$<br>$P_{barnH}$: farm worker<br>$P_{barnH}$: veterinarian | Proportion of day a companion animal, farm worker, and veterinarian spent in the barns | 0<br>0.33<br>0.005 | Yes | Assumption |
| $C_{tranA}$<br>$C_{tranE}$ | Proportion of *Acinobacter* transferred from fomite to finger (A) and from finger to fomite (E) | Log-normal (0.24, 0.14)<br>Log-normal (0.06, 0.06) | Yes | [59] |
| $P_T$ | The probability of Dutch travelers visiting 16 world regions in 2013 | Table S5 | Yes | [41] |
| $P_{holiday}$: broiler and pig farm worker<br>$P_{holiday}$: veal calf farm worker<br>$P_{holiday}$: veterinarian | Probability of farm worker on farm *i* taking holiday abroad annually | 0.53<br>0.33<br>0.64 | Yes | [41,61,91] |
| $Avg_{farmers}$ | The average number of farm workers in all farm types | Pert (1, 2, 4) | Yes | Assumption |

Table 4. Cont.

| Input * | Description | Value Distribution ** | Value in Sensitivity Analysis | References |
|---|---|---|---|---|
| $P_{admit}$ $P_{admit\,NL}$ | Probability of hospital admission while traveling overseas and in The Netherlands | 0.04 0.054 | Yes | [41,90,92] |

Footnotes: * Type of farm is indicated by subscript *i* and source country by *j*. ** Parameters for input distributions given in brackets: beta (α,β), where α equals the number of positives plus one, and β the number of negatives plus one; log-normal (mean, SD); normal (mean, SD); pert (minimum, most likely, maximum); uniform (minimum, maximum). Parameters with an empty *Value Distribution* are parameters calculated from the raw input.

*4.3. Sensitivity Analysis*

4.3.1. Spearman Rank Correlation on Baseline Simulations

Sensitivity analysis was applied to the risk model to assess the impact of uncertain and highly variable input parameters that were inputted as probability distributions on the estimated number of CPE introductions ($N_{intro_s}$). Spearman rank correlation was used to analyze the impact of these input parameters. Only input parameters with a correlation coefficient > |0.1| with $N_{intro_s}$ were included in the result.

4.3.2. One-at-a-Time Sensitivity Analysis

In an additional one-at-a-time (OAT) sensitivity analysis, the most input parameters (non-inferred) (Table 4) were either decreased or increased by 50%. The result of each input adjustment was compared to the baseline result to determine which parameter had the most effect on the expected number of colonized farms. Results were calculated per CPE source (imported livestock, livestock feed, companion animals, hospital patients, and returning travelers). To analyze the effect of changes in input parameters on the ranking of sources for the expected number of farms with CPE introduction, outcomes of each input adjustment were compared to the outcomes of all other input adjustments, including the baseline model, and the frequency of changes in the ranking were counted.

*4.4. What-If Analysis*

Three what-if scenarios were analyzed for their impact on the estimated number of CPE introductions ($N_{intro_s}$). The first scenario simulated the effect of less sanitary measures in livestock feed production by increasing the bacteria number in feed ($Ecoli_{concF}$) to the maximum limit for rejecting feed according to GMP+. The second scenario modeled the effect of banning livestock importation from EU member states with insufficient CPE surveillance. In the calculations for this scenario, livestock imports from countries that sampled less than 100 animals for CPE surveillance were excluded from the model calculations. The third scenario evaluated weak compliance with biosecurity protocols on farms. This affected both the risk of introduction from humans and companion animals. The lower biosecurity was mimicked by assuming farm workers did not wash their hands after toilet use, resulting in a higher number of CPE on their hands, and by adjusting the proportion of time a companion animal was present in the animal area $P_{barnC}$. This parameter was set to 0.1 in broiler and pig farms and 0.3 in veal calf farms. All other input parameters were kept at their baseline values in the what-if scenarios.

## 5. Conclusions

Feed and imported livestock are expected to pose the highest risk of CPE introduction to pig, broiler, and veal calf farms. Our risk assessment shows that CPE surveillance should focus on broiler and fattening pig farms, given the highest probability of introduction per farm and the highest total number of introductions, respectively. Our model clearly indicates that we currently do not have sufficient information on the CPE presence in sources, i.e., CPE prevalence in humans, animals, and feed, and the CPE concentration in feed, and that this information is essential for the reliability of this risk estimate and for effective risk mitigation. Therefore, the calculated numbers of exposure and introduction cannot be considered as accurate quantitative estimates of the risk. The ranking of farm types for the total number of introductions in each farm type and for the probability of introduction in individual farm types is, however, robust despite the huge uncertainties in input parameters. More surveillance of CPE prevalence in feed and imported animals, especially veal calves, is essential to improve the certainty of the risk assessment. Banning livestock importation from countries that put little effort into CPE surveillance could reduce the risk from imported livestock.

**Supplementary Materials:** The following are available online at https://www.mdpi.com/article/10.3390/antibiotics11020281/s1, Supplementary File S1: Literature review [6,12,37,58,76,93–152]. Supplementary File S2: Report expert elicitation in projects "Risk assessment CPE" and "BEWARE". Supplementary File S3: veal calves' CPE sample size inference [9]. Supplementary File S4: Community: Clinical prevalence. Supplementary File S5: Estimated CPE in local and imported companion animal [49–53]. Supplementary File S6: Model input and queries [41,62–71,73–83,85,86,90,144,153]. Supplementary File S7: Queries to retrieve import data from cbs.nl. Supplementary File S8: One-at-a-time sensitivity analysis on introduction. Supplementary File S9: One-at-a-time sensitivity analysis on introduction compared between sources. Supplementary File S10: Introduction from imported livestock to veal calf farms. Figure S1: PRISMA chart indicates the literature review of potential CPE sources, Figure S2: One-at-a-time sensitivity analysis from livestock import source, Figure S3: One-at-a-time additional parameters sensitivity analysis of feed source, Figure S4: number of veal calves sampled in the import origin countries reported by EARS-Net 2018, Table S1: Proportion ESBL positive in bovine meat and in calves and their ratio for 4 UN regions in EU, Table S2: CPE sample size in veal calves inferred from ESBL samples, Table S3: ESBL prevalence in community and clinical setting collected from literatures review, Table S4: Components for calculation of companion animal in livestock farm colonized with CPE $N_{colC_l}$, Table S5: inputs to estimate the number of farms exposed to CPE, Table S6: Total number of test runs in which one parameters were discounted or increased two-fold, Table S7: Comparison of introduction between livestock feed and import livestock, Table S8: Comparison of introduction between import and returning traveler sources, Table S9: Comparison of introduction between import and companion animal sources, Table S10: Top six countries with the highest number of introduction from imported livestock to veal calf farm.

**Author Contributions:** Conceptualization, N.D., C.J.d.V., M.S. and A.J.S.; methodology, N.D., C.J.d.V., E.A.J.F. and A.J.S.; software, N.D. and C.J.d.V.; validation, C.J.d.V., E.A.J.F., M.S., A.J.S. and J.A.W.; formal analysis, N.D., C.J.d.V. and E.A.J.F.; investigation, N.D., C.J.d.V., M.S. and A.J.S.; resources, N.D., C.J.d.V., E.A.J.F., M.S., A.J.S. and J.A.W.; data curation, N.D.; writing—original draft preparation, N.D., C.J.d.V., E.A.J.F. and A.J.S.; writing—review and editing, N.D., C.J.d.V., E.A.J.F., A.J.S., J.A.W. and M.S.; visualization, N.D., C.J.d.V. and E.A.J.F.; supervision, C.J.d.V., E.A.J.F., M.S., A.J.S. and J.A.W.; project administration, A.J.S.; funding acquisition, A.J.S. All authors have read and agreed to the published version of the manuscript.

**Funding:** This research was funded by The Netherlands Organisation for Health Research and Development (ZonMw), grant number 541002004.

**Informed Consent Statement:** Not applicable.

**Data Availability Statement:** Data retrieved from publicly available sources are provided in the references. All other data are provided in the Supplementary Information.

**Acknowledgments:** We would like to thank feed expert Arjan van Dijk (Nevedi) and veal calf expert Peter Mölder (Denkavit) for providing information to estimate input parameters of the model. We highly appreciate the contribution from Nedzib Tafro (NVWA), Heike Schmidt (RIVM), Engeline van Duijkeren (RIVM), Arjan van Dijk (Nevedi), Alex Spieker (Avined), and Dik Mevius (WBVR) in the expert elicitation on CPE sources.

**Conflicts of Interest:** The authors declare no conflict of interest.

# References

1. Davies, J.; Davies, D. Origins and Evolution of Antibiotic Resistance. *Microbiol. Mol. Biol. Rev.* **2010**, *74*, 417–433. [CrossRef] [PubMed]
2. EFSA. *Scientific Opinion on Carbapenem Resistance in Food Animal Ecosystems*; EFSA: Parma, Italy, 2013; p. 18314732.

3. Jacob, J.; Klein, E.; Laxminarayan, R.; Lynfield, R.; Kallen, A.; Ricks, P.; Edwards, J.; Srinivasan, A.; Fridkin, S.; Rasheed, J.K.; et al. Vital Signs: Carbapenem-Resistant Enterobacteriaceae. *Cent. Dis. Control. Prev.* **2013**, *62*, 165.
4. Albiger, B.; Glasner, C.; Struelens, M.J.; Grundmann, H.; Monnet, D.L.; European Survey of Carbapenemase-Producing Enterobacteriaceae (EuSCAPE) Working Group. Carbapenemase-producing Enterobacteriaceae in Europe: Assessment by national experts from 38 countries, May 2015. *Eurosurveillance* **2015**, *20*, 30062. [CrossRef] [PubMed]
5. Kelly, A.M.; Mathema, B.; Larson, E.L. Carbapenem-resistant Enterobacteriaceae in the community: A scoping review. *Int. J. Antimicrob. Agents* **2017**, *50*, 127–134. [CrossRef]
6. Nordmann, P.; Naas, T.; Poirel, L. Global Spread of Carbapenemase-producingEnterobacteriaceae. *Emerg. Infect. Dis.* **2011**, *17*, 1791–1798. [CrossRef]
7. Köck, R.; Daniels-Haardt, I.; Becker, K.; Mellmann, A.; Friedrich, A.W.; Mevius, D.; Schwarz, S.; Jurke, A. Carbapenem-resistant Enterobacteriaceae in wildlife, food-producing, and companion animals: A systematic review. *Clin. Microbiol. Infect.* **2018**, *24*, 1241–1250. [CrossRef]
8. Mughini-Gras, L.; Barrucci, F.; Smid, J.H.; Graziani, C.; Luzzi, I.; Ricci, A.; Barco, L.; Rosmini, R.; Havelaar, A.H.; van Pelt, W.; et al. Attribution of human Salmonella infections to animal and food sources in Italy (2002–2010): Adaptations of the Dutch and modified Hald source attribution models. *Epidemiol. Infect.* **2014**, *142*, 1070–1082. [CrossRef]
9. Authority, E.F.S. The European Union summary report on antimicrobial resistance in zoonotic and indicator bacteria from humans, animals and food in 2017. *EFSA J.* **2019**, *17*, e05598.
10. ECDC. *Annual Report of The European Antimicrobial Resistance Surveillance Network (EARS-Net)*; Surveillance Report; ECDC: Stockholm, Sweeden, 2017.
11. Veldman, K.; Mevius, D.; Pelt, W.; Heederik, D.; Geijlswijk, M.; Wagenaar, J.; Mouton, W.; Jacobs, J.; Sanders, P.; Veldman, K.T.; et al. *Monitoring of Antimicrobial Resistance and Antibiotic Usage in Animals in The Netherlands in 2016*; MARAN: Amsterdam, The Netherlands, 2017.
12. Blaak, H.; de Kruijf, P.; Hamidjaja, R.A.; van Hoek, A.H.A.M.; de Roda Husman, A.M.; Schets, F.M. Prevalence and characteristics of ESBL-producing *E. coli* in Dutch recreational waters influenced by wastewater treatment plants. *Vet. Microbiol.* **2014**, *171*, 448–459. [CrossRef]
13. Blaak, H.; van Rooijen, S.; Schuijt, M.; van Leeuwen, D.; van den Berg, L.; Lodder-Verschoor, F.; Schets, F.; de Roda Husman, A. *Prevalence of Antibiotic Resistant Bacteria in the Rivers Meuse, Rhine, and New Meus*; RIVM Report; National Institute for Public Health and the Environment: Amsterdam, The Netherlands, 2011.
14. Wit, B.; Veldman, K.; Hordijk, J.; Wagnaar, J.; Heuvelink, A.; Vellema, P.; Dierikx, C.M.; Backer, J.A.; Takumi, K.; van Duijkeren, E. *Inventarisatie Screening Carbapenemase-Producerende Bacteriën In Dieren En Dierlijke Producten: Is De Huidige Screening Toereikend? RIVM Briefrappor*; National Institute for Public Health and the Environment: Amsterdam, The Netherlands, 2017.
15. Biedenbach, D.J.; Bouchillon, S.K.; Hoban, D.J.; Hackel, M.; Phuong, D.M.; Nga, T.T.T.; Phuong, N.T.M.; Phuong, T.T.L.; Badal, R.E. Antimicrobial susceptibility and extended-spectrum beta-lactamase rates in aerobic gram-negative bacteria causing intra-abdominal infections in Vietnam: Report from the Study for Monitoring Antimicrobial Resistance Trends (SMART 2009–2011). *Diagn. Microbiol. Infect. Dis.* **2014**, *79*, 463–467. [CrossRef]
16. Cameron, S.; Baldock, F. Two-stage sampling in surveys to substantiate freedom from disease. *Prev. Vet. Med.* **1998**, *34*, 19–30. [CrossRef]
17. Dodd, C.C.; Sanderson, M.W.; Sargeant, J.M.; Nagaraja, T.G.; Oberst, R.D.; Smith, R.A.; Griffin, D.D. Prevalence of Escherichia coli O157 in Cattle Feeds in Midwestern Feedlots. *Appl. Environ. Microbiol.* **2003**, *69*, 5243–5247. [CrossRef] [PubMed]
18. Sargeant, J.M.; Sanderson, M.W.; Griffin, D.D.; Smith, R.A. Factors associated with the presence of Escherichia coli O157 in feedlot-cattle water and feed in the Midwestern USA. *Prev. Vet. Med.* **2004**, *66*, 207–237. [CrossRef]
19. Dargatz, D.; Strohmeyer, R.M.P.; Hyatt, D.; Salman, M. Characterization of Escherichia coli and Salmonella enterica from Cattle Feed Ingredients. *Foodborne Pathog. Dis.* **2005**, *2*, 341–347. [CrossRef] [PubMed]
20. Hancock, D.R.D.; Thomas, L.; Dargatz, D.; Besser, T. Epidemiology of Escherichia coli 0157 in Feedlot Cattle. *J. Food Prot.* **1997**, *60*, 462–465. [CrossRef] [PubMed]
21. Andreoletti, O.B.; Buncic, S.; Colin, P.; Collins, J.D.; De Koeijer, A.; Griffin, J.; Havelaar, A.; Hope, J.; Klein, G.; Kruse, H.; et al. *Microbiological Risk Assessment in Feedingstuffs for Food-Producing Animals*; European Food Safety Authority: Parma, Italy, 2008.
22. Ge, B.; Lafon, P.C.; Carter, P.J.; McDermott, S.D.; Abbott, J.; Glenn, A.; Ayers, S.L.; Friedman, S.L.; Paige, J.C.; Wagner, D.D.; et al. Retrospective Analysis of Salmonella, Campylobacter, Escherichia coli, and Enterococcus in Animal Feed Ingredients. *Foodborne Pathog. Dis.* **2013**, *10*, 684–691. [CrossRef]
23. da Costa, P.M.; Oliveira, M.; Bica, A.; Vaz-Pires, P.; Bernardo, F. Antimicrobial resistance in Enterococcus spp. and Escherichia coli isolated from poultry feed and feed ingredients. *Vet. Microbiol.* **2007**, *120*, 122–131. [CrossRef]
24. European Food Safety Authority; European Centre for Disease Prevention and Control. The European Union summary report on antimicrobial resistance in zoonotic and indicator bacteria from humans, animals and food in 2016. *EFSA J.* **2018**, *16*, e05182.
25. EFSA. *Scientific Opinion on the Public Health Risks of Bacterial Strains Producing Extended-Spectrum B-Lactamases and/or Ampc B-Lactamases in Food and Food-Producing Animals*; EFSA: Parma, Italy, 2011; p. 18314732.
26. Ibrahim, D.R.; Dodd, C.E.; Stekel, D.J.; Ramsden, S.J.; Hobman, J.L. Multidrug resistant, extended spectrum beta-lactamase (ESBL)-producing Escherichia coli isolated from a dairy farm. *FEMS Microbiol. Ecol.* **2016**, *92*, fiw013. [CrossRef]

27. Pickering, A.J.; Davis, J.; Walters, S.P.; Horak, H.M.; Keymer, D.P.; Mushi, D.; Strickfaden, R.; Chynoweth, J.; Liu, J.; Blum, A.; et al. Hands, Water, and Health: Fecal Contamination in Tanzanian Communities with Improved, Non-Networked Water Supplies. *Environ. Sci. Technol.* **2010**, *44*, 3267–3272. [CrossRef]
28. de Aceituno, A.F.; Bartz, F.E.; Hodge, D.W.; Shumaker, D.J.; Grubb, J.E.; Arbogast, J.W.; Dávila-Aviña, J.; Venegas, F.; Heredia, N.; García, S.; et al. Ability of Hand Hygiene Interventions Using Alcohol-Based Hand Sanitizers and Soap to Reduce Microbial Load on Farmworker Hands Soiled during Harvest. *J. Food Prot.* **2015**, *78*, 2024–2032. [CrossRef] [PubMed]
29. Van Dijk, A. *Programmamanager Diervoeder En Sectoren*; De Nederlandse Vereniging Diervoederindustrie: Rijswijk, The Netherlands, 2020.
30. Edmonds, S.L.; McCormack, R.R.; Zhou, S.S.; Macinga, D.R.; Fricker, C.M. Hand Hygiene Regimens for the Reduction of Risk in Food Service Environments. *J. Food Prot.* **2012**, *75*, 1303–1309. [CrossRef] [PubMed]
31. WIN/Gallup International Association. *One in Three across the World Don't Always Wash Their Hands Properly after Going to the Toilet*; WIN/Gallup International Association: Washington, DC, USA, 2015.
32. World Organization for Animal Health (OIE). Terrestrial Animal Health Code. 2021, Chapter 6.7 to 6.11. Available online: https://www.oie.int/en/what-we-do/standards/codes-and-manuals/terrestrial-code-online-access/ (accessed on 1 January 2022).
33. OIE. *Handbook on Import Risk Analysis for Animals and Animal Products*; The World Organisation for Animal Health (OIE): Paris, France, 2010.
34. De Vos, C.J.; Saatkamp, H.W.; Nielen, M.; Huirne, R.B.M. Scenario Tree Modeling to Analyze the Probability of Classical Swine Fever Virus Introduction into Member States of the European Union. *Risk Anal.* **2004**, *24*, 237–253. [CrossRef] [PubMed]
35. Haas, C.N.; Rose, J.B.; Gerba, C.P. *Quantitative Microbial Risk Assessment*, 2nd ed.; John Wiley & Sons: New York, NY, USA, 2014.
36. WHO. *Principles and Guidelines for The Conduct of Microbiological Risk Assessment Cac/Gl 30-1999*; CODEX Alimentarius; WHO: Geneva, Switzerland, 2014.
37. Schmitt, H.B.; Kemper, M.; van Passel, H.; Leuken, J.; Husman, A.M.R.; Grinten, E.M.; Rutgers, J.S.; Man, H.; Hoeksma, P.; Zuidema, T. *Sources of Antibiotic Resistance in the Environment and Possible Measures*; RIVM Report; RIVM: Utrecht, The Netherlands, 2017.
38. Smeets, P.W.M.H.; Medema, G.J.; van Dijk, J.C. The Dutch secret: How to provide safe drinking water without chlorine in The Netherlands. *Drink. Water Eng. Sci.* **2009**, *2*, 1–14. [CrossRef]
39. Vemin, A.D. *Dutch Drinking Water Statistics 2017*; Vemin: Hague, The Netherlands, 2017.
40. Vose Software. @*ModelRISK. 6.1.89.0*; Vose Software: Ghent, Belgium, 2022.
41. Statistiek, C.B. Statline. Available online: https://opendata.cbs.nl/statline#/CBS/nl/ (accessed on 1 May 2019).
42. European Union. On the Protection of Animals During Transport and Related Operations and Amending Directives 64/432/EEC and 93/119/EC and Regulation (EC) No 1255/9. *Off. J. Eur. Union* **2005**. Available online: https://www.fao.org/faolex/results/details/en/c/LEX-FAOC186519/ (accessed on 1 January 2022).
43. Dame-Korevaar, A.; Fischer, E.A.; van der Goot, J.; Stegeman, A.; Mevius, D. Transmission routes of ESBL/pAmpC producing bacteria in the broiler production pyramid, a literature review. *Prev. Vet. Med.* **2018**, *162*, 136–150. [CrossRef]
44. Robe, C.; Blasse, A.; Merle, R.; Friese, A.; Roesler, U.; Guenther, S. Low Dose Colonization of Broiler Chickens With ESBL-/AmpC-Producing Escherichia coli in a Seeder-Bird Model Independent of Antimicrobial Selection Pressure. *Front. Microbiol.* **2019**, *10*, 2124. [CrossRef]
45. Hansen, K.H.; Damborg, P.; Andreasen, M.; Nielsen, S.S.; Guardabassi, L. Carriage and Fecal Counts of Cefotaxime M-Producing Escherichia coli in Pigs: A Longitudinal Study. *Appl. Environ. Microbiol.* **2013**, *79*, 794–798. [CrossRef]
46. Mir, R.A.; Weppelmann, T.A.; Teng, L.; Kirpich, A.; Elzo, M.A.; Driver, J.D.; Jeong, K.C. Colonization Dynamics of Cefotaxime Resistant Bacteria in Beef Cattle Raised Without Cephalosporin Antibiotics. *Front. Microbiol.* **2018**, *9*, 500. [CrossRef]
47. Nations, U. Standard Country or Area Codes for Statistical Use (M49). Available online: https://unstats.un.org/unsd/methodology/m49/ (accessed on 1 November 2021).
48. Nederland, R.O. Statistieken Marktinformatie. Available online: https://www.rvo.nl/onderwerpen/internationaal-ondernemen/handel-planten-dieren-producten/marktinformatie/statistieken (accessed on 2 November 2021).
49. Husickova, V.; Cekanova, L.; Chroma, M.; Htoutou-Sedlakova, M.; Hricova, K.; Kolar, M. Carriage of ESBL- and AmpC-positive Enterobacteriaceae in the gastrointestinal tract of community subjects and hospitalized patients in the Czech Republic. *Biomed. Pap. Med. Fac. Univ. Palacky Olomouc. Czech. Repub.* **2012**, *156*, 348–353. [CrossRef]
50. Stapleton, J.P.; O'Kelly, F.; Lundon, J.D.; Lynch, M.; McWade, R.; Scanlon, N.; Hannan, M. Antibiotic resistance patterns of Escherichia coli urinary isolates and comparison with antibiotic consumption data over 10 years, 2005–2014. *Ir. J. Med.Sci.* **2017**, *186*, 733–741. [CrossRef]
51. Smet, A.; Martel, A.; Persoons, D.; Dewulf, J.; Heyndrickx, M.; Claeys, G.; Lontie, M.V.M.B.; Herman, L.; Haesebrouck, F.; Butaye, P. Characterization of Extended-Spectrum b-Lactamases Produced by Escherichia coli Isolated from Hospitalized and Nonhospitalized Patients. Emergence of CTX-M-15-Producing Strains Causing Urinary Tract Infections. *Microb. Drug Resist.* **2010**, *16*, 129–134. [CrossRef] [PubMed]
52. Schoevaerdts, D.; Bogaerts, P.; Grimmelprez, A.; De Saint-Hubert, M.; Delaere, B.; Jamart, J.; Swine, C.; Glupczynski, Y. Clinical profiles of patients colonized or infected with extended-spectrum beta-lactamase producing Enterobacteriaceae isolates: A 20 month retrospective study at a Belgian University Hospital. *BMC Infect. Dis.* **2011**, *11*, 12. [CrossRef] [PubMed]

53. Olesen, B.; Hansen, S.D.; Nilsson, F.; Frimodt-Møller, J.; Leihof, F.; Struve, C.; Scheutz, F.; Johnston, B.; Krogfelt, K.; Johnsond, R.J. Prevalence and Characteristics of the Epidemic Multiresistant Escherichia coli ST131 Clonal Group among Extended-Spectrum BetaLactamase-Producing E. coli Isolates in Copenhagen, Denmark. *J. Clin. Microbiol.* **2013**, *51*, 1779–1785. [CrossRef] [PubMed]
54. GMP+. *GMP+ Community Sample*; GMP+ International: Rijswijk, The Netherlands, 2019.
55. Veldman, K.; Mevius, D.; Pelt, W.; Wit, I.; Hordijk, J. Monitoring of Antimicrobial Resistance and Antibiotic Usage in Animals in The Netherlands in 2017. 2018. Available online: https://www.wur.nl/nl/Onderzoek-Resultaten/Onderzoeksinstituten/Bioveterinary-Research/Publicaties/MARAN-Rapporten.htm (accessed on 1 October 2020).
56. Moran, N.E.; Ferketich, A.K.; Wittum, T.E.; Stull, J.W. Dogs on livestock farms: A cross-sectional study investigating potential roles in zoonotic pathogen transmission. *Zoonoses Public Health* **2017**, *65*, 80–87. [CrossRef]
57. Scrumbles Healthy Dog Poop Chart: In Search of the Perfect Poop. Available online: https://www.scrumbles.co.uk/healthy-dog-poop-chart/ (accessed on 2 November 2021).
58. Wright, M.E.; Solo-Gabriele, H.M.; Elmir, S.; Fleming, L.E. Microbial load from animal feces at a recreational beach. *Mar. Pollut. Bull.* **2009**, *58*, 1649–1656. [CrossRef]
59. Greene, C.; Vadlamudi, G.; Eisenberg, M.; Foxman, B.; Koopman, J.; Xi, C. Fomite-fingerpad transfer efficiency (pick-up and deposit) of Acinetobacter baumannii—with and without a latex glove. *Am. J. Infect. Control* **2015**, *43*, 928–934. [CrossRef]
60. Baede, V.O.; Wagenaar, J.A.; Broens, E.M.; Duim, B.; Dohmen, W.; Nijsse, R.; Timmerman, A.J.; Hordijk, J. Longitudinal study of extended-spectrum-beta-lactamase- and AmpC-producing Enterobacteriaceae in household dogs. *Antimicrob. Agents Chemother.* **2015**, *59*, 3117–3124. [CrossRef]
61. Welink, M. Meeste Boeren Wel Met Zomervakantie. Available online: https://www.boerderij.nl/meeste-boeren-wel-met-zomervakantie (accessed on 1 May 2020).
62. WHO. *Antimicrobial Resistance Global Report on Surveillance*; WHO: Geneva, Switzerland, 2014.
63. Iregui, A.; Ha, K.; Meleney, K.; Landman, D.; Quale, J. Carbapenemases in New York City: The continued decline of KPC-producing Klebsiella pneumoniae, but a new threat emerges. *J. Antimicrob. Chemother.* **2018**, *73*, 2997–3000. [CrossRef]
64. Patel, G.; Huprikar, S.; Factor, S.H.; Jenkins, S.G.; Calfee, D.P. Outcomes of Carbapenem-Resistant Klebsiella pneumoniae Infection and the Impact of Antimicrobial and Adjunctive Therapies. *Infect. Control Hosp. Epidemiol.* **2008**, *29*, 1099–1106. [CrossRef]
65. Khan, E.; Ejaz, M.; Zafar, A.; Jabeen, K.; Shakoor, S.; Inayat, R.; Hasan, R. Increased isolation of ESBL producing Klebsiella pneumoniae with emergence of carbapenem resistant isolates in Pakistan: Report from a tertiary care hospital. *J. Pak. Med. Assoc.* **2010**, *60*, 186–190.
66. Castanheira, M.; Deshpande, L.M.; Mathai, D.; Bell, J.M.; Jones, R.N.; Mendes, R.E. Early Dissemination of NDM-1- and OXA-181-Producing Enterobacteriaceae in Indian Hospitals: Report from the SENTRY Antimicrobial Surveillance Program, 2006-2007. *Antimicrob. Agents Chemother.* **2011**, *55*, 1274–1278. [CrossRef] [PubMed]
67. Mohanty, S.; Gaind, R.; Ranjan, R.; Deb, M. Prevalence and phenotypic characterisation of carbapenem resistance in Enterobacteriaceae bloodstream isolates in a tertiary care hospital in India. *Int. J. Antimicrob. Agents* **2011**, *37*, 273–275. [CrossRef] [PubMed]
68. Ben-David, D.; Kordevani, R.; Keller, N.; Tal, I.; Marzel, A.; Gal-Mor, O.; Maor, Y.; Rahav, G. Outcome of carbapenem resistant Klebsiella pneumoniae bloodstream infections. *Clin. Microbiol. Infect.* **2012**, *18*, 54–60. [CrossRef] [PubMed]
69. Liu, S.-W.; Chang, H.-J.; Chia, J.-H.; Kuo, A.-J.; Wu, T.-L.; Lee, M.-H. Outcomes and characteristics of ertapenem-nonsusceptible Klebsiella pneumoniae bacteremia at a university hospital in Northern Taiwan: A matched case-control study. *J. Microbiol. Immunol. Infect.* **2012**, *45*, 113–119. [CrossRef]
70. Rimrang, B.; Chanawong, A.; Lulitanond, A.; Wilailuckana, C.; Charoensri, N.; Sribenjalux, P.; Phumsrikaew, W.; Wonglakorn, L.; Kerdsin, A.; Chetchotisakd, P. Emergence of NDM-1- and IMP-14a-producing Enterobacteriaceae in Thailand. *J. Antimicrob. Chemother.* **2012**, *67*, 2626–2630. [CrossRef]
71. Balm, M.N.D.; La, M.-V.; Krishnan, P.; Jureen, R.; Lin, R.T.P.; Teo, J.W.P. Emergence of Klebsiella pneumoniae co-producing NDM-type and OXA-181 carbapenemases. *Clin. Microbiol. Infect.* **2013**, *19*, E421–E423. [CrossRef]
72. Koh, T.H.; Cao, D.; Shan, Q.Y.; Bacon, A.; Hsu, L.-Y.; Ooi, E.E. Acquired carbapenemases in Enterobactericeae in Singapore, 1996–2012. *Pathology* **2013**, *45*, 600–603. [CrossRef]
73. Khajuria, A.; Praharaj, A.K.; Kumar, M.; Grover, N. Emergence of Escherichia coli, Co-Producing NDM-1 and OXA-48 Carbapenemases, in Urinary Isolates, at a Tertiary Care Centre at Central India. *J. Clin. Diagn. Res.* **2014**, *8*, DC01–DC04. [CrossRef]
74. Alagesan, M.; Gopalakrishnan, R.; Panchatcharam, S.N.; Dorairajan, S.; Ananth, T.M.; Venkatasubramanian, R. A decade of change in susceptibility patterns of Gram-negative blood culture isolates: A single center study. *Germs* **2015**, *5*, 65–77. [CrossRef]
75. Tran, H.H.; Ehsani, S.; Shibayama, K.; Matsui, M.; Suzuki, S.; Nguyen, M.B.; Tran, D.N.; Tran, V.P.; Nguyen, H.T.; Dang, D.A.; et al. Common isolation of New Delhi metallo-beta-lactamase 1-producing Enterobacteriaceae in a large surgical hospital in Vietnam. *Eur. J. Clin. Microbiol.* **2015**, *34*, 1247–1254. [CrossRef]
76. Hsu, L.-Y.; Apisarnthanarak, A.; Khan, E.; Suwantarat, N.; Ghafur, A.; Tambyah, P.A. Carbapenem-Resistant Acinetobacter baumannii and Enterobacteriaceae in South and Southeast Asia. *Clin. Microbiol. Rev.* **2017**, *30*, 1–22. [CrossRef] [PubMed]
77. Liu, J.; Yu, J.; Chen, F.; Yu, J.; Simner, P.; Tamma, P.; Liu, Y.; Shen, L. Emergence and establishment of KPC-2-producing ST11 Klebsiella pneumoniae in a general hospital in Shanghai, China. *Eur. J. Clin. Microbiol.* **2017**, *37*, 293–299. [CrossRef] [PubMed]
78. CPE Thailand. *Percentage of Susceptible Organisms Isolated from All Specimen, 85 Hospitals*; CPE Thailand: Bangkok, Thailand, 2018.

79. Singh-Moodley, A.; Perovic, O. Antimicrobial susceptibility testing in predicting the presence of carbapenemase genes in Enterobacteriaceae in South Africa. *BMC Infect. Dis.* **2016**, *16*, 536. [CrossRef]
80. Correa, L.; Martino, M.D.V.; Siqueira, I.; Pasternak, J.; Gales, A.C.; Silva, C.V.; Camargo, T.Z.S.; Scherer, P.F.; Marra, A.R. A hospital-based matched case–control study to identify clinical outcome and risk factors associated with carbapenem-resistant Klebsiella pneumoniae infection. *BMC Infect. Dis.* **2013**, *13*, 80. [CrossRef] [PubMed]
81. Schwaber, M.J.; Klarfeld-Lidji, S.; Navon-Venezia, S.; Schwartz, D.; Leavitt, A.; Carmeli, Y. Predictors of Carbapenem-Resistant Klebsiella pneumoniae Acquisition among Hospitalized Adults and Effect of Acquisition on Mortality. *Antimicrob. Agents Chemother.* **2008**, *52*, 1028–1033. [CrossRef] [PubMed]
82. Al Johani, S.M.; Akhter, J.; Balkhy, H.; El-Saed, A.; Younan, M.; Memish, Z. Prevalence of antimicrobial resistance among gram-negative isolates in an adult intensive care unit at a tertiary care center in Saudi Arabia. *Ann. Saudi Med.* **2010**, *30*, 364–369. [CrossRef] [PubMed]
83. Nahid, F.; Khan, A.A.; Rehman, S.; Zahra, R. Prevalence of metallo-beta-lactamase NDM-1-producing multi-drug resistant bacteria at two Pakistani hospitals and implications for public health. *J. Infect. Public Health* **2013**, *6*, 487–493. [CrossRef]
84. Turner, J.; Garcés, L.; Smith, W.; Stevensont, P. *The Welfare of Broiler Chickens in The European Union*; CWFT: Hampshire, UK, 2005.
85. Rönnqvist, M.; Välttilä, V.; Heinola, K.; Ranta, J.; Niemi, J.; Tuominen, P. *Risk Assessment and Cost–Benefit Analysis of Salmonella in Feed and Animal Production*; Ministry of Agriculture and Forestry: Helsinki, Finland, 2018.
86. Bussel, V. Veal Farm. Available online: https://vanbusselbv.nl/en/veal-farm/ (accessed on 1 January 2022).
87. Espinosa-Gongora, C.; Shah, S.Q.; Jessen, L.R.; Bortolaia, V.; Langebaek, R.; Bjornvad, C.R.; Guardabassi, L. Quantitative assessment of faecal shedding of beta-lactam-resistant Escherichia coli and enterococci in dogs. *Vet. Microbiol.* **2015**, *181*, 298–302. [CrossRef]
88. Dame-Korevaar, A.; Fischer, E.A.J.; van der Goot, J.; Velkers, F.; van den Broek, J.; Veldman, K.; Ceccarelli, D.; Mevius, D.; Stegeman, A. Effect of challenge dose of plasmid-mediated extended-spectrum beta-lactamase and AmpC beta-lactamase producing Escherichia coli on time-until-colonization and level of excretion in young broilers. *Vet. Microbiol.* **2019**, *239*, 108446. [CrossRef]
89. Cornick, N.A.; Helgerson, A.F. Transmission and Infectious Dose of Escherichia coli O157:H7 in Swine. *Appl. Environ. Microbiol.* **2004**, *70*, 5331–5335. [CrossRef]
90. Arcilla, M.S.; van Hattem, J.M.; Haverkate, M.R.; Bootsma, M.C.J.; van Genderen, P.J.J.; Goorhuis, A.; Grobusch, M.P.; Lashof, A.M.O.; Molhoek, N.; Schultsz, C.; et al. Import and spread of extended-spectrum β-lactamase-producing Enterobacteriaceae by international travellers (COMBAT study): A prospective, multicentre cohort study. *Lancet Infect. Dis.* **2017**, *17*, 78–85. [CrossRef]
91. Molder, P. *Pathways for Import of Veal Calves*; Denkavit: Voorthuizen, The Netherlands, 2019.
92. Ministerie van Volksgezondheid, W.S. Indicatie Zorg Zonder En Met Verblijf. Available online: https://www.monitorlangdurigezorg.nl/kerncijfers/indicatie/indicatie-zorg-zonder-en-met-verblijf (accessed on 1 January 2022).
93. Lien, L.T.Q.; Lan, P.T.; Chuc, N.T.K.; Hoa, N.Q.; Nhung, P.H.; Thoa, N.T.M.; Diwan, V.; Tamhankar, A.J.; Lundborg, C.S. Antibiotic Resistance and Antibiotic Resistance Genes in Escherichia coli Isolates from Hospital Wastewater in Vietnam. *Int. J. Environ. Res. Public Heal.* **2017**, *14*, 699. [CrossRef]
94. Kleinkauf, N.; Hausemann, A.; Kempf, V.A.; Gottschalk, R.; Heudorf, U. Burden of carbapenem-resistant organisms in the Frankfurt/Main Metropolitan Area in Germany 2012/2013—First results and experiences after the introduction of legally mandated reporting. *BMC Infect. Dis.* **2014**, *14*, 1471–2334. [CrossRef] [PubMed]
95. Lamba, M.; Gupta, S.; Shukla, R.; Graham, D.W.; Sreekrishnan, T.R.; Ahammad, S.Z. Carbapenem resistance exposures via wastewaters across New Delhi. *Environ. Int.* **2018**, *119*, 302–308. [CrossRef]
96. Poirel, L.; Nordmann, P. Carbapenem resistance in Acinetobacter baumannii: Mechanisms and epidemiology. *Clin. Microbiol. Infect.* **2006**, *12*, 826–836. [CrossRef] [PubMed]
97. Djenadi, K.; Zhang, L.; Murray, A.K.; Gaze, W.H. Carbapenem resistance in bacteria isolated from soil and water environments in Algeria. *J. Glob. Antimicrob. Resist.* **2018**, *15*, 262–267. [CrossRef]
98. Morrison, B.J.; Rubin, J.E. Carbapenemase Producing Bacteria in the Food Supply Escaping Detection. *PLoS ONE* **2015**, *10*, e0126717. [CrossRef] [PubMed]
99. Poirel, L.; Bercot, B.; Millemann, Y.; Bonnin, R.A.; Pannaux, G.; Nordmann, P. Carbapenemase-producing *Acinetobacter* spp. In Cattle, France. *Emerg. Infect. Dis.* **2012**, *18*, 523–525. [CrossRef] [PubMed]
100. Woodford, N.; Wareham, D.W.; Guerra, B.; Teale, C. Carbapenemase-producing Enterobacteriaceae and non-Enterobacteriaceae from animals and the environment: An emerging public health risk of our own making? *J. Antimicrob. Chemother.* **2014**, *69*, 287–291. [CrossRef] [PubMed]
101. White, L.; Hopkins, K.; Meunier, D.; Perry, C.; Pike, R.; Wilkinson, P.; Pickup, R.W.; Cheesbrough, J.; Woodford, N. Carbapenemase-producing Enterobacteriaceae in hospital wastewater: A reservoir that may be unrelated to clinical isolates. *J. Hosp. Infect.* **2016**, *93*, 145–151. [CrossRef]
102. Oteo, J.; Saez, D.; Bautista, V.; Fernandez-Romero, S.; Hernandez-Molina, J.M.; Perez-Vazquez, M.; Aracil, B.; Campos, J. Spanish Collaborating Group for the Antibiotic Resistance Surveillance, P. Carbapenemase-producing enterobacteriaceae in Spain in 2012. *Antimicrob. Agents Chemother.* **2013**, *57*, 6344–6347. [CrossRef] [PubMed]

103. Ceccarelli, D.; van Essen-Zandbergen, A.; Veldman, K.T.; Tafro, N.; Haenen, O.; Mevius, D.J. Chromosome-Based blaOXA-48-Like Variants in Shewanella Species Isolates from Food-Producing Animals, Fish, and the Aquatic Environment. *Antimicrob. Agents Chemother.* **2017**, *61*. [CrossRef] [PubMed]
104. Yousfi, M.; Touati, A.; Muggeo, A.; Mira, B.; Asma, B.; Brasme, L.; Guillard, T.; de Champs, C. Clonal dissemination of OXA-48-producing Enterobacter cloacae isolates from companion animals in Algeria. *J. Glob. Antimicrob. Resist.* **2018**, *12*, 187–191. [CrossRef]
105. Falgenhauer, L.; Ghosh, H.; Guerra, B.; Yao, Y.; Fritzenwanker, M.; Fischer, J.; Helmuth, R.; Imirzalioglu, C.; Chakraborty, T. Comparative genome analysis of IncHI2 VIM-1 carbapenemase-encoding plasmids of Escherichia coli and Salmonella enterica isolated from a livestock farm in Germany. *Vet. Microbiol.* **2015**, *200*, 114–117. [CrossRef] [PubMed]
106. Nadimpalli, M.; Fabre, L.; Yith, V.; Sem, N.; Gouali, M.; Delarocque-Astagneau, E.; Sreng, N.; Le Hello, S. CTX-M-55-type ESBL-producing Salmonella enterica are emerging among retail meats in Phnom Penh, Cambodia. *J. Antimicrob. Chemother.* **2019**, *74*, 342–348. [CrossRef]
107. Szczepanowski, R.; Linke, B.; Krahn, I.; Gartemann, K.-H.; Gützkow, T.; Eichler, W.; Pühler, A.; Schlüter, A. Detection of 140 clinically relevant antibiotic-resistance genes in the plasmid metagenome of wastewater treatment plant bacteria showing reduced susceptibility to selected antibiotics. *Microbiology* **2009**, *155*, 2306–2319. [CrossRef]
108. Furlan, J.P.R.; Stehling, E.G. Detection of beta-lactamase encoding genes in feces, soil and water from a Brazilian pig farm. *Environ. Monit. Assess.* **2018**, *190*, 76. [CrossRef]
109. Walsh, T.R.; Weeks, J.; Livermore, D.M.; Toleman, M.A. Dissemination of NDM-1 positive bacteria in the New Delhi environment and its implications for human health: An environmental point prevalence study. *Lancet Infect. Dis.* **2011**, *11*, 355–362. [CrossRef]
110. Stolle, I.; Prenger-Berninghoff, E.; Stamm, I.; Scheufen, S.; Hassdenteufel, E.; Guenther, S.; Bethe, A.; Pfeifer, Y.; Ewers, C. Emergence of OXA-48 carbapenemase-producing Escherichia coli and Klebsiella pneumoniae in dogs. *J. Antimicrob. Chemother.* **2013**, *68*, 2802–2808. [CrossRef]
111. Guerra, B.; Fischer, J.; Helmuth, R. An emerging public health problem: Acquired carbapenemase-producing microorganisms are present in food-producing animals, their environment, companion animals and wild birds. *Vet. Microbiol.* **2014**, *171*, 290–297. [CrossRef]
112. Poirel, L.; Barbosa-Vasconcelos, A.; Simões, R.R.; Da Costa, P.M.; Liu, W.; Nordmann, P. Environmental KPC-Producing Escherichia coli Isolates in Portugal. *Antimicrob. Agents Chemother.* **2011**, *56*, 1662–1663. [CrossRef] [PubMed]
113. Fischer, J.; Rodríguez, I.; Schmoger, S.; Friese, A.; Roesler, U.; Helmuth, R.; Guerra, B. Escherichia coli producing VIM-1 carbapenemase isolated on a pig farm. *J. Antimicrob. Chemother.* **2012**, *67*, 1793–1795. [CrossRef] [PubMed]
114. Rubin, J.E.; Pitout, J.D. Extended-spectrum β-lactamase, carbapenemase and AmpC producing Enterobacteriaceae in companion animals. *Vet. Microbiol.* **2014**, *170*, 10–18. [CrossRef]
115. Schijven, J.F.; Blaak, H.; Schets, F.M.; de Roda Husman, A.M. Fate of Extended-Spectrum beta-Lactamase-Producing Escherichia coli from Faecal Sources in Surface Water and Probability of Human Exposure through Swimming. *Environ. Sci. Technol.* **2015**, *49*, 11825–11833. [CrossRef]
116. Pulss, S.; Semmler, T.; Prenger-Berninghoff, E.; Bauerfeind, R.; Ewers, C. First report of an Escherichia coli strain from swine carrying an OXA-181 carbapenemase and the colistin resistance determinant MCR-1. *Int. J. Antimicrob. Agents* **2017**, *50*, 232–236. [CrossRef] [PubMed]
117. Yousfi, M.; Mairi, A.; Bakour, S.; Touati, A.; Hassissen, L.; Hadjadj, L.; Rolain, J.-M. First report of NDM-5-producing Escherichia coli ST1284 isolated from dog in Bejaia, Algeria. *New Microbes New Infect.* **2015**, *8*, 17–18. [CrossRef]
118. Manges, A.R.; Johnson, J.R. Food-Borne Origins of Escherichia coli Causing Extraintestinal Infections. *Clin. Infect. Dis.* **2012**, *55*, 712–719. [CrossRef] [PubMed]
119. Pantel, A.; on behalf of the CARB-LR group; Boutet-Dubois, A.; Jean-Pierre, H.; Marchandin, H.; Sotto, A.; Lavigne, J.-P. French regional surveillance program of carbapenemase-producing Gram-negative bacilli: Results from a 2-year period. *Eur. J. Clin. Microbiol.* **2014**, *33*, 2285–2292. [CrossRef]
120. Davido, B.; Moussiegt, A.; Dinh, A.; Bouchand, F.; Matt, M.; Senard, O.; Deconinck, L.; Espinasse, F.; Lawrence, C.; Fortineau, N.; et al. Germs of thrones—Spontaneous decolonization of Carbapenem-Resistant Enterobacteriaceae (CRE) and Vancomycin-Resistant Enterococci (VRE) in Western Europe: Is this myth or reality? *Antimicrob. Resist. Infect. Control.* **2018**, *7*, 100. [CrossRef]
121. Seiffert, S.N.; Carattoli, A.; Tinguely, R.; Lupo, A.; Perreten, V.; Endimiani, A. High prevalence of extended-spectrum beta-lactamase, plasmid-mediated AmpC, and carbapenemase genes in pet food. *Antimicrob. Agents Chemother.* **2014**, *58*, 6320–6323. [CrossRef]
122. Gentilini, F.; Turba, M.E.; Pasquali, F.; Mion, D.; Romagnoli, N.; Zambon, E.; Terni, D.; Peirano, G.; Pitout, J.D.D.; Parisi, A.; et al. Hospitalized Pets as a Source of Carbapenem-Resistance. *Front. Microbiol.* **2018**, *9*, 2872. [CrossRef]
123. Ahammad, Z.S.; Sreekrishnan, T.R.; Hands, C.L.; Knapp, C.W.; Graham, D.W. Increased Waterborne blaNDM-1 Resistance Gene Abundances Associated with Seasonal Human Pilgrimages to the Upper Ganges River. *Environ. Sci. Technol.* **2014**, *48*, 3014–3020. [CrossRef]
124. Huang, T.D.; Bogaerts, P.; Berhin, C.; Hoebeke, M.; Bauraing, C.; Glupczynski, Y.; on behalf of a multicentre study group. Increasing proportion of carbapenemase-producing Enterobacteriaceae and emergence of a MCR-1 producer through a multicentric study among hospital-based and private laboratories in Belgium from September to November 2015. *Eurosurveillance* **2017**, *22*. [CrossRef] [PubMed]

125. Milanović, V.; Osimani, A.; Roncolini, A.; Garofalo, C.; Aquilanti, L.; Pasquini, M.; Tavoletti, S.; Vignaroli, C.; Canonico, L.; Ciani, M.; et al. Investigation of the Dominant Microbiota in Ready-to-Eat Grasshoppers and Mealworms and Quantification of Carbapenem Resistance Genes by qPCR. *Front. Microbiol.* **2018**, *9*, 3036. [CrossRef]
126. Abraham, S.; O'Dea, M.; Trott, D.J.; Abraham, R.J.; Hughes, D.; Pang, S.; McKew, G.; Cheong, E.Y.L.; Merlino, J.; Saputra, S. Isolation and plasmid characterization of carbapenemase (IMP-4) producing Salmonella enterica Typhimurium from cats. *Sci. Rep.* **2016**, *6*, 1–7. [CrossRef] [PubMed]
127. Buelow, E.; Bayjanov, J.R.; Majoor, E.; Willems, R.; Bonten, M.J.M.; Schmitt, H.; van Schaik, W. Limited influence of hospital wastewater on the microbiome and resistome of wastewater in a community sewerage system. *FEMS Microbiol. Ecol.* **2018**, *94*. [CrossRef] [PubMed]
128. El Garch, F.; Sauget, M.; Hocquet, D.; LeChaudee, D.; Woehrle, F.; Bertrand, X. mcr-1 is borne by highly diverse Escherichia coli isolates since 2004 in food-producing animals in Europe. *Clin. Microbiol. Infect.* **2017**, *23*, 51.e1–51.e4. [CrossRef]
129. Grøntvedt, C.A.; Elstrøm, P.; Stegger, M.; Skov, R.L.; Andersen, P.S.; Larssen, K.W.; Urdahl, A.M.; Angen, Ø.; Larsen, J.; Åmdal, S.; et al. Methicillin-ResistantStaphylococcus aureusCC398 in Humans and Pigs in Norway: A "One Health" Perspective on Introduction and Transmission. *Clin. Infect. Dis.* **2016**, *63*, 1431–1438. [CrossRef]
130. Pulss, S.; Stolle, I.; Stamm, I.; Leidner, U.; Heydel, C.; Semmler, T.; Prenger-Berninghoff, E.; Ewers, C. Multispecies and Clonal Dissemination of OXA-48 Carbapenemase in Enterobacteriaceae From Companion Animals in Germany, 2009—2016. *Front. Microbiol.* **2018**, *9*, 1265. [CrossRef]
131. Fischer, J.; Schmoger, S.; Jahn, S.; Helmuth, R.; Guerra, B. NDM-1 carbapenemase-producing Salmonella enterica subsp. enterica serovar Corvallis isolated from a wild bird in Germany. *J. Antimicrob. Chemother.* **2013**, *68*, 2954–2956. [CrossRef]
132. Girlich, D.; Poirel, L.; Nordmann, P. Novel ambler class A carbapenem-hydrolyzing beta-lactamase from a Pseudomonas fluorescens isolate from the Seine River, Paris, France. *Antimicrob. Agents Chemother.* **2010**, *54*, 328–332. [CrossRef] [PubMed]
133. Haller, L.; Chen, H.; Ng, C.; Le, T.H.; Koh, T.H.; Barkham, T.; Sobsey, M.; Gin, K.Y. Occurrence and characteristics of extended-spectrum beta-lactamase- and carbapenemase- producing bacteria from hospital effluents in Singapore. *Sci. Total Environ.* **2018**, *615*, 1119–1125. [CrossRef] [PubMed]
134. Chouchani, C.; Marrakchi, R.; Henriques, I.; Correia, A. Occurrence of IMP-8, IMP-10, and IMP-13 metallo-beta-lactamases located on class 1 integrons and other extended-spectrum beta-lactamases in bacterial isolates from Tunisian rivers. *Scand J. Infect. Dis.* **2013**, *45*, 95–103. [CrossRef]
135. Liu, X.; Thungrat, K.; Boothe, D.M. Occurrence of OXA-48 Carbapenemase and Other beta-Lactamase Genes in ESBL-Producing Multidrug Resistant Escherichia coli from Dogs and Cats in the United States, 2009–2013. *Front. Microbiol.* **2016**, *7*, 1057. [PubMed]
136. Smet, A.; Boyen, F.; Pasmans, F.; Butaye, P.; Martens, A.; Nemec, A.; Deschaght, P.; Vaneechoutte, M.; Haesebrouck, F. OXA-23-producing Acinetobacter species from horses: A public health hazard? *J. Antimicrob. Chemother.* **2012**, *67*, 3009–3010. [CrossRef]
137. Vergara, A.; Pitart, C.; Montalvo, T.; Roca, I.; Sabate, S.; Hurtado, J.C.; Planell, R.; Marco, F.; Ramirez, E.; Peracho, V.; et al. Prevalence of Extended-Spectrum-beta-Lactamase- and/or Carbapenemase-Producing Escherichia coli Isolated from Yellow-Legged Gulls from Barcelona, Spain. *Antimicrob. Agents Chemother.* **2017**, *61*, e02071-16. [CrossRef] [PubMed]
138. Baede, V.O.; Broens, E.M.; Spaninks, M.P.; Timmerman, A.J.; Graveland, H.; Wagenaar, J.A.; Duim, B.; Hordijk, J. Raw pet food as a risk factor for shedding of extended-spectrum beta-lactamase-producing Enterobacteriaceae in household cats. *PLoS ONE* **2017**, *12*, e0187239. [CrossRef]
139. Huijbers, P.M.C.; Blaak, H.; de Jong, M.C.M.; Graat, E.A.M.; Vandenbroucke-Grauls, C.M.J.E.; de Roda Husman, A.M. Role of the Environment in the Transmission of Antimicrobial Resistance to Humans: A Review. *Environ. Sci. Technol.* **2015**, *49*, 11993–12004. [CrossRef]
140. Wang, J.; Ma, Z.-B.; Zeng, Z.-L.; Yang, X.-W.; Huang, Y.; Liu, J.-H. Response to Comment on "The role of wildlife (wild birds) in the global transmission of antimicrobial resistance genes". *Zool. Res.* **2017**, *38*, 212. [CrossRef]
141. Fischer, J.; Rodríguez, I.; Schmoger, S.; Friese, A.; Roesler, U.; Helmuth, R.; Guerra, B. Salmonella enterica subsp. enterica producing VIM-1 carbapenemase isolated from livestock farms. *J. Antimicrob. Chemother.* **2012**, *68*, 478–480. [CrossRef]
142. Grönthal, T.; Österblad, M.; Eklund, M.; Jalava, J.; Nykäsenoja, S.; Pekkanen, K.; Rantala, M. Sharing more than friendship—Transmission of NDM-5 ST167 and CTX-M-9 ST69 Escherichia coli between dogs and humans in a family, Finland, 2015. *Eurosurveillance* **2018**, *23*, 1700497. [CrossRef] [PubMed]
143. Hellweger, F.L.; Ruan, X.; Sanchez, S. A Simple Model of Tetracycline Antibiotic Resistance in the Aquatic Environment (with Application to the Poudre River). *Int. J. Environ. Res. Public Heal.* **2011**, *8*, 480–497. [CrossRef] [PubMed]
144. Van Doremalen, N.; Bushmaker, T.; Karesh, W.; Munster, V.J. Stability of Middle East Respiratory Syndrome Coronavirus in Milk. *Emerg. Infect. Dis.* **2014**, *20*, 1263–1264. [CrossRef] [PubMed]
145. Summary ESBL-Attribution-Analysis (ESBLAT). 2018. Available online: https://www.uu.nl/sites/default/files/summary_esbl_attribution_en.pdf (accessed on 1 January 2022).
146. Rhomberg, P.; Jones, R.N. Summary trends for the Meropenem Yearly Susceptibility Test Information Collection Program: A 10-year experience in the United States (1999–2008). *Diagn. Microbiol. Infect. Dis.* **2009**, *65*, 414–426. [CrossRef]
147. González-Torralba, A.; Oteo, J.; Asenjo, A.; Bautista, V.; Fuentes, E.; Alós, J.-I. Survey of Carbapenemase-Producing Enterobacteriaceae in Companion Dogs in Madrid, Spain. *Antimicrob. Agents Chemother.* **2016**, *60*, 2499–2501. [CrossRef]

148. Levast, M.; Deiber, M.; Decroisette, E.; Mallaval, F.-O.; LeComte, C.; Poirel, L.; Carrër, A.; Nordmann, P. Transfer of OXA-48-positive carbapenem-resistant Klebsiella pneumoniae from Turkey to France. *J. Antimicrob. Chemother.* **2011**, *66*, 944–945. [CrossRef]
149. Høg, B.B.; Ellis-Iversen, J.; Sönksen, U.W. Use of Antimicrobial Agents and Occurrence of Antimicrobial Resistance in Bacteria from Food Animals, Food and Humans in Denma. DANMAP 2017. Available online: https://backend.orbit.dtu.dk/ws/files/161713656/Rapport_DANMAP_2017.pdf (accessed on 1 January 2022).
150. Vittecoq, M.; Laurens, C.; Brazier, L.; Durand, P.; Elguero, E.; Arnal, A.; Thomas, F.; Aberkane, S.; Renaud, N.; Prugnolle, F.; et al. VIM-1 carbapenemase-producing Escherichia coli in gulls from southern France. *Ecol. Evol.* **2017**, *7*, 1224–1232. [CrossRef]
151. Zurfluh, K.; Bagutti, C.; Brodmann, P.; Alt, M.; Schulze, J.; Fanning, S.; Stephan, R.; Nüesch-Inderbinen, M. Wastewater is a reservoir for clinically relevant carbapenemase- and 16s rRNA methylase-producing Enterobacteriaceae. *Int. J. Antimicrob. Agents* **2017**, *50*, 436–440. [CrossRef]
152. Fernandes, M.R.; Sellera, F.P.; Moura, Q.; Carvalho, M.P.N.; Rosato, P.N.; Cerdeira, L.; Lincopan, N. Zooanthroponotic Transmission of Drug-Resistant Pseudomonas aeruginosa, Brazil. *Emerg. Infect. Dis.* **2018**, *24*, 1160–1162. [CrossRef]
153. The European Coalition for Farm Animals. The Welfare of Broiler Chickens in the European Union. 2005. Available online: https://www.ciwf.org.uk/research/species-meat-chickens/the-welfare-of-broiler-chickens-in-the-european-union (accessed on 1 January 2022).

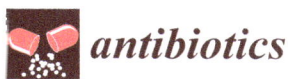 

Article

# Antimicrobial Resistance in Isolates from Cattle with Bovine Respiratory Disease in Bavaria, Germany

Alexander Melchner [1], Sarah van de Berg [1], Nelly Scuda [1], Andrea Feuerstein [1], Matthias Hanczaruk [1], Magdalena Schumacher [1], Reinhard K. Straubinger [2], Durdica Marosevic [1] and Julia M. Riehm [1,*]

[1] Bavarian Health and Food Safety Authority, 85764 Oberschleissheim, Germany; alexander.melchner@t-online.de (A.M.); Sarah.vandeBerg@lgl.bayern.de (S.v.d.B.); Nelly.Scuda@lgl.bayern.de (N.S.); heubeck.a95@gmail.com (A.F.); Matthias.Hanczaruk@lgl.bayern.de (M.H.); Magdalena.Schumacher@lgl.bayern.de (M.S.); Durdica.Marosevic@lgl.bayern.de (D.M.)

[2] Institute of Infectious Diseases and Zoonoses, Department of Veterinary Sciences, Faculty of Veterinary Medicine, Ludwig-Maximilians-University, 80539 Munich, Germany; Reinhard.Straubinger@micro.vetmed.uni-muenchen.de

* Correspondence: Julia.Riehm@lgl.bayern.de

**Abstract:** Patterns of antimicrobial resistance (AMR) regarding *Pasteurella multocida* (n = 345), *Mannheimia haemolytica* (n = 273), *Truperella pyogenes* (n = 119), and *Bibersteinia trehalosi* (n = 17) isolated from calves, cattle and dairy cows with putative bovine respiratory disease syndrome were determined. The aim of this study was to investigate temporal trends in AMR and the influence of epidemiological parameters for the geographic origin in Bavaria, Germany, between July 2015 and June 2020. Spectinomycin was the only antimicrobial agent with a significant decrease regarding not susceptible isolates within the study period (*P. multocida* 88.89% to 67.82%, *M. haemolytica* 90.24% to 68.00%). Regarding *P. multocida*, significant increasing rates of not susceptible isolates were found for the antimicrobials tulathromycin (5.56% to 26.44%) and tetracycline (18.52% to 57.47%). The proportions of multidrug-resistant (MDR) *P. multocida* isolates (n = 48) increased significantly from 3.70% to 22.90%. The proportions of MDR *M. haemolytica* and *P. multocida* isolates (n = 62) were significantly higher in fattening farms (14.92%) compared to dairy farms (3.29%) and also significantly higher on farms with more than 300 animals (19.49%) compared to farms with 100 animals or less (6.92%). The data underline the importance of the epidemiological farm characteristics, here farm type and herd size regarding the investigation of AMR.

**Keywords:** bovine respiratory disease; antimicrobial resistance; multidrug-resistance; *Pasteurella multocida*; *Mannheimia haemolytica*; *Truperella pyogenes*; dairy farm

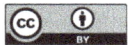

## 1. Introduction

Bovine respiratory disease (BRD) is one of the most significant health problems in bovine medicine worldwide [1]. The syndrome causes significant economic losses in both beef and dairy production farms [2,3]. Regarding its impact on US feedlots, BRD is the most important disease, with an annual incidence of up to 44%, resulting in economic losses of 13.90 USD per animal regarding treatment costs and lower weight gains [3]. Preweaned calves are most affected by BRD in dairy farms [2]. Furthermore, the pregnancy rates, milk yield, and longevity of dairy cows are also negatively influenced by this syndrome [4–6]. The etiology of BRD is multifactorial, as it is caused by infectious and non-infectious factors [7,8]. Stressful conditions are involved in the development of BRD, such as commingling of calves from different sources or transports over long distances [7,9]. Further, viral agents, such as bovine parainfluenza virus type 3 (PI-3), bovine respiratory syncytial virus (BRSV), bovine herpes virus type 1 (BHV-1), bovine viral diarrhea virus (BVDV) and bovine coronavirus (BCoV) are associated with BRD and may promote secondary bacterial infections by impairing the animals' immune system [8,10–12].

Lastly, bacterial pathogens, such as *Mannheimia haemolytica*, *Pasteurella multocida*, *Bibersteinia trehalosi*, *Histophilus somni*, *Mycoplasma bovis* and *Truperella pyogenes* contribute to the clinical picture [8,10,13,14]. These may cause various forms of pneumonia with an acute, subacute, or chronic course. The different forms of disease representation include mainly fibrinous pleuropneumonia, which is the most common form of acute pneumonia in weaned, stressed beef cattle, and suppurative bronchopneumonia often seen in young dairy calves [15,16].

Suitable preventive measures start from the management of young calves and comprise an adequate colostrum supply [17]. Optimized housing conditions with appropriate ventilation that provide adequate air exchange also show preventive effects on BRD [18–20]. Vaccination against both bacterial and viral pathogens is a valuable prevention measure and leads to improved animal health and fewer economic losses [21–23]. However, antibiotic treatment is indicated for controlling acute bacterial infection and the emerged BRD syndrome [23]. In Germany, the approved classes of antibiotic agents aiming at the treatment of respiratory diseases with bacterial origin include ß-lactam antibiotics, fluoroquinolones, phenicols, tetracyclines, trimethoprim-sulphonamides, aminoglycosides, lincosamides, and macrolides, respectively [24]. Besides the treatment of individual diseased animals, metaphylactic medication of all animals within one epidemiological flock is important in this context [25–27]. Metaphylaxis may include antibiotic treatment of clinically healthy animals, if they had close contact with already infected animals, as these are likely to be infected [28].

Worldwide studies indicate that there is a trend towards increasing bacterial resistance towards certain antimicrobial agents, especially multidrug-resistance (MDR) when pathogens of BRD are investigated [29–37]. In the context of the BRD complex, *P. multocida* and *M. haemolytica* isolates are categorized as MDR if they are not susceptible (resistant or intermediate) to at least one agent in at least three antimicrobial classes [38]. Exposure, overuse, or even misuse of antimicrobial substances do provide evolutionary advantages and may result in resistant bacteria [39–41]. Resistance genes spread between pathogens from the bovine respiratory tract. Two forms of horizontal gene transfer appear to play a key role, namely plasmids and so-called integrative and conjugative elements (ICEs) [30,33,42]. The latter contains an entire collection of resistance genes that may transfer horizontally within one single event between strains, species, and even different bacterial genera [43–45].

The alarming increase of antimicrobial resistance (AMR) in both, human and veterinary medicine, as well as the fact that antimicrobial resistant strains do circulate between humans and animals, set the impulse for the World Health Organization (WHO) to adopt a global action plan against increasing antimicrobial resistance in 2015 [46,47]. The primary goal was to ensure that the treatment and therapy of infectious diseases in both human and veterinary medicine will remain effective in the future. Therefore, WHO statements plead for responsible and prudent use of antimicrobial substances [46]. In Germany, this global action plan of the WHO was implemented in the so-called German Antibiotic Resistance Strategy (DARTS) in 2008, and thoroughly followed since then. Important elements of this strategy were the establishment of monitoring systems for the detection of AMR as well as new legal regulations, such as the documentation of antibiotic consumption levels, the determination of therapy frequency in fattening farms, as well as the obligation of antimicrobial resistance testing under certain conditions for veterinarians [48,49].

The aim of this study was to complement the already existing resistance monitoring programs, to record current trends in the development of AMR and MDR with regard to bacterial pathogens of BRD in Bavaria over the last 5 years and finally to derive treatment recommendations from this. Furthermore, the influence of epidemiological parameters, such as farm type and farm size on the resistance pattern were investigated.

## 2. Results
*2.1. Bacterial Isolates*

Between July 2015 and June 2020, a total of 754 isolates were collected from 662 animals with suspected BRD syndrome, origination from 519 farms were included in the present study. *P. multocida* was the most frequently isolated pathogen with 345 (45.76%), followed by 273 *M. haemolytica* (36.21%), 119 *T. pyogenes* (15.78%), and 17 *B. trehalosi* (2.25%) isolates (Table 1 and Figure 1).

**Table 1.** Species, absolute and (relative) number of isolates investigated in the present study over the five-year period 2015–2020 in Bavaria, Germany.

|  | 2015/2016 n (%) | 2016/2017 n (%) | 2017/2018 n (%) | 2018/2019 n (%) | 2019/2020 n (%) | Total |
|---|---|---|---|---|---|---|
| *P. multocida* | 54 (49.09) | 43 (34.96) | 70 (46.36) | 91 (46.19) | 87 (50.29) | 345 (45.76) |
| *M. haemolytica* | 41 (37.27) | 52 (42.28) | 57 (37.75) | 73 (37.06) | 50 (28.90) | 273 (36.21) |
| *T. pyogenes* | 14 (12.73) | 28 (22.76) | 21 (13.90) | 27 (13.70) | 29 (16.76) | 119 (15.78) |
| *B. trehalosi* | 1 (0.91) | 0 (0.00) | 3 (1.99) | 6 (3.05) | 7 (4.05) | 17 (2.25) |
| Total isolates | 110 (100) | 123 (100) | 151 (100) | 197 (100) | 173 (100) | 754 (100) |

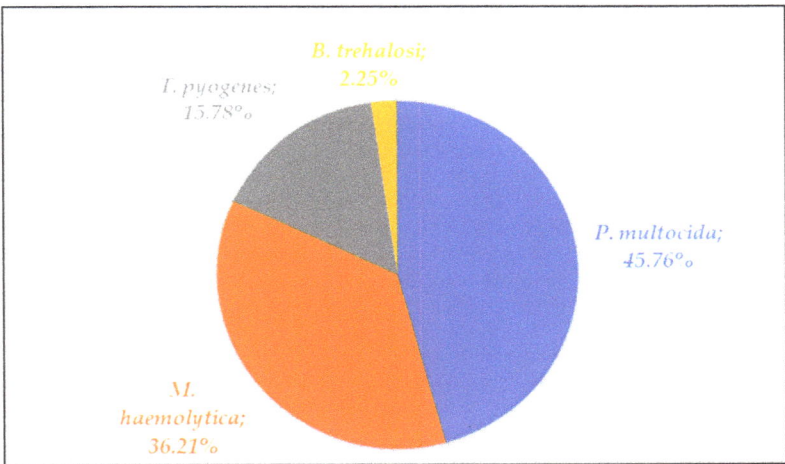

**Figure 1.** Overall proportion (%) of pathogens detected among the total number of analyzed samples.

*2.2. Five-Year Antimicrobial Susceptibility*

Low resistance rates with a proportion of not susceptible isolates of less than five percent were found for *P. multocida* isolates (n = 345) in the case of cephalosporin class (ceftiofur), penicillin class (penicillin G), phenicol class (florfenicol), and fluoroquinolone class (enrofloxacin) (Table 2 and Supplementary Table S1). The fraction of not susceptible isolates was higher for the macrolide antibiotic tulathromycin (15.65%) (Tables 2 and S1). The highest proportion of not susceptible *P. multocida* isolates was found for tetracycline (39.42%), and spectinomycin (78.84%) (Tables 2 and S1).

The proportion of not-susceptible *M. haemolytica* isolates (n = 273) collected over the five-year range was below five percent for ceftiofur, for penicillin G, for enrofloxacin, for florfenicol, and for tulathromycin. It was slightly higher for the macrolide compound tilmicosin with 6.59% (Table 2 and Supplementary Table S2). The highest not susceptibility rates were found when isolates were tested with tetracycline (21.25%), and the aminocyclitol class compound spectinomycin, 80.95% (Tables 2 and S2).

For *T. pyogenes* isolates (n = 119) and *B. trehalosi* isolates (n = 17) no defined species-specific minimum inhibitory concentration (MIC) breakpoints according to CLSI VET guidelines are available to categorize these into susceptible and not susceptible (intermediate and resistant) [50–52]. The distribution of MIC values of these two pathogens is shown in Tables S3 and S4.

**Table 2.** Five-year not susceptible rates of bacterial pathogens with defined species-specific breakpoints according to CLSI VET guidelines.

| Antimicrobial Class | Antimicrobial Agent | P. multocida % (n) | M. haemolytica % (n) | Recommendation for Therapy [1] |
|---|---|---|---|---|
| cephalosporin | ceftiofur | 0.87 (3/345) | 0.00 (0/273) | (+/−) |
| penicillin | penicillin_G | 3.48 (12/345) | 4.76 (13/273) | (+) |
| phenicol | florfenicol | 4.06 (14/345) | 1.10 (3/273) | (+) |
| fluorochinolone | enrofloxacin | 0.29 (1/345) | 2.93 (8/273) | (+/−) |
| macrolide | tilmicosin | no breakpoint [2] | 6.59 (18/273) | (+/−) |
|  | tulathromycin | 15.65 (54/345) | 2.93 (8/273) | (+/−) |
| tetracycline | tetracycline | 39.42 (136/345) | 21.25 (58/273) | (−) |
| aminocyclitol | spectinomycin | 78.84 (272/345) | 80.95 (221/273) | (−) |

[1] recommendation for therapy: (+): suitable for therapy, (+/−): partly suitable for therapy, (−): not suitable for therapy; [2] no breakpoint according to CLSI VET guidelines.

### 2.3. Trends in Not Susceptibility

The trend analysis of the annual not susceptibility rates pertaining to the species *P. multocida* and *M. haemolytica* revealed a decreasing tendency only for the aminocyclitol agent spectinomycin (Tables 3 and S5, Figure 2a,b). The proportion of not susceptible isolates regarding *P. multocida* isolates decreased from 88.89% in the first study year (July 2015 to June 2016) to 67.82% in the last study year (July 2019 to June 2020; OR = 0.70; 95% CI: 0.56–0.86; $p < 0.001$). Regarding *M. haemolytica* isolates it decreased from 90.24% in the first study year to 68.00% in the last study year (OR = 0.71; 95% CI: 0.55–0.90; $p = 0.005$; Tables 3 and S5; Figure 2a,b). For the investigated *P. multocida* isolates significantly increasing rates of not susceptible isolates were found within the study period for the antimicrobial agents tulathromycin (5.56% to 26.44%; OR = 1.60; 95% CI: 1.25–2.08; $p < 0.001$) and tetracycline (18.52% to 57.47%; OR = 1.62; 95% CI: 1.36–1.94; $p < 0.001$; Tables 3 and S5; Figure 2a).

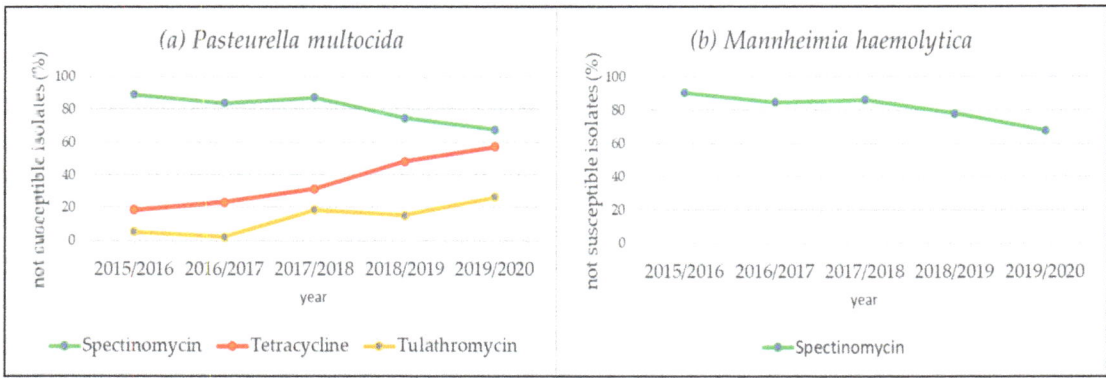

**Figure 2.** Statistically significant trends regarding the not susceptibility of *P. multocida* (a) and *M. haemolytica* (b) over the five-year period in Bavaria, Germany. For spectinomycin a significant decrease in not susceptibility could be observed in *P. multocida* (OR = 0.70; 95% CI: 0.56–0.86; $p < 0.001$) (a) and in *M. haemolytica* isolates (OR = 0.71; 95% CI: 0.55–0.90; $p = 0.005$) (b). For tetracycline (OR = 1.62; 95% CI: 1.36–1.94; $p < 0.001$) and tulathromycin (OR = 1.60; 95% CI: 1.25–2.08; $p < 0.001$) a significant increase in not susceptible *P. multocida* isolates could be observed (a).

**Table 3.** Statistically significant trends, decrease or increase, regarding the not susceptibility of bacterial pathogens investigated in this study over the five-year period 2015–2020 in Bavaria, Germany.

| Pathogen | Antimicrobial Class | Antimicrobial Agent | 2015/2016 % (n) | 2016/2017 % (n) | 2017/2018 % (n) | 2018/2019 % (n) | 2019/2020 % (n) | OR (95% CI) | p-Value |
|---|---|---|---|---|---|---|---|---|---|
| P. multocida | Aminocyclitol | Spectinomycin | 88.89 (48/54) | 83.72 (36/43) | 87.14 (61/70) | 74.73 (68/91) | 67.82 (59/87) | 0.70 (0.56–0.86) | <0.001 |
| | Tetracycline | Tetracycline | 18.52 (10/54) | 23.26 (10/43) | 31.43 (22/70) | 48.35 (44/91) | 57.47 (50/87) | 1.62 (1.36–1.94) | <0.001 |
| | Macrolide | Tulathromycin | 5.56 (3/54) | 2.33 (1/43) | 18.57 (13/70) | 15.38 (14/91) | 26.44 (23/87) | 1.60 (1.25–2.08) | <0.001 |
| M. haemolytica | Aminocyclitol | Spectinomycin | 90.24 (37/41) | 84.62 (44/52) | 85.96 (49/57) | 78.08 (57/73) | 68.00 (34/50) | 0.71 (0.55–0.90) | =0.005 |

## 2.4. Multidrug-Resistance

In veterinary medicine, *P. multocida* and *M. haemolytica* isolates of BRD are classified as multidrug-resistant (MDR) if they are not susceptible to at least one agent in at least three antimicrobial classes [38]. Following this definition, the prevalence of MDR *P. multocida* and *M. haemolytica* isolates was determined in this study. The eight antibiotic agents penicillin G, ceftiofur, florfenicol, enrofloxacin, tilmicosin (only for *M. haemolytica*), tulathromycin, tetracycline and spectinomycin from the seven antimicrobial classes penicillins, cephalosporins, phenicols, fluoroquinolones, macrolides, tetracyclines, and aminocyclitols were included in this MDR analysis. The highest proportion of MDR-isolates was found for *P. multocida* (13.91%), whereas of the *M. haemolytica* isolates only 5.13% were categorized as MDR (Tables 4 and S6). The analysis of annual MDR rates of the bacterial pathogens showed a significant increase over the five-year period for *P. multocida* from 3.70% (first year) to 22.99% (final year) (OR = 1.61; 95% CI: 1.25–2.14; $p < 0.001$) (Figure 3 and Table S6).

**Table 4.** Amongst the investigated bacterial species, the absolute and (relative) number of isolates was ranked into the characteristic pan-susceptible, if these were susceptible towards all agents tested. Not susceptible isolates revealed to be resistant against at least two tested antimicrobial classes (shaded in light grey), and multidrug-resistant (MDR) isolates revealed to be resistant against three or more tested antimicrobial classes (shaded in grey).

| Pathogen | Number of Isolates | Category/Number of Antimicrobial Classes towards Isolates Were Not Susceptible | | | | | | | |
|---|---|---|---|---|---|---|---|---|---|
| | | Pan-Susceptible 0 | Not Susceptible | | MDR | | | | |
| | | | 1 | 2 | 3 | 4 | 5 | 6 | 7 |
| *P. multocida* | 345 (100%) | 52 (15.07%) | 159 (46.09%) | 86 (24.93%) | 37 (10.72%) | 6 (1.74%) | 4 (1.16%) | 1 (0.29%) | 0 (0%) |
| *M. haemolytica* | 273 (100%) | 33 (12.09%) | 176 (64.47%) | 50 (18.32%) | 11 (4.03%) | 3 (1.10%) | 0 (0%) | 0 (0%) | 0 (0%) |

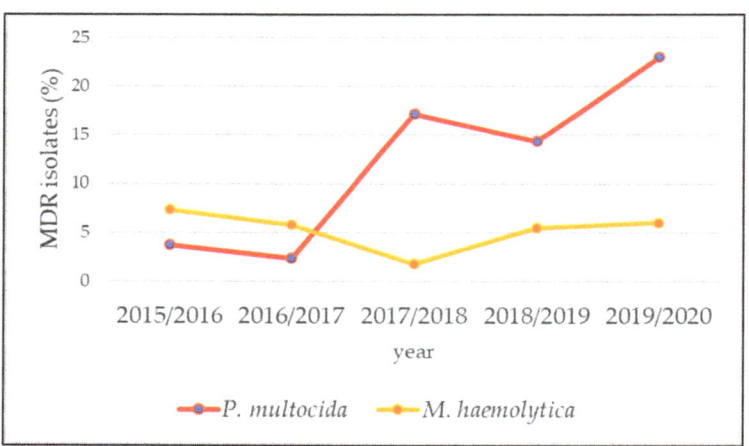

**Figure 3.** Annual multidrug-resistance (MDR) rates of the bacterial pathogens *P. multocida* and *M. haemolytica* from cattle with bovine respiratory disease (BRD) in Bavaria, Germany. A significant increase of MDR *P. multocida* isolates could be observed over the five-year period 2015–2020 (OR = 1.61; 95% CI: 1.25–2.14; $p < 0.001$).

## 2.5. Additional Epidemiological Investigations

Further epidemiological investigations were carried out including the 618 MDR *P. multocida* and *M. haemolytica* isolates. Information on the distribution of animal and farm characteristics is displayed in Tables S7 and S8. Most isolates originated from male animals (56.63%), one to two months old (34.95%) and diseased due to BRD (44.98%). PI-3, *My-*

*coplasma* species and BRSV were detected in 4.05%, 15.37% and 12.94% of the isolates. Most isolates are derived from farms in Upper Bavaria (30.58%), with 101 to 300 animals (58.41%), fattening farms (50.97%) and farms with a therapy frequency of five or less (20.06%).

The results of the univariable and multivariable logistic regression to determine the association of occurrence of MDR *P. multocida* and *M. haemolytica* isolates with certain farm or animal characteristics are shown in Table S7. Regarding the individual animal characteristics, neither sex and age nor the detection of *M. bovis* or PI-3 and BRSV were statistically significantly associated with the occurrence of MDR (Table S7). Additionally, the odds of the occurrence of MDR were not significantly higher among animals, which had died due to the BRD complex as compared to animals that had survived the disease (Table S7). Among the farm characteristics, neither the geographical location in one of the seven administrative districts nor the farm antibiotic therapy frequency was statistically significantly associated with the occurrence of MDR isolates (Table S7). There was a significant association between the occurrence of MDR *P. multocida* and *M. haemolytica* isolates and the size of a farm (Figure 4a). In farms with more than 300 animals, the odds for MDR isolates were significantly higher as compared to farms with a size of 100 animals or less (Adjusted OR = 2.89; 95% CI: 1.26–7.29; $p$ = 0.017; Table S7). Our analysis showed that in farms with 100 animals or less, 6.92% of all isolates were MDR, on farms with 101 to 300 animals 8.31% were MDR, while on farms with more than 300 animals 19.49% of all isolates were MDR (Figure 4a).

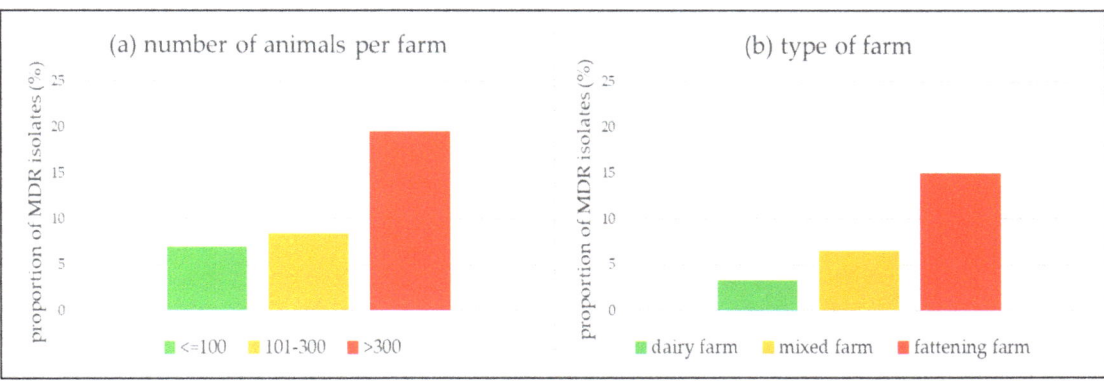

**Figure 4.** Proportion of multidrug-resistant (MDR) *P. multocida* and *M. haemolytica* isolates depending on farm size (number of animals per farm) (**a**) and type of farm (**b**). In farms with more than 300 animals, the odds for isolating MDR isolates were significantly higher than in farms with 100 or less animals (Adjusted OR = 2.89; 95% CI: 1.26–7.29; $p$ = 0.017). In addition, the odds for isolating MDR isolates were significantly lower in dairy (aOR = 0.23; 95% CI: 0.08–0.54; $p$ = 0.002) and mixed farms (aOR = 0.46; 95% CI: 0.20–0.93; $p$ = 0.042) than in fattening farms.

In addition, the odds for isolating MDR isolates were significantly lower in dairy farms (aOR = 0.23; 95% CI: 0.08–0.54; $p$ = 0.002) and mixed farms (aOR = 0.46; 95% CI: 0.20–0.93; $p$ = 0.042) as compared to in pure fattening farms (Table S7). Only 3.29% of isolates in dairy farms were MDR, 6.52% were MDR in mixed farms, while in fattening farms 14.92% were MDR (Figure 4b).

## 3. Discussion

### 3.1. New Legal Regulations and Increase in Tested Isolates

As a response to the increasing trend in the emergence of resistant pathogens and WHO's global action plan on AMR, the German Antibiotic Resistance Strategy (DARTS) was developed and numerous legal changes have been made [46,48]. Out of these, the amendment to the 2018 "Tierärztliche Hausapothekenverordnung", a national German law, obliges veterinarians to ensure the efficacy regarding antimicrobial therapy applying prior resistance testing under certain conditions [49]. This legal change is visible, in our study, as the number of all tested bacterial isolates sent to our laboratory has increased since the third investigation year with 151 isolates compared to 197 isolates in the following observation period (Table 1).

### 3.2. Therapy Guide for the Practitioner

With AMR of bacterial isolates on the rise, precise knowledge of the resistance situation at hand is essential for the targeted treatment of bacterial infections [29,30,32,34]. Since there is only an obligation to determine resistance in certain cases and antibiotic therapy must be started immediately in acute cases of the disease, the practicing veterinarian has to rely on existing data and studies on the local resistance situation [49,53]. Currently, the Germany-wide resistance monitoring program GERM-Vet as well as the Swiss therapy guide for veterinarians advises valuable treatment recommendations considering pharmacological aspects [34,54]. The present study was evaluated on reappraising these guidelines with up-to-date clinical data from Bavaria, Germany (Table 2).

### 3.3. Antimicrobial Agents with a Favourable Resistance Situation

The Swiss therapy guideline recommends the phenicol agent florfenicol as a first-line antibiotic for the treatment of acutely ill animals with BRD [54]. This compound offers several advantages: firstly, it has a bactericidal effect and thus has advantages over bacteriostatic agents that only inhibit growth and replication and thus depend on good immunocompetence, which may no longer be present in cattle suffering from BRD [53–56]. Secondly, one shot preparations are approved and very practical to use, as a single subcutaneous injection is sufficient [24]. In our analysis, florfenicol showed excellent efficacies for all pathogens (Table 2). However, nine of 14 florfenicol not susceptible *P. multocida* isolates were isolated in the final study year, which might indicate a tendency of upcoming resistance of this bacterial species against florfenicol and needs to be observed in detail in the future (Table S5). Similar increasing trends towards florfenicol-resistant *M. haemolytica* have been reported by the GERM-Vet data in recent years. That underlines the importance of continuous monitoring of resistance trends [34]. We conclude that the benefits of florfenicol outweigh the above-mentioned upcoming risk of resistance development and still recommend florfenicol for therapy in cattle suffering from BRD.

As second-line antibiotics, the Swiss therapy guideline recommends, among others, the use of all compounds of the ß-lactam antimicrobials, with the exception of third-generation cephalosporins, as ceftiofur [54]. In the present study, the proportion of not susceptible isolates for penicillin G regarding the investigated bacterial species was below five percent (Table 2). Consequently, we recommend penicillin G, a member of the ß-lactams, for the therapy of BRD.

At the third-line position, the Swiss therapy guide lists the 3rd and 4th generation cephalosporins, which include the antimicrobial agent ceftiofur and the fluoroquinolone antimicrobial class, including enrofloxacin [54]. It should be noted that these represent important therapeutic reserve antibiotics in human medicine against (MDR) germs, such as methicillin/oxacillin-resistant staphylococci. The WHO classifies these substances, therefore, as "highest priority critically important antimicrobials" and calls on veterinarians to use them prudently, if at all necessary [53,57]. In Germany, too, the cephalosporins of the 3rd and 4th generation as well as the fluoroquinolones are classified as reserve antibiotics and should only be used as antibiotics of last resort if no other effective compounds are available [53]. The legislator, therefore, requires resistance testing or a known resistance situation in the respective farm, which is known from previous antimicrobial susceptibility testing, for every use of these reserve antibiotics [49,53]. Given that ceftiofur is an antimicrobial of last resort, it is quite encouraging that the fraction of not susceptible isolates for *P. multocida* and *M. haemolytica* in our study was less than one percent (Table 2). Data originating from a current North American study regarding feedlot cattle show that the resistance rates for ceftiofur, which are between 3% and 33% for *P. multocida* and between 0% and 4% for *M. haemolytica*, were substantially higher compared to our study from Bavaria (Table 2) [30]. The outcome of the resistance situation regarding the fluoroquinolone agent enrofloxacin is also favorable (Table 2). Given that both ceftiofur and enrofloxacin are important therapeutic reserves, these two antimicrobial agents can only be recommended for therapy to a limited and well-considered extent (Table 2).

*3.4. Antimicrobial Agents with Unfavorable Resistance Situation*

In the Swiss therapy guidelines, the agent tetracycline is mentioned as a second-line antibiotic for the treatment of acutely ill animals and as an antimicrobial substance for metaphylaxis. However, it is pointed out that its efficacy is limited due to a considerable AMR rate [54]. The latter has been described for BRD pathogens already since the 1990s and was confirmed since then in studies from all over the world [29,30,34,35]. The unfavorable resistance situation was also reflected in the present study. 39.42% of *P. multocida* and 21.25% of *M. haemolytica* isolates were revealed to be not susceptible (Table 2). For *P. multocida*, a significant increase of the portion of not susceptible isolates from 18.52% in the first study year up to 57.47% in the last study year was found (Tables 3 and S5, Figure 2a). Reasons for the decrease in efficacy could be the high use of this compound. In North American feedlots, tetracycline is one of the most frequently used antibiotics for the treatment of BRD, but also for the prevention of liver abscesses [30,31]. In Germany, tetracycline is in terms of volume the most frequently used antibiotic for calves and cattle kept in fattening farms [58]. Due to the demonstrated increase in resistance levels and very poor efficacy, the general use of tetracycline in calf and cattle fattening should be reconsidered and can, therefore, not be recommended for the therapy of BRD (Table 2).

Antibiotics from the macrolide class are also listed as agents for metaphylactic treatment in the Swiss therapy guidelines [54]. We observed a significant increase in not susceptible *P. multocida* isolates from 5.56% in the first study year up to 26.44% in the last study year regarding tulathromycin (Tables 3 and S5, Figure 2a). Within the scope of the Germany-wide resistance monitoring GERM-Vet, an increase of resistant *P. multocida* isolates from 3% in 2016 up to 14% in 2018 was also detected and currently confirms the trend towards a higher resistance rate against tulathromycin [34]. It is of particular concern that although this compound has been authorized in Europe by the European Medicines Agency only since 2003, its resistance situation has increased so rapidly within only few years [59]. This fact is furthermore worrying, as tulathromycin is not only approved and used for therapy but also for metaphylactic treatment [24,30,33]. There is a strong accumulation in inflamed lung tissue and also accomplishes a concentration above the minimum inhibitory concentration (MIC) of over seven days after a single subcutaneous injection [24,60]. Such one-shot preparations, therefore, offer enormous advantages purely from a hands-on point of view, since an animal only needs to be treated once at a time. Nevertheless, it should be emphasized that this antimicrobial class also belongs to the "highest priority critically important antimicrobials" defined by the WHO and represent one of a few available therapeutic options for serious bacterial infections [57]. In this context, the use of tulathromycin in metaphylaxis should also be reconsidered (Table 2).

Spectinomycin from the aminocyclitol class cannot be recommended for the treatment of BRD due to an unfavorable resistance situation (Table 2). With a proportion of 78.84% not susceptible *P. multocida* and 80.95 % not susceptible *M. haemolytica* isolates, spectinomycin represents the antimicrobial agent with the highest proportion of not susceptible isolates in our analysis (Table 2). Moreover, spectinomycin is not among the most frequently used compounds in calf and cattle fattening, and the consumption quantities did not increase in recent years [30,58]. However, a significant decrease of not susceptible isolates against spectinomycin from 88.89% to 67.82% and 90.24% to 68.00% could be seen in *P. multocida* and *M. haemolytica* isolates (Tables 3 and S5, Figure 2a,b).

*3.5. Multidrug-Resistance*

As described above, eight antibiotic agents from seven antimicrobial classes were included in the MDR analysis because they have species-specific breakpoints according to the CLSI VET guidelines [50]. However, it must be mentioned that there are other antibiotic agents from these seven classes with species-specific minimum inhibitory concentration (MIC) breakpoints for respiratory diseases in cattle. For example, the agent tildipirosin and gamithromycin from the macrolide class or danofloxacin from the fluoroquinolone class were not tested for susceptibility in our laboratory despite the presence of species-specific breakpoints and thus could not be included in the MDR analysis. Ampicillin could also not be included in the analysis because the inhibitory concentrations on the microtiter plate we used were in a higher range than the breakpoints set by CLSI [50]. Since we did not test all antibiotic agents with defined breakpoints for susceptibility, it must be assumed that even more isolates in our data set could be characterized as MDR. A notable finding in our study was the higher rate of MDR *P. multocida* isolates (13.91%) compared to *M. haemolytica* isolates (5.13%) (Tables 4 and S6). This effect was explained in prior publications by different gene transfer and integration rates, or the persistence of ICEs hosting resistance genes and regarding diverse bacterial species [30]. However, the rate of MDR *P. multocida* isolates increased significantly from 3.70% in 2015/2016 to 22.99% in 2019/2020 in the present study (Figure 3, Table S6). This most alarming result was observed also in isolates from North America and illustrates that increasing AMR is a worldwide problem [30,37]. Resistance levels in North America appear high, with proportions of MDR *P. multocida* isolates exceeding 90% and proportions of MDR *M. haemolytica* isolates exceeding 80%, respectively [30]. These numbers exceed those determined in the present study for Bavarian farms (Figure 2, Table S7). It must be mentioned, however, that it is difficult to compare MDR prevalences from different studies, as MIC breakpoints other than those specific to veterinary medicine are often used to divide isolates into susceptible, intermediate and resistant [38].

*3.6. Additional Epidemiological Investigations*

The investigation of further epidemiological parameters concluded that no animal characteristics were associated with a higher probability of occurrence of MDR *P. multocida* and *M. haemolytica* isolates (Table S7). However, it was seen that the odds for MDR isolates were significantly lower in dairy farms (aOR = 0.23; 95% CI: 0.08–0.54; $p$ = 0.002) and mixed farms (aOR = 0.46; 95% CI: 0.20–0.93; $p$ = 0.042) compared to fattening farms (Table S7, Figure 4b). The reasons why the resistance problem mainly affects fattening farms can only be speculated and requires further research. However, it is known that the stressful transport from a dairy farm, birthplace, to the fattening farm, as well as the assortment of calves from many individual farms of origin, increases the risk of BRD and thus the need for antimicrobial treatment [7,9,23]. In the U.S., such groups of animals at increased risk for BRD are treated metaphylactically upon arrival in the feedlot to reduce morbidity and mortality rates and achieve better fattening results [25–27,30,31]. In Germany, metaphylactic treatment of an entire group of animals is also permitted. However, it requires diseased animals within this group that show clinical signs and the concern that the healthy animals in the group will also rapidly become ill [28,53]. In prior studies investigating the metaphylactic use of antimicrobial agents in groups of animals, it was shown that the administration of antimicrobial agents favored the shedding of MDR isolates and increased the likelihood of finding such MDR isolates in stablemates after contagious spreading [61,62]. Equally important to mention in this context is the small farm structure of dairy farms within Bavaria with an average herd size of 40 dairy cows per farm [63]. On these farms, calves are often kept individually in calf hutches during the first weeks of life. On the one hand, this is associated with a lower risk of developing BRD and possibly results in a more targeted individual antimicrobial treatment for various diseases compared to the situation in fattening farms [64–66]. There, the beef cattle are kept in groups and subsequently treated possibly as an epidemiologic unit [25–27,30,31]. In order to limit antimicrobial metaphylaxis and the resulting development of AMR, German law requires laboratory diagnostics including pathogen identification and AMR testing in the case of repeated use of antibiotics in certain age groups and production steps [49].

In addition to the type of farm, the size of the farm is also a critical variable (Figure 4a). In the present study, the odds for MDR isolates were significantly higher on farms with more than 300 animals than on farms with 100 animals or less (aOR = 2.89; 95% CI: 1.26–7.29; $p$ = 0.017; Table S7, Figure 4a). At the same time, data from the Federal Ministry of Agriculture and Food show that the frequency of antimicrobial treatment in recent years has been higher for farms with a larger number of animals, and thus more frequently treated with antimicrobials, than on farms with a smaller number of animals [58]. It remains speculative why antimicrobials are used more frequently on farms with a higher number of animals and whether this influenced the higher probability of the presence of MDR isolates. One possible explanation could be that farms with smaller animal numbers have better control of infectious diseases resulting in better individual animal treatment [66]. Other studies have shown that a smaller number of individual animals per group in the animal husbandry departments is advantageous, as the risk of BRD infection increases with the number of animals per group [64,65].

In the present study, there was no statistically significant association between the frequency of therapy and the occurrence of MDR isolates (Table S7). It needs to be mentioned, however, that the values of the treatment frequency only refer to the respective half-year of sampling, but the fattening period lasts more than six months and the values in the preceding or following half-year could differ markedly from the one considered in the analysis. Furthermore, the treatment frequency refers to the entire farm, so it is possible that the animals in our analysis were kept in a barn compartment where fewer antimicrobials were applied. In addition, the treatment frequency refers to all antimicrobials used in the half-year and thus also includes treatments against other diseases. The value of the farm treatment frequency in our study is, therefore, maybe less suitable as an indicator of antimicrobial consumption.

### 3.7. Limits of the Study

The samples analyzed in the study include samples from the upper respiratory tract, such as nasal swabs but also samples from the lower respiratory tract, such as organ samples from necropsy or bronchoalveolar lavage fluid. However, there is evidence that cultures of nasal swabs from the upper airways are not representative of the pathogen in the lower airways [67]. One study revealed that although samples from both the upper and lower airways were positive for *M. haemolytica*, only 77% showed an identical pulse field gel electrophoresis type [67]. We cannot rule out that the isolates originating from nasal swabs in our study may not be responsible for the clinical picture of BRD.

Another disadvantage of the study is that it is not known whether or how often antimicrobial treatment was applied before sampling. The extent to which immediate antimicrobial treatment before sampling influences the resistance pattern is also controversially discussed in other studies [30,33,61,62]. However, it could be that a previous antimicrobial treatment exerts a selection pressure towards more resistant strains and that the original microbial flora is not represented in these samples.

Another important point to mention is that our study is not an analysis with a clearly defined sampling plan, as is the case, for example, in the national resistance monitoring GERM-Vet, but is a retrospective evaluation of all isolates sent in [34]. Therefore, and following previous publications, only a single individual of each species was included per quarter of a year per farm in our analysis to prevent bias and overrepresentation of clonal isolates [36,68]. Nevertheless, there could also be a potential geographical bias in our dataset, as described in other studies, because our study only includes isolates from Bavaria, a single state of Germany, and even within Bavaria, more samples in our analysis originate from the southern districts than from the northern ones (Supplementary Materials Tables S7 and S8) [30,36,37].

Finally, it should be mentioned that additional molecular screening for AMR genes, as also carried out in recent publications, could provide further insights, especially with regard to the role of ICEs in the spread of MDR isolates and should be part of future endeavors [30,33].

## 4. Materials and Methods

### 4.1. Study Design and Origin of Animals

Data included in the present study were collected within the scope of the state veterinary laboratory diagnostics at the Bavarian Health and Food Safety Authority. In the present study, the investigated samples originated from calves, cattle, or dairy cows with putative symptoms of BRD in Bavaria, Germany, from July 2015 to June 2020. In the present study, cows were kept in dairy farms solely for the purpose of milk production, in fattening farms, cattle were kept for meat production, and finally, in mixed farms, both categories of animals were kept. In order to prevent bias and over-representation of clonal isolates, only one isolate of a species per farm per quarter year was included in the data set, following previous publications [36,68].

### 4.2. Bacterial Isolates

The specimens, here nasal swabs, bronchoalveolar lavage fluid, or lung tissue samples, were analyzed in the ISO 17025 accredited laboratory at the Bavarian Health and Food Safety Authority. Samples were initially inoculated on Columbia sheep blood agar (Oxoid, Wesel, Germany) and incubated at 37 °C for 24 to 48 h under aerobic conditions as well as under a microaerophilic atmosphere, at 10% $CO_2$. To isolate pure suspicious colonies of *P. multocida*, *M. haemolytica*, *B. trehalosi* or *T. pyogenes*, fresh subcultures were incubated under the above-described conditions. Identification of bacterial species was carried out using MALDI-TOF MS (Bruker, Bremen, Germany).

Regarding the isolation of *Mycoplasma* species, animal samples were inoculated in specific Thermo Scientific™ Mycoplasma/Ureaplasma Broth that inhibits the growth of most gram-negative, gram-positive bacteria, as well as yeasts (Thermo Scientific, Schwerte, Germany), and incubated microaerophilic for 120 h at 37 °C with 10% $CO_2$.

### 4.3. Antimicrobial Susceptibility Testing

Antimicrobial susceptibility testing was carried out according to the protocols published in VET01 5th edition, VET01S 5th edition and VET06 1st edition, by the Clinical and Laboratory Standards Institute (CLSI), Wayne, PA, USA [50–52]. The microbroth dilution method was carried out on 16 different antibiotic substances as commercially available and according to the manufacturer's instructions (Micronaut-S, Grosstiere 4, Merlin, Bruker, Bornheim, Germany). This panel was designed to test on recommended antibiotics for the treatment of farm animals in Germany. The minimum inhibitory concentration (MIC) of each isolate and antimicrobial substance was metered using a photometric plate reader system (Micronaut scan, MCN6 software, Merlin, Bruker, Bornheim, Germany). Subsequently, the MIC value was reconciled with determined species-specific breakpoints to categorize the respective *M. haemolytica* and *P. multocida* isolates into "susceptible", "intermediate" and "resistant" for the tested antimicrobial agents: ceftiofur, penicillin G, florfenicol, enrofloxacin, tilmicosin (only *M. haemolytica*), tulathromycin, tetracyclin and spectinomycin [50]. For the antibiotic agent amoxicillin clavulanic acid, cephalotin, trimethoprim-sulfamethoxazole, colistin, tiamulin, erythromycin and gentamicin, no species-specific breakpoints for bovines with BRD are available. Specific breakpoints for *T. pyogenes* and *B. trehalosi* have not been published by the CLSI for any of the tested antibiotic agents for veterinary medicine either, so that only the distribution of the MIC can be given [50–52].

Regarding the BRD syndrome, *P. multocida* and *M. haemolytica* were termed MDR isolates if they were not susceptible (intermediate and resistant) to at least one antibiotic substance in three or more antimicrobial classes [38]. Following this definition, our study investigated the prevalence of MDR *P. multocida* and *M. haemolytica* isolates under epidemiological aspects.

*4.4. Viral Isolates*

Within the scope of the diagnostic services at the Bavarian Health and Food Safety Authority, Germany, results on further viral pathogens were incorporated regarding BRSV and PI-3.

*4.5. Epidemiological Data*

In addition to the isolated pathogens and respective resistance, epidemiological data on the isolated was collected, including sex of the animal, age of the animal, geographical location of the farm, type of farm, herd size of the farm and antimicrobial therapy frequency of the farm, respectively. Furthermore, it was investigated whether the animal died because of BRD. Data were obtained from the German database "Herkunftssicherungs- und Informationssystem für Tiere" (HIT). The HIT database contains comprehensive data on every single animal, including date of birth, sex, date of death and the status of animal diseases, such as BHV-1. For reasons of animal traceability, the database minutely reveals dates and addresses of trading procedures. Extra data pertaining to farms, such as the geographical location, the age and sex statistics on herds, the number of animals and the corresponding antimicrobial therapy frequency were also be downloaded. All results on animals were connected to the unique ear tag number that is assigned to each animal in the HIT database. It further allowed linking the respective farm characteristics from the HIT database, even beyond the death of an animal. Death due to BRD was defined as death within 14 days after diagnosis, assuming a median recovery time from BRD of 14 days [8]. All data on farms included in the study were determined retrospectively for the initial sampling date. The geographical location of the farm was extracted on administrative district level in Bavaria, here, North Bavaria (Upper, Middle, Lower Franconia and Upper Palatinate), Lower Bavaria, Upper Bavaria, or Swabia. The classification into the type of farm was made by us on the basis of the age and gender statistics in the HIT database. A farm was defined as a dairy farm if it had female animals with calving and male animals only up to the age of four months. If male animals over four months of age were recorded in addition to female animals with calving, we assumed that this farm with cows and female offspring also kept male animals for fattening and, therefore, the farm is categorized as a mixed farm with milk production and beef production. Farms were defined as fattening farms if they kept only male animals or female animals that had not reached first calving age and were, therefore, not used for milk production. Therapy frequency per half-year represents an indicator of the use of antibiotics. It is calculated by multiplying the number of animals treated by the number of treatment days for each active substance used. The sum of all these multiplications per half-year is then divided by the average number of animals kept in the corresponding half-year. In Germany, this parameter is notified officially regarding fattening farms with more than 20 animals since the 16th Amendment to the Medicinal Products Act in 2014 [58,69].

*4.6. Statistical Analysis*

First, the proportion of isolates containing *M. haemolytica* and *P. multocida*, respectively, per year and for the whole study period was determined. Next, the proportion of not susceptible/MDR isolates was calculated. To investigate whether to proportion of not susceptible/MDR isolates changed over the course of the study period, univariable logistic regression analyses were conducted using the year of sampling as an independent variable. To determine what animal and farm factors are associated with MDR, we conducted multivariable logistic regression analyses. Therefore, the univariable effects of the year the sample was taken, the presence of other pathogens in the isolate (*Mycoplasma* species, BRSV and PI-3), age, sex and disease outcome (diseased vs. deceased) of the animal, as well as region, type (dairy vs. fattening farm), size and therapy frequency of the farm were assessed. Factors with a $p$-value $\geq 0.2$ were considered for the multivariable model. The most parsimonious model was determined in a stepwise, forward-selection process. All analyses were conducted in R Statistical Software (R Core Team, R: A language and environment for statistical computing. R Foundation for Statistical Computing, Vienna, Austria, 2021).

**Supplementary Materials:** The following are available online at https://www.mdpi.com/article/10.3390/antibiotics10121538/s1, Table S1: Distribution of minimum inhibitory concentration (MIC) values over the five-year period 2015–2020 for *Pasteurella multocida* in Bavaria, Germany, Table S2: Distribution of minimum inhibitory concentration (MIC) values over the five-year period 2015–2020 for *Mannhemia haemolytica* in Bavaria, Germany, Table S3: Distribution of minimum inhibitory concentration (MIC) values over the five-year period 2015–2020 for *Truperella pyogenes* in Bavaria, Germany, Table S4: Distribution of minimum inhibitory concentration (MIC) values over the five-year period 2015–2020 for *Bibersteinia trehalosi* in Bavaria, Germany, Table S5: Annual not susceptibility rates of *Pasteurella multocida* and *Mannheimia haemolytica* over the five-year period 2015–2020 in Bavaria, Germany, Table S6: Annual multidrug-resistance (MDR) rates of *P. multocida* and *M. haemolytica* over the five-year period 2015–2020 in Bavaria, Germany, Table S7: Association between the occurrence of multidrug-resistant (MDR) *Pasteurella multocida* and *Mannheimia haemolytica* isolates and certain animal and farm characteristics over the five-year period 2015–2020 in Bavaria, Germany, Table S8: Overview of *Pasteurella multocida* and *Mannheimia haemolytica* isolates included in the study with corresponding resistance pattern, animal characteristics and farm characteristics.

**Author Contributions:** Conceptualization, A.M., R.K.S. and J.M.R., methodology, M.H. and M.S.; software, S.v.d.B., M.H., M.S., D.M. and J.M.R.; validation, A.M., S.v.d.B., N.S., A.F., R.K.S., D.M. and J.M.R.; formal analysis, A.M., S.v.d.B., D.M. and J.M.R.; investigation, A.M., S.v.d.B., A.F., D.M. and J.M.R.; resources, M.H., M.S. and J.M.R.; data curation, A.M., M.H., M.S. and J.M.R.; writing—original draft preparation, A.M., A.F. and J.M.R.; writing—review and editing, S.v.d.B., N.S., R.K.S. and D.M.; visualization, A.M. and J.M.R.; supervision, R.K.S. and J.M.R.; project administration, J.M.R.; funding acquisition, M.H. and J.M.R. All authors have read and agreed to the published version of the manuscript.

**Funding:** This research received no external funding.

**Institutional Review Board Statement:** Not applicable.

**Informed Consent Statement:** Not applicable.

**Acknowledgments:** The authors are grateful to the veterinary bacteriology staff members for technical assistance. Furthermore, the authors are grateful to the staff of the StabLab, Ludwig-Maximilians-University Munich, for a basic teaching class in statistical analyses.

**Conflicts of Interest:** The authors declare no conflict of interest.

## References

1. Hilton, W.M. BRD in 2014: Where have we been, where are we now, and where do we want to go? *Anim. Health Res. Rev.* **2014**, *15*, 120–122. [CrossRef]
2. Dubrovsky, S.A.; Van Eenennaam, A.L.; Karle, B.M.; Rossitto, P.V.; Lehenbauer, T.W.; Aly, S.S. Bovine respiratory disease (BRD) cause-specific and overall mortality in preweaned calves on California dairies: The BRD 10K study. *J. Dairy Sci.* **2019**, *102*, 7320–7328. [CrossRef]
3. Snowder, G.D.; Van Vleck, L.D.; Cundiff, L.V.; Bennett, G.L. Bovine respiratory disease in feedlot cattle: Environmental, genetic, and economic factors. *J. Anim. Sci.* **2006**, *84*, 1999–2008. [CrossRef]
4. Teixeira, A.G.V.; McArt, J.A.A.; Bicalho, R.C. Thoracic ultrasound assessment of lung consolidation at weaning in Holstein dairy heifers: Reproductive performance and survival. *J. Dairy Sci.* **2017**, *100*, 2985–2991. [CrossRef] [PubMed]
5. Dunn, T.R.; Ollivett, T.L.; Renaud, D.L.; Leslie, K.E.; LeBlanc, S.J.; Duffield, T.F.; Kelton, D.F. The effect of lung consolidation, as determined by ultrasonography, on first-lactation milk production in Holstein dairy calves. *J. Dairy Sci.* **2018**, *101*, 5404–5410. [CrossRef] [PubMed]
6. Bach, A. Associations between several aspects of heifer development and dairy cow survivability to second lactation. *J. Dairy Sci.* **2011**, *94*, 1052–1057. [CrossRef]
7. Sanderson, M.W.; Dargatz, D.A.; Wagner, B.A. Risk factors for initial respiratory disease in United States' feedlots based on producer-collected daily morbidity counts. *Can. Vet. J.* **2008**, *49*, 373–378.

8. Grissett, G.P.; White, B.J.; Larson, R.L. Structured literature review of responses of cattle to viral and bacterial pathogens causing bovine respiratory disease complex. *J. Vet. Intern. Med.* **2015**, *29*, 770–780. [CrossRef] [PubMed]
9. Ishizaki, H.; Kariya, Y. Road transportation stress promptly increases bovine peripheral blood absolute NK cell counts and cortisol levels. *J. Vet. Med. Sci.* **2010**, *72*, 747–753. [CrossRef]
10. Headley, S.A.; Okano, W.; Balbo, L.C.; Marcasso, R.A.; Oliveira, T.E.; Alfieri, A.F.; Negri Filho, L.C.; Michelazzo, M.Z.; Rodrigues, S.C.; Baptista, A.L.; et al. Molecular survey of infectious agents associated with bovine respiratory disease in a beef cattle feedlot in southern Brazil. *J. Vet. Diagn. Investig.* **2018**, *30*, 249–251. [CrossRef]
11. Lopez, A.; Thomson, R.G.; Savan, M. The pulmonary clearance of Pasteurella hemolytica in calves infected with bovine parainfluenza-3 virus. *Can. J. Comp. Med.* **1976**, *40*, 385–391. [PubMed]
12. Gershwin, L.J.; Gunther, R.A.; Hornof, W.J.; Larson, R.F. Effect of infection with bovine respiratory syncytial virus on pulmonary clearance of an inhaled antigen in calves. *Am. J. Vet. Res.* **2008**, *69*, 416–422. [CrossRef] [PubMed]
13. Kishimoto, M.; Tsuchiaka, S.; Rahpaya, S.S.; Hasebe, A.; Otsu, K.; Sugimura, S.; Kobayashi, S.; Komatsu, N.; Nagai, M.; Omatsu, T.; et al. Development of a one-run real-time PCR detection system for pathogens associated with bovine respiratory disease complex. *J. Vet. Med. Sci.* **2017**, *79*, 517–523. [CrossRef] [PubMed]
14. Anton, B.P.; Harhay, G.P.; Smith, T.P.; Blom, J.; Roberts, R.J. Comparative Methylome Analysis of the Occasional Ruminant Respiratory Pathogen Bibersteinia trehalosi. *PLoS ONE* **2016**, *11*, e0161499. [CrossRef]
15. Panciera, R.J.; Confer, A.W. Pathogenesis and pathology of bovine pneumonia. *Vet. Clin. N. Am. Food Anim. Pract.* **2010**, *26*, 191–214. [CrossRef] [PubMed]
16. Andrews, G.A.; Kennedy, G.A. Respiratory diagnostic pathology. *Vet. Clin. N. Am. Food Anim. Pract.* **1997**, *13*, 515–547. [CrossRef]
17. Virtala, A.M.; Gröhn, Y.T.; Mechor, G.D.; Erb, H.N. The effect of maternally derived immunoglobulin G on the risk of respiratory disease in heifers during the first 3 months of life. *Prev. Vet. Med.* **1999**, *39*, 25–37. [CrossRef]
18. Ollivett, T.L. How Does Housing Influence Bovine Respiratory Disease in Dairy and Veal Calves? *Vet. Clin. N. Am. Food Anim. Pract.* **2020**, *36*, 385–398. [CrossRef] [PubMed]
19. Lago, A.; McGuirk, S.M.; Bennett, T.B.; Cook, N.B.; Nordlund, K.V. Calf respiratory disease and pen microenvironments in naturally ventilated calf barns in winter. *J. Dairy Sci.* **2006**, *89*, 4014–4025. [CrossRef]
20. Nordlund, K.V.; Halbach, C.E. Calf Barn Design to Optimize Health and Ease of Management. *Vet. Clin. N. Am. Food Anim. Pract.* **2019**, *35*, 29–45. [CrossRef]
21. Wildman, B.K.; Perrett, T.; Abutarbush, S.M.; Guichon, P.T.; Pittman, T.J.; Booker, C.W.; Schunicht, O.C.; Fenton, R.K.; Jim, G.K. A comparison of 2 vaccination programs in feedlot calves at ultra-high risk of developing undifferentiated fever/bovine respiratory disease. *Can. Vet. J.* **2008**, *49*, 463–472. [PubMed]
22. Schunicht, O.C.; Booker, C.W.; Jim, G.K.; Guichon, P.T.; Wildman, B.K.; Hill, B.W. Comparison of a multivalent viral vaccine program versus a univalent viral vaccine program on animal health, feedlot performance, and carcass characteristics of feedlot calves. *Can. Vet. J.* **2003**, *44*, 43–50.
23. Edwards, T.A. Control methods for bovine respiratory disease for feedlot cattle. *Vet. Clin. N. Am. Food Anim. Pract.* **2010**, *26*, 273–284. [CrossRef]
24. Universität Leipzig. Veterinärmedizinischer Informationsdienst für Arzneimittelanwendung, Toxikologie und Arzneimittelrecht. Available online: https://vetidata.de/public/quicksearch/do.php (accessed on 14 December 2021).
25. Baptiste, K.E.; Kyvsgaard, N.C. Do antimicrobial mass medications work? A systematic review and meta-analysis of randomised clinical trials investigating antimicrobial prophylaxis or metaphylaxis against naturally occurring bovine respiratory disease. *Pathog. Dis.* **2017**, *75*, ftx083. [CrossRef]
26. Abell, K.M.; Theurer, M.E.; Larson, R.L.; White, B.J.; Apley, M. A mixed treatment comparison meta-analysis of metaphylaxis treatments for bovine respiratory disease in beef cattle. *J. Anim. Sci.* **2017**, *95*, 626–635. [CrossRef] [PubMed]
27. Tennant, T.C.; Ives, S.E.; Harper, L.B.; Renter, D.G.; Lawrence, T.E. Comparison of tulathromycin and tilmicosin on the prevalence and severity of bovine respiratory disease in feedlot cattle in association with feedlot performance, carcass characteristics, and economic factors. *J. Anim. Sci.* **2014**, *92*, 5203–5213. [CrossRef] [PubMed]
28. European Medicines Agency (EMA). Guideline for the Demonstration of Efficacy for Veterinary Medicinal Products Containing Antimicrobial Substances. Available online: https://www.ema.europa.eu/en/documents/scientific-guideline/final-guideline-demonstration-efficacy-veterinary-medicinal-products-containing-antimicrobial_en.pdf (accessed on 7 December 2020).
29. El Garch, F.; de Jong, A.; Simjee, S.; Moyaert, H.; Klein, U.; Ludwig, C.; Marion, H.; Haag-Diergarten, S.; Richard-Mazet, A.; Thomas, V.; et al. Monitoring of antimicrobial susceptibility of respiratory tract pathogens isolated from diseased cattle and pigs across Europe, 2009-2012: VetPath results. *Vet. Microbiol.* **2016**, *194*, 11–22. [CrossRef]
30. Klima, C.L.; Holman, D.B.; Cook, S.R.; Conrad, C.C.; Ralston, B.J.; Allan, N.; Anholt, R.M.; Niu, Y.D.; Stanford, K.; Hannon, S.J.; et al. Multidrug Resistance in Pasteurellaceae Associated With Bovine Respiratory Disease Mortalities in North America From 2011 to 2016. *Front. Microbiol.* **2020**, *11*, 606438. [CrossRef] [PubMed]
31. Anholt, R.M.; Klima, C.; Allan, N.; Matheson-Bird, H.; Schatz, C.; Ajitkumar, P.; Otto, S.J.; Peters, D.; Schmid, K.; Olson, M.; et al. Antimicrobial Susceptibility of Bacteria That Cause Bovine Respiratory Disease Complex in Alberta, Canada. *Front. Vet. Sci.* **2017**, *4*, 207. [CrossRef] [PubMed]

32. Holschbach, C.L.; Aulik, N.; Poulsen, K.; Ollivett, T.L. Prevalence and temporal trends in antimicrobial resistance of bovine respiratory disease pathogen isolates submitted to the Wisconsin Veterinary Diagnostic Laboratory: 2008–2017. *J. Dairy Sci.* **2020**, *103*, 9464–9472. [CrossRef]
33. Stanford, K.; Zaheer, R.; Klima, C.; McAllister, T.; Peters, D.; Niu, Y.D.; Ralston, B. Antimicrobial Resistance in Members of the Bacterial Bovine Respiratory Disease Complex Isolated from Lung Tissue of Cattle Mortalities Managed with or without the Use of Antimicrobials. *Microorganisms* **2020**, *8*, 288. [CrossRef]
34. Bundesamt für Verbraucherschutz und Lebensmittelsicherheit (BVL). Resistenzsituation bei Klinisch Wichtigen Tierpathogenen Bakterien. Available online: https://www.bvl.bund.de/SharedDocs/Berichte/07_Resistenzmonitoringstudie/Bericht_Resistenzmonitoring_2018.pdf?__blob=publicationFile&v=4 (accessed on 29 December 2020).
35. Welsh, R.D.; Dye, L.B.; Payton, M.E.; Confer, A.W. Isolation and antimicrobial susceptibilities of bacterial pathogens from bovine pneumonia: 1994–2002. *J. Vet. Diagn. Investig.* **2004**, *16*, 426–431. [CrossRef]
36. Portis, E.; Lindeman, C.; Johansen, L.; Stoltman, G. A ten-year (2000–2009) study of antimicrobial susceptibility of bacteria that cause bovine respiratory disease complex–Mannheimia haemolytica, Pasteurella multocida, and Histophilus somni–in the United States and Canada. *J. Vet. Diagn. Investig.* **2012**, *24*, 932–944. [CrossRef] [PubMed]
37. Lubbers, B.V.; Hanzlicek, G.A. Antimicrobial multidrug resistance and coresistance patterns of Mannheimia haemolytica isolated from bovine respiratory disease cases–a three-year (2009-2011) retrospective analysis. *J. Vet. Diagn. Investig.* **2013**, *25*, 413–417. [CrossRef]
38. Sweeney, M.T.; Lubbers, B.V.; Schwarz, S.; Watts, J.L. Applying definitions for multidrug resistance, extensive drug resistance and pandrug resistance to clinically significant livestock and companion animal bacterial pathogens. *J. Antimicrob. Chemother.* **2018**, *73*, 1460–1463. [CrossRef] [PubMed]
39. Bell, B.G.; Schellevis, F.; Stobberingh, E.; Goossens, H.; Pringle, M. A systematic review and meta-analysis of the effects of antibiotic consumption on antibiotic resistance. *BMC Infect. Dis.* **2014**, *14*, 13. [CrossRef]
40. World Health Organisation (WHO). WHO Global Strategy for Containment of Antimicrobial Resistance. Available online: https://www.who.int/drugresistance/WHO_Global_Strategy_English.pdf (accessed on 28 August 2021).
41. The World Organisation for Animal Health (OIE). The OIE Strategy on Antimicrobial Resistance and the Prudent Use of Antimicrobials. Available online: https://www.oie.int/fileadmin/Home/eng/Media_Center/docs/pdf/PortailAMR/EN_OIE-AMRstrategy.pdf (accessed on 14 January 2021).
42. Kadlec, K.; Watts, J.L.; Schwarz, S.; Sweeney, M.T. Plasmid-located extended-spectrum β-lactamase gene blaROB-2 in Mannheimia haemolytica. *J. Antimicrob. Chemother.* **2019**, *74*, 851–853. [CrossRef]
43. Michael, G.B.; Kadlec, K.; Sweeney, M.T.; Brzuszkiewicz, E.; Liesegang, H.; Daniel, R.; Murray, R.W.; Watts, J.L.; Schwarz S. ICEPmu1, an integrative conjugative element (ICE) of Pasteurella multocida: Analysis of the regions that comprise 12 antimicrobial resistance genes. *J. Antimicrob. Chemother.* **2012**, *67*, 84–90. [CrossRef] [PubMed]
44. Michael, G.B.; Kadlec, K.; Sweeney, M.T.; Brzuszkiewicz, E.; Liesegang, H.; Daniel, R.; Murray, R.W.; Watts, J.L.; Schwarz, S. ICEPmu1, an integrative conjugative element (ICE) of Pasteurella multocida: Structure and transfer. *J. Antimicrob. Chemother.* **2012**, *67*, 91–100. [CrossRef]
45. Eidam, C.; Poehlein, A.; Leimbach, A.; Michael, G.B.; Kadlec, K.; Liesegang, H.; Daniel, R.; Sweeney, M.T.; Murray, R.W.; Watts, J.L.; et al. Analysis and comparative genomics of ICEMh1, a novel integrative and conjugative element (ICE) of Mannheimia haemolytica. *J. Antimicrob. Chemother.* **2015**, *70*, 93–97. [CrossRef]
46. World Health Organisation (WHO). Global Action Plan on Antimicrobial Resistance. Available online: https://www.who.int/publications/i/item/9789241509763 (accessed on 28 August 2021).
47. Berendonk, T.U.; Manaia, C.M.; Merlin, C.; Fatta-Kassinos, D.; Cytryn, E.; Walsh, F.; Bürgmann, H.; Sørum, H.; Norström, M.; Pons, M.N.; et al. Tackling antibiotic resistance: The environmental framework. *Nat. Rev. Microbiol.* **2015**, *13*, 310–317. [CrossRef]
48. Federal Ministry of Health Federal Ministry of Food and Agriculture Federal Ministry of Education and Research. DART 2020 Fighting Antibiotic Resistance for the Good of Both Humans and Animals. Available online: https://www.bmel.de/SharedDocs/Downloads/EN/Publications?DART2020.pdf;jsessionid=42432EA3DD38EA0D58BFF1DD601CCC04.live842?_blob=publicationFile&v=3 (accessed on 29 December 2020).
49. Bundesministerium der Justiz und für Verbraucherschutz. Verordnung über tierärztliche Hausapotheken (TÄHAV). Available online: https://www.gesetze-im-internet.de/t_hav/BJNR021150975.html (accessed on 15 December 2020).
50. Clinical and Laboratory Standards Institute (CSLI). *Performance Standards for Antimicrobial Disk and Dilution Susceptibility Tests for Bacteria Isolated from Animals*, 5th ed.; CLSI supplement VET01S; Clinical and Laboratory Standards Institute: Wayne, PA, USA, 2020.
51. Clinical and Laboratory Standards Institute (CLSI). *Methods for Antimicrobial Susceptibility Testing of Infrequently Isolated o fastidous Bacteria Isolated From Animals*, 1st ed.; CLSI supplement VET06; Clinical and Laboratory Standards Institute: Wayne, PA, USA, 2017.
52. Clinical and Laboratory Standards Institute (CLSI). *Performance Standards for Antimicrobial Disc and Dilution Susceptibility Tests fo Bacteria isolated from Animals*, 5th ed.; CLSI standard VET01; Clinical and Laboratory Standards Institute: Wayne, PA, USA, 2018.
53. Bundestierärztekammer e.V. Leitlinien für den Sorgsamen Umgang Mit Antibakteriell Wirksamen Tierarzneimitteln. Available online: https://www.bundestieraerztekammer.de/tieraerzte/leitlinien/ (accessed on 14 December 2020).

54. Vetsuisse Fakultät Gesellschaft Schweizer Tierärztinnen und Tierärzte (GST) Bundesamt Lebensmittelsicherheit und Veterinärwesen. Umsichtiger Einsatz von Antibiotika bei Rindern, Schweinen und kleinen Wiederkäuern. Available online: https://www.blv.admin.ch/blv/de/home/tiere/tierarzneimittel/antibiotika/nationale-strategie-antibiotikaresistenzen--star--/sachgemaesser-antibiotikaeinsatz.html (accessed on 12 December 2020).
55. Coetzee, J.F.; Cernicchiaro, N.; Sidhu, P.K.; Kleinhenz, M.D. Association between antimicrobial drug class selection for treatment and retreatment of bovine respiratory disease and health, performance, and carcass quality outcomes in feedlot cattle. *J. Anim. Sci.* **2020**, *98*, skaa109. [CrossRef]
56. Coetzee, J.F.; Magstadt, D.R.; Sidhu, P.K.; Follett, L.; Schuler, A.M.; Krull, A.C.; Cooper, V.L.; Engelken, T.J.; Kleinhenz, M.D.; O'Connor, A.M. Association between antimicrobial drug class for treatment and retreatment of bovine respiratory disease (BRD) and frequency of resistant BRD pathogen isolation from veterinary diagnostic laboratory samples. *PLoS ONE* **2019**, *14*, e0219104. [CrossRef] [PubMed]
57. World Health Organisation (WHO). Critically Important Antimicrobials for Human Medicine. Available online: https://apps.who.int/iris/bitstream/handle/10665/312266/9789241515528-eng.pdf (accessed on 15 December 2020).
58. Federal Ministry of Food and Agriculture. Report of the Federal Ministry of Food and Agriculture on the Evaluation of the Antibiotics Minimisation Concept Introduced with the 16th Act to Amend the Medicinal Products Act (16th AMG Amendment). Available online: https://www.bmel.de/SharedDocs/Downloads/EN/_Animals/16-AMG-Novelle.pdf;jsessionid=8FFAF96307741BA3063F4AE3A8D379A2.live842?__blob=publicationFile&v=3 (accessed on 29 December 2020).
59. European Medicines Agency (EMA). Available online: https://www.ema.europa.eu/en/medicines/veterinary/EPAR/draxxin (accessed on 5 June 2021).
60. Giguère, S.; Huang, R.; Malinski, T.J.; Dorr, P.M.; Tessman, R.K.; Somerville, B.A. Disposition of gamithromycin in plasma, pulmonary epithelial lining fluid, bronchoalveolar cells, and lung tissue in cattle. *Am. J. Vet. Res.* **2011**, *72*, 326–330. [CrossRef]
61. Noyes, N.R.; Benedict, K.M.; Gow, S.P.; Booker, C.W.; Hannon, S.J.; McAllister, T.A.; Morley, P.S. Mannheimia haemolytica in feedlot cattle: Prevalence of recovery and associations with antimicrobial use, resistance, and health outcomes. *J. Vet. Intern. Med.* **2015**, *29*, 705–713. [CrossRef] [PubMed]
62. Woolums, A.R.; Karisch, B.B.; Frye, J.G.; Epperson, W.; Smith, D.R.; Blanton, J., Jr.; Austin, F.; Kaplan, R.; Hiott, L.; Woodley, T.; et al. Multidrug resistant Mannheimia haemolytica isolated from high-risk beef stocker cattle after antimicrobial metaphylaxis and treatment for bovine respiratory disease. *Vet. Microbiol.* **2018**, *221*, 143–152. [CrossRef]
63. Milchreporte Bayern. Available online: https://www.lfl.bayern.de/iba/tier/020223/index.php (accessed on 5 October 2021).
64. Svensson, C.; Liberg, P. The effect of group size on health and growth rate of Swedish dairy calves housed in pens with automatic milk-feeders. *Prev. Vet. Med.* **2006**, *73*, 43–53. [CrossRef] [PubMed]
65. Maier, G.U.; Love, W.J.; Karle, B.M.; Dubrovsky, S.A.; Williams, D.R.; Champagne, J.D.; Anderson, R.J.; Rowe, J.D.; Lehenbauer, T.W.; Van Eenennaam, A.L.; et al. Management factors associated with bovine respiratory disease in preweaned calves on California dairies: The BRD 100 study. *J. Dairy Sci.* **2019**, *102*, 7288–7305. [CrossRef] [PubMed]
66. McEwen, S.A.; Fedorka-Cray, P.J. Antimicrobial use and resistance in animals. *Clin. Infect. Dis.* **2002**, *34* (Suppl. 3), S93–S106. [CrossRef]
67. Timsit, E.; Christensen, H.; Bareille, N.; Seegers, H.; Bisgaard, M.; Assié, S. Transmission dynamics of Mannheimia haemolytica in newly-received beef bulls at fattening operations. *Vet. Microbiol.* **2013**, *161*, 295–304. [CrossRef]
68. Watts, J.L.; Yancey, R.J., Jr.; Salmon, S.A.; Case, C.A. A 4-year survey of antimicrobial susceptibility trends for isolates from cattle with bovine respiratory disease in North America. *J. Clin. Microbiol.* **1994**, *32*, 725–731. [CrossRef] [PubMed]
69. Bundesamt für Verbraucherschutz und Lebensmittelsicherheit (BVL). Die Bestimmung der Kennzahlen zu den Therapiehäufigkeiten. Available online: https://www.bvl.bund.de/DE/Arbeitsbereiche/05_Tierarzneimittel/01_Aufgaben/05_AufgAntibiotikaResistenz/02_KennzahlenTherapiehaeufigkeit/KennzahlenTherapiehaeufigkeit_node.html (accessed on 28 August 2021).

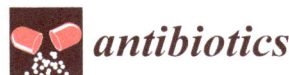 

Article

# Antimicrobial Resistance Patterns in Organic and Conventional Dairy Herds in Sweden

Karin Sjöström [1], Rachel A. Hickman [2], Viktoria Tepper [2,3], Gabriela Olmos Antillón [1], Josef D. Järhult [4], Ulf Emanuelson [1], Nils Fall [1] and Susanna Sternberg Lewerin [5,*]

1. Department of Clinical Sciences, Swedish University of Agricultural Sciences, 750 07 Uppsala, Sweden; karin.sjostrom@slu.se (K.S.); gabriela.olmos.antillon@slu.se (G.O.A.); ulf.emanuelson@slu.se (U.E.); nils.fall@slu.se (N.F.)
2. Department of Medical Biochemistry and Microbiology, Zoonosis Science Center, Uppsala University, 751 23 Uppsala, Sweden; rachel.hickman@medsci.uu.se (R.A.H.); vtepper05@gmail.com (V.T.)
3. Institute of Environmental Engineering, ETH, Stefano-Franscini-Platz 5, 8093 Zürich, Switzerland
4. Department of Medical Sciences, Zoonosis Science Center, Uppsala University Hospital, 751 85 Uppsala, Sweden; josef.jarhult@medsci.uu.se
5. Department of Biomedical Sciences and Veterinary Public Health, Swedish University of Agricultural Sciences, 750 07 Uppsala, Sweden
* Correspondence: susanna.sternberg-lewerin@slu.se

Received: 3 November 2020; Accepted: 17 November 2020; Published: 21 November 2020

**Abstract:** Monitoring antimicrobial resistance (AMR) and use (AMU) is important for control. We used *Escherichia coli* from healthy young calves as an indicator to evaluate whether AMR patterns differ between Swedish organic and conventional dairy herds and whether the patterns could be related to AMU data. Samples were taken twice, in 30 organic and 30 conventional dairy herds. Selective culturing for *Escherichia coli*, without antibiotics and with nalidixic acid or tetracycline, was used to estimate the proportions of resistant isolates. Microdilution was used to determine the minimum inhibitory concentrations (MICs) for thirteen antimicrobial substances. AMU data were based on collection of empty drug packages. Less than 8% of the bacterial growth on non-selective plates was also found on selective plates with tetracycline, and 1% on plates with nalidixic acid. Despite some MIC variations, resistance patterns were largely similar in both periods, and between organic and conventional herds. For most substances, only a few isolates were classified as resistant. The most common resistances were against ampicillin, streptomycin, sulfamethoxazole, and tetracycline. No clear association with AMU could be found. The lack of difference between organic and conventional herds is likely due to a generally good animal health status and consequent low AMU in both categories.

**Keywords:** antibiotic; antibiotic resistance; livestock; antibiotic use; AMR; MDR; environment

## 1. Introduction

Antimicrobial resistance (AMR) in bacteria is a natural phenomenon that is accelerated by the selection pressure caused by antimicrobial use (AMU). Antibacterial drugs are important tools in human and veterinary medicine, necessary to combat bacterial infections, conduct advanced surgical and immunosuppressive treatments as well as ensure global food security [1]. Overuse and misuse of antibacterial drugs in humans, companion animals and livestock promote antimicrobial resistance worldwide, leading to an increased risk of treatment failures [1]. Both veterinarians and physicians face the challenge of balancing the need to treat infections against the risk of promoting AMR. Historically, Sweden has been a strong advocate for developing and implementing strategies to reduce the selection pressure by reducing AMU and closely monitoring AMU and AMR across all sectors [2–4]. Monitoring AMU in animals is challenging in many ways, as regards legislative framework, data sources and methods for data collection and analysis [5–7]. The quality and availability of data on livestock AMU vary between different regions of the world but many countries have spent a considerable effort on the development of data collection systems [5]. In Sweden, as in the rest of the European Union, antibiotics for animals are available on veterinary prescription only. Swedish AMU statistics stem from sales data from pharmacies, based on veterinary prescriptions [8]. Generally, farm-based data are not available in national statistics. In the Swedish dairy sector, however, detailed statistics on animal health and veterinary treatments are available and continuously evaluated.

The main reason for studying AMU is to monitor strategies to contain AMR, and to assess associations with AMR prevalence. Harada and Asai [9] reviewed data on AMR prevalence in bacteria from cattle in several countries around the world. Out of the included countries, Sweden presented the lowest prevalence figures, whereas countries such as Japan, France and Germany had medium levels and the Netherlands had the highest prevalence. AMR monitoring entails many methodological challenges. In the EU, data on AMR in zoonotic and indicator bacteria from humans, selected animal species and food are collected annually and jointly analyzed [6,7]. The AMR figures are based on epidemiological cut offs, so-called ECOFFs [10]. According to Commission Decision 213/652/EU, antimicrobial susceptibility testing of *Escherichia coli* from fecal samples taken at slaughter from calves <1 year of age should be included in AMR monitoring. This, however, applies only to countries where the total amount of meat from calf slaughter exceeds 10,000 tones/year and there is not sufficient longitudinal data to evaluate temporal trends in those countries that participate in harmonized monitoring [7]. In Sweden, indicator bacteria such as *E. coli* are isolated from the intestinal content of healthy pigs and poultry sampled at slaughter within the monitoring framework, or from feces collected from live animals in other projects [8]. In 2017, *E. coli* isolated from rectal swabs taken in a project, from 85 calves <2 months old, were included in the monitoring report [11]. Approximately half of the isolates in this study were susceptible to all substances tested while less than one-third were resistant to three or more substances. The most common resistance traits were against streptomycin, sulfamethoxazole, tetracycline or ampicillin. No isolate was resistant to cefotaxime, ceftazidime, colistin, florfenicol or gentamicin. Currently, these are the only available data on indicator *E. coli* from cattle in the national monitoring program.

There are no published papers that compare AMR prevalence in different dairy production systems in Sweden. Due to the link between AMU and AMR, it would be assumed that herd types with lower AMU would also have a lower prevalence of AMR. There are some international studies comparing AMU and AMR in organic and conventional herds. In the United States, organic farms are not allowed to treat with antibiotics at all, as was confirmed in a study on AMU [12,13]. In the European regulation for organic dairy herds (Council Regulation (EC) No 834/2007), AMU is restricted to a maximum number of three treatments per cow and year. The rules of the Swedish organic certification association are in some respects stricter than the EU regulations, such as requiring double withdrawal periods for milk from treated cows [14]. Whether these strict regulations are reflected in the prevalence of AMR in Swedish organic dairy herds is not known.

The aim of this study was to estimate the prevalence of AMR in Swedish dairy herds, using susceptibility testing of *E. coli* from healthy young calves as an indicator to evaluate whether AMR patterns differ between organic and conventional dairy herds and whether they could be related to AMU data.

## 2. Materials and Methods

### 2.1. Study Population

A convenience sampling design was used, where 30 organic and 30 conventional dairy herds were selected. The herds were located throughout Sweden, with an equal number of organic and conventional farms in each geographic area, and with herd sizes reflecting the overall population of Swedish dairy herds. Each farm was visited by the first author (KS) during the indoor season, February to May in 2016 and November 2016 to March in 2017.

*2.2. Faecal Sampling*

At the beginning of each study period, fecal samples from healthy calves (i.e., calves with no signs of disease) were collected by the first author. The aim was to sample 5 calves less than two months old, but if this was not possible at the time of the visit, the farmer took the remaining samples according to instructions provided and sent the samples to the laboratory. The fecal samples were collected from rectum with Amie's charcoal culture swabs (Copan diagnostics Inc., Murrieta, CA, USA) and either brought directly to the laboratory by the first author, or sent by standard mail. The samples were, upon arrival to the lab, stored in a refrigerator and analyzed within 48 h from sampling.

At the beginning of the second study period, the first author also collected fecal samples from the farm environment. Two fecal swab samples were collected: one from an indoor drainage site and one from the manure pit. E-swabs (Copan diagnostics Inc., Murrieta, CA, USA) were used for sampling, and the samples were brought to the laboratory by the first author and stored as described above.

*2.3. Collection of AMU Data*

In a parallel study, information about AMU was collected from the study herds during three months following each initial sampling visit [15]. On-farm data collection was performed according to the so-called BIN method, where empty drug containers were collected on each farm as described by Olmos Antillón et al. [15]. Briefly, the farm staff/owners were instructed to place discarded packaging of any drug used on farm (administered by them or a visiting veterinarian) into plastic bags throughout the observation period. The bags were collected one day after the end of each observation period. In the current study, these data were used as a proxy for AMU in the study herds.

*2.4. Antimicrobial Susceptibility Testing*

We used *E. coli* as the AMR indicator bacteria and the quality accredited laboratory methods described in detail by Duse et al. [16]. In summary, the samples were diluted in 3 mL of 0.9% NaCl and, subsequently, 50 µL of 10-fold dilutions ($10^{-2}$ and $10^{-4}$ for calf samples, $10^{-1}$ and $10^{-3}$ for environmental samples) were streaked on Petrifilm$^{TM}$ (3M$^{TM}$, St Paul, MN, USA) Select *E. coli* count (SEC) plates (3M Microbiology Products) and cultured overnight at 42 °C. The colony-forming units (CFUs) were counted the next day and calculated back to CFU/mL in the original sample.

The proportion of *E. coli* that were resistant to nalidixic acid and tetracycline was determined by parallel plating of the diluted fecal samples on SEC plates supplemented with 50 µL of 672 µg/mL nalidixic acid or 1344 µg/mL tetracycline, respectively. The plates were incubated overnight at 42 °C and the CFUs were counted on the next day. Isolates growing on these plates were regarded as resistant. Based on the estimated CFU/mL in the original sample, it was possible to estimate the proportion of tetracycline-resistant and nalidixic acid-resistant *E. coli*.

Subsequently, one random colony from each sample on the plates without antibiotics was selected, subcultured and identified as *E. coli* by morphology and the indole test. The antimicrobial susceptibility of these *E. coli* isolates was then determined with a VetMIC$^{TM}$ (SVA, Uppsala, Sweden) panel of 13 antimicrobial substances. Epidemiological cut-off values for the minimum inhibitory concentration (MIC), determined according to the European Committee on Antimicrobial Susceptibility Testing [10], were used to classify isolates as susceptible or resistant. An isolate was defined as resistant if the MIC value was above the cut off for an antimicrobial substance and as multidrug resistant (MDR) if the MIC values were above the cut off for at least three substances from different antimicrobial classes.

All isolates with an MIC for colistin >2 mg/L were examined with PCR targeting *mcr* 1–5, according to Rebelo et al. [17]. Similarly, isolates that were resistant to third-generation cephalosporines (MIC for ceftazidime >0.5 mg/L), were examined further for extended spectrum beta-lactamase (ESBL) production and ESBL genes. Phenotypic confirmatory tests for production of ESBL in *E. coli* were performed with and without clavulanic acid in Sensititre EUVSEC2 (Thermo Fisher Scientific Inc., Waltham, MA, USA) microdilution panels and interpreted according to EUCAST [10]. PCR for identification of ESBL-encoding genes was performed on ESBL-producing isolates as previously described [18].

All analyses during the first period were performed by the accredited laboratory in the Swedish National Veterinary Institute (SVA), while analyses during period 2 were performed at the Zoonosis Science Center, Uppsala University. To ensure equal procedures in both periods, the researchers performing the analyses in the second period carried out the laboratory work and interpretations of the VetMIC plates on some samples together with SVA staff. These samples included isolates where the interpretation of MIC values was difficult as well as isolates where the results were more evident.

*2.5. Antimicrobial Resistance Patterns and Herd Production System*

The difference in the proportion of resistant isolates (for each antimicrobial substance as well as MDR) between organic and conventional herds was tested with Fisher's exact test. The difference in the proportion of *E. coli* growing on media supplemented with tetracycline or nalidixic acid, as compared to non-supplemented medium, between organic and conventional herds was assessed by the Mann Whitney U test for unpaired samples.

The mean and median MIC values and proportion of isolates classified as resistant for each substance, from herds treated or not treated with the same class of drug, were also assessed. In addition, the proportion of resistant isolates for each substance and the herd AMU for the corresponding substance, expressed as the total number of defined course doses (DCD/animal/year, see Olmos Antillón et al., 2020 for details on DCD calculations), was assessed for organic and conventional herds.

Heatmaps illustrating AMR patterns in calf isolates from each herd were generated in Python (www.python.org) using the matplotlib, pandas and seaborn packages. All Python scripts are available on request.

*2.6. Ethical Statement*

All animals in this study were treated according to the ethical standards of the Swedish regulations. The competent authorities stated that no ethical permission was required for this sampling. Participation in this study was voluntary, and the farmers were informed about the purpose and methods of this study. They were assured that all information would be treated anonymously and that they could withdraw from this study at any time.

## 3. Results

In total, 293 calves from 60 herds were sampled during the first period. During the second period, 258 calves from 54 herds were sampled (3 organic and 3 conventional farms did not participate in the second round). A total of 103 fecal environmental samples (54 from manure drainage and 49 from manure pit) were also taken from these 54 herds at the start of the second period. The herd size ranged from 48 to 230 cows, with a median of 80 cows in the organic herds and 110 in the conventional herds. The number of sampled calves per herd and time point varied from 2 to 6, with a median of 5. The age of the sampled calves ranged from 0 to 46 days, with a median of 15 days in both herd types in the first sampling round, while the median age was 18 days in organic herds and 26 days in conventional herds in the second sampling round.

*3.1. Proportion of Tetracycline- and Nalidixic Acid-Resistant E. Coli*

In the calf samples from organic herds in the first period, 7.3% of the bacterial growth on non-selective plates was also found on selective plates with tetracycline; the corresponding proportion for selective plates with nalidixic acid was 0.8%. In samples from conventional herds, 4.9% of the growth on non-selective plates was also found on selective plates with tetracycline and 1.0% on selective plates with nalidixic acid. The difference was significant ($p < 0.05$) for nalidixic acid but not for tetracycline. The results from the calf samples for period 2 had to be discarded due to methodological errors that could not be resolved. In the environmental samples from organic herds, 6.4% of the bacterial growth on non-selective plates was also found on selective plates with tetracycline, the corresponding proportion for selective plates with nalidixic acid was 2.6%. In samples from conventional herds, 9.5% of the growth on non-selective plates was also found on selective plates with tetracycline and 3.8% on selective plates with nalidixic acid. The differences observed were not significant.

### 3.2. Antimicrobial Susceptibility

Figures 1–3 show the distribution of MIC values for substances in the VetMIC$^{TM}$ panel for calf isolates in period 1 and 2, and for environmental isolates, respectively. Some variations were seen but the resistance patterns were largely similar in period 1 and 2, and between organic and conventional herds. For most of the antimicrobial agents, only a few isolates had MIC values above the epidemiological cut offs. All isolates from calves and environment were susceptible to florfenicol. All but two isolates in period 2 (one from a calf and one from a manure drainage) were susceptible to gentamicin, with the resistant isolates having MICs just above the cut off. The proportions of isolates with MICs above the epidemiological cut offs were highest for ampicillin, streptomycin, tetracycline and sulfamethoxazole (Figures 1–3).

The proportions of isolates with AMR and MDR in the different samples are illustrated in Figure 4. There were no clear differences between calf samples in period 1 and period 2, whereas the proportions of both AMR and MDR were lower in the environmental samples. In period 1, 52% of the calf isolates were resistant to at least one of the tested antimicrobial substances, the corresponding figure for period 2 was 44%, and for environmental samples 27%. There was no significant difference between organic and conventional herds. In both periods, 28% of the calf isolates were MDR and in environmental samples 12% of the isolates were MDR (7% of isolates from manure drainage and 16% of isolates from manure pit). There was no significant difference between organic and conventional herds. There were very few significant differences between the herd types for single antimicrobial substances, and no consistent pattern over the two sampling occasions (Figures 1–3). The most common resistances were against ampicillin, streptomycin, sulfamethoxazole, and tetracycline. Most herds had a rather high proportion of isolates that were resistant to at least one antimicrobial, but the majority had no, or very few, samples that were MDR (Figure 4). In the first period, five herds had >60% of calf isolates with MDR, while three other herds had >60% of calf isolates with MDR in the second period.

In period 1, 31 *E. coli* isolates had a colistin MIC of >2 mg/L, but no *mcr* genes were detected. Three isolates were resistant to third-generation cephalosporins, where one was confirmed as ESBL producing and carried CTX-M-1.

In period 2, 11 *E. coli* isolates from calf samples had a colistin MIC above cut off, but at the time of PCR testing, pure cultures could not be obtained from four of these. The remaining seven were subjected to the *mcr*-PCR and all were negative. Five calf *E. coli* isolates were resistant to third-generation cephalosporins, but none of these were ESBL producing and were therefore not further analyzed for resistance genes. Four isolates from environmental samples had a colistin MIC above cut off but three could not be pure cultured for the PCR, the remaining one was negative in the *mcr*-PCR. When the microdilution tests were performed, all cultures were checked for purity and hence it was concluded that the contamination had occurred after this step, in the process of storing the isolates.

The resistance patterns in calf isolates from each herd and for each substance are illustrated in the heatmaps in Figure 5. No consistent pattern could be discerned between herd type or sampling period and the heatmaps confirm the generally low resistance prevalence in the sampled herds.

**Figure 1.** Minimum inhibitory concentration (MIC) distribution of *Escherichia coli* isolates from calves, sampled in period 1, in 30 (148 isolates) organic (Org) and 30 (145 isolates) conventional (Conv) Swedish dairy herds, in a panel of 13 antimicrobial agents. Blue color indicates the range of concentrations tested. Vertical black lines are the epidemiological cut-off points, according to EUCAST. $p$ values test the difference between organic and conventional herds with Fisher's exact test. Yellow color denotes isolates from conventional herds and pink color shows MIC values.

Distribution (isolates) of MICs (mg/L)

| Antimicrobial agent | 0.008 | 0.016 | 0.03 | 0.06 | 0.12 | 0.25 | 0.5 | 1 | 2 | 4 | 8 | 16 | 32 | 64 | 128 | 256 | 512 | 1024 | >1024 | %R | p |
|---|---|---|---|---|---|---|---|---|---|---|---|---|---|---|---|---|---|---|---|---|---|
| Ampicillin Conv. | | | | | | | | 57 | 52 | 1 | 1 | 0 | 0 | 1 | 8 | 25 | | | | 23% | 0.59 |
| Ampicillin Org. | | | | | | | | 73 | 34 | 2 | 0 | 1 | 0 | 2 | 6 | 30 | | | | 26% | |
| Cefotaxime Conv. | | | 30 | 97 | 16 | 2 | 0 | 0 | | | | | | | | | | | | 0 | 0.50 |
| Cefotaxime Org. | | | 22 | 107 | 17 | 0 | 0 | 0 | | | | | | | | | | | | 1% | |
| Ceftazidime Conv. | | | | 2 | 36 | 105 | 3 | 0 | 1 | | | | | | | | | | | 0.7% | 1 |
| Ceftazidime Org. | | | | 2 | 47 | 94 | 3 | 0 | 1 | | | | | | | | | | | 1% | |
| Chloramphenicol Conv. | | | | | | | | 1 | | 108 | 32 | 0 | 1 | 4 | | | | | | 3% | 0.09 |
| Chloramphenicol Org. | | | | | | | | | | 113 | 22 | 0 | 0 | 13 | | | | | | 9% | |
| Ciprofloxacin Conv. | 21 | 95 | 20 | 7 | 2 | 0 | 0 | 0 | 2 | | | | | | | | | | | 6% | 1 |
| Ciprofloxacin Org. | 19 | 106 | 14 | 3 | 4 | 0 | 2 | | | | | | | | | | | | | 6% | |
| Colistin Conv. | | | | | | | 21 | 46 | 54 | 22 | 2 | | | | | | | | | 17% | 0.001 |
| Colistin Org. | | | | | | | 32 | 61 | 48 | 7 | | | | | | | | | | 5% | |
| Florfenicol Conv. | | | | | | 37 | 87 | 19 | 2 | 63 | 78 | 4 | | | | | | | | 0 | NA |
| Florfenicol Org. | | | | | | 35 | 101 | 11 | 1 | 84 | 63 | 1 | | | | | | | | 0 | |
| Gentamicin Conv. | | | | | | | | 19 | 2 | | | 1 | 3 | 2 | 0 | | | | | 0 | NA |
| Gentamicin Org. | | | | | | | | 11 | 1 | | | 1 | 4 | 1 | | | | | | 0 | |
| Nalidixic acid Conv. | | | | | | | | 5 | 75 | 58 | 1 | 1 | 3 | 2 | 0 | | | | | 3% | 0.29 |
| Nalidixic acid Org. | | | | | | | | 4 | 89 | 44 | 1 | 0 | 4 | 1 | 3 | 2 | | | | 7% | |
| Streptomycin Conv. | | | | | | | | | | 29 | 55 | 9 | 8 | 12 | 4 | 13 | 10 | 5 | | 30% | 0.70 |
| Streptomycin Org. | | | | | | | | | | 40 | 49 | 6 | 12 | 6 | 8 | 13 | 10 | 4 | | 28% | |
| Sulfamethoxazole Conv. | | | | | | | | | | | 11 | 42 | 43 | 2 | 0 | 0 | 0 | 2 | 45 | 32% | 0.62 |
| Sulfamethoxazole Org. | | | | | | | | | | | 20 | 46 | 26 | 3 | 0 | 0 | 1 | 3 | 49 | 36% | |
| Tetracycline Conv. | | | | | | | | 60 | 49 | 0 | 0 | 1 | 22 | 9 | 4 | | | | | 25% | 0.51 |
| Tetracycline Org. | | | | | | | | 69 | 37 | 0 | 0 | 2 | 19 | 16 | 5 | | | | | 28% | |
| Trimethoprim Conv. | | | | | 14 | 64 | 52 | 1 | 0 | 0 | 0 | 14 | | | | | | | | 10% | 0.69 |
| Trimethoprim Org. | | | | | 12 | 76 | 47 | 1 | 2 | 0 | 0 | 12 | | | | | | | | 8% | |

## Distribution (isolates) of MICs (mg/L)

| Antimicrobial agent | 0.008 | 0.016 | 0.03 | 0.06 | 0.12 | 0.25 | 0.5 | 1 | 2 | 4 | 8 | 16 | 32 | 64 | 128 | 256 | 512 | 1024 | >1024 | %R | p |
|---|---|---|---|---|---|---|---|---|---|---|---|---|---|---|---|---|---|---|---|---|---|
| Ampicillin Conv. | | | | | | | | 40 | 66 | 1 | 0 | 1 | 0 | 0 | 2 | 21 | | | | 18% | |
| Ampicillin Org. | | | | | | | | 25 | 65 | 5 | 1 | 0 | 0 | 1 | 2 | 28 | | | | 25% | 0.17 |
| Cefotaxime Conv. | | | 7 | 89 | 31 | 3 | 0 | | | | | | | | | | | | | 0.8% | |
| Cefotaxime Org. | | | 1 | 76 | 42 | 8 | | | | | | | | | | | | | | 0 | 1 |
| Ceftazidime Conv. | | | | | | 119 | 10 | 0 | 1 | 0 | 0 | 1 | | | | | | | | 2% | |
| Ceftazidime Org. | | | | | | 109 | 15 | 3 | | | | | | | | | | | | 2% | 0.68 |
| Chloramphenicol Conv. | | | | | | | | | 1 | 62 | 67 | 0 | 0 | 0 | 1 | | | | | 0.8% | |
| Chloramphenicol Org. | | | | | | | | | 3 | 56 | 60 | 0 | 0 | 1 | 7 | | | | | 6% | 0.02 |
| Ciprofloxacin Conv. | 4 | 111 | 10 | 0 | 6 | | | | | | | | | | | | | | | 5% | |
| Ciprofloxacin Org. | 4 | 107 | 12 | 1 | 3 | | | | | | | | | | | | | | | 3% | 0.75 |
| Colistin Conv. | | | | | | | 98 | 29 | 2 | 1 | 1 | | | | | | | | | 2% | |
| Colistin Org. | | | | | | | 79 | 35 | 4 | 3 | 6 | | | | | | | | | 7% | 0.06 |
| Florfenicol Conv. | | | | | | | | | | 41 | 85 | 5 | | | | | | | | 0 | |
| Florfenicol Org. | | | | | | | | | | 38 | 87 | 2 | | | | | | | | 0 | NA |
| Gentamicin Conv. | | | | | | 2 | 117 | 11 | 0 | 1 | | 0 | 0 | 0 | 3 | | | | | 0.8% | |
| Gentamicin Org. | | | | | | 1 | 108 | 14 | 4 | | | 0 | 0 | 0 | 2 | 1 | | | | 0 | 1 |
| Nalidixic acid Conv. | | | | | | | | 3 | 78 | 43 | 1 | 0 | 0 | 20 | 10 | 7 | 7 | | | 5% | |
| Nalidixic acid Org. | | | | | | | | 2 | 73 | 44 | 5 | 0 | 9 | 20 | 10 | 7 | | | | 3% | 0.50 |
| Streptomycin Conv. | | | | | | | | | | 49 | 28 | 1 | 9 | 4 | 9 | 13 | 5 | | | 40% | |
| Streptomycin Org. | | | | | | | | | 2 | 50 | 32 | 5 | 7 | | | | | | | 30% | 0.09 |
| Sulfamethoxazole Conv. | | | | | | | | | | | 37 | 33 | 16 | 1 | 0 | 0 | 0 | 1 | 43 | 34% | |
| Sulfamethoxazole Org. | | | | | | | | | | | 31 | 39 | 18 | 2 | 0 | 0 | 0 | | 36 | 29% | 0.50 |
| Tetracycline Conv. | | | | | | 50 | 56 | 60 | 36 | 7 | 0 | 3 | 20 | 5 | | | | | | 21% | |
| Tetracycline Org. | | | | | | 37 | 50 | 55 | 40 | 6 | 0 | 6 | 10 | 10 | | | | | | 20% | 0.88 |
| Trimethoprim Conv. | | | | | 10 | 8 | 56 | 8 | 1 | 0 | 0 | 0 | 6 | | | | | | | 5% | |
| Trimethoprim Org. | | | | | 6 | 24 | 50 | 1 | 1 | 0 | 0 | 0 | 9 | | | | | | | 7% | 0.40 |
| | 0.008 | 0.016 | 0.03 | 0.06 | 0.12 | 0.25 | 0.5 | 1 | 2 | 4 | 8 | 16 | 32 | 64 | 128 | 256 | 512 | 1024 | >1024 | | |

**Figure 2.** Minimum inhibitory concentration (MIC) distributions of *Escherichia coli* isolates from calves, sampled in period 2, in 27 (127 isolates) organic (Org) and 27 (131 isolates) conventional (Conv) Swedish dairy herds, in a panel of 13 antimicrobial agents. Blue color indicates the range of concentrations tested. Vertical black lines are the epidemiologic cut-off points according to EUCAST. *p* values test the difference between organic and conventional herds with Fisher's exact test. Yellow color denotes isolates from conventional herds and pink color shows MIC values.

**Figure 3.** Minimum inhibitory concentration (MIC) distributions of *Escherichia coli* isolates from environmental samples of farm manure (drainage and manure pit) at the beginning of period 2, in 27 (50 isolates) organic (Org) and 27 (53 isolates) conventional (Conv) Swedish dairy herds, in a panel of 13 antimicrobial agents. Blue color indicates the range of concentrations tested. Vertical thicker black lines are the epidemiologic cut-off points according to EUCAST. *p* values test the difference between organic and conventional herds with Fisher's exact test. Yellow color denotes isolates from conventional herds and pink color shows MIC values.

Distribution (isolates) of MICs (mg/L)

| Antimicrobial agent | 0.008 | 0.016 | 0.03 | 0.06 | 0.12 | 0.25 | 0.5 | 1 | 2 | 4 | 8 | 16 | 32 | 64 | 128 | 256 | 512 | 1024 | >1024 | %R | P |
|---|---|---|---|---|---|---|---|---|---|---|---|---|---|---|---|---|---|---|---|---|---|
| Ampicillin Conv. | | | | | | | | 8 | 36 | 5 | 0 | 1 | 0 | 0 | 1 | 2 | | | | 9% | |
| Ampicillin Org. | | | | | | | | 9 | 31 | 3 | 1 | 1 | 0 | 0 | 0 | 5 | | | | 12% | 0.52 |
| Cefotaxime Conv. | | | 2 | 30 | 20 | 1 | 0 | | | | | | | | | | | | | 0 | NA |
| Cefotaxime Org. | | | 2 | 30 | 20 | 0 | 0 | 0 | | | | | | | | | | | | 0 | NA |
| Ceftazidime Conv. | | | | | | 44 | 7 | 0 | | | | | | | | | | | | 0 | NA |
| Ceftazidime Org. | | | | | | 42 | 8 | 0 | | | | | | | | | | | | 0 | NA |
| Chloramphenicol Conv. | | | | | | | | | | 21 | 31 | 0 | 0 | 1 | | | | | | 2% | 1 |
| Chloramphenicol Org. | | | | | | | | | | 24 | 26 | 0 | 0 | | | | | | | 0 | |
| Ciprofloxacin Conv. | 1 | 42 | 9 | 0 | | 1 | | 0 | 0 | | | | | | | | | | | 2% | 1 |
| Ciprofloxacin Org. | | 44 | 6 | | 0 | 1 | | | | | | | | | | | | | | 0 | |
| Colistin Conv. | | | | | | | | 17 | 2 | 0 | 0 | 1 | | | | | | | | 2% | 0.35 |
| Colistin Org. | | | | | | | | 10 | 0 | 0 | 3 | | | | | | | | | 6% | |
| Florfenicol Conv. | | | | | | | 33 | | 9 | 43 | 1 | | | | | | | | | 0 | NA |
| Florfenicol Org. | | | | | | | 37 | | 19 | 31 | 1 | | | | | | | | | 0 | |
| Gentamicin Conv. | | | | | | 1 | 45 | 6 | 0 | 1 | | 0 | 0 | 1 | | | | | | 2% | 1 |
| Gentamicin Org. | | | | | | 2 | 40 | 8 | 0 | 1 | | 0 | 0 | | | | | | | 0 | |
| Nalidixic acid Conv. | | | | | | | | 1 | 22 | 27 | 1 | 0 | 0 | 0 | 1 | 1 | | | | 4% | 0.50 |
| Nalidixic acid Org. | | | | | | | | | 24 | 26 | | 0 | 0 | 0 | | | | | | 0 | |
| Streptomycin Conv. | | | | | | | | | 3 | 21 | 22 | 0 | 2 | 2 | 1 | 2 | | | | 13% | 1 |
| Streptomycin Org. | | | | | | | | | | 23 | 20 | 0 | 1 | 0 | 0 | 0 | 2 | | | 14% | |
| Sulfamethoxazole Conv. | | | | | | | | | | | 20 | 16 | 8 | 0 | 0 | 0 | 0 | 0 | 9 | 17% | 1 |
| Sulfamethoxazole Org. | | | | | | | | | | | 22 | 11 | 10 | 1 | 0 | 0 | 0 | 0 | 6 | 12% | 0.58 |
| Tetracycline Conv. | | | | | | | | 24 | 20 | 3 | 0 | 2 | 3 | 1 | | | | | | 11% | |
| Tetracycline Org. | | | | | | | | 21 | 16 | 6 | 0 | 1 | 5 | 1 | | | | | | 14% | 0.77 |
| Trimethoprim Conv. | | | | 2 | 23 | 16 | 7 | 1 | 0 | 0 | | | 4 | | | | | | | 8% | |
| Trimethoprim Org. | | | | 6 | 15 | 17 | 7 | 1 | 0 | 0 | | | 4 | | | | | | | 8% | 1 |
| | 0.008 | 0.016 | 0.03 | 0.06 | 0.12 | 0.25 | 0.5 | 1 | 2 | 4 | 8 | 16 | 32 | 64 | 128 | 256 | 512 | 1024 | >1024 | | |

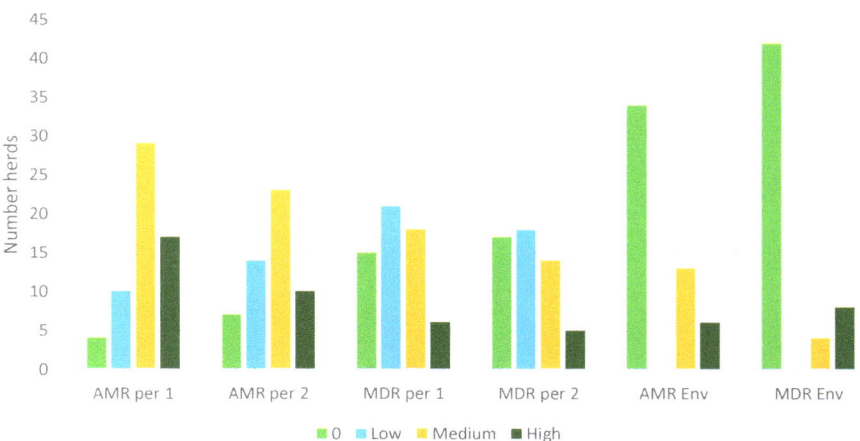

**Figure 4.** Number of sampled herds with zero (0), low (1–25%), medium (26–60%) and high (>60%) proportions of *Escherichia coli* with antimicrobial resistance to any antimicrobial class (AMR) or to three or more antimicrobial classes (MDR) in Swedish organic and conventional dairy herds. Isolates from calf samples in period 1 (per 1) and period 2 (per 2) and environmental samples in period 2 (env).

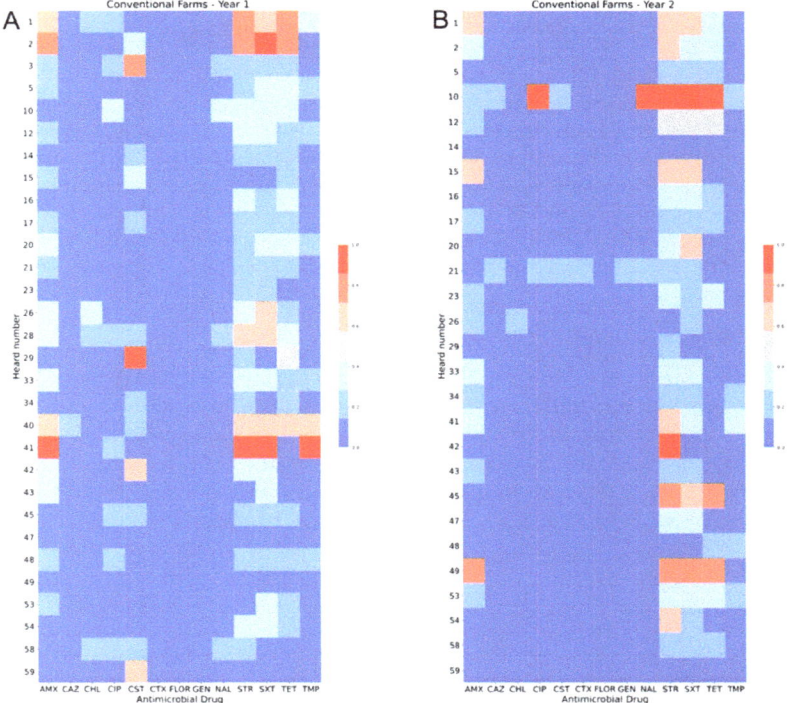

**Figure 5.** *Cont.*

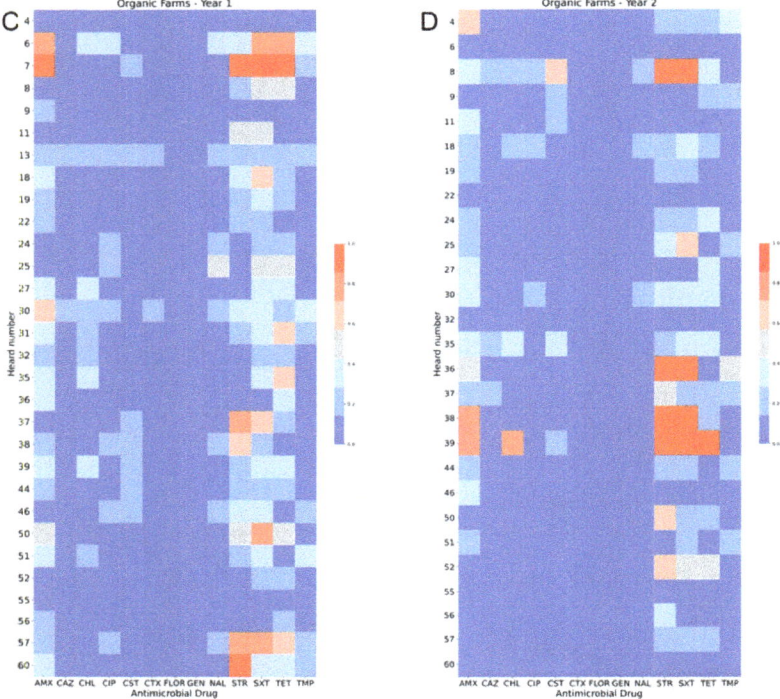

**Figure 5.** Heatmaps showing the patterns of resistant and susceptible *Escherichia coli* isolates from Swedish organic and conventional dairy herds sampled in two different time periods. (**A**) conventional herds 1st sampling (**B**) conventional herds 2nd sampling (**C**) organic herds 1st sampling (**D**) organic herds 2nd sampling. Color scale illustrates average value for each herd and each antimicrobial substance tested, where 1 = resistant and 0 = susceptible. AMX = ampicillin, CAZ = ceftazidime, CHL = chloramphenicol, CIP = ciprofloxacin, CST = colistin, CTX = cefotaxime, FLOR = florfenicol, GEN = gentamycin, NAL = nalidixic acid, STR = streptomycin, SXT = sulfamethoxazole, TET = tetracycline, and TMP = trimethoprim.

### 3.3. Association between AMU and AMR

All herds but one had used some antibiotic treatment during the observation periods. Table 1 shows the average and median MICs as well as the proportions of resistant isolates of each sample type, in herds with or without records of having used the corresponding antimicrobial substance. For most substances, the average MIC and the proportion of resistant isolates was lower in herds with low or no recorded treatments, while for others the opposite, or no difference, was seen. There was little or no difference in median MIC values, and the observed differences correspond to one dilution step.

**Table 1.** Summary of antimicrobial susceptibility test results for *Escherichia coli* isolates from fecal samples from calves and environment (manure drainage and manure pit) in 27 organic and 27 conventional Swedish dairy herds (sampling period 2) and the corresponding use of antimicrobial treatments in these herds, as determined by collection of empty drug packages. Treated=use of the corresponding substance recorded for the herd. Not treated=no use of the corresponding substance recorded.

| Substance | Calf Isolates | | Environmental Isolates | |
|---|---|---|---|---|
| | Herd Treated [a] | Herd Not Treated | Herd Treated | Herd Not Treated |
| **Ampicillin** [a1] | N = 53 | N = 1 | N = 53 | N = 1 |
| Average MIC | 54 | 2 | 22 | 3 |
| Median MIC | 2 | 2 | 2 | 2 |
| %resistant | 22 | 0 | 12 | 0 |
| **Ciprofloxacin** [a2] | N = 6 | N = 48 | N = 6 | N = 48 |
| Average MIC | 0.055 [b] | 0.036 | 0.040 | 0.035 |
| Median MIC | 0.030 | 0.030 | 0.030 | 0.030 |
| %resistant | 14 | 2 | 7 | 2 |
| **Nalidixic acid** [a2] | N = 6 | N = 48 | N = 6 | N = 48 |
| Average MIC | 21 | 7 | 3 | 6 |
| Median MIC | 4 | 2 | 5 | 4 |
| %resistant | 10 | 2 | 0 | 2 |
| **Gentamicin** [a3] | N = 20 | N = 34 | N = 20 | N = 34 |
| Average MIC | 0.60 | 0.56 | 0.58 | 0.71 |
| Median MIC | 0.50 | 0.50 | 0.50 | 0.50 |
| %resistant | 0.5 | 0 | 0 | 4 |
| **Streptomycin** [a3] | N = 20 | N = 34 | N = 20 | N = 34 |
| Average MIC | 69 | 67 | 42 | 10 |
| Median MIC | 8 | 8 | 8 | 6 |
| %resistant | 32 | 44 | 20 | 10 |
| **Tetracycline** [a4] | N = 10 | N = 44 | N = 10 | N = 44 |
| Average MIC | 7 | 10 | 5 | 3 |
| Median MIC | 2 | 2 | 2 | 2 |
| %resistant | 19 | 23 | 16 | 13 |
| **Sulfamethoxazole** [a5] | N = 8 | N = 46 | N = 8 | N = 46 |
| Average MIC | 850 | 590 | 463 | 264 |
| Median MIC | 320 | 160 | 80 | 160 |
| %resistant | 42 | 29 | 22 | 14 |
| **Trimethoprim** [a5] | N = 8 | N = 46 | N = 8 | N = 46 |
| Average MIC | 2.22 | 2.31 | 5.86 | 2.32 |
| Median MIC | 0.50 | 0.50 | 0.50 | 0.50 |
| %resistant | 6 | 6 | 17 | 8 |

[a] Treatments represent the following corresponding substances: [a1] benzylpenicillin/amoxicillin/kloxacillinbensatin; [a2] enrofloxacin; [a3] dihydrostreptomycin; [a4] oxytetracycline; [a5] sulfadiazin-trimethoprim/sulfadoxine-trimethoprim, N = number of herds with recorded treatment of the corresponding substance, and [b] number of decimal points reflect the number of decimal points in the MIC values (i.e., depending on the concentration/degree of dilution in the test panel).

The overall proportions of resistant *E. coli* isolates from calf and environmental samples and the corresponding use of antimicrobial treatments in these herds, expressed as the average of the total number of defined course doses per animal per year for the corresponding antimicrobial substance, are shown in Table 2. Some variation but no clear association between the proportion of resistant isolates and recorded AMU or herd management category could be found.

**Table 2.** Proportion of resistant *Escherichia coli* isolates from fecal samples from calves and environment (manure drainage and manure pit) in 27 organic and 27 conventional Swedish dairy herds (sampling period 2) and the corresponding use of antimicrobial treatments in these herds, as determined by collection of empty drug packages. Organic = organic herds, conventional = conventional herds, %R = proportion of resistant isolates (%), and DCD = total number of defined course doses per animal per year for the corresponding antimicrobial substance, expressed as the average figure for all herds in the category during the two data collection periods.

| Substance | Calf Isolates | | Environmental Isolates | |
|---|---|---|---|---|
| | Organic | Conventional | Organic | Conventional |
| Ampicillin %R | 25 | 18 | 12 | 9 |
| DCD penicillins | 0.584 | 1.170 | 0.584 | 1.170 |
| Ciprofloxacin %R | 3 | 5 | 0 | 2 |
| Nalidixic acid %R | 3 | 5 | 0 | 4 |
| DCD enrofloxacin | 0.002 | 0.002 | 0.002 | 0.002 |
| Gentamicin %R | 0 | 0.8 | 0 | 2 |
| Streptomycin %R | 30 | 40 | 14 | 13 |
| DCD dihydrostreptomycin | 0.102 | 0.167 | 0.102 | 0.167 |
| Tetracycline %R | 20 | 21 | 14 | 11 |
| DCD oxitetracycline | 0.010 | 0.005 | 0.010 | 0.005 |
| Sulfamethoxazole %R | 29 | 34 | 12 | 17 |
| Trimethoprim %R | 7 | 5 | 8 | 8 |
| DCD trimethoprim/sulfa | 0.021 | 0.012 | 0.021 | 0.012 |

From the available data, there was no indication of higher AMU in herds with higher proportions of MDR isolates.

## 4. Discussion

To the best of our knowledge, potential differences in AMR patterns between organic and conventional dairy herds in Sweden have not been previously studied. Some studies indicate that AMU is lower in organic herds [19,20], and AMR has been reported to be lower in organic pig herds, although the difference between organic and conventional production was less in Sweden than in some other countries [21]. Previous studies indicate that the differences in health status (that would affect AMU) between organic and conventional dairy herds in Sweden are small [22,23]. This is supported by the data from the herds in the present study that revealed no statistical difference in overall AMU between the two production systems, although some minor difference in patterns of AMU could be noted [15].

We chose to sample calves because previous data indicate that the prevalence of AMR decreases with the age of the animals [13,24,25] and we wanted to maximize the detection of AMR in the study herds. Sampling older animals might underestimate the levels of AMR, which should be taken into account when comparing data from different studies [24]. The environmental manure samples collected at the start of period 2 can be assumed to represent older animals (as cows produce most of the manure in the herd) and reflect a previous time period. The lower proportion of isolates classified as resistant in these samples, in comparison to the calf samples, support the assumption that herd-level AMR might be underestimated in samples from older animals. On the other hand, the storage time for the manure in the farm environment may also affect the composition and resistance pattern of the *E. coli* population in the samples.

In Europe, the prevalence of ESBL-producing *E. coli* in food-producing animals varies by country and animal species. In 2017, the prevalence in individual veal calves ranged from 7.1% in Denmark to 89.0% in Italy, with an EU mean of 44.5% [6]. Overall, in the eight EU countries supplying data on resistance in *E. coli* from calves to ampicillin, cefotaxime, ciprofloxacin and tetracycline for the period 2009–2017, there were 10 decreasing and 8 increasing trends [7]. A study in Spanish cattle herds tested *E. coli* isolated from healthy animals of all ages and found a significantly higher prevalence of resistance in dairy herds than in beef herds [26]. As much as 97.8% of all isolates were resistant to fourth-generation cephalosporins, 87.4% were resistant to third-generation cephalosporins, 70.4% to tetracycline, 70.4% to sulfamethoxazole, 47.4% to trimethoprim, 41.5% to ciprofloxacin, 28.9% to chloramphenicol and 23.7% to gentamicin.

In a Chilean study, *E. coli* isolated from healthy dairy calves, calves with diarrhoea and their environment (bedding) showed 92% resistance to amoxicillin, 18.3% to ceftiofur, 27.5% to enrofloxacin, 25.5% to florfenicol, 7.2% to gentamicin, 53.6% to oxytetracycline and 37.5% to trim-sulfa [27]. Nearly half of the isolates (49%) were resistant to three or more substances. In a case-control study from 2012 in healthy and diarrheic calves in Swedish dairy herds, the corresponding figures were 25% resistant to ampicillin, 0% to ceftiofur, 14% to enrofloxacin, 0% to florfenicol, 0% to gentamicin and 32% to tetracycline, with 28% resistant to 3 or more substances [28].

From an international perspective, AMR levels are low in Sweden [8] and this was also confirmed in our study, with AMR figures well below the levels found in the studies cited above. As seen in Figure 5, the overall pattern in the sampled herds reflect a low level of AMR. The highest number of isolates with MIC values above epidemiological cut offs were seen for ampicillin, streptomycin, sulfamethoxazole and tetracycline. However, only a small percentage of colonies grew on the plates supplemented by tetracycline at the cut-off concentration, indicating that the selected isolates with higher MIC values constituted a minority of the *E. coli* present in the samples.

The most common cause for AMU in Swedish dairy herds is mastitis [29]. In 2018/2019, the reported treatment incidence for clinical mastitis in dairy cows was 9.0 recorded treatments per 100 lactations [29]. Benzylpenicillin is the most common drug used and is recorded for more than 90% of reported treatments in the period 2018–2019 [29]. Historically, tetracycline was one of the most commonly used antimicrobial substances in Swedish livestock. In the last decade, the overall sale of tetracycline for veterinary use in Sweden has halved [8]. Still, tetracycline, together with sulfonamides and trimethoprim are among the most frequently used substances in dairy herds, although with treatment incidences at less than 10% of the beta lactam use [29]. Nalidixic acid is a representative for quinolones, enrofloxacin is the only quinolone used in Swedish animals. Enrofloxacin is only recommended for treatment of mastitis if *Klebisella* spp. is confirmed, while for *E. coli* mastitis only supportive therapy is recommended [30]. Since 2012, legislation restricts the use of quinolones and third- and fourth-generation cephalosporins in animals to situations when bacterial culture and susceptibility testing demonstrate that there is no other effective treatment option [30]. The level of quinolone-resistant isolates was low in this study, and the results from selective culturing indicate that the resistant isolates constituted a minority of the *E. coli* in the samples. No treatment of dairy cattle with cephalosporins was reported in the last available statistics from the Swedish dairy association [29]. Only one ESBL-producing isolate out of eight cephalosporin-resistant *E. coli* was detected in this study, which supports the absence of a selective pressure (i.e., exposure to third- or fourth-generation cephalosporins) in the studied herds. Chloramphenicol is not allowed in food-producing animals in Sweden, but florfenicol is registered for use in cattle [31]. Veterinary treatment guidelines, however, do not recommend its use [29], and no treatment of dairy cattle with florfenicol is reported in the available statistics [29]. A total of 28 isolates had MICs above cut off for chloramphenicol. Chloramphenicol can be produced by *Streptomyces venezuelae* in soil and absorbed by grass and crops. If animals are fed roughage and crops/grains that have grown in soil where *Str. venezuelae* is present, it may be a source for chloramphenicol exposure of these animals [32]. Another reason for chloramphenicol resistance in the absence of a selective pressure could be the location of chloramphenicol resistance genes on transferable genetic elements that carry other resistance genes, causing co-resistance to other drugs where a selective pressure may exist. Co-resistance to chloramphenicol and other drug classes commonly used in cattle, such as dihydrostreptomycin and trimethoprim, was reported in bovine *E. coli* in a Japanese study [33] and co-resistance to tetracycline was found in >92% of chloramphenicol resistant *E. coli* from humans and animals in a US survey [34].

A total of 46 isolates were defined as colistin resistant according to MIC values but no *mcr* gene was detected. Colistin is not used in Swedish cattle [29] and there is no colistin-containing drug preparation registered for use in cattle in Sweden [31]. So far, *mcr* genes constitute the only known transferable genetic element conferring colistin resistance, so the high MIC values may be caused by chromosomal mutations or a yet unidentified mobile genetic element [35], or may be due to the inherent difficulties in MIC analysis for colistin. The microdilution method for colistin MIC determination is challenging, as the concentration of free colistin may be affected by adherence to organic or inorganic material, or the presence of polysorbate in the dilution broth [36]. Within the scope of this study, we cannot determine whether some of the high MIC values were due to a lower than expected concentration of colistin in the MIC plates or whether the isolates were indeed colistin resistant.

The differences in average and median MIC values (see Table 1) are not surprising as the susceptibility testing method uses a series of 2-fold dilutions of the antimicrobial substance and hence a difference in one dilution step will cause a 2-fold difference in MIC. Repeated testing of the same isolate may result in a one-step change in MIC [10] and this should be kept in mind when interpreting results that are close to the cut-off value, regardless of whether ECOFFs or clinical breakpoints are used. AMR levels can be presented in various ways, but the most transparent is showing the MIC distributions, as in Figures 1–3. By showing the distribution of the obtained MIC values when testing a number of non-clinical isolates collected in a systematic manner, it might be possible to discern two phenotypic populations with varying levels of MIC. The epidemiological cut-off points provided by EUCAST are based on a large number of samples and aim to differentiate between the wild type of a bacterial population and isolates with acquired resistance, but there may be overlap in the MIC distributions of these two types of isolates [10]. Hence, cut offs or breakpoints may be regarded as guidance, not an absolute divider between wild-type isolates and isolates with acquired resistance (potentially due to exposure to antimicrobials). The representativeness of the isolates is also an issue, although single isolates from a few animals per herd are regularly used as a basis for illustrating the herd-level AMR pattern, or for national monitoring [7]. The results from our selective culturing, where the resistant isolates constituted a minority of the *E. coli* population in most of the samples, illustrate the challenge of obtaining representative isolates. Methodological variation caused by differences in sample transportation time or different people taking the samples was not expected to have affected the results, and no systematic differences related to these aspects were observed.

AMU contributes to AMR by exerting a selective pressure on bacterial populations, favoring clones carrying resistance traits that protect them from the antimicrobial substances used. The varying patterns of phenotypic resistance traits and sometimes contradictory relationship between AMR and AMU for specific substances seen in this study illustrate the complexity of AMR dynamics. The optimal timeframe for assessing the selective effect of AMU is difficult to pinpoint. We chose to use on farm-collected AMU information for two time periods during the indoor season in order to reflect the overall pattern of AMU in the study herds. The AMU data did not cover the entire time period before sampling but were deemed to be the most accurate reflection of actual on-farm use, not hampered by challenges in reporting [15]. One of the study farms stated to not have used any antibiotics for at least five, maybe as much as 10 years, either in animals (pets included) or people living on the farm. Still, resistant isolates of *E. coli* were found in the samples from this farm, demonstrating the unpredictability of temporal AMR patterns. The association between AMU and AMR may be apparent on a larger scale, although not easily demonstrated on an individual farm level. A recent European study in poultry, pigs and veal calves detected significant associations between on-farm AMR and national AMU for some substances in some herd types but not all [37].

AMR has been detected in bacteria isolated from flies, rats and other animals in farm environments [38], further illustrating the challenges in determining the associations between AMU and AMR. Similar patterns of ESBL-producing *E. coli* have been demonstrated in wild gulls and humans, and it has been suggested that the humans might have served as the source for AMR in animals [39]. A possible route for cattle is from people excreting antimicrobial residues (and resistant bacteria) into effluent [40] and further into surface water that is subsequently consumed by grazing livestock.

In the present study, there was no obvious difference in AMR patterns in organic and conventional herds, indicating that a generally good animal health status and consequent low AMU may have the same effect in controlling AMR as the specific AMU rules for organic production. Although the number of farms and sampling occasions were limited and small differences may have been difficult to discern, the strict regulation of AMU in both production systems in Sweden prompts the question whether other herd-level factors exert a higher influence on AMR patterns in this context. Further studies of the entire farm environment are needed to disentangle the complex web of AMR and its drivers on livestock farms.

## 5. Conclusions

No obvious difference in AMR patterns between organic and conventional herds could be detected in this study, most likely due to a generally good animal health status and consequent low AMU in both herd types. The results illustrate the general variation in AMR patterns on a farm level and the challenges in detecting associations with herd management or AMU. Further studies of the entire farm environment are needed to disentangle the complex web of AMR and its drivers on livestock farms.

**Author Contributions:** Conceptualization, K.S., U.E., N.F. and S.S.L.; investigation (fieldwork), K.S., (laboratory methodology and performance), V.T., R.A.H. and J.D.J.; data curation, K.S.; formal analyses, K.S., S.S.L., G.O.A.; writing—original draft preparation and editing, S.S.L.; manuscript review, K.S., V.T., R.A.H., J.D.J., U.E., N.F., G.O.A., S.S.L.; visualization, R.A.H.; supervision, U.E., S.S.L., J.D.J.; project administration, U.E.; funding acquisition, U.E. All authors have read and agreed to the published version of the manuscript.

**Funding:** This research was funded by Formas—The Swedish Research Council for Environment, Agricultural Sciences and Spatial Planning, grant No. 2014-281.

**Acknowledgments:** The authors wish to acknowledge Helle Unnerstad, who contributed significantly to this study with her expertise in antimicrobial susceptibility testing and AMR issues. Sadly, she passed away before the writing of the manuscript. We are grateful to the farmers for taking the time to assist in data collection and allowing access to their farms.

**Conflicts of Interest:** The authors declare no conflict of interest.

## References

1. O'Neill, J. Tackling Drug Resistance Globally: Final Report. Wellcome Trust: London, UK, 2016. Available online: https://amr-review.org/sites/default/files/160525_Final%20paper_with%20cover.pdf (accessed on 1 September 2020).
2. Mölstad, S.; Löfmark, S.; Carlin, K.; Erntell, M.; Aspevall, O.; Blad, L.; Hanberger, H.; Hedin, K.; Hellman, J.; Norman, C.; et al. Lessons learnt during 20 years of the Swedish strategic programme against antibiotic resistance. *Bull. World Health Organ.* **2017**, *95*, 764–773. [CrossRef]
3. Grundin, J.; Blanco-Penedo, I.; Fall, N.; Sternberg-Lewerin, S. The Swedish Experience—A Summary of the Swedish Efforts towards a Low and Prudent Use of Antibiotics in Animal Production. SLU Future Animals, Nature and Health Report No. 5. 2020. Available online: https://www.slu.se/en/Collaborative-Centres-and-Projects/slu-future-animals-nature-and-health/forskning/publications/rapporter/the-swedish-experience/ (accessed on 1 September 2020).
4. Swedish Public Health Agency, Swedish Board of Agriculture. Swedish Work against Antibiotic Resistance—A One Health Approach. 2020. Available online: https://www2.jordbruksverket.se/download/18.693595921700d430c72b254f/1580906107699/ovr524.pdf (accessed on 1 September 2020).
5. OIE Annual Report on Antimicrobial Agents Intended for Use in Animals. 2018. Available online: https://rr-africa.oie.int/wp-content/uploads/2019/09/annual_report_amr_3.pdf (accessed on 1 September 2020).
6. European Food Safety Authority, European Centre for Disease Prevention and Control. The European Union summary report on antimicrobial resistance in zoonotic and indicator bacteria from humans, animals and food in 2017. *EFSA J.* **2019**, *17*, 5598. [CrossRef]

7. European Food Safety Authority and European Centre for Disease Prevention and Control: The European Union Summary Report on Antimicrobial Resistance in zoonotic and indicator bacteria from humans, animalsand food in 2017/2018. *EFSA J.* **2020**, *18*, 6007. [CrossRef]
8. Swedres-Svarm 2019. Sales of Antibiotics and Occurrence of Resistance in Sweden. Solna/Uppsala ISSN1650-6332. Available online: https://www.folkhalsomyndigheten.se/contentassets/fb80663bc7c94d678be785e3360917d1/swedres-svarm-2019.pdf (accessed on 1 September 2020).
9. Harada, K.; Asai, T. Role of antimicrobial selective pressure and secondary factors on antimicrobial resistance prevalence in *Escherichia coli* from food-producing animals in Japan. *J. Biomed. Biotechnol.* **2010**, 180682. [CrossRef]
10. EUCAST. The European Committee on Antimicrobial Susceptibility Testing. MIC and Zone Diameter Distributions and ECOFFs. 2018. Available online: https://www.eucast.org/mic_distributions_and_ecoffs/ (accessed on 1 September 2020).
11. Swedres-Svarm 2017. Sales of Antibiotics and Occurrence of Resistance in Sweden. Solna/Uppsala ISSN1650-6332. Available online: https://www.sva.se/media/103hg3vh/swedres_svarm2017.pdf (accessed on 1 September 2020).
12. USDA National Organic Program. 2002. Available online: https://www.ams.usda.gov/about-ams/programs-offices/national-organic-program (accessed on 1 September 2020).
13. Sato, K.; Bartlett, P.C.; Saeed, M.A. Antimicrobial susceptibility of *Escherichia coli* isolates from dairy farms using organic versus conventional production methods. *J. Am. Vet. Med. Assoc.* **2005**, *226*, 589–594. [CrossRef] [PubMed]
14. KRAV (Kontrollföreningen för Ekologisk Produktion). KRAV Regler. 2018. Available online: https://www.krav.se/regler/ (accessed on 1 September 2020). (In Swedish).
15. Olmos Antillón, G.; Sjöström, K.; Fall, N.; Sternberg Lewerin, S.; Emanuelson, U. Antibiotic Use in Organic and Non-Organic Swedish Dairy Farms: A Comparison of Three Recording Methods. *Front. Vet. Sci.* **2020**, *7*, 843. [CrossRef]
16. Duse, A.; Waller, K.P.; Emanuelson, U.; Unnerstad, H.E.; Persson, Y.; Bengtsson, B. Risk factors for antimicrobial resistance in fecal *Escherichia coli* from preweaned dairy calves. *J. Dairy Sci.* **2015**, *98*, 500–516. [CrossRef]
17. Rebelo, A.R.; Bortolaia, V.; Kjeldgaard, J.S.; Pedersen, S.K.; Leekitcharoenphon, P.; Hansen, I.M.; Guerra, B.; Malorny, B.; Borowiak, M.; Hammerl, J.A.; et al. Multiplex PCR for detection of plasmid-mediated colistin resistance determinants, *mcr*-1, *mcr*-2, *mcr*-3, *mcr*-4 and *mcr*-5 for surveillance purposes. *Eurosurveillance* **2018**, *23*, 1–11. [CrossRef]
18. Woodford, N.; Fagan, E.J.; Ellington, M.J. Multiplex PCR for rapid detection of genes encoding CTX-M extended-spectrum β-lactamases. *J. Antimicrob. Chemother.* **2006**, *57*, 154–155. [CrossRef]
19. Krogh, M.A.; Nielsen, C.L.; Sørensen, J.T. Antimicrobial use in organic and conventional dairy herds. *Animal* **2020**, *14*, 2187–2193. [CrossRef]
20. Pol, M.; Ruegg, P.L. Treatment practices and quantification of antimicrobial drug usage in conventional and organic dairy farms in Wisconsin. *J. Dairy Sci.* **2007**, *90*, 249–261. [CrossRef]
21. Österberg, J.; Wingstrand, A.; Jensen, A.N.; Kerouanton, A.; Cibin, V.; Barco, L.; Denis, M.; Aabo, S.; Bengtsson, B. Antibiotic resistance in *Escherichia coli* from pigs in organic and conventional farming in four European countries. *PLoS ONE* **2016**, *11*, 1–12. [CrossRef] [PubMed]
22. Fall, N.; Forslund, K.; Emanuelson, U. Reproductive performance, general health, and longevity of dairy cows at a Swedish research farm with both organic and conventional production. *Livest. Sci.* **2008**, *118*, 11–19. [CrossRef]
23. Fall, N.; Emanuelson, U. Milk yield, udder health and reproductive performance in Swedish organic and conventional dairy herds. *J. Dairy Res.* **2009**, *76*, 402–410. [CrossRef] [PubMed]
24. Hoyle, D.V.; Shaw, D.J.; Knight, H.I.; Davison, H.C.; Pearce, M.C.; Low, C.; Gunn, G.J.; Woolhouse, M.E.J. Age-related decline in carriage of ampicillin-resistant *Escherichia coli* in young calves. *Appl. Environ. Microbiol.* **2004**, *70*, 6927–6930. [CrossRef] [PubMed]
25. Duse, A.; Waller, K.P.; Emanuelson, U.; Unnerstad, H.E.; Persson, Y.; Bengtsson, B. Risk factors for quinolone-resistant *Escherichia coli* in feces from preweaned dairy calves and postpartum dairy cows. *J. Dairy Sci.* **2015**, *9*, 6387–6398. [CrossRef] [PubMed]

26. Tello, M.; Ocejo, M.; Oporto, B.; Hurtado, A. Prevalence of Cefotaxime-Resistant *Escherichia coli* Isolates from Healthy Cattle and Sheep in Northern Spain: Phenotypic and Genome-Based Characterization of Antimicrobial Susceptibility. *Appl. Environ. Microbiol.* **2020**, *86*, e00742. [CrossRef]
27. Astorga, F.; Navarrete-Talloni, M.J.; Miro, M.P.; Bravo, V.; Toro, M.; Blondel, C.J.; Herve-Claude, L.P. Antimicrobial resistance in *E. coli* isolated from dairy calves and bedding material. *Heliyon* **2019**, *5*, e02773. [CrossRef]
28. De Verdier, K.; Nyman, A.; Greko, C.; Bengtsson, B. Antimicrobial resistance and virulence factors in *Escherichia coli* from swedish dairy calves. *Acta Vet. Scand.* **2012**, *54*, 2. [CrossRef]
29. Nyman, A. Treatment Incidence with Antibacterial Substances for Systemic Use in Controlled Herds 2001–2018. Available online: https://www.vxa.se/globalassets/dokument/statistik/antibiotikaforbrukning-2001-2018.pdf (accessed on 1 September 2020). (In Swedish).
30. Swedish Veterinary Association. Guidelines for the Use of Antibiotics in Production Animals. Available online: https://svf.se/media/vd5ney4l/svfs-riktlinje-antibiotika-till-produktionsdjur-eng-2017.pdf (accessed on 1 September 2020).
31. LIF (Swedish Association of the Pharmaceutical Industry). FASS Djurläkemedel (Approved Veterinary Drugs in Sweden). 2020. Available online: https://www.fass.se/LIF/startpage?userType=1 (accessed on 1 September 2020). (In Swedish).
32. Berendsen, B.; Pikkemaat, M.; Römkens, P.; Wegh, R.; Van Sisseren, M.; Stolker, L.; Nielen, M. Occurrence of chloramphenicol in crops through natural production by bacteria in soil. *J. Agric. Food Chem.* **2013**, *61*, 4004–4010. [CrossRef]
33. Harada, K.; Asai, T.; Kojima, A.; Ishihara, K.; Takahashi, T. Role of coresistance in the development of resistance to chloramphenicol in *Escherichia coli* isolated from sick cattle and pigs. *Am. J. Vet. Res.* **2006**, *67*, 230–235. [CrossRef] [PubMed]
34. Tadesse, D.A.; Zhao, S.; Tong, E.; Ayers, S.; Singh, A.; Bartholomew, M.J.; McDermott, P.F. Antimicrobial drug resistance in *Escherichia coli* from humans and food animals, United States, 1950–2002. *Emerg. Infect. Dis.* **2012**, *18*, 741–749. [CrossRef] [PubMed]
35. Aghapour, Z.; Gholizadeh, P.; Ganbarov, K.; Zahedi Bialvaei, A.; Saad Mahmood, S.; Tanomand, A.; Yousefi, M.; Asgharzadeh, M.; Yousefi, B.; Samadi Kafilet, H. Molecular mechanisms related to colistin resistance in *Enterobacteriaceae*. *Infect Drug Resist.* **2019**, *12*, 965–975. [CrossRef] [PubMed]
36. Albur, M.; Noel, A.; Bowker, K.; MacGowan, A. Colistin susceptibility testing: Time for a review. *J. Antimicr. Chemother.* **2014**, *69*, 1432–1434. [CrossRef] [PubMed]
37. Ceccarelli, D.; Hesp, A.; Van Der Goot, J.; Joosten, P.; Sarrazin, S.; Wagenaar, J.A.; Dewulf, J.; Mevius, D.J. Antimicrobial resistance prevalence in commensal *Escherichia coli* from broilers, fattening turkeys, fattening pigs and veal calves in European countries and association with antimicrobial usage at country level. *J. Med. Microbiol.* **2020**, *69*, 4. [CrossRef]
38. Literak, I.; Dolejska, M.; Rybarikova, J.; Cizek, A.; Strejckova, P.; Vyskocilova, M.; Friedman, M.; Klimes, J. Highly variable patterns of antimicrobial resistance in commensal *Escherichia coli* isolates from pigs, sympatric rodents, and flies. *Microb. Drug Resist.* **2009**, *15*, 229–237. [CrossRef]
39. Atterby, C.; Börjesson, S.; Ny, S.; Järhult, J.D.; Byfors, S.; Bonnedahl, J. ESBL-producing *Escherichia coli* in Swedish gulls—A case of environmental pollution from humans? *PLoS ONE* **2017**, *12*, 1–13. [CrossRef]
40. Hirsch, R.; Ternes, T.; Haberer, K.; Kratz, K.L. Occurrence of antibiotics in the aquatic environment. *Sci. Total Environ.* **1999**, *225*, 109–118. [CrossRef]

**Publisher's Note:** MDPI stays neutral with regard to jurisdictional claims in published maps and institutional affiliations.

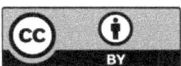

© 2020 by the authors. Licensee MDPI, Basel, Switzerland. This article is an open access article distributed under the terms and conditions of the Creative Commons Attribution (CC BY) license (http://creativecommons.org/licenses/by/4.0/).

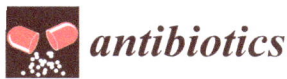

Article

# Antimicrobial Resistance Profile of *Staphylococcus hyicus* Strains Isolated from Brazilian Swine Herds

Andrea Micke Moreno [1,*], Luisa Zanolli Moreno [1], André Pegoraro Poor [1], Carlos Emilio Cabrera Matajira [2], Marina Moreno [1], Vasco Túlio de Moura Gomes [1], Givago Faria Ribeiro da Silva [1], Karine Ludwig Takeuti [3] and David Emilio Barcellos [3]

[1] Department of Preventive Veterinary Medicine and Animal Health, Faculty of Veterinary Medicine and Animal Science, University of São Paulo, São Paulo 05508-270, Brazil; luzanolli@gmail.com (L.Z.M.); andrepegoraro21@gmail.com (A.P.P.); marinamo@gmail.com (M.M.); gomesvtm@gmail.com (V.T.d.M.G.); givagofaria@yahoo.com.br (G.F.R.d.S.)
[2] Facultad de Ciencias Básicas, Universidad Santiago de Cali, Cali 760042, Colombia; k.rlos89.cabrera@gmail.com
[3] Setor de Suínos, Faculdade de Veterinária, Universidade Federal do Rio Grande do Sul (UFRGS), Porto Alegre 91501-970, Brazil; karinelt87@yahoo.com.br (K.L.T.); davidbarcellos@terra.com.br (D.E.B.)
* Correspondence: morenoam@usp.br; Tel.: +55-11-3091-1377

**Abstract:** *Staphylococcus hyicus* is the causative agent of porcine exudative epidermitis. This disorder affects animals in all producing countries and presents a widespread occurrence in Brazil. This study evaluated strains from a historical collection in order to detect the presence of exfoliative-toxin-encoding genes (SHETB, ExhA, ExhB, ExhC, ExhD), characterize the strains using PFGE, and determine their respective antimicrobial resistance profiles. The results obtained from the evaluation of 77 strains from 1982 to 1987 and 103 strains from 2012 reveal a significant change in resistance profiles between the two periods, especially regarding the antimicrobial classes of fluoroquinolones, amphenicols, lincosamides, and pleuromutilins. The levels of multidrug resistance observed in 2012 were significantly higher than those detected in the 1980s. It was not possible to correlate the resistance profiles and presence of genes encoding toxins with the groups obtained via PFGE. Only 10.5% of the strains were negative for exfoliative toxins, and different combinations of toxins genes were identified. The changes observed in the resistance pattern of this bacterial species over the 30-year period analyzed indicate that *S. hyicus* could be a useful indicator in resistance monitoring programs in swine production. In a country with animal protein production such as Brazil, the results of this study reinforce the need to establish consistent monitoring programs of antimicrobial resistance in animals, as already implemented in various countries of the world.

**Keywords:** *Staphylococcus hyicus*; antimicrobial resistance; PFGE; exudative epidermitis; swine

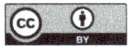

## 1. Introduction

*Staphylococcus hyicus* is the causative agent of exudative epidermitis in pigs, a generalized cutaneous infection characterized by skin exfoliation, excessive sebaceous secretion, and the formation of a brownish coat of exudate that may cover the entire body [1]. The disease is a widely recognized condition in pigs, especially in suckling and weaned piglets. It has been sporadically reported to cause significant morbidity that can be up to 90% in infected herds, and moderate mortality in naïve herds [2].

*S. hyicus* strains may be considered pathogenic or nonpathogenic according to their ability to induce exudative epidermitis in pigs and their ability to produce the exfoliative toxins, which are the main virulence factors necessary to induce the disease [3]. Until now, five exfoliative toxins from *S. hyicus* were described. SHETB was characterized in Japan [4], and ExhA, ExhB, ExhC, and ExhD were characterized in Denmark [5]. The Exh toxins have been shown to cause a loss of cell adhesion in the epidermis of porcine skin by cleaving desmoglein-1, while human desmoglein-1 is resistant to *S. hyicus* exfoliative toxins [3,6,7].

The disease is frequently treated with antimicrobial agents, but treatment is a problem because of the frequent occurrence of antimicrobial resistance in pig strains and subsequent treatment failure. The frequent occurrence of antimicrobial resistance has been previously reported among *S. hyicus* in different countries [1]; in contrast, there is limited information regarding the distribution of different resistance profiles of *S. hyicus* originating in Brazilian swine.

This investigation evaluated *S. hyicus* strains from Brazilian pigs with exudative epidermitis, examined in two different periods with an interval of 30 years, for the purpose of detecting the presence of genes encoding exfoliative toxins, characterizing the strains using PFGE, and determining the minimal inhibitory concentration of antimicrobial agents against each strain.

## 2. Materials and Methods

### 2.1. Bacterial Isolation and Culture Conditions

A total of 77 *S. hyicus* strains isolated in the 1980s and 103 strains isolated in 2012 were evaluated. The strains were isolated from skin lesions of pigs presenting with exudative epidermitis in 27 swine herds from two states, Rio Grande do Sul and São Paulo. Skin swabs were inoculated onto Tween 80 agar plates and aerobically incubated for 18–24 h at 37 °C [8]. Colonies with morphological characteristics of *S. hyicus* were selected and identified using standard biochemical procedures [9] and polymerase chain reaction (PCR). Historical strains were stored in a lyophilized form following isolation, whereas recent strains were stored at −86 °C until characterization.

### 2.2. Detection of Genes Encoding Superoxide Dismutase A and Toxins SHETB, ExhA, ExhB, ExhC, and ExhD

All strains were subjected to species-specific PCR with partial amplification of the *sodA* gene that encodes superoxide dismutase A, as previously described [10], to confirm the identification of *S. hyicus*. Genes encoding toxins SHETB, ExhA, ExhB, ExhC, and ExhD were detected as described in [5,11].

Purified DNA was recovered according to the protocol of Boom et al. [12], with previous enzymatic treatment for 60 min at 37 °C, with 100 mg of lysozyme and 20 mg of proteinase K (USBiological, Swampscott, MA, USA). Samples were stored at −20 °C until processing.

Polymerase chain reactions (50 µL) comprised 5 µL of genomic DNA, ultrapure water, 10× PCR buffer, 1.5 mM $MgCl_2$, 200 µM of dNTPs, 10 pmol of each primer, and 1.25 U of Taq-DNA-polymerase (Fermentas Inc., Rockville, MD, USA). The amplified products were stained with BlueGreen® (LGC Biotecnologia, São Paulo, Brazil) and separated by electrophoresis using 1.5% agarose gel, using the 100 bp DNA Ladder® (New England Biolabs Inc., Ipswich, MA, USA).

### 2.3. Molecular Typing by PFGE

*S. hyicus* strains were grown in brain heart infusion broth for 18–24 h at 37 °C. Plug preparation and DNA extraction followed a previously described protocol [13]. The restriction enzyme *Sma*I (New England Biolabs, Ipswich, MA, USA) was used for DNA digestion at 30 °C for 24 h. Electrophoresis was performed using 1% SeaKem Gold® agarose (Cambrex Bio Science Rockland, East Rutherford, NJ, USA) and a CHEF-DR III System (Bio-Rad Laboratories, Hercules, CA, USA) with 0.5× TBE at 14 °C. DNA fragments were separated at 6 V/cm at a 120° fixed angle, with pulse times from 3 to 33 s ramping for 20 h. Gels were stained with a fluorescent DNA stain (SYBR® Safe, Invitrogen Corporation, Carlsbad, CA, USA) for 30 min and imaged under UV transillumination. Lambda DNA-PFGE marker (New England Biolabs, Ipswich, MA, USA) was used for fragment size determination.

*2.4. Broth Microdilution*

The minimal inhibitory concentration (MIC) was determined by the broth microdilution technique as recommended by the Clinical and Laboratory Standards Institute [14], using Sensititre™ Standard Susceptibility MIC Plates BOPO6F (TREK Diagnostic Systems/Thermo Fisher Scientific, Waltham, MA, USA). *Staphylococcus aureus* (ATCC 29213) was used as a quality control. The applied breakpoints for interpretation of results were obtained mainly from the CLSI supplement VET08 [14] and are described in Table 1. If interpretive criteria were not present in the VET08 dataset [14], applied breakpoints were calculated using the twenty-eighth edition of the CLSI performance standard M100 [15], and the literature [16,17]. The reported breakpoints were selected with the following order of preference: those described for swine species were favored, then those for *Staphylococcus* spp. (regardless of the animal species or human indication), and in cases where there was no description in the CLSI or EUCAST datasets, a literature reference was used.

Table 1. Antimicrobials' MIC range evaluated, and breakpoints applied to *S. hyicus*.

| Antimicrobial | MIC Range (µg/mL) | MIC Breakpoints | | |
|---|---|---|---|---|
| | | Susceptible | Intermediary | Resistant |
| Ampicillin | ≤0.25–1.0 | ≤0.25 | 0.5 | ≥1 |
| Ceftiofur | ≤0.25–2.0 | ≤2 | 4 | ≥8 |
| Penicillin | ≤0.12–2.0 | ≤0.12 | - | ≥0.25 |
| Chlortetracycline | ≤0.5–>8.0 | ≤0.5 | 1 | ≥2 |
| Oxitetracycline | ≤0.5–>8.0 | ≤0.5 | 1 | ≥2 |
| Danofloxacin | 0.5–>1.0 | ≤0.25 | 0.5 | ≥1 |
| Enrofloxacin | 0.5–>2.0 | ≤0.5 | 1 | ≥2 |
| Florfenicol | 1.0–>8.0 | ≤2 | 4 | ≥8 |
| Spectinomycin | 16.0–>64.0 | ≤32 | 64 | ≥128 |
| Gentamycin | ≤1.0–>16.0 | ≤2 | 4 | ≥8 |
| Neomycin | ≤4.0–>32.0 | ≤8 | - | - |
| Sulfadimethoxine | >256.0 | ≤256 | - | ≥512 |
| Trimethoprim/sulfamethoxazole | >2/38 | ≤2/38 | - | ≥4/76 |
| Clindamycin | ≤0.25–>16.0 | ≤0.5 | 1–2 | ≥4 |
| Tylosin | ≤0.5–>32.0 | ≤1 | 2–4 | >4 |
| Tilmicosin | ≤4.0–>64.0 | ≤16 | - | ≥32 |
| Tulathromycin | ≤1.0–>64.0 | ≤16 | 32 | ≥64 |
| Tiamulin | 1.0–>32.0 | ≤16 | - | ≥32 |

*2.5. Statistical Analysis*

The association analysis between resistance profile and strain origin was performed with SPSS 16.0 (SPSS Inc., Chicago, IL, USA), using chi-square and Fisher's exact tests. Statistical significance was considered when $p$-values were less than 0.05. The PFGE fingerprint patterns were analyzed by a comprehensive pairwise comparison of restriction fragment sizes, using the Dice coefficient. The mean values obtained from the Dice coefficient were employed in UPGMA, using BioNumerics 7.6 (Applied Maths NV, Sint-Martens-Latem, Belgium). The isolates were considered from different pulsotypes when they differed by four or more bands [18]. Resistance profiles were analyzed as categorical data with the Dice coefficient, using BioNumerics 7.6 software (Applied Maths NV, Sint-Martens-Latem, Belgium).

## 3. Results

All strains from this study were confirmed as *S. hyicus* by PCR. The detection of exfoliative-toxin-encoding genes resulted in the following frequencies: shetB 0%, exhA 34.4% (62/180), exhB 24.4% (44/180), exhC 76.1% (137/180), and exhD 54.4% (98/180). By considering the distribution of toxin genes according to the year of isolation, it was possible to observe a significant increase in the occurrence of the ExhA toxin and a significant reduction in the occurrence of the ExhB toxin between strains from the 1980s and 2012 (Table 2). Only 10.5% (19/180) of strains were negative for all toxin genes, and 13 different profiles were identified according four toxins detected.

Table 2. Frequency of strains positive for exfoliative toxins in the two periods evaluated (1980s and 2012).

| Toxins | 1980 | | 2012 | | p |
|---|---|---|---|---|---|
| | N | % | N | % | |
| ExhA | 17 | 22.08 | 45 | 43.68 | <0.001 |
| ExhB | 31 | 40.26 | 13 | 12.62 | <0.001 |
| ExhC | 55 | 71.40 | 82 | 79.61 | 0.150 |
| ExhD | 48 | 62.30 | 50 | 48.54 | 0.087 |

p—probability of the chi-square test or Fisher's exact test (£).

Tests of 180 strains yielded 123 profiles through PFGE with the SmaI enzyme, presenting 9 to 20 fragments with sizes ranging from 40 to 300 kb. Strains showed a similarity greater than 70%, and it was possible to identify 28 pulsotypes. In several cases, pulsotypes grouped strains from the same farm, period of isolation, or state of origin. The dendrogram shown in Figure 1a,b illustrates the results observed in the PFGE analysis.

The observed pulsotypes were denoted as C1 to C28. Several pulsotypes clearly grouped the strains isolated in 2012, such as clusters C1, C2, C18, C19, C20, C23, C25, and C27. Other pulsotypes grouped strains isolated in the 1980s, such as clusters C7, C8, and C21. By considering the farm of origin, it was possible to observe the presence of strains from the same farm clustering into certain groups, such as cluster C17, which contained six strains from farm 18. However, other strains from this farm can also be found in groups C2, C10, and C16. This behavior is repeated in strains from different farms and can be observed most clearly at extreme points of the dendrogram, where strains from farm 15 are allocated into clusters C1, C6, C11, C13, C15, C26, and C27. It was not possible to correlate the resistance profiles, the presence of toxin-encoding genes, and the state of origin with the PFGE clusters.

All strains were subjected to the determination of the minimum inhibitory concentration; the observed resistance rates are presented in Table 3 and Figure 2. It is possible to observe that the resistance pattern changed when comparing strains from the 1980s to 2012 (a period of 30 years), particularly when considering the antimicrobial classes of fluoroquinolones, lincosamides, pleuromutilins, and amphenicols. According to the resistance phenotype, strains were classified into 86 resistance profiles, with 103 strains from 2012 classified into 55 profiles, and 77 strains from 1982 to 1987 into 31 profiles.

Multidrug-resistant strains (resistant to three or more different antimicrobial classes) were found in both assessed groups. However, we observed that the frequency of multidrug-resistant strains isolated in 2012 was significantly higher ($p < 0.001$) than that of those isolated between 1982 and 1987 (Table 4). Among multidrug-resistant strains, there was wide variation in the number of antimicrobial classes against which the strains presented resistance between the studied periods. Among the strains from 1982 to 1987, there were no strains which were resistant to more than six antimicrobial classes, whereas in the 2012 group, 25% of tested strains were resistant to more than seven antimicrobial classes. The distribution of MIC values (MIC50 and MIC90) from the historic and 2012 strains is presented in the Supplementary Material (Tables S1 and S2).

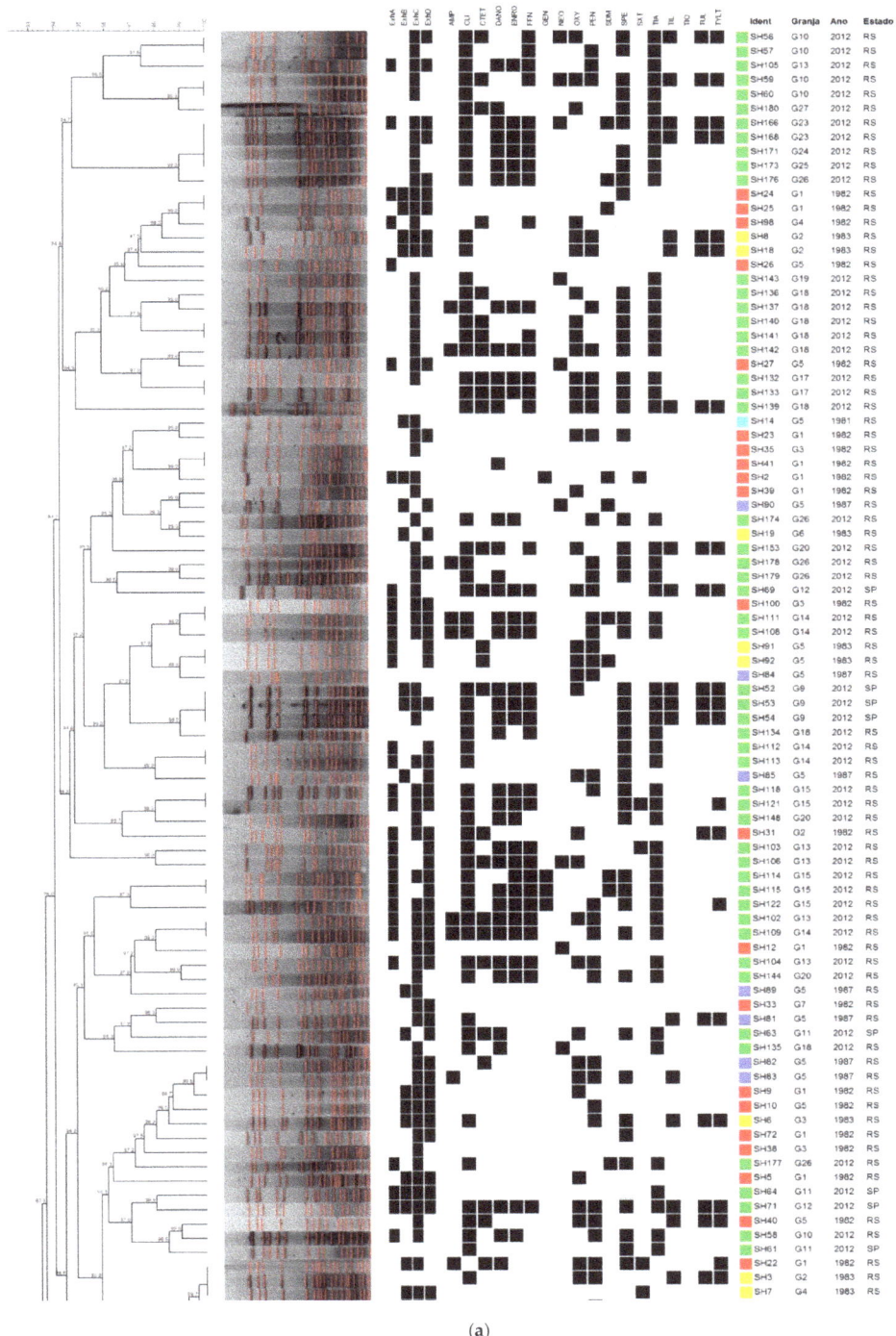

**Figure 1.** *Cont.*

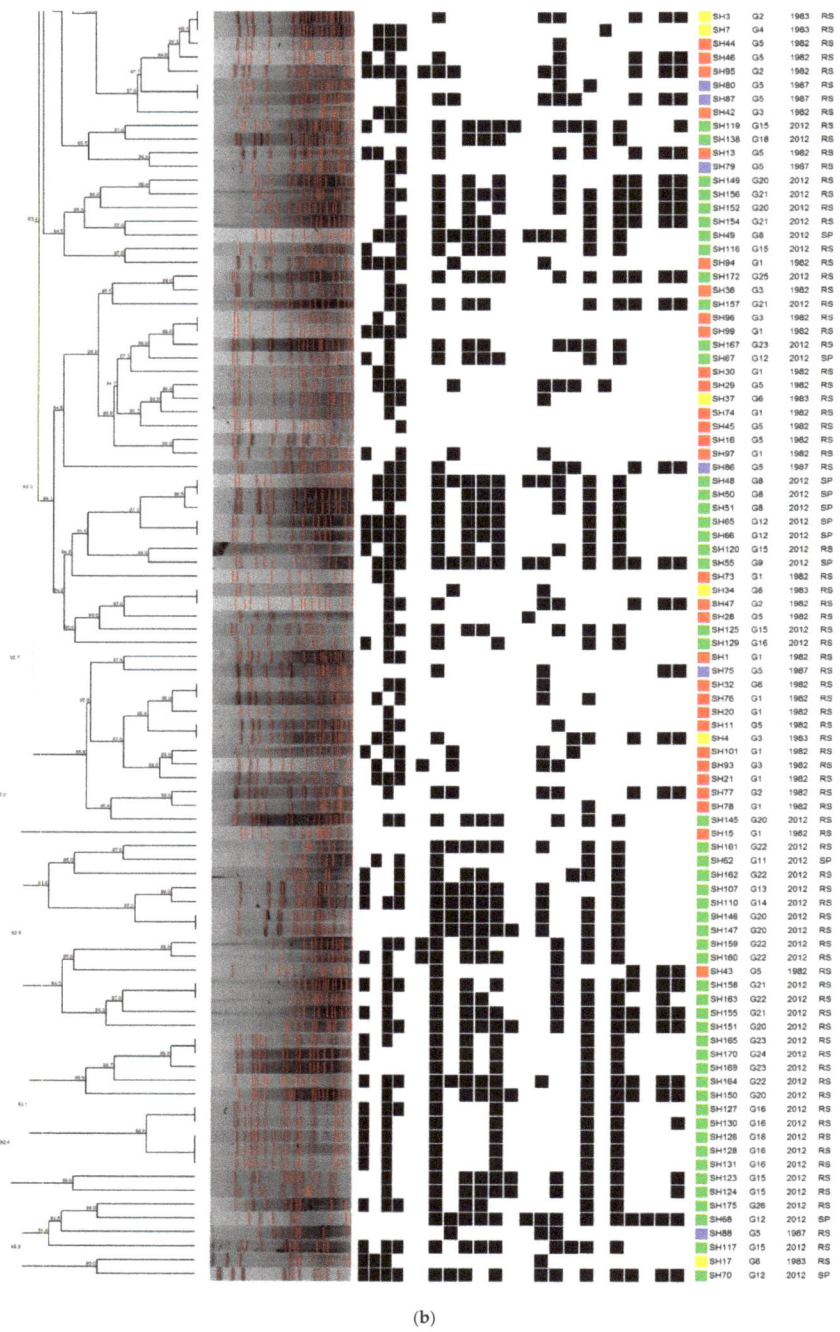

(b)

**Figure 1.** (a) Dendrogram showing the relationship among the *S. hyicus* pulsotypes, resistance profiles, and detection of toxin genes (Part I). (b) Dendrogram showing the relationship among the *S. hyicus* pulsotypes, resistance profiles, and detection of toxin genes (Part II).

Table 3. Resistance rates of *S. hyicus* from the 1980s and 2012 against tested antimicrobials.

| Class | Antimicrobial | 1980 N | 1980 (%) | 2012 N | 2012 (%) | p |
|---|---|---|---|---|---|---|
| Beta-lactams | Ampicillin | 16 | 20.77 | 29 | 28.15 | 0.258 |
| | Ceftiofur | 0 | 0.00 | 1 | 0.97 | 0.386 |
| | Penicillin | 28 | 36.36 | 46 | 44.66 | 0.263 |
| Tetracycline | Oxitetracycline | 33 | 42.86 | 29 | 28.16 | 0.040 |
| | Chlortetracycline | 34 | 44.15 | 30 | 29.12 | 0.037 |
| Fluoroquinolones | Danofloxacin | 2 | 2.60 | 81 | 78.64 | <0.001 |
| | Enrofloxacin | 0 | 0.00 | 67 | 65.05 | <0.001 |
| Aminoglycosides | Gentamycin | 1 | 1.30 | 9 | 8.74 | 0.045 |
| | Neomycin | 4 | 5.19 | 10 | 9.71 | 0.263 |
| | Spectinomycin | 8 | 10.4 | 99 | 96.1 | <0.001 |
| Fenicois | Florfenicol | 1 | 1.30 | 77 | 74.76 | <0.001 |
| Sulfas | Sulfadimethoxine | 9 | 11.69 | 10 | 9.71 | 0.669 |
| | Trimethoprim/sulfamethoxazole | 4 | 5.19 | 2 | 1.94 | 0.229 |
| Lincosamides | Clindamycin | 17 | 22.08 | 102 | 99.03 | <0.001 |
| Pleuromutilins | Tiamulin | 0 | 0.00 | 103 | 100.00 | <0.001 |
| Macrolides | Tilmicosin | 16 | 20.78 | 25 | 24.27 | 0.580 |
| | Tylosin | 18 | 23.38 | 31 | 30.10 | 0.316 |
| | Tulathromycin | 17 | 22.08 | 26 | 25.24 | 0.622 |

*p*—probability of chi-square or Fisher's exact (£) tests.

Table 4. Frequency of *S. hyicus* strains presenting multidrug resistance to antimicrobials according to isolation period.

| Classification | 1980 N | 1980 % | 2012 N | 2012 % | p |
|---|---|---|---|---|---|
| Resistant to 2 classes or less | 47 | 61.0 | 1 | 1.0 | <0.001 |
| Multidrug resistant (3 classes or more) | 30 | 39.0 | 102 | 99.0 | |

*p*—probability of the chi-square test.

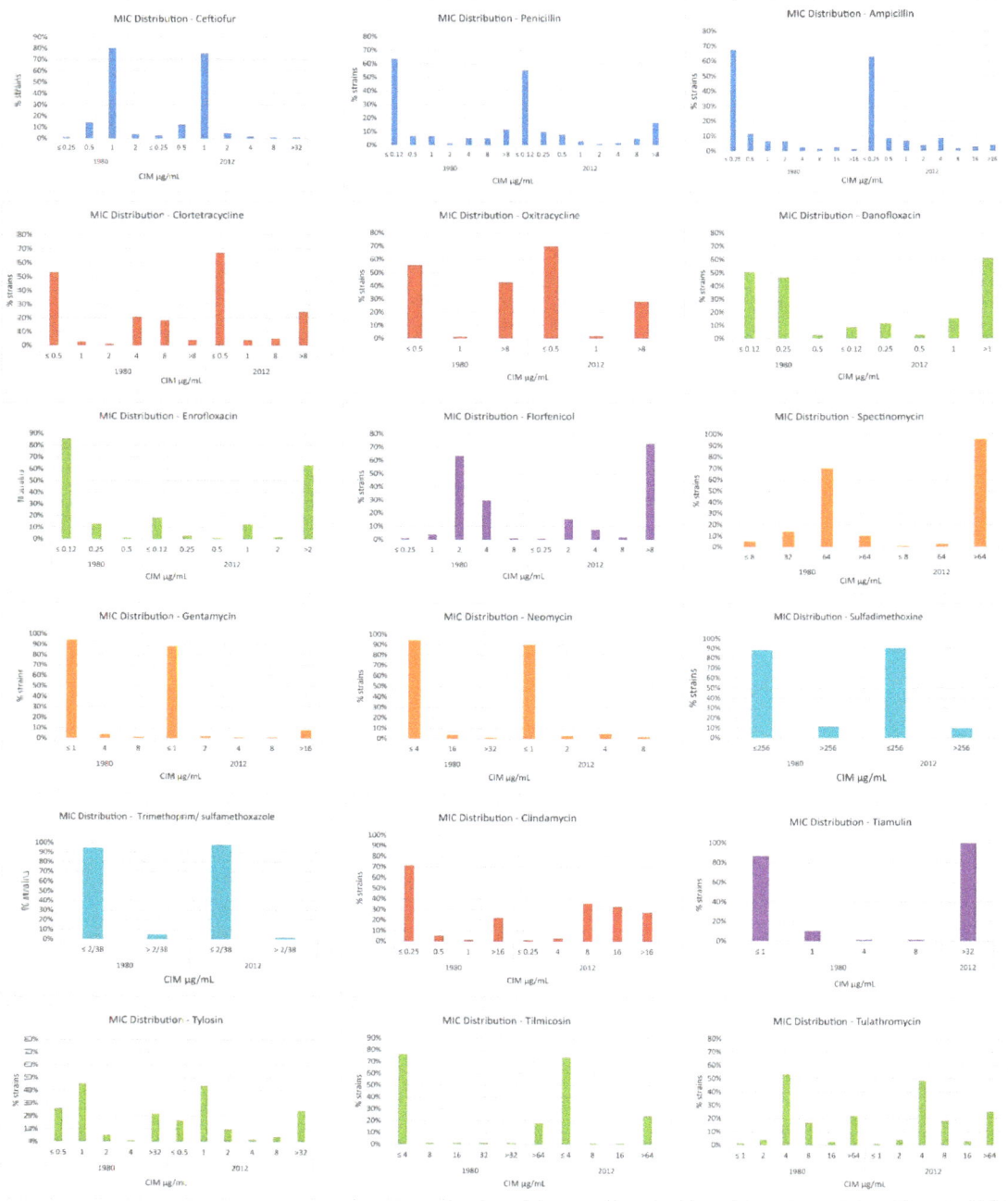

**Figure 2.** Distribution of MIC values according to antimicrobial tested and period evaluated (1980s or 2012).

## 4. Discussion

Exudative epidermitis has been described in swine for over 170 years, and its impact on pig production is observed to this day in different countries worldwide. The analysis of genes encoding exfoliative toxins presented here revealed a high frequency of positive samples for one or more toxins. Few studies have described the frequency of *S. hyicus* toxigenic strains. In a study carried out in Japan, Futagawa-Saito et al. [19] described the following rates: ExhA 35.7% (74/207), ExhB 19.3% (40/207), ExhC 0.5% (1/207), and ExhD 16.9% (35/207). Their results are similar to those observed in this study, except for the ExhC toxin, whose gene was detected more frequently in Brazilian strains (76.1%). Andresen [20] described the detection of genes in 218 *S. hyicus* strains from different countries (across Europe, Japan, and EUA), observing the following frequencies: ExhA 10.6% (23/218), ExhB 5.5% (12/218), ExhC 3.2% (7/218), and ExhD 14.2% (31/218). The increase in the frequency of the ExhA toxin and the reduction in the ExhB toxin observed between the periods evaluated in this study have no similar descriptions in the literature.

Through PFGE, the evaluated strains showed a high genetic diversity, which is characteristic of well-adapted agents which are widely disseminated in the population. *S. hyicus* strains constitute part of the microbiota of healthy animals, even if these strains have been isolated from animals with a clinical picture of epidermitis. Few studies report the application of PFGE in the characterization of *S. hyicus* strains. The most striking association in the different clusters formed in this study is related to the period of isolation. Some pulsotypes stand out for grouping strains isolated in 2012, such as clusters C1 (six strains), C2 (six strains), C18 (five strains), C19 (six strains), C20 (four strains), C22 (six strains), C23 (six strains), C25 (eight strains), and C27 (six strains). That is, 53 of 103 strains from 2012 (51.4%) were clustered according to the isolation period. Other pulsotypes contained only those strains isolated in the 1980s, such as clusters C7 (8 strains), C8 (9 strains), and C21 (4 strains), totaling 21 of 77 strains from the 1980s (27.2%), grouped in common clusters.

It was also possible to observe some groups such as C3, C4, C12, and C15 in which there was a predominance of strains from the 1980s, but with the presence of some recent strains. The strains from certain farms tend to be grouped into specific pulsotypes; however, in all cases, specific isolates from each farm are dispersed at different points on the dendrogram. It was not possible to correlate the resistance profiles and presence of genes encoding toxins with the groups obtained in PFGE.

The MICs of the 180 studied strains were evaluated against 9 antimicrobial classes, and the rising resistance level in several of these classes certainly reflects the increase in antibiotic use in intensive pig production systems in Brazil in recent decades [21]. This indicates that *S. hyicus* could be an important bacterial species for use in antimicrobial resistance monitoring programs in pig production in Brazil, as has been achieved in Denmark [1].

Among the tested beta-lactams, we saw a slight increase in ampicillin and penicillin resistance rates over the 30 years evaluated. The frequency of ceftiofur resistance was low in both groups. This may be related to the high cost of ceftiofur what restricted its use via parenteral administration until 2012. Nevertheless, higher rates of ceftiofur resistance have been described in Canada, where Park et al. [22] described 71% (101/142) of assessed *S. hyicus* strains as ceftiofur resistant in a study conducted on 30 herds. The occurrence of *S. hyicus* resistance to penicillin and ampicillin, or to ampicillin, penicillin, and ceftiofur, and positivity for the presence of the *mecA* gene was also described in the same study and has been considered a risk for swine and human health [22].

A slight decrease in tetracycline resistance rates was also observed in the studied strains. The culmination of the use of tetracyclines in Brazilian swine production was in the 1980s and 1990s. However, a study conducted in 2017 [21] showed that this class was the third most used among 25 Brazilian swine herds, despite the widespread resistance genes among several bacterial species.

The tetracycline resistance rates are quite varied in the literature, according to different countries and studied periods. In Denmark, Wegener et al. [23] reported that 44% (44/100) of *S. hyicus* strains were tetracycline resistant between 1991 and 1992, while Aarestrup and

Jensen [1] reported that only 28.9% (109/377) of Danish *S. hyicus* strains were tetracycline resistant in 2002. In Canada, 55% (79/142) of *S. hyicus* strains were resistant to tetracycline [22], whereas only 1.4% (3/207) of strains were resistant to doxycycline in a Japanese study [19].

The fluoroquinolone resistance levels found were low but represented a significant increase among the studied strains. This change probably reflects the introduction of these antimicrobial in swine production in the 1990s and the selection of resistant strains since then. Our results corroborate previous reports of low levels of enrofloxacin (5.6%) and ciprofloxacin (4.8%) resistance described in Danish *S. hyicus* [1].

The tested aminoglycosides exhibited two distinct resistance patterns: gentamicin and neomycin had low levels of resistance in the 1980s, and these rates have not increased significantly since then, but spectinomycin presented a low resistance rate in the 1980s which has significantly increased as of 2012. Spectinomycin has been added to in-feed formulations for several years to aid the control of enteric infections; this does not occur with neomycin and gentamicin, which are mostly restricted to individual treatments in oral or injectable formulations in Brazil. High resistance rates against spectinomycin (45.1%) have also been described in Canada [22].

The amphenicols currently permitted for use in swine production in Brazil are florfenicol and thiamphenicol. The use of florfenicol in the country began in the 2000s and has intensified since then, especially in in-feed treatment formulations. Resistance levels of the strains isolated in the 1980s were extremely low but demonstrated a large increase in 2012. In a Danish study conducted in 2003, resistance rates to florfenicol were 0% [24]. The sulfonamides, represented by sulfadimethoxine and a combination of trimethoprim/sulfamethoxazole, presented low levels of resistance in strains from the 1980s compared to a slight reduction in 2012. The drop in resistance is probably due to the reduction in the use of sulfonamides in feed production animals in Brazil during some years.

The studied macrolides (tilmicosin, tylosin, and tulathromycin) presented only a slight increase in resistance levels, despite their wide use in the treatment of respiratory and enteric infections in intensive swine production. In the literature, among the macrolides, erythromycin resistance rates were most frequently described with a variation of 15% to 62% between 1991 and 2001, in *S. hyicus* isolated in Denmark [1,23].

For clindamycin, we found high resistance rates in both studied periods. Regarding lincosamide resistance, a 59% (59/100) lincomycin resistance rate was reported in Denmark in 1990 [25]. The combination of lincomycin and spectinomycin has been widely used in recent years to control and prevent respiratory and enteric infections in Brazilian swine production. This could explain the high resistance rates to both of these antimicrobial classes during the studied periods.

The pleuromutilin class, represented by tiamulin, was approved for use in pigs in 1979 in Europe and the United States and was introduced in Brazil in late 1990. The drug is the second most used during the weaning and growing phases, as described by Dutra et al. [21], reinforcing the observed result that tiamulin resistance rates have increased from 0% in the 1980s to 100% of the strains in 2012. In staphylococci, the transferable resistance mechanisms of pleuromutilins have been linked to vga genes, which codify the ABC transporter that exports pleuromutilins, streptogramin A, and lincosamides. There are seven vga resistance genes described thus far (vga A, B, C, D, and E) and all of them are located in plasmids [26]. It is suggested that the use of pleuromutilins may have also favored the selection of cfr-positive *Staphylococcus* of animal origin, and a high frequency of multidrug resistance in strains resistant to pleuromutilins has been observed. Mobile elements containing pleuromutilin resistance genes often contain genes encoding resistance to other antimicrobial classes. Not only does the use of pleuromutilins select strains with this set of resistance genes, but also the use of other antimicrobial classes can select pleuromutilin-resistant strains in a mutual selection process [27]. Considering these risks of cross-selection, in January 2020, the Brazilian government prohibited the use of lincomycin, tiamulin, and tylosin as growth promoters in animals [28].

Given the genetic components related to resistance against the multiple antimicrobial classes tested in this study, and the associations described in the literature among different genes and mobile elements, it becomes easier to understand the observed changes in the resistance profiles of *S. hyicus* strains over the 30-year period studied and the significant increase in the phenomenon of multidrug resistance.

## 5. Conclusions

The results described here expand current knowledge about porcine exudative epidermitis in Brazil, as well as painting a portrait of the change in the antimicrobial resistance profiles that can occur over time in a bacterial population. The selection of multidrug-resistant *S. hyicus* strains in swine in this 30-year interval suggests that this phenomenon may also be occurring in other Gram-positive bacterial species of greater zoonotic potential such as *S. aureus, Enterococcus faecalis,* or *E. faecium*.

**Supplementary Materials:** The following supporting information can be downloaded at https://www.mdpi.com/article/10.3390/antibiotics11020205/s1, Table S1: Distribution of MIC values observed in *S. hyicus* strains isolated in 1980 decade. Table S2: Distribution of MIC values observed in *S. hyicus* strains isolated in 2012.

**Author Contributions:** Conceptualization, A.M.M. and L.Z.M.; methodology, A.M.M., D.E.B., C.E.C.M. and L.Z.M.; formal analysis, L.Z.M. and V.T.d.M.G.; investigation, A.M.M., M.M., G.F.R.d.S. and K.L.T.; resources, A.M.M. and D.E.B.; writing—original draft preparation, A.M.M. and L.Z.M.; writing—review and editing, L.Z.M., D.E.B., C.E.C.M. and A.P.P.; supervision, A.M.M. and D.E.B.; project administration, A.M.M. and L.Z.M.; funding acquisition, A.M.M. and D.E.B. All authors have read and agreed to the published version of the manuscript.

**Funding:** This study was supported by FAPESP - Fundação de Amparo à Pesquisa do Estado de São Paulo (grant 2011/08541-5). C.E.C.M., V.T.d.M.G., and L.Z.M. are recipients of FAPESP PhD fellowships (grants 2015/26159-1, 2013/16946-0, and 2013/17136-2). A.M.M. is a CNPq fellow (grant 310736/2018-8). L.Z.M. is supported by CNPq (grant 151908/2020-6).

**Institutional Review Board Statement:** This study was approved by the FMVZ-USP ethics committee (protocol code 3083/2013, 07/05/2014).

**Informed Consent Statement:** Not applicable.

**Acknowledgments:** The authors would like to thank all the farm owners, employees, and veterinarians who allowed access to the studied herds for their support.

**Conflicts of Interest:** The authors declare no conflict of interest.

## References

1. Aarestrup, F.M.; Jensen, L.B. Trends in antimicrobial susceptibility in relation to antimicrobial usage and presence of resistance genes in *Staphylococcus hyicus* isolated from exudative epidermitis in pigs. *Vet. Microbiol.* **2002**, *89*, 83–94. [CrossRef]
2. Foster, A.P. Staphylococcal skin disease in livestock. *Vet. Dermatol.* **2012**, *23*, 342–351.e63. [CrossRef] [PubMed]
3. Leekitcharoenphon, P.; Pamp, S.J.; Andresen, L.O.; Aarestrup, F.M. Comparative genomics of toxigenic and non-toxigenic *Staphylococcus hyicus*. *Vet. Microbiol.* **2016**, *185*, 34–40. [CrossRef] [PubMed]
4. Sato, H.; Watanabe, T.; Higuchi, K.; Teruya, K.; Ohtake, A.; Murata, Y.; Saito, H.; Aizawa, C.; Danbara, H.; Maehara, N. Chromosomal and Extrachromosomal Synthesis of Exfoliative Toxin from *Staphylococcus hyicus*. *J. Bacteriol.* **2000**, *182*, 4096–4100. [CrossRef]
5. Andresen, L.; Ahrens, P. A multiplex PCR for detection of genes encoding exfoliative toxins from *Staphylococcus hyicus*. *J. Appl. Microbiol.* **2004**, *96*, 1265–1270. [CrossRef]
6. Fudaba, Y.; Nishifuji, K.; Andresen, L.O.; Yamaguchi, T.; Komatsuzawa, H.; Amagai, M.; Sugai, M. *Staphylococcus hyicus* exfoliative toxins selectively digest porcine desmoglein 1. *Microb. Pathog.* **2005**, *39*, 171–176. [CrossRef] [PubMed]
7. Nishifuji, K.; Fudaba, Y.; Yamaguchi, T.; Iwasaki, T.; Sugai, M.; Amagai, M. Cloning of swine desmoglein 1 and its direct proteolysis by *Staphylococcus hyicus* exfoliative toxins isolated from pigs with exudative epidermitis. *Vet. Dermatol.* **2005**, *16*, 315–323. [CrossRef]
8. Devriese, L.A. Isolation and identification of *Staphylococcus hyicus*. *Am. J. Vet. Res.* **1977**, *38*, 787–792.
9. Quinn, P.J.; Carter, M.E.; Markey, B.; Carter, G.R. *Clinical Veterinary Microbiology*; Wolfe: London, UK, 1994; pp. 137–143.

10. Voytenko, A.; Kanbar, T.; Alber, J.; Lammler, C.; Weiss, R.; Prenger-Berninghoff, E.; Zschöck, M.; Akineden, O.; Hassan, A.; Dmitrenko, O. Identification of *Staphylococcus hyicus* by polymerase chain reaction mediated amplification of species specific sequences of superoxide dismutase A encoding gene sodA. *Vet. Microbiol.* **2006**, *116*, 211–216. [CrossRef]
11. Kanbar, T.; Voytenko, A.V.; Alber, J.; Lämmler, C.; Weiss, R.; Skvortzov, V.N. Distribution of the putative virulence factor encoding gene sheta in *Staphylococcus hyicus* strains of various origins. *J. Vet. Sci.* **2008**, *9*, 327–329. [CrossRef]
12. Boom, R.; Sol, C.J.; Salimans, M.M.; Jansen, C.L.; Dillen, P.M.W.-V.; van der Noordaa, J. Rapid and simple method for purification of nucleic acids. *J. Clin. Microbiol.* **1990**, *28*, 495–503. [CrossRef] [PubMed]
13. Hassler, C.; Nitzsche, S.; Iversen, C.; Zweifel, C.; Stephan, R. Characteristics of *Staphylococcus hyicus* strains isolated from pig carcasses in two different slaughterhouses. *Meat Sci.* **2008**, *80*, 505–510. [CrossRef]
14. Clinical and Laboratory Standards Institute (CLSI). *Performance Standards for Antimicrobial Disk and Dilution Susceptibility Tests for Bacteria Isolated from Animals*, 4th ed.; CLSI Supplement VET08. CLSI Document VET08; Clinical and Laboratory Standards Institute (CLSI): Wayne, PA, USA, 2018.
15. Clinical and Laboratory Standards Institute (CLSI). *Performance Standards for Antimicrobial Susceptibility Testing*, 28th ed.; CLSI Document M100S; Clinical and Laboratory Standards Institute: Wayne, PA, USA, 2018.
16. Hu, Y.; Liu, L.; Zhang, X.; Feng, Y.; Zong, Z. In Vitro Activity of Neomycin, Streptomycin, Paromomycin and Apramycin against Carbapenem-Resistant Enterobacteriaceae Clinical Strains. *Front. Microbiol.* **2017**, *8*, 2275. [CrossRef]
17. Rønne, H.; Szancer, J. In vitro susceptibility of Danish field isolates of Treponema hyodysenteriae to chemotherapeutics in swine dysentery (SD) therapy. Interpretation of MIC results based on the pharmacokinetic properties of the antibacterial agents. In Proceedings of the 11th International Pig Veterinary Society Congress, Swiss Association of Swine Medicine, Berne, Switzerland, 1–5 July 1990; p. 1126.
18. van Belkum, A.; Tassios, P.T.; Dijkshoorn, L.; Haeggman, S.; Cookson, B.; Fry, N.; Fussing, V.; Green, J.; Feil, E.; Gerner-Smidt, P.; et al. Guidelines for the validation and application of typing methods for use in bacterial epidemiology. *Clin. Microbiol. Infect.* **2007**, *13* (Suppl. 3), 1–46. [CrossRef]
19. Futagawa-Saito, K.; Ba-Thein, W.; Fukuyasu, T. Antimicrobial Susceptibilities of Exfoliative Toxigenic and Non-Toxigenic *Staphylococcus hyicus* Strains in Japan. *J. Vet. Med. Sci./Jpn. Soc. Vet. Sci.* **2009**, *71*, 681–684. [CrossRef]
20. Andresen, L.O. Production of exfoliative toxin by isolates of *Staphylococcus hyicus* from different countries. *Vet. Rec.* **2005**, *157*, 376–378. [CrossRef] [PubMed]
21. Dutra, M.; Moreno, L.; Dias, R.; Moreno, A. Antimicrobial Use in Brazilian Swine Herds: Assessment of Use and Reduction Examples. *Microorganisms* **2021**, *9*, 881. [CrossRef] [PubMed]
22. Park, J.; Friendship, R.M.; Weese, J.S.; Poljak, Z.; Dewey, C.E. An investigation of resistance to β-lactam antimicrobials among staphylococci isolated from pigs with exudative epidermitis. *BMC Vet. Res.* **2013**, *9*, 211. [CrossRef] [PubMed]
23. Wegener, H.C.; Watts, J.L.; Salmon, S.A.; Yancey, R.J. Antimicrobial Susceptibility of *Staphylococcus hyicus* Isolated from Exudative Epidermitis in Pigs. *J. Clin. Microbiol.* **1994**, *32*, 793–795. Available online: http://www.pubmedcentral.nih.gov/articlerender.fcgi?artid=263126&tool=pmcentrez&rendertype=abstract (accessed on 26 January 2022). [CrossRef]
24. Aarestrup, F.M.; Duran, C.O.; Burch, D.G.S. Antimicrobial resistance in swine production. *Anim. Health Res. Rev./Conf. Res. Work. Anim. Dis.* **2008**, *9*, 135–148. [CrossRef]
25. Wegener, H.C.; Schwarz, S. Antibiotic-resistance and plasmids in *Staphylococcus hyicus* isolated from pigs with exudative epidermitis and from healthy pigs. *Vet. Microbiol.* **1993**, *34*, 363–372. [CrossRef]
26. Li, B.; Wendlandt, S.; Yao, J.; Liu, Y.; Zhang, Q.; Shi, Z.; Wei, J.; Shao, D.; Schwarz, S.; Wang, S.; et al. Detection and new genetic environment of the pleuromutilin-lincosamide-streptogramin A resistance gene lsa(E) in methicillin-resistant *Staphylococcus aureus* of swine origin. *J. Antimicrob. Chemother.* **2013**, *68*, 1251–1255. [CrossRef] [PubMed]
27. Witte, W.; Cuny, C. Emergence and spread of cfr-mediated multiresistance in staphylococci: An interdisciplinary challenge. *Future Microbiol.* **2011**, *6*, 925–931. [CrossRef] [PubMed]
28. MAPA. Ministério da Agricultura Pecuária e Abastecimento. Instrução Normativa N° 1, de 13 de Janeiro de 2020. Available online: https://pesquisa.in.gov.br/imprensa/jsp/visualiza/index.jsp?jornal=515&pagina=6&data=23/01/2020 (accessed on 23 January 2021).

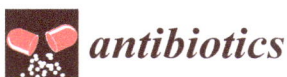 

Article

# Multidrug-Resistant Methicillin-Resistant Coagulase-Negative Staphylococci in Healthy Poultry Slaughtered for Human Consumption

Vanessa Silva [1,2,3,4], Manuela Caniça [5,6], Eugénia Ferreira [5,6], Madalena Vieira-Pinto [7], Cândido Saraiva [7], José Eduardo Pereira [1,7,8], José Luis Capelo [9,10], Gilberto Igrejas [2,3,4] and Patrícia Poeta [1,4,7,8,*]

[1] Microbiology and Antibiotic Resistance Team (MicroART), Department of Veterinary Sciences, University of Trás-os-Montes and Alto Douro (UTAD), 5000-801 Vila Real, Portugal; vanessasilva@utad.pt (V.S.); jeduardo@utad.pt (J.E.P.)

[2] Department of Genetics and Biotechnology, University of Trás-os-Montes and Alto Douro, 5000-801 Vila Real, Portugal; gigrejas@utad.pt

[3] Functional Genomics and Proteomics Unit, University of Trás-os-Montes and Alto Douro (UTAD), 5000-801 Vila Real, Portugal

[4] LAQV-REQUIMTE, Department of Chemistry, NOVA School of Science and Technology, Universidade Nova de Lisboa, 2829-516 Caparica, Portugal

[5] National Reference Laboratory of Antibiotic Resistances and Healthcare Associated Infections (NRL-AMR/HAI), Department of Infectious Diseases, National Institute of Health Dr Ricardo Jorge, Av. Padre Cruz, 1649-016 Lisbon, Portugal; manuela.canica@insa.min-saude.pt (M.C.); eugenia.ferreira@insa.min-saude.pt (E.F.)

[6] Centre for the Studies of Animal Science, Institute of Agrarian and Agri-Food Sciences and Technologies, Oporto University, 4051-401 Oporto, Portugal

[7] CECAV—Veterinary and Animal Research Centre, University of Trás-os-Montes and Alto Douro (UTAD), 5000-801 Vila Real, Portugal; mmvpinto@utad.pt (M.V.-P.); candido.ls95@gmail.com (C.S.)

[8] Associate Laboratory for Animal and Veterinary Sciences (AL4AnimalS), 5000-801 Vila Real, Portugal

[9] BIOSCOPE Group, LAQV-REQUIMTE, Chemistry Department, Faculty of Science and Technology, NOVA University of Lisbon, 2825-466 Almada, Portugal; jlcm@fct.unl.pt

[10] Proteomass Scientific Society, 2825-466 Costa de Caparica, Portugal

* Correspondence: ppoeta@utad.pt

**Citation:** Silva, V.; Caniça, M.; Ferreira, E.; Vieira-Pinto, M.; Saraiva, C.; Pereira, J.E.; Capelo, J.L.; Igrejas, G.; Poeta, P. Multidrug-Resistant Methicillin-Resistant Coagulase-Negative Staphylococci in Healthy Poultry Slaughtered for Human Consumption. *Antibiotics* **2022**, *11*, 365. https://doi.org/10.3390/antibiotics11030365

Academic Editors: Clair L. Firth and Marc Maresca

Received: 18 January 2022
Accepted: 3 March 2022
Published: 9 March 2022

**Publisher's Note:** MDPI stays neutral with regard to jurisdictional claims in published maps and institutional affiliations.

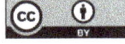

**Copyright:** © 2022 by the authors. Licensee MDPI, Basel, Switzerland. This article is an open access article distributed under the terms and conditions of the Creative Commons Attribution (CC BY) license (https://creativecommons.org/licenses/by/4.0/).

**Abstract:** Coagulase-negative staphylococci are commensals that are known to be prevalent in most environments, and they are also an important reservoir of antimicrobial-resistant genes. Staphylococcal infections in animal husbandry are a high economic burden. Thus, we aimed to determine the prevalence and species diversity of methicillin-resistant coagulase-negative staphylococci (MRCoNS) in poultry slaughtered for human consumption and to study the antimicrobial resistance of the isolates. Swab samples were recovered from 220 commercial chickens, homebred chickens and quails. Species identification was performed using MALDI-TOF. Antimicrobial susceptibility testing was performed by the disc diffusion method against 14 antimicrobials. The presence of antimicrobial-resistant genes was investigated by polymerase chain reaction. Totals of 11 (19.6%), 13 (20.3%), and 51 (51%) MRCoNS were isolated from commercial chickens, homebred chickens and quails, respectively. *S. lentus* was isolated from all homebred chickens, whereas 11 *S. lentus* and 2 *S. urealyticus* were isolated from commercial chickens. As for quails, the most prevalent MRCoNS were *S. urealyticus*. Almost all isolates had a multidrug-resistant profile and carried the *mecA* gene. Most isolates showed resistance to erythromycin, clindamycin, penicillin, tetracycline, ciprofloxacin and fusidic acid and harbored the *ermA*, *ermB*, *ermC*, *mphC tetK*, *tetL*, *tetM* and *tetO* genes. This study showed a frequent occurrence of multidrug resistance in MRCoNS isolated from healthy poultry in Portugal.

**Keywords:** coagulase-negative *Staphylococcus*; CoNS; antimicrobial resistance; poultry; quails; broilers

## 1. Introduction

Staphylococci colonize the skin and mucous membranes of humans and are considered commensals or opportunistic pathogens [1]. By 2018, 45 species and 24 subspecies of *Staphylococcus* had been described [2]. Staphylococci are divided into two groups, coagulase-positive (CoPS) and coagulase-negative staphylococci (CoNS), according to their ability to coagulate plasma. CoPS are pathogenic species which have the coagulase enzyme that converts plasma fibrinogen into fibrin [3]. CoNS lack this enzyme and were considered, until recently, to be minor pathogens or apathogenic [4]. CoNS possess fewer virulence factors that participate in the pathogenesis of infection when compared to CoPS, such as *S. aureus*, but, in the last few decades, CoNS have emerged as common causes of nosocomial infections [4]. Within the CoNS species, *S. epidermidis*, *S. haemolyticus* and *S. saprophyticus* are examples of the most significant types of CoNS in human infections [5]. As opportunistic pathogens, CoNS generally cause infection in colonized immunocompromised individuals, patients with catheters and prosthetic implants, dialysis and oncologic patients and neonates [6]. CoNS are responsible for a broad spectrum of infections, such as invasive endocarditis, bacteremia and bone infections [6,7]. In addition, increasing rates of antibiotic resistance have been detected in CoNS, in some cases even greater than for *S. aureus*, which limits the therapeutic options available [5]. Methicillin resistance in CoNS is usually due to the expression of the *mecA* gene, which encodes an alternative binding protein 2a (PBP2a) that has a low affinity for β-lactam antibiotics, although some studies have reported the presence the *mecC* gene, a homologue of *mecA* [8–10]. The *mec* genes are located on a mobile genetic element called the Staphylococcal Cassette Chromosome *mec* (SCC*mec*). SCC*mec* elements are more diverse in methicillin-resistant CoNS when compared to *S. aureus*, and many SCC*mec* elements could not be typed using multiplex PCR [10]. Tetracycline resistance is also frequently detected in different CoNS species [11].

CoNS also colonize and infect other mammals besides humans, with *S. chromogenes*, *S. simulans* and *S. xylosus* being the principal cause of infection [11]. CoNS are frequently responsible for arthritis, cow mastitis and, less often, systemic infections in animals [12]. The presence of CoNS has been reported in pets, livestock and wild animals [13–15]. It has been shown that food of animal origin can carry CoNS and other foodborne pathogens and, besides being able to cause infection, CoNS can also cause food poisoning [16]. Both CoPS and CoNS have been associated with avian pathologies such as arthritis, osteomyelitis, pododermatitis, septicemia and blepharitis [17,18]. Nevertheless, the presence of CoPS and CoNS has also been observed in healthy poultry and poultry meat, which may act as reservoirs and vehicles of zoonotic pathogens and antimicrobial resistance [16,19]. The spread of antimicrobial resistance among commensal CoNS in healthy poultry may represent a hazard for human and animal health [11]. Studies reporting the monitorization of antimicrobial-resistant pathogens in poultry and poultry meat have been published, but most studies focus only on *S. aureus* species [20–24]. The prevalence of antimicrobial-resistant pathogens in poultry, particularly staphylococci, may be due to their high consumption of antimicrobials. According to the ESVAC report, in Portugal the population-weighted mean consumption (expressed in milligrams per kilogram of estimated biomass) of antimicrobials was 175.8 mg/Kg in food-producing animals in 2020 [25]. In Portugal, the biomass-corrected consumption of third- and fourth-generation cephalosporins, quinolones, penicillin, macrolides and tetracyclines in food-producing animals was around 0.4, 7.3, 38.9, 20 and 60.4 mg/Kg [25]. Furthermore, all these antimicrobial classes were used in poultry production. Therefore, we aimed to investigate the presence of methicillin-resistant CoNS (MRCoNS) in healthy poultry for human consumption as well as the antimicrobial-resistant phenotypes and genotypes of the isolates.

## 2. Results

In this study, the presence of methicillin-resistant CoNS (MRCoNS) was detected in 71 (32.3%) of the 220 birds tested (Table 1). The co-carriage of two different species was identified in four animals, and 67 birds carried only one staphylococcal species. Co-carriage of MRCoNS species was identified only among quail samples, and the pattern of co-carriage was as follows: *Staphylococcus sciuri/S. urealyticus* (n = 2), *Staphylococcus lentus/S. urealyticus* and *Staphylococcus lentus/Staphylococcus haemolyticus*. A total of 75 MRCoNS were recovered and identified as *S. lentus* (n = 26), *S. urealyticus* (n = 21), *S. sciuri* (n = 15) and *S. haemolyticus* (n = 3). *S. haemolyticus* was exclusively isolated from quails. Chickens, both commercial and homebred, were mainly colonized by *S. lentus*, while *S. urealyticus* was the most frequently detected species in quails, followed by *S. lentus*. Quails were colonized significantly more frequently by MRCoNS than homebred chickens. Furthermore, the prevalence of *S. lentus* and *S. urealyticus* was significantly higher than that of *S. haemolyticus*. Results of the prevalence of each staphylococcal species are shown in Supplementary Figure S1.

**Table 1.** Number of animals sampled, frequency and diversity of CoNS species detected among healthy poultry.

| Animal | Number of Animals Sampled | Number of CoNS Carriers (%) | Isolates Recovered | S. lentus | S. urealyticus | S. sciuri | S. haemolyticus |
|---|---|---|---|---|---|---|---|
| Quails | 100 | 47 (47) | 51 | 15 | 19 | 14 | 3 |
| Commercial chickens | 50 | 13 (26) | 13 | 11 | 2 | - | - |
| Homebred chickens | 70 | 11 (15.7) | 11 | 10 | - | 1 | - |
| Total | 220 | 71 (32.3) | 75 | 36 | 21 | 15 | 3 |

Table 2 shows the antimicrobial-resistant phenotypes and genotypes of MRCoNS, while the detailed characterization of each isolate is summarized in Supplementary Table S1. The percentage of resistance to each antibiotic is shown in Figure 1. All isolates showed phenotypic and genotypic resistance to antibiotics, with 73 (97.3%) isolates displaying a multidrug-resistant profile since they showed resistance to at least three different classes of antimicrobials. The multidrug-resistance pattern was as follows: 15 (20%) isolates were resistant to 3 classes, 27 (26%) to 4 classes, 17 (22.7%) to 5 classes, 12 (16%) to 6 classes and 2 (2.7%) to 7 classes of antimicrobials. The non-multiresistant isolates were both *S. lentus* and were isolated from chickens. Both isolates showing resistance to seven antimicrobial classes were isolated from quails. The *mec*A gene was detected in all isolates, including those that were susceptible to cefoxitin. Totals of 11 *S. lentus*, 21 *S. urealyticus*, 14 *S. sciuri* and 3 *S. haemolyticus* were phenotypically resistant to penicillin, but the mechanism of penicillin resistance could not be identified. Resistance to aminoglycosides was detected in 40% of the isolates and was mediated by the $aph(3')$-IIIa, $ant(4')$-Ia and *str* genes in different combinations. All *S. lentus* and *S. urealyticus* were resistant to macrolides and lincosamides, while 14 *S. sciuri* and 2 *S. haemolyticus* showed resistance to this antimicrobial class. Macrolide-lincosamide resistant isolates harbored the *ermA*, *ermB*, *ermC* and *mphC* genes alone or in different combinations: *ermB* (n = 5); *ermC* (n = 11); *mphC* (n = 3); *ermC* and *mphC* (n = 27); *ermA*, *ermC* and *mphC* (n = 6); *ermB*, *ermC* and *mphC* (n = 10); *ermB* and *mphC* (n = 8); *ermA* and *ermC* (n = 1); *ermA*, *ermB*, *ermC* and *mphC* (n = 1); and *ermA*, *ermB* and *mphC* (n = 1). Tetracycline resistance, which was detected in all *S. urealyticus*, *S. sciuri* and *S. haemolyticus*, and in 25 (69.4%) *S. lentus*, was mediated by the *tet*K, tetL, tetM and/or *tetO* genes. The *tetL* gene was the most frequent, followed by the *tetK*. The $cat_{p194}$ encoding resistance to chloramphenicol was detected in one *S. lentus* isolate. Resistance to trimethoprim-sulfamethoxazole was detected in 10 isolates. Some *S. lentus* isolates harbored a combination of *dfrK* and *dfrD* genes, while *S. sciuri* and *S. haemolyticus* carried only the *dfrK*. One *S. sciuri* exhibited resistance to linezolid, mediated by the *cfr* gene. None of the isolates showed resistance to vancomycin.

Table 2. Antimicrobial-resistant genes identified among the CoNS isolated from poultry.

| Species | Number of Isolates | Antimicrobial Resistance | |
|---|---|---|---|
| | | Phenotype | Genotype |
| S. lentus | 36 | PEN[11], FOX[4], CIP[11], CN[2], TOB[14], KAN[9], ERY[35], CD[36], TET[25], C[4], FD[12], SXT[6] | mecA[36], ermA[8], ermB[8], ermC[28], mphC[29], aph(3′)-IIIa[9], ant(4′)-Ia[12], str[2], tetL[19], tetK[14], tetO[1], tetM[2], cat$_{p194}$[1], dfrK[6], dfrD[2] |
| S. urealyticus | 21 | PEN[21], FOX[18], CIP[3], CN[4], TOB[6], KAN[5], ERY[21], CD[21], TET[21], C[3], FD[17] | mecA[21], ermA[1], ermB[7], ermC[19], mphC[16], aph(3′)-IIIa[5], ant(4′)-Ia[2], str[2], tetL[17], tetK[18], tetO[13], tetM[4] |
| S. sciuri | 15 | PEN[14], FOX[6], LNZ[1], CIP[3], TOB[8], KAN[4], ERY[14], CD[14], TET[15], C[2], FD[10], SXT[2] | mecA[15], cfr[1], ermB[9], ermC[7], mphC[9], aph(3′)-IIIa[3], ant(4′)-Ia[7], str[1], tetL[11], tetK[12], tetO[2], tetM[3], dfrK[1] |
| S. haemolyticus | 3 | PEN[3], FOX[1], CIP[2], TOB[2], KAN[1], ERY[2], CD[2], TET[3], FD[2], SXT[2] | mecA[3], ermB[1], ermC[2], mphC[2], aph(3′)-IIIa[2], ant(4′)-Ia[1], str[1], tetL[3], tetK[1], dfrK[1] |

Abbreviations. C: chloramphenicol; CD: clindamycin; CIP: ciprofloxacin; ERY: erythromycin; FD: fusidic acid; FOX: cefoxitin; PEN: penicillin; SXT: trimethoprim-sulfamethoxazole; TET: tetracycline; CN: gentamicin; KAN: kanamycin; TOB: tobramycin; LNZ: linezolid. Note: the superscript number after each antibiotic and gene indicates the number of strains showing resistance to that antibiotic and harboring that gene, respectively.

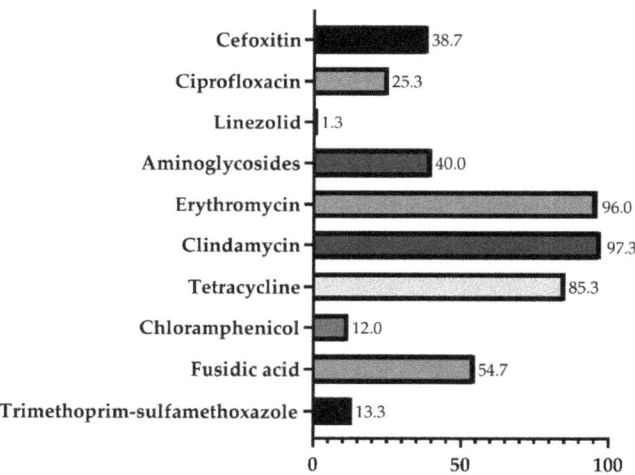

Figure 1. Percentage of resistance to each antibiotic by MRCoNS isolated from poultry.

## 3. Discussion

MRCoNS in livestock was first reported in healthy chickens in Japan in 1996. Despite the increasing interest in CoNS in recent years, there is very limited information on their prevalence and resistance profiles in poultry production, and information is even more limited regarding MRCoNS. In our study, we investigated the presence of MRCoNS in healthy quails and commercial and homebred chickens. Among the 220 birds tested, 71 (32.3%) carried at least one CoNS, which is in accordance with the results obtained by Marek et al. [26]. CoNS colonized 47% and 20% of the quails and chickens, respectively. This carriage frequency was higher than the one obtained by Younis et al., who found a prevalence of CoNS in quails and chickens of 8.75% and 7.14%, respectively [27]. A study conducted with turkey samples found a frequency of CoNS of 15.6%, which is also lower than the one obtained in this study [28]. Other studies found a higher frequency of CoNS in poultry [18,29]. Nevertheless, it is important to point out that in our study all samples were only screened for the presence of MRCoNS, which may have contributed to a higher frequency of CoNS. Furthermore, some studies focused only on diseased animals that would most likely have been discarded in the slaughterhouse and would not have reached the final consumer. In our study, only four different species of CoNS were detected: *S. lentus* (n = 26), *S. urealyticus* (n = 21), *S. sciuri* (n = 15) and *S. haemolyticus* (n = 3). The predominant CoNS species found in our study included those commonly found in skin microbiota in chickens [29,30]. The occurrence of the staphylococci species among poultry samples appears to vary widely. *Pyzik* et al. detected a high number of CoNS species in diseased broiler chickens and turkeys, with *S. cohnii* being the most frequent followed by *S. saprophyticus* and *S. epidermidis* [29]. In accordance with our results, Saha et al. found a higher occurrence of *S. lentus* in poultry samples [30]. Boamah et al. reported a frequency of 42.97% *S. sciuri*, 35.94% *S. lentus*, 4.30% *S. xylosus*, 3.91%, *S. haemolyticus* 3.91%, 1.95% *S. saprophyticus* and 0.39% *S. cohnii* [31]. A study conducted in Brazil found that most CoNS from chickens were *S. gallinarum* followed by *S. simulans* [18]. In a report by El-Nagar et al., the majority of CoNS were *S. xylosus* [32]. Marek et al. found a higher occurrence of *S. epidermidis* in poultry in Poland [26]. Finally, *S. hominis* followed by *S. xylosus* and *S. lentus* were the most frequently detected species in quail eggs [33]. Yet, most studies have reported the presence of *S. sciuri*, *S. lentus* and *S. cohnii*. It has been shown that some species of CoNS, such as *S. sciuri*, *S. xylosus* or *S. cohnii*, are considered important poultry pathogens, particularly when associated with antimicrobial resistance [29]. Furthermore, most of these CoNS species are considered an issue of meat safety rather than the classical poultry pathogens [29].

The most common species found among poultry in this study was *S. lentus*. This species is considered an animal pathogen and has been detected among livestock, pets, wild animals and retail meats [13,16,34,35]. Nevertheless, *S. lentus* has also been responsible for a wide range of human infections and its clinical relevance seems to be increasing [36]. *S. urealyticus* was the second most common CoNS species found in poultry and it was mostly detected in quail samples. This CoNS species has been regarded as a commensal organism and is not usually involved in severe infections [37]. *S. urealyticus* strains of animal origin were shown to have multiple phenotypic resistances and carry several antimicrobial resistance genes [38]. All CoNS isolated in this study harbored the *mecA* gene, and the methicillin resistance of the isolates was confirmed. However, most *S. lentus* and *S. sciuri* isolates were phenotypically susceptible to cefoxitin. It has been shown that the staphylococcal species belonging to the *S. sciuri* group, which include *S. sciuri*, *S. fleurettii*, *S. lentus*, *S. stepanovicii* and *S. vitulinus*, carry a close homologue to the *mecA* gene, which does not confer resistance to β-lactam antibiotics [39]. Accordingly, almost all *S. urealyticus* had phenotypic resistance to cefoxitin. Multidrug resistance was exhibited in almost all isolates, which is in accordance with other studies conducted with poultry samples [27–29]. Although the European Union banned the use of antibiotics for growth promotion in livestock in 2006, and several other measures have been taken since then, it is estimated that over 60% of all antimicrobials produced are used in livestock comprising poultry [40]. Higher resistance levels were detected among quails, including two isolates resistant to seven antimicrobial classes, which may be explained by the fact that in Portugal the legislation for antibiotics administration in quails is not as well-regulated as that for other poultry, such as chickens; thus, antibiotics may be administered indiscriminately to quails, leading to an increase in antimicrobial resistance [20]. Only one isolate, *S. sciuri*, was resistant to linezolid and carried the *cfr* gene. This gene was first detected in a bovine *S. sciuri* [41]. Although uncommon, resistance to linezolid mediated by the *cfr* gene is worrisome, since this gene confers cross-resistance to phenicols, lincosamides, oxazolidinones, pleuromutilins and streptogramin A antibiotics [42,43]. Studies reporting the *cfr* gene in poultry identified it in *S. lentus*, *S. urealyticus*, *S. arlettae*. *sciuri* and *S. simulans* [39,44,45]. Furthermore, a low frequency of this gene has been reported in CoNS from poultry [39]. Resistance to macrolides and lincosamides was detected in all isolates, except for one *S. sciuri* and one *S. haemolyticus*, and it was mediated by the *ermA*, *ermB*, *ermC* and *mphC* genes. Both *ermC* and *mphC* genes were carried by 56 isolates. Phosphotransferases are encoded by the *mphC* gene which confers resistance to erythromycin and other macrolides but not to lincosamides [46]. Nevertheless, the *erm* genes confer cross-resistance to macrolides, lincosamides and streptogramins B [46]. Although the *ermA* and *ermC* genes are the most frequent *erm* genes in staphylococci, the *ermA* gene was only detected in the *S. lentus* and *S. urealyticus* isolates, while *ermB* was identified in all MRCoNS species in this study. Other studies reported similar results for the frequency of *erm* genes in poultry [28,39]. A study by Syed et al. investigated the resistance of staphylococci in poultry intestines and reported a lower frequency of resistance to macrolides and lincosamides, but the *ermC* gene was also the most prevalent [47]. In the same study, resistance to tetracycline was detected in more than half of the isolates encoded by the *tetK* and *tetM* genes [47]. In our study, resistance to tetracycline was detected in 85.3% of the isolates, including all *S. sciuri*, *S. urealyticus* and *S. haemolyticus*, and in 25 out of 36 *S. lentus*, which was similar to the findings of other studies [28,31,48]. The high frequency of tetracycline resistance in poultry samples may be due to the fact that, according to the ECDC/EFSA/EMA report, tetracycline and penicillin were the most prescribed antibiotics for food-producing animals in 2017 [49]. Among the genes that confer resistance to tetracycline, *tetL* ($n = 50$) was the most prevalent, followed by *tetK* ($n = 45$), *tetO* ($n = 16$) and *tetM* ($n = 9$). Similar results were obtained by Lee et al. in a study that investigated the *tet* genes in poultry meat [16]. In contrast, in a study by Nemeghaire et al. *tetM* was the most common gene among *S. sciuri* from healthy chickens [39]. However, due to the lack of studies investigating the prevalence of resistant genes in CoNS from poultry, it is difficult to make a direct comparison. Fusidic acid was detected in 54.6% of the isolates but none of the resistance genes tested were found, which suggests the presence of other resistant genes. Indeed, in a study by Chen et al. none of the fusidic acid-resistant *S. urealyticus* possessed *fusB*, *fusC* or *fusD* genes; instead, *S. urealyticus* isolates carried the novel *fusF* gene, which seems to be an intrinsic factor in *S. urealyticus* and may not be conserved in another subspecies [50]. Resistance to vancomycin was not detected in this study, which was unsurprising since vancomycin-resistant staphylococci are rare and, as far as we know, in Portugal there is only one study reporting a vancomycin intermediate-resistant *S. aureus* isolated from a human infection [51].

In general, penicillin and tetracycline are extensively used for the treatment of staphylococcal infections in poultry [52]. In our study, we also found higher levels of resistance to those antimicrobial agents. The ingestion of poultry meat contaminated with staphylococci may lead to food poisoning. Furthermore, the handling or ingesting of staphylococci contaminated meat is a potential risk factor for colonization by methicillin-resistant staphylococci [53]. Our findings show that the frequency of multidrug-resistant staphylococci in poultry is alarming and may represent a public health problem.

## 4. Materials and Methods

### 4.1. Sample Collection and Bacterial Isolates

During the month of February 2020, a total of 220 samples were collected from poultry in a Portuguese slaughterhouse. Swab samples were collected from the cloaca and trachea of 100 quails, 50 commercial chickens and 70 homebred chickens. Batches of quails, homebred and commercial chickens arrived at the slaughterhouse 3 days a week and around 36,000 quails, 3500 homebred and 8000 commercial chickens were slaughtered each day. Four samples were recovered from each batch. The swabs were inserted into tubes containing brain heart infusion (BHI) broth with 6.5% of NaCl and incubated at 37 °C under aerobic conditions for 24 h. The inoculum was then seeded onto ORSAB agar plates supplemented with 2 mg/mL of oxacillin, incubated at 37 °C and examined after 24 h to 48 h. Up to three colonies per plate with different colors and morphology were recovered and further investigated. The staphylococci species identification was performed by matrix-assisted laser desorption/ionization time-of-flight coupled to time-of-flight mass spectrometry (MALDI-TOF MS) (Bruker Daltonics, Bremen, Germany) as described by Dubois et al. [54].

## 4.2. Phenotypic Antibiotic Resistance Testing

Antibiotic susceptibility profiles were determined for all of isolates by the Kirby–Bauer disc diffusion method on Mueller Hinton agar. The tested antibiotics included: cefoxitin (30 μg), chloramphenicol 132 (30 μg), ciprofloxacin (5 μg), clindamycin (2 μg), erythromycin (15 μg), fusidic acid (10 133 μg), gentamicin (10 μg), kanamycin (30 μg), linezolid (10 μg), mupirocin (200 μg), penicillin (1 U), tetracycline (30 μg), tobramycin (10 μg), and trimethoprim/sulfamethoxazole 135 (1.25/23.75 μg). The diameter of the inhibition zones was measured for each antibiotic disk and recorded in millimeters. The interpretation of results followed the recommendations given in the European Committee on Antimicrobial Susceptibility Testing (EUCAST) 2019 guidelines with the exception of kanamycin that followed the Clinical and Laboratory Standards Institute (CLSI) 2017 recommendations. The minimal inhibitory concentrations (MICs) of vancomycin were determined by a standard broth microdilution method in sterile 96-well microplates according to the EUCAST guidelines. Briefly, bacterial suspension was adjusted to 0.5 McFarland standards and then diluted 1:20. Then, 50 μL of Mueller–Hinton broth, 50 μL of the antibiotic dilutions, and 5 μL of the inoculum were mixed and incubated at 37 °C for 24 h. Isolates showing a vancomycin MIC $\leq 4$ μg/mL were considered susceptible and those showing an MIC > 4 μg/mL were classified as resistant. The reference strain *S. aureus* ATCC 25923 was used for quality control.

## 4.3. DNA Extraction

DNA extraction was performed as previously described. Briefly, 2 staphylococci colonies were suspended in 45 μL of Milli-Q water and 5 μL of lysostaphin (1 mg/mL) was added. The samples were incubated at 37 °C for 10 min, after which 45 μL of Milli-Q water, 150 μL of Tris-HCl (0.1 M) and 5 μL of proteinase K (2 mg/mL) were added. After 10 min of incubation at 67 °C, the samples were boiled at 100 °C for 5 min. The DNA was stored at −20 °C until use. The spectrophotometric quantification of DNA was carried out through the NanoDrop 1000 (Thermo Fisher Scientific, Waltham, MA, USA) [55].

## 4.4. Antimicrobial-Resistant Genes

The presence of antimicrobial-resistant genes was investigated in each isolate according to the phenotypic resistance. The detection of the following antimicrobial-resistant genes was performed in a ProFlex™ PCR system (Applied Biosystems, Waltham, MA, USA): beta-lactams (*blaZ*, *mecA* and *mecC*), linezolid (*cfr*), aminoglycosides (*aac(6′)*-aph(2″), *aph(3′)*-IIIa, *ant(4′)*-Ia and *str*), macrolides and lincosamide (*ermA*, *ermB*, *ermC*, *ermT*, *msr(A/B)*, mphC, lnuA, lnuB, vgaA and vgaB), tetracycline (*tetK*, tetM, *tetL* and *tetO*), chloramphenicol (*fexA*, *fexB*, *cat*$_{pC194}$, *cat*$_{pC221}$ and *cat*$_{pC223}$), fusidic acid (*fusB*, *fusC* and *fusD*) and trimethoprim/sulfamethoxazole (*dfrA*, *dfrG*, *dfrK* and *dfrD*). The protocol used for DNA amplification was as follows: a final volume of 50 μL contained 39.7 μL of ultra-pure water, 5 μL 10× complete buffer (Bioron, Römerberg, Germany), 1 μL 25 mM MgCl2, 1 μL deoxynucleotides triphosphate, 1 μL of each primer, 0.3 μL DFS Taq DNA polymerase (Bioron) and 1 μL DNA sample at 10 pg/μL. Primer sequences and PCR programs for the same are given in Table S2. The concentration and purity of the extracted DNA was measured using a spectrophotometer and Nano-Drop™ software (Thermo Scientific™, Waltham, MA, USA). Positive and negative controls used in all the experiments belonged to the strain collection of the University of Trás-os-Montes and Alto Douro.

## 4.5. Statistical Analysis

Pearson's chi-square test was used compare the carriage of *S. sciuri*, *S. lentus*, *S. urealyticus* and *S. haemolyticus* between the quails, the homebred chickens and the commercial chickens. The analyses were carried out using IBM SPSS Statistics, Version 26.0 (IBM Corp., Armonk, NY, USA) and significance was set at $p \leq 0.05$.

## 5. Conclusions

MRCoNS are common bacteria found in healthy poultry in Portugal. *S. urealyticus* seems to be more prevalent in quails, while broiler chickens are more often colonized by *S. lentus*, indicating a separate epidemiology. The high frequency of MRCoNS isolates in this study may be due to the fact that these bacteria are colonizers of the normal skin flora of animals. However, the multidrug resistance found in almost all isolates indicates that MRCoNS in poultry may be an important reservoir of antimicrobial-resistant genes. This is of great concern for public health, since most antimicrobial resistances detected were antimicrobials commonly used in human medicine. Some measures to overcome antimicrobial resistance in poultry in Portugal should be taken into consideration, such as the education of poultry producers, limiting the availability of antibiotics and the application of strict legislation concerning antimicrobial prescription.

**Supplementary Materials:** The following supporting information can be downloaded at https://www.mdpi.com/article/10.3390/antibiotics11030365/s1: Table S1: Antimicrobial-resistant phenotype and genotype and SCC*mec* typing of CoNS isolated from poultry. Table S2: Primer pairs used for molecular typing and detection of antimicrobial resistance genes in MRSA strains. Figure S1: Prevalence of each staphylococci specie in poultry samples. References [56–71] are cited in the Supplementary Materials.

**Author Contributions:** Conceptualization, V.S., M.V.-P. and P.P.; methodology, V.S.; validation, V.S., M.C. and P.P.; investigation, V.S.; resources, M.V.-P. and C.S.; data curation, V.S. and E.F.; writing—original draft preparation, V.S.; writing—review and editing, V.S., M.C. and P.P.; visualization, J.E.P.; supervision, J.L.C., G.I. and P.P.; funding acquisition, P.P. All authors have read and agreed to the published version of the manuscript.

**Funding:** This work was funded by the R&D Project CAREBIO2: Comparative assessment of antimicrobial resistance in environmental biofilms through proteomics—towards innovative theranostic biomarkers, with reference NORTE-01-0145-FEDER-030101 and PTDC/SAU-INF/30101/2017, financed by the European Regional Development Fund (ERDF) through the Northern Regional Operational Program (NORTE 2020) and the Foundation for Science and Technology (FCT). This work was supported by the Associate Laboratory for Green Chemistry-LAQV, which is financed by national funds from FCT/MCTES (UIDB/50006/2020 and UIDP/50006/2020) and by the projects UIDB/CVT/00772/2020 and LA/P/0059/2020 funded by the Portuguese Foundation for Science and Technology (FCT). Vanessa Silva is grateful to FCT (Fundacão para a Ciência e a Tecnologia) for financial support through the PhD grant SFRH/BD/137947/2018.

**Institutional Review Board Statement:** The study was conducted according to the Helsinki Declaration (ICH-GCP principles), compliance with Schedule Y/ICMR Guidelines, the Oviedo Convention, and approved by the Ethics Committee of the University of Trás-os-Montes e Alto Douro (EC-UTAD, 8 November 2019).

**Informed Consent Statement:** Not applicable.

**Conflicts of Interest:** The authors declare no conflict of interest.

## References

1. Parlet, C.P.; Brown, M.M.; Horswill, A.R. Commensal staphylococci influence Staphylococcus aureus skin colonization and disease. *Trends Microbiol.* **2019**, *27*, 497–507. [CrossRef] [PubMed]
2. Gherardi, G.; Di Bonaventura, G.; Savini, V. Chapter 1—Staphylococcal Taxonomy. In *Pet-to-Man Travelling Staphylococci*; Academic Press: Cambridge, MA, USA, 2018; pp. 1–10, ISBN 978-0-12-813547-1.
3. Smith, J.T.; Andam, C.P. Extensive horizontal gene transfer within and between species of coagulase-negative Staphylococcus. *Genome Biol. Evol.* **2021**, *13*, evab206. [CrossRef] [PubMed]
4. Heilmann, C.; Ziebuhr, W.; Becker, K. Are coagulase-negative staphylococci virulent? *Clin. Microbiol. Infect.* **2019**, *25*, 1071–1080. [CrossRef] [PubMed]
5. Becker, K.; Heilmann, C.; Peters, G. Coagulase-negative staphylococci. *Clin. Microbiol. Rev.* **2014**, *27*, 870–926. [CrossRef]
6. Michalik, M.; Samet, A.; Podbielska-Kubera, A.; Savini, V.; Międzobrodzki, J.; Kosecka-Strojek, M. Coagulase-negative staphylococci (CoNS) as a significant etiological factor of laryngological infections: A review. *Ann. Clin. Microbiol. Antimicrob.* **2020**, *19*, 1–10. [CrossRef]

7. Noshak, M.A.; Rezaee, M.A.; Hasani, A.; Mirzaii, M. The role of the coagulase-negative staphylococci (CoNS) in infective endocarditis; a narrative review from 2000 to 2020. *Curr. Pharm. Biotechnol.* **2020**, *21*, 1140–1153. [CrossRef]
8. MacFadyen, A.C.; Harrison, E.M.; Drigo, I.; Parkhill, J.; Holmes, M.A.; Paterson, G.K. A mecC allotype, mecC3, in the CoNS *Staphylococcus caeli*, encoded within a variant SCCmecC. *J. Antimicrob. Chemother.* **2019**, *74*, 547–552. [CrossRef]
9. Loncaric, I.; Kübber-Heiss, A.; Posautz, A.; Ruppitsch, W.; Lepuschitz, S.; Schauer, B.; Feßler, A.T.; Krametter-Frötscher, R.; Harrison, E.M.; Holmes, M.A.; et al. Characterization of mecC gene-carrying coagulase-negative *Staphylococcus* spp. isolated from various animals. *Vet. Microbiol.* **2019**, *230*, 138–144. [CrossRef]
10. Zong, Z.; Peng, C.; Lü, X. Diversity of SCCmec Elements in Methicillin-Resistant Coagulase-Negative Staphylococci Clinical Isolates. *PLoS ONE* **2011**, *6*, e20191. [CrossRef]
11. Chajęcka-Wierzchowska, W.; Zadernowska, A.; Nalepa, B.; Sierpińska, M.; Łaniewska-Trokenheim, Ł. Coagulase-negative staphylococci (CoNS) isolated from ready-to-eat food of animal origin—Phenotypic and genotypic antibiotic resistance. *Food Microbiol.* **2015**, *46*, 222–226. [CrossRef]
12. Argemi, X.; Hansmann, Y.; Prola, K.; Prévost, G. Coagulase-negative staphylococci pathogenomics. *Int. J. Mol. Sci.* **2019**, *20*, 1215. [CrossRef] [PubMed]
13. Silva, V.; Pereira, J.E.; Maltez, L.; Ferreira, E.; Manageiro, V.; Caniça, M.; Capelo, J.L.; Igrejas, G.; Poeta, P. Diversity of methicillin-resistant staphylococci among wild Lepus granatensis: First detection of mecA-MRSA in hares. *FEMS Microbiol. Ecol.* **2019**, *96*, fiz204. [CrossRef] [PubMed]
14. Roberts, M.C.; Garland-Lewis, G.; Trufan, S.; Meschke, S.J.; Fowler, H.; Shean, R.C.; Greninger, A.L.; Rabinowitz, P.M. Distribution of *Staphylococcus* species in dairy cows, workers and shared farm environments. *FEMS Microbiol. Lett.* **2018**, *365*, fny146. [CrossRef] [PubMed]
15. Suepaul, S.; Georges, K.; Unakal, C.; Boyen, F.; Sookhoo, J.; Ashraph, K.; Yusuf, A.; Butaye, P. Determination of the frequency, species distribution and antimicrobial resistance of staphylococci isolated from dogs and their owners in Trinidad. *PLoS ONE* **2021**, *16*, e0254048. [CrossRef] [PubMed]
16. Lee, S.I.; Kim, S.D.; Park, J.H.; Yang, S.-J. Species Distribution, Antimicrobial Resistance, and Enterotoxigenicity of Non-aureus Staphylococci in Retail Chicken Meat. *Antibiotics* **2020**, *9*, 809. [CrossRef] [PubMed]
17. Huynh, M.; Carnaccini, S.; Driggers, T.; Shivaprasad, H.L. Ulcerative Dermatitis and Valvular Endocarditis Associated with *Staphylococcus aureus* in a Hyacinth Macaw (*Anadorhynchus hyacinthinus*). *Avian Dis.* **2014**, *58*, 223–227. [CrossRef] [PubMed]
18. Pimenta, R.L.; de Melo, D.A.; Bronzato, G.F.; Souza, V.R.d.S.; Holmström, T.C.N.; de Mattos de Oliveira Coelho, S.; de Silva Coelho, I.; de Souza, M.M.S. Characterization of *Staphylococcus* spp. isolates and β-lactam resistance in broiler chicken production. *Braz. J. Vet. Med.* **2021**, *43*, e00720. [CrossRef]
19. Bhargava, K.; Zhang, Y. Characterization of methicillin-resistant coagulase-negative staphylococci (MRCoNS) in retail meat. *Food Microbiol.* **2014**, *42*, 56–60. [CrossRef]
20. Silva, V.; Vieira-Pinto, M.; Saraiva, C.; Manageiro, V.; Reis, L.; Ferreira, E.; Caniça, M.; Capelo, J.L.; Igrejas, G.; Poeta, P. Prevalence and Characteristics of Multidrug-Resistant Livestock-Associated Methicillin-Resistant *Staphylococcus aureus* (LA-MRSA) CC398 Isolated from Quails (Coturnix Coturnix Japonica) Slaughtered for Human Consumption. *Animals* **2021**, *11*, 2038. [CrossRef]
21. Bernier-Lachance, J.; Arsenault, J.; Usongo, V.; Parent, É.; Labrie, J.; Jacques, M.; Malouin, F.; Archambault, M. Prevalence and characteristics of Livestock-Associated Methicillin-Resistant *Staphylococcus aureus* (LA-MRSA) isolated from chicken meat in the province of Quebec, Canada. *PLoS ONE* **2020**, *15*, e0227183. [CrossRef]
22. Tang, Y.; Larsen, J.; Kjeldgaard, J.; Andersen, P.S.; Skov, R.; Ingmer, H. Methicillin-resistant and -susceptible *Staphylococcus aureus* from retail meat in Denmark. *Int. J. Food Microbiol.* **2017**, *249*, 72–76. [CrossRef] [PubMed]
23. Okorie-Kanu, O.J.; Anyanwu, M.U.; Ezenduka, E.V.; Mgbeahuruike, A.C.; Thapaliya, D.; Gerbig, G.; Ugwuijem, E.E.; Okorie-Kanu, C.O.; Agbowo, P.; Olorunleke, S.; et al. Molecular epidemiology, genetic diversity and antimicrobial resistance of *Staphylococcus aureus* isolated from chicken and pig carcasses, and carcass handlers. *PLoS ONE* **2020**, *15*, e0232913. [CrossRef] [PubMed]
24. Bala, H.K.; Igwe, J.C.; Olayinka, B.O.; Olonitola, O.S.; Onaolapo, J.A.; Okafo, C.N. Antibiotic susceptibility profile of *Staphylococcus aureus* isolated from healthy chickens in poultry farms in Kano state, Nigeria. *Sky J. Microbiol. Res.* **2016**, *4*, 42–46.
25. European Medicines Agency European Surveillance of Veterinary Antimicrobial Consumption. *'Sales of Veterinary Antimicrobial Agents in 31 European Countries in 2019 and 2020'* EMA/58183/2021; Publications Office of the European Union: Luxembourg, 2021.
26. Marek, A.; Pyzik, E.; Stępień-Pyśniak, D.; Dec, M.; Jarosz, Ł.S.; Nowaczek, A.; Sulikowska, M. Biofilm-Formation Ability and the Presence of Adhesion Genes in Coagulase-Negative Staphylococci Isolates from Chicken Broilers. *Animals* **2021**, *11*, 728. [CrossRef] [PubMed]
27. Younis, W.; Sabra, M.; Sayed, H.H. Occurrence and characterization of coagulase positive and negative Staphylococci isolated from Japanese quails and broiler chickens at Qena Governorate, Egypt. *SVU-Int. J. Vet. Sci.* **2021**, *4*, 1–15. [CrossRef]
28. Moawad, A.A.; Hotzel, H.; Awad, O.; Roesler, U.; Hafez, H.M.; Tomaso, H.; Neubauer, H.; El-Adawy, H. Evolution of Antibiotic Resistance of Coagulase-Negative Staphylococci Isolated from Healthy Turkeys in Egypt: First Report of Linezolid Resistance. *Microorganisms* **2019**, *7*, 476. [CrossRef]
29. Pyzik, E.; Marek, A.; Stępień-Pyśniak, D.; Urban-Chmiel, R.; Jarosz, Ł.S.; Jagiełło-Podębska, I. Detection of antibiotic resistance and classical enterotoxin genes in coagulase-negative staphylococci isolated from poultry in Poland. *J. Vet. Res.* **2019**, *63*, 183. [CrossRef]

30. Saha, O.; Rakhi, N.N.; Istiaq, A.; Islam, I.; Sultana, M.; Hossain, M.A.; Rahaman, M.M. Evaluation of Commercial Disinfectants against *Staphylococcus lentus* and *Micrococcus* spp. of Poultry Origin. *Vet. Med. Int.* **2020**, *2020*, 8811540. [CrossRef]
31. Boamah, V.E.; Agyare, C.; Odoi, H.; Adu, F.; Gbedema, S.Y.; Dalsgaard, A. Prevalence and antibiotic resistance of coagulase-negative Staphylococci isolated from poultry farms in three regions of Ghana. *Infect. Drug Resist.* **2017**, *10*, 175–183. [CrossRef]
32. El-Nagar, S.; Abd El-Azeem, M.W.; Nasef, S.A.; Sultan, S. Prevalence of toxigenic and methicillin resistant staphylococci in poultry chain production. *J. Adv. Vet. Res.* **2017**, *7*, 33–38.
33. Pyzik, E.; Marek, A. Characterization of bacteria of the genus Staphylococcus isolated from the eggs of Japanese quail (*Coturnix japonica*). *Pol. J. Vet. Sci.* **2012**, *15*, 791–792. [CrossRef] [PubMed]
34. Ruzauskas, M.; Couto, N.; Kerziene, S.; Siugzdiniene, R.; Klimiene, I.; Virgailis, M.; Pomba, C. Prevalence, species distribution and antimicrobial resistance patterns of methicillin-resistant staphylococci in Lithuanian pet animals. *Acta Vet. Scand.* **2015**, *57*, 27. [CrossRef] [PubMed]
35. Dhaouadi, S.; Soufi, L.; Campanile, F.; Dhaouadi, F.; Sociale, M.; Lazzaro, L.; Cherif, A.; Stefani, S.; Elandoulsi, R.B. Prevalence of meticillin-resistant and -susceptible coagulase-negative staphylococci with the first detection of the mecC gene among cows, humans and manure in Tunisia. *Int. J. Antimicrob. Agents* **2020**, *55*, 105826. [CrossRef] [PubMed]
36. Wu, C.; Zhang, X.; Liang, J.; Li, Q.; Lin, H.; Lin, C.; Liu, H.; Zhou, D.; Lu, W.; Sun, Z.; et al. Characterization of florfenicol resistance genes in the coagulase-negative Staphylococcus (CoNS) isolates and genomic features of a multidrug-resistant *Staphylococcus lentus* strain H29. *Antimicrob. Resist. Infect. Control* **2021**, *10*, 9. [CrossRef] [PubMed]
37. Seni, J.; Mshana, S.E.; Msigwa, F.; Iddi, S.; Mazigo, H.; Parkhill, J.; Holmes, M.A.; Paterson, G.K. Draft genome sequence of a multidrug-resistant caprine isolate of *Staphylococcus cohnii* subsp. urealyticus from Tanzania encoding ermB, tet(K), dfrG, fusF and fosD. *J. Glob. Antimicrob. Resist.* **2019**, *18*, 163–165. [CrossRef]
38. Lienen, T.; Schnitt, A.; Hammerl, J.A.; Marino, S.F.; Maurischat, S.; Tenhagen, B.-A. Multidrug-resistant *Staphylococcus cohnii* and *Staphylococcus urealyticus* isolates from German dairy farms exhibit resistance to beta-lactam antibiotics and divergent penicillin-binding proteins. *Sci. Rep.* **2021**, *11*, 6075. [CrossRef]
39. Nemeghaire, S.; Argudín, M.A.; Haesebrouck, F.; Butaye, P. Molecular epidemiology of methicillin-resistant Staphylococcus sciuri in healthy chickens. *Vet. Microbiol.* **2014**, *171*, 357–363. [CrossRef]
40. Agyare, C.; Boamah, V.E.; Zumbi, C.N.; Osei, F.B. Antibiotic use in poultry production and its effects on bacterial resistance. In *Antimicrobial Resistance—A Global Threat*; IntechOpen: London, UK, 2018; pp. 33–50.
41. Schwarz, S.; Werckenthin, C.; Kehrenberg, C. Identification of a plasmid-borne chloramphenicol-florfenicol resistance gene in *Staphylococcus sciuri*. *Antimicrob. Agents Chemother.* **2000**, *44*, 2530–2533. [CrossRef]
42. Wendlandt, S.; Shen, J.; Kadlec, K.; Wang, Y.; Li, B.; Zhang, W.-J.; Feßler, A.T.; Wu, C.; Schwarz, S. Multidrug resistance genes in staphylococci from animals that confer resistance to critically and highly important antimicrobial agents in human medicine. *Trends Microbiol.* **2015**, *23*, 44–54. [CrossRef]
43. Schoenfelder, S.M.K.; Dong, Y.; Feßler, A.T.; Schwarz, S.; Schoen, C.; Köck, R.; Ziebuhr, W. Antibiotic resistance profiles of coagulase-negative staphylococci in livestock environments. *Vet. Microbiol.* **2017**, *200*, 79–87. [CrossRef]
44. Wang, Y.; He, T.; Schwarz, S.; Zhao, Q.; Shen, Z.; Wu, C.; Shen, J. Multidrug resistance gene cfr in methicillin-resistant coagulase-negative staphylococci from chickens, ducks, and pigs in China. *Int. J. Med. Microbiol.* **2013**, *303*, 84–87. [CrossRef] [PubMed]
45. He, T.; Wang, Y.; Schwarz, S.; Zhao, Q.; Shen, J.; Wu, C. Genetic environment of the multi-resistance gene cfr in methicillin-resistant coagulase-negative staphylococci from chickens, ducks, and pigs in China. *Int. J. Med. Microbiol.* **2014**, *304*, 257–261. [CrossRef] [PubMed]
46. Petinaki, E. Resistance of Staphylococci to Macrolides-Lincosamides-Streptogramins B (MLSB): Epidemiology and Mechanisms of Resistance. In *Staphylococcus Aureus*; Hemeg, H., Ozbak, H., Afrin, F., Eds.; IntechOpen: Rijeka, Croatia, 2019.
47. Syed, M.A.; Ullah, H.; Tabassum, S.; Fatima, B.; Woodley, T.A.; Ramadan, H.; Jackson, C.R. Staphylococci in poultry intestines: A comparison between farmed and household chickens1. *Poult. Sci.* **2020**, *99*, 4549–4557. [CrossRef] [PubMed]
48. Hamed, E.A.; Abdelaty, M.F.; Sorour, H.K.; Roshdy, H.; AbdelRahman, M.A.A.; Magdy, O.; Ibrahim, W.A.; Sayed, A.; Mohamed, H.; Youssef, M.I.; et al. Monitoring of Antimicrobial Susceptibility of Bacteria Isolated from Poultry Farms from 2014 to 2018. *Vet. Med. Int.* **2021**, *2021*, 6739220. [CrossRef]
49. European Centre for Disease Prevention and Control (ECDC); European Food Safety Authority (EFSA); European Medicines Agency (EMA). Third joint inter-agency report on integrated analysis of consumption of antimicrobial agents and occurrence of antimicro. *EFSA J.* **2021**, *19*, e06712.
50. Chen, H.-J.; Hung, W.-C.; Lin, Y.-T.; Tsai, J.-C.; Chiu, H.-C.; Hsueh, P.-R.; Teng, L.-J. A novel fusidic acid resistance determinant, fusF, in *Staphylococcus cohnii*. *J. Antimicrob. Chemother.* **2015**, *70*, 416–419. [CrossRef]
51. Gardete, S.; Aires-De-Sousa, M.; Faustino, A.; Ludovice, A.M.; de Lencastre, H. Identification of the First Vancomycin Intermediate-Resistant *Staphylococcus aureus* (VISA) Isolate from a Hospital in Portugal. *Microb. Drug Resist.* **2008**, *14*, 1–6. [CrossRef]
52. Ali, Y.; Islam, M.A.; Muzahid, N.H.; Sikder, M.O.F.; Hossain, M.A.; Marzan, L.W. Characterization, prevalence and antibiogram study of *Staphylococcus aureus* in poultry. *Asian Pac. J. Trop. Biomed.* **2017**, *7*, 253–256. [CrossRef]
53. Bortolaia, V.; Espinosa-Gongora, C.; Guardabassi, L. Human health risks associated with antimicrobial-resistant enterococci and *Staphylococcus aureus* on poultry meat. *Clin. Microbiol. Infect.* **2016**, *22*, 130–140. [CrossRef]

54. Damien, D.; David, L.; Paul, C.J.; Markus, K.; Olivier, S.P.; Régine, T.; Richard, B.; Julien, D. Identification of a Variety of Staphylococcus Species by Matrix-Assisted Laser Desorption Ionization-Time of Flight Mass Spectrometry. *J. Clin. Microbiol.* **2010**, *48*, 941–945. [CrossRef]
55. Silva, V.; Almeida, F.; Carvalho, J.A.; Castro, A.P.; Ferreira, E.; Manageiro, V.; Tejedor-Junco, M.T.; Caniça, M.; Igrejas, G.; Poeta, P. Emergence of community-acquired methicillin-resistant *Staphylococcus aureus* EMRSA-15 clone as the predominant cause of diabetic foot ulcer infections in Portugal. *Eur. J. Clin. Microbiol. Infect. Dis.* **2020**, *39*, 179–186. [CrossRef] [PubMed]
56. Zhang, K.; Sparling, J.; Chow, B.L.; Elsayed, S.; Hussain, Z.; Church, D.L.; Gregson, D.B.; Louie, T.; Conly, J.M. New quadriplex PCR assay for detection of methicillin and mupirocin resistance and simultaneous discrimination of *Staphylococcus aureus* from coagulase-negative staphylococci. *J. Clin. Microbiol.* **2004**, *42*, 4947–4955. [CrossRef] [PubMed]
57. Schnellmann, C.; Gerber, V.; Rossano, A.; Jaquier, V.; Panchaud, Y.; Doherr, M.G.; Thomann, A.; Straub, R.; Perreten, V. Presence of new mecA and mph(C) variants conferring antibiotic resistance in *Staphylococcus* spp. isolated from the skin of horses before and after clinic admission. *J. Clin. Microbiol.* **2006**, *44*, 4444–4454. [CrossRef] [PubMed]
58. Sutcliffe, J.; Grebe, T.; Tait-Kamradt, A.; Wondrack, L. Detection of erythromycin-resistant determinants by PCR. *Antimicrob. Agents Chemother.* **1996**, *40*, 2562–2566. [CrossRef]
59. Shopsin, B.; Mathema, B.; Alcabes, P.; Said-Salim, B.; Lina, G.; Matsuka, A.; Martinez, J.; Kreiswirth, B.N. Prevalence of agr specificity groups among *Staphylococcus aureus* strains colonizing children and their guardians. *J. Clin. Microbiol.* **2003**, *41*, 456–459. [CrossRef]
60. Gomez-Sanz, E.; Torres, C.; Lozano, C.; Fernandez-Perez, R.; Aspiroz, C.; Ruiz-Larrea, F.; Zarazaga, M. Detection, molecular characterization, and clonal diversity of methicillin-resistant *Staphylococcus aureus* CC398 and CC97 in Spanish slaughter pigs of different age groups. *Foodborne Pathog. Dis.* **2010**, *7*, 1269–1277. [CrossRef]
61. Wondrack, L.; Massa, M.; Yang, B.V.; Sutcliffe, J. Clinical strain of *Staphylococcus aureus* inactivates and causes efflux of macrolides. *Antimicrob. Agents Chemother.* **1996**, *40*, 992–998. [CrossRef]
62. Lina, G.; Quaglia, A.; Reverdy, M.E.; Leclercq, R.; Vandenesch, F.; Etienne, J. Distribution of genes encoding resistance to macrolides, lincosamides, and streptogramins among staphylococci. *Antimicrob. Agents Chemother.* **1999**, *43*, 1062–1066. [CrossRef]
63. Bozdogan, B.; Berrezouga, L.; Kou, M.S.; Yurek, D.A.; Farley, K.A.; Stockman, B.J.; Leclercq, R. A new resistance gene, linB, conferring resistance to lincosamides by nucleotidylation in *Enterococcus faecium* HM1025. *Antimicrob. Agents Chemother.* **1999**, *43*, 925–929. [CrossRef]
64. Lozano, C.; Aspiroz, C.; Rezusta, A.; Gómez-Sanz, E.; Simon, C.; Gómez, P.; Ortega, C.; Revillo, M.J.; Zarazaga, M.; Torres, C. Identification of novel vga(A)-carrying plasmids and a Tn5406-like transposon in meticillin-resistant *Staphylococcus aureus* and *Staphylococcus epidermidis* of human and animal origin. *Int. J. Antimicrob. Agents* **2012**, *40*, 306–312. [CrossRef]
65. Hammerum, A.M.; Jensen, L.B.; Aarestrup, F.M. Detection of the satA gene and transferability of virginiamycin resistance in *Enterococcus faecium* from food- animals. *FEMS Microbiol. Lett.* **1998**, *168*, 145–151. [CrossRef] [PubMed]
66. Aarestrup, F.M.; Agers, L.Y.; Ahrens, P.; JŁrgensen, J.L.; Madsen, M.; Jensen, L.B. Antimicrobial susceptibility and presence of resistance genes in staphylococci from poultry. *Vet. Microbiol.* **2020**, *74*, 353–364. [CrossRef]
67. Van de Klundert, J.A.M.; Vliegenthart, J.S. PCR detection of genes coding for aminoglycoside-modifying enzymes. In *Diagnostic Molecular Microbiology: Principles and Applications*; Persing, D.H., Smith, T.F., Tenover, F.C., White, T.J., Eds.; American Society for Microbiology: Washington, DC, USA, 1993; pp. 547–552.
68. Kehrenberg, C.; Schwarz, S. Distribution of Florfenicol Resistance Genes fexA and cfr among Chloramphenicol-Resistant *Staphylococcus* Isolates. *Antimicrob. Agents Chemother.* **2006**, *50*, 1156–1163. [CrossRef] [PubMed]
69. Liu, H.; Wang, Y.; Wu, C.; Schwarz, S.; Shen, Z.; Jeon, B.; Ding, S.; Zhang, Q.; Shen, J. A novel phenicol exporter gene, fexB, found in enterococci of animal origin. *J. Antimicrob. Chemother.* **2012**, *67*, 322–325. [CrossRef]
70. Mclaws, F.; Chopra, I.; O'Neill, A.J. High prevalence of resistance to fusidic acid in clinical isolates of *Staphylococcus epidermidis*. *J. Antimicrob. Chemother.* **2008**, *61*, 1040–1043. [CrossRef]
71. Chen, H.J.; Hung, W.C.; Tseng, S.P.; Tsai, J.C.; Hsueh, P.R.; Teng, L.J. Fusidic acid resistance determinants in *Staphylococcus aureus* clinical isolates. *Antimicrob. Agents Chemother.* **2010**, *54*, 4985–4991. [CrossRef]

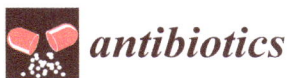 

Article

# Antimicrobial Resistance (AMR) of Bacteria Isolated from Dogs with Canine Parvovirus (CPV) Infection: The Need for a Rational Use of Antibiotics in Companion Animal Health

Giorgia Schirò [†], Delia Gambino [†], Francesco Mira *, Maria Vitale, Annalisa Guercio, Giuseppa Purpari, Francesco Antoci, Francesca Licitra, Gabriele Chiaramonte, Maria La Giglia, Vincenzo Randazzo and Domenico Vicari

Istituto Zooprofilattico Sperimentale della Sicilia "A. Mirri", Via Gino Marinuzzi n. 3, 90129 Palermo, Italy; giorgia.schiro91@gmail.com (G.S.); deliagamb@gmail.com (D.G.); maria.vitale@izssicilia.it (M.V.); annalisa.guercio@izssicilia.it (A.G.); giuseppa.purpari@izssicilia.it (G.P.); francesco.antoci@izssicilia.it (F.A.); francescalicitra15@gmail.com (F.L.); gabrielechiaramonte90@gmail.com (G.C.); maria.lagiglia@izssicilia.it (M.L.G.); vincenzorandazzo78@gmail.com (V.R.); domenico.vicari@izssicilia.it (D.V.)
* Correspondence: dottoremira@gmail.com; Tel.: +39-091-6565447
† These authors contributed equally to this work.

**Citation:** Schirò, G.; Gambino, D.; Mira, F.; Vitale, M.; Guercio, A.; Purpari, G.; Antoci, F.; Licitra, F.; Chiaramonte, G.; La Giglia, M.; et al. Antimicrobial Resistance (AMR) of Bacteria Isolated from Dogs with Canine Parvovirus (CPV) Infection: The Need for a Rational Use of Antibiotics in Companion Animal Health. *Antibiotics* **2022**, *11*, 142. https://doi.org/10.3390/antibiotics11020142

Academic Editor: Clair L. Firth

Received: 23 November 2021
Accepted: 19 January 2022
Published: 23 January 2022

**Publisher's Note:** MDPI stays neutral with regard to jurisdictional claims in published maps and institutional affiliations.

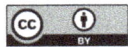

**Copyright:** © 2022 by the authors. Licensee MDPI, Basel, Switzerland. This article is an open access article distributed under the terms and conditions of the Creative Commons Attribution (CC BY) license (https://creativecommons.org/licenses/by/4.0/).

**Abstract:** Canine parvovirus type 2 (CPV-2) represents a major viral threat to dogs. Considering the potential effects of pets on antimicrobial resistance, information on the CPV and associated bacterial co-infections is limited. The aim of this study was to analyze the antimicrobial susceptibility and multidrug-resistance profiles of bacterial species from tissue samples of dogs with canine parvovirus infection. A set of PCR assays and sequence analyses was used for the detection and the molecular characterization of the CPV strains and other enteric viruses. Bacterial isolation, the determination of antimicrobial susceptibility via the disk diffusion method, and the determination of the minimum inhibitory concentration were performed. The detection of β-lactamase genes and toxin genes for specific bacteria was also carried out. CPV infection was confirmed in 23 dogs. Forty-three bacterial strains were isolated and all showed phenotypic resistance. Seventeen multidrug-resistant bacteria and bacteria with high resistance to third- and fourth-generation cephalosporins and metronidazole were detected. Almost 50% of the isolated *Enterobacteriaceae* were positive for at least one β-lactamase gene, with the majority carrying more genes as well. The evidence for multi-resistant bacteria with the potential for intra- or cross-species transmission should be further considered in a One Health approach.

**Keywords:** dog; canine parvovirus; *Carnivore protoparvovirus 1*; antimicrobial resistance; multidrug resistance; One Health; *Enterobacteriaceae*

## 1. Introduction

Canine parvovirus type 2 (CPV-2) emerged as a dog pathogen in early 1978 and rapidly spread worldwide, causing a pandemic event [1]. Despite the widespread use of effective vaccines, after forty years, CPV remains a significant pathogen, still representing a major threat to young dogs [2–4].

Canine parvovirus (CPV) is a small (about 25 nm in diameter), non-enveloped DNA virus, recently included with other related parvoviruses in the unique species *Carnivore protoparvovirus 1*, within the *Protoparvovirus* genus (family *Parvoviridae*, subfamily *Parvovirinae*) [5–7]. Soon after its emergence, two antigenic variants (CPV-2a and CPV-2b) were identified, replacing the original CPV-2 type [8,9]. In 2000, a third antigenic variant (CPV-2c) rapidly spread, and all three variants are currently distributed worldwide with different prevalence rates [5,10].

Parvoviral infection is characterized by depression, anorexia, vomiting, and severe enteritis; mucoid or bloody diarrhea, dehydration, leukopenia, fever, and shock are also detected [5,11]. No specific therapy exists for CPV, and therefore, treatment is primarily supportive and symptomatic, mainly based on rehydration and antimicrobial and antiemetic therapies [11–13].

Alterations of the intestinal mucosa have been associated with CPV infection [14], leading to the disruption of gut barrier function and microbiota dysbiosis [15–17]. These changes can result in bacterial and endotoxin translocation, with the consequent development of systemic inflammatory responses and multiple organ dysfunction syndromes [11]. A broad spectrum of antibiotics is used in the therapy of CPV infection, although the use of antibiotics may cause an increase in the release of endotoxins and/or the exacerbation of the systemic inflammatory response [14,18]. Despite the close relationship between CPV infection and the bacterial population, few studies on these co-infections are currently available [19–22].

Moreover, the diffuse and sometimes uncontrolled use of antibiotics in veterinary medicine has increased concerns related to the high diffusion of antimicrobial resistance (AMR), a real threat to public health in all countries. For the efficacious control of AMR spread worldwide, a One Health perspective has been suggested by the international authorities for public health [23]. Particularly, attention is focused on those critically important antimicrobials (CIAs) for human medicine [24]. Indeed, there is considerable evidence that their use in animals can also contribute to antimicrobial resistance among some common enteric human pathogens [25,26]. Most of this renewed attention is focused on food-producing animals, as well as their potential role in environmental contamination with AMR strains; however, a small—but increasing—amount of the current research is also looking at the potential role of pets.

The aim of this study was the evaluation of the antimicrobial susceptibility and multidrug resistance (MDR) profiles of bacterial species from the tissue samples of 23 dogs with canine parvovirus infection. Co-infection with other viruses was also analyzed.

## 2. Results

### 2.1. Clinical Cases

All 23 sampled dog carcasses, with a modal age value of 2 months (ranging from 40 days to 2 years), were submitted for suspected infectious gastrointestinal disease. Most of them (n = 16) were young dogs (<12 months) and mixed breed stray (n = 15) dogs (Supplementary Materials Table S1). Anamnesis, the clinical history, and the vaccination statuses of most of the analyzed dogs were unavailable.

At necropsy, the common anatomopathological lesions characteristic of CPV infection were observed: hyperemia of the gastric mucosa and catarrhal-hemorrhagic fluids in the stomach, hyperemia, and hemorrhage of the serous membrane of the small intestine, and congestion and enlargement of mesenteric lymph nodes. In some dogs, further lesions (brain edema and hemorrhage, paleness of and focal fibrous lesions on the myocardium, ecchymoses, petechiae and necrosis on the lungs, subcutaneous petechiae, and icterus and hepatic lipidosis) in different organs were observed (Supplementary Materials Figure S1).

### 2.2. Viral Detection and Molecular Characterization of CPV

All the tissue samples tested positive for CPV by conventional PCR assay. Positive samples were obtained both from commonly and from less tested tissues, such as the brain and cerebellum, bone marrow [27], and spinal cord. The tissue samples tested negative for canine distemper virus (CDV), canine adenovirus (CAdV) type 2, and canine rotavirus (CRoV), with the exception of five intestines, which tested positive for canine coronavirus (CCoV), and the tissues of dog id. 19, which tested positive for CAdV type 1 (Supplementary Materials Table S1).

Based on the analysis of the VP2 amino acid residues, 9, 3, and 11 CPV strains were typed as CPV2a, CPV-2b, and CPV-2c variants, respectively.

The phylogenetic analysis (Supplementary Materials Figure S2) evidenced the relationship with CPV-2a/2b/2c strains previously reported in Italy [28,29], as well as with CPV-2c strains more recently circulating in Italy and in Asia [30,31]. The viral variants are listed in Supplementary Materials Table S1.

### 2.3. Bacterial Detection

The bacteriological examination was carried out on 161 tissue samples. One or more bacterial species were isolated from all the dogs, for a total of 43 strains, mainly from the intestine but also frequently from the brain, liver, spleen, heart, kidney, and, less frequently, lung and lymph nodes (Table 1, Supplementary Materials Table S1). The most isolated bacterial species (n = 31) belong to the Gram-negative group (72%), with the highest prevalence at the species level represented by *Escherichia coli* (19/43, 44%). *Klebsiella pneumoniae* (4/43, 9.3%), *Enterobacter* spp. (4/43, 9.3%), *Escherichia fergusonii* (1/43, 2.3%), *Salmonella enterica* subsp. *Enterica* serovar Schleissheim (1/43, 2.3%), *Proteus mirabilis* (1/43, 2.3%), and *Pseudomonas aeruginosa* (1/43, 2.3%) were also detected. Among the Gram-positive bacteria (n = 12), equal amounts of strains belonging to the genuses *Enterococcus* (3/43, 6.9%), *Staphylococcus* (3/43, 6.9%), *Streptococcus* (3/43, 6.9%), and *Clostridium* (3/43, 6.9%) were isolated.

**Table 1.** Bacteria isolated from dogs with canine parvovirus infection.

| Species | Family | Order | Number of Isolates | Tissue Sample |
| --- | --- | --- | --- | --- |
| **Gram-negative** | | | | |
| *Escherichia coli* | | | 19 | Brain, heart, intestine, kidney, lymph nodes, liver, spleen |
| *Klebsiella pneumoniae* | | | 4 | Brain, intestine, liver, spleen |
| *Enterobacter cloacae* | Enterobacteriaceae | Enterobacteriales | 2 | Brain, intestine |
| *Enterobacter gergoviae* | | | 2 | Brain, intestine |
| *Escherichia fergusonii* | | | 1 | Intestine |
| *Proteus mirabilis* | | | 1 | Intestine |
| *Salmonella enterica* | | | 1 | Intestine |
| *Pseudomonas aeruginosa* | Pseudomonadaceae | Pseudomonadales | 1 | Intestine |
| **Gram-positive** | | | | |
| *Clostridium perfringens* | Clostridiaceae | Clostridiales | 3 | Intestine, liver, spleen |
| *Enterococcus faecium* | Enterococcaceae | Lactobacillales | 2 | Brain, lymph nodes |
| *Enterococcus faecalis* | | | 1 | Intestine |
| *Streptococcus canis* | Streptococcaceae | Lactobacillales | 2 | Brain, lung |
| *Streptococcus pseudoporcinus* | | | 1 | Intestine |
| *Staphylococcus lentus* | | | 1 | Lung |
| *Staphylococcus sciuri* | Staphylococcaceae | Bacillales | 1 | Brain |
| *Staphylococcus xylosus* | | | 1 | Brain |

A unique bacterial species was isolated in 43% (10/23) of the dogs, whereas in 22% (5/23) and 26% (6/23), two and three bacterial species were simultaneously isolated, respectively. The coexistence of four different bacterial species was detected only in one dog (id. 20). Although they are normally present in the intestinal microbiota, *E. coli* strains were isolated from the intestines of only 7/23 dogs. In 12/23, *E. coli* was also isolated from other organs. The isolated bacterial species are listed in Table 1 and Supplementary Materials Table S1.

### 2.4. Antimicrobial Susceptibility According to the Disk Diffusion Method

The results obtained with the Kirby-Bauer method showed the presence of resistance in all 43 isolated strains. All the Gram-negative strains (31/43, 72%) were resistant to cefquinome (fourth gen. cephalosporin), methicillin, and metronidazole. Some strains were resistant to antibiotics considered the last line of defense against resistant infections in human health: *Escherichia fergusonii* was resistant to colistin sulphate, one *E. coli* to imipenem, and three *E. coli* were resistant to chloramphenicol. Two more *E. coli* with two

*Klebsiella pneumoniae* strains and one *Enterobacter cloacae* strain were resistant to ceftriaxone. Two *E. coli* isolated from dogs 19 and 22 were simultaneously resistant to chloramphenicol/ceftriaxone and chloramphenicol/imipenem, respectively. Additionally, another five bacteria (four *E. coli* and a *Pseudomonas aeruginosa*) showed intermediate sensitivity to imipenem, and one more *E. coli* isolate to chloramphenicol. In addition, many of the strains of *Enterobacteriaceae* were resistant to cefadroxil and cephalexin (first gen. cephalosporin). All the *Klebsiella pneumoniae* (4/31), one of two *Enterobacter gergoviae* (2/31), and *Salmonella enterica* (1/31) were found to be resistant to cefadroxil and cephalexin, and one *Enterobacter gergoviae* (2/31) was resistant to cefadroxil and sensitive to cefalexin, while of the 19 *E. coli* isolated, 15 were resistant to cephalexin and 14 to cefadroxil.

On the other hand, most of the Gram-negative strains were sensitive to marbofloxacin (24/31, 77.4%), enrofloxacin, and sulfamethoxazole/trimethoprim (19/31, 61.2%). Despite the reported intrinsic resistance [32], one *Enterobacter cloacae* and the *Pseudomonas aeruginosa* strains tested sensitive to penicillin, chloramphenicol, and doxycycline. The antibiotic sensitivity results for the Gram-negative strains are shown in Table 2.

Most of the Gram-positive strains were resistant to metronidazole (10/12, 83.3%), cefquinome (fourth gen. cephalosporin) (9/12, 75%), and cefuroxime (second gen. cephalosporin) (6/12, 50%) and sensitive to vancomycin (12/12, 100%), amoxicillin/clavulanic acid, and imipenem (10/12, 83.3%), marbofloxacin (8/12, 66.6%), cephalexin, cefadroxil, and ceftriaxone (first and third gen. cephalosporin, respectively) (7/12, 58.3%). The antibiotic sensitivity results for the Gram-positive strains are shown in Table 3.

*2.5. Antimicrobial Susceptibility According to the Minimum Inhibitory Concentration (MIC)*

To quantitatively assess the bacterial sensitivity to some of the antibiotics previously tested with the Kirby–Bauer test, five sets of antibiotics were used to determine the MICs; additional molecules were selected by the manufacturer according to the bacterial species. The MICs are reported in Supplementary Materials Tables S2 and S3.

The set used for the 28 Gram-negative bacteria confirmed the higher incidence of resistance to cephalexin (77.7% of the 27 strains tested) and ampicillin (47.3% of the 19 strains tested): 15/28 *E. coli*, 2/28 *Enterobacter cloacae*, 2/28 *Enterobacter gergoviae*, and 2 *Klebsiella pneumoniae* were resistant to cephalexin (first gen. cephalosporin) and 9/28 *E. coli* to ampicillin. Some antibiotics were tested only by the MIC assay, and the following results were derived: 8/28 *E. coli*, 4/28 *Klebsiella pneumoniae*, and 1/28 *Enterobacter cloacae* were found to be resistant to piperacillin (46.4%); 6/28 *E. coli*, 4/28 *Klebsiella pneumoniae*, 2/28 *Enterobacter cloacae*, and 1/28 *Proteus mirabilis* to tetracycline (48.1% of the 27 strains tested). All of them were sensitive to amikacin, and many, to marbofloxacin (24/28, 85.7%), tobramycin (22/28, 78.5%), enrofloxacin, and gentamicin (21/28, 75%) as well. The two isolates, *E. fergusonii* and *S. enterica*, showed sensitivity to all the tested antibiotics.

Among the Gram-positive strains, the MICs determined for 1/8 *Streptococcus pseudoporcinus* showed sensitivity to all the tested antibiotics, whereas 1/8 *Streptococcus canis* was resistant to tetracycline only. However, resistance was found in the strains of *Enterococcus faecium* and *Staphylococcus xylosus*: both *Enterococcus faecium* strains tested were resistant to enrofloxacin, marbofloxacin, and doxycycline, and one of them, also to erythromycin, while the *Staphylococcus xylosus* strain tested was resistant to clindamycin, enrofloxacin, marbofloxacin, doxycycline, and minocycline. Moreover, all the Gram-positive strains have been found to be sensitive to chloramphenicol and florphenicol.

Table 2. Antibiotic sensitivity results derived with the Kirby-Bauer method for the Gram-negative strains (n = 31).

| Bacterial Isolates | Dog ID. | AMC | AMP | CFR | CL | CXM | CVN | CRO | CEQ | MET | ATM | IPM | SP | DA | CN | VA | CT | ENR | MAR | MPZ | C | DO | SXT |
|---|---|---|---|---|---|---|---|---|---|---|---|---|---|---|---|---|---|---|---|---|---|---|---|
| Escherichia coli (n = 19) | 1 | I | R | R | R | R | R | I | R | R | S | S | R[a] | R[a] | R | R[a] | S | S | S | R | S | I | R |
| | 3 | I | R | R | R | R | R | S | R | R | S | I | R[a] | R[a] | R | R[a] | I | S | S | R | S | S | S |
| | 4 | I | R | R | R | R | R | R | R | R | R | I | R[a] | R[a] | R | R[a] | I | I | S | R | S | S | R |
| | 5 | S | S | S | R | R | I | S | R | R | I | S | R[a] | R[a] | I | R[a] | S | S | S | R | S | I | S |
| | 6 | S | S | R | R | R | I | S | R | R | S | S | R[a] | R[a] | R | R[a] | S | S | S | R | S | S | S |
| | 7 | S | R | R | R | R | I | S | R | R | I | S | R[a] | R[a] | R | R[a] | S | S | S | R | R | S | R |
| | 8 | S | R | R | R | R | R | S | R | R | S | S | R[a] | R[a] | R | R[a] | S | S | S | R | S | S | R |
| | 9 | I | S | R | R | R | I | S | R | R | I | S | R[a] | R[a] | I | R[a] | S | S | S | R | S | S | S |
| | 10 | R | R | R | R | R | R | S | R | R | S | S | R[a] | R[a] | R | R[a] | S | R | R | R | R | R | R |
| | 11 | I | R | R | R | R | I | S | R | R | I | S | R[a] | R[a] | R | R[a] | S | R | R | R | R | R | R |
| | 13 | S | I | R | R | R | R | S | R | R | S | S | R[a] | R[a] | R | R[a] | S | I | S | R | S | S | R |
| | 14 | S | R | S | R | R | R | S | R | R | R | S | R[a] | R[a] | R | R[a] | I | S | S | R | I | R | S |
| | 15 | S | S | S | S | R | S | S | R | R | S | I | R[a] | R[a] | S | R[a] | S | S | S | R | S | S | R |
| | 16 | S | S | S | R | R | R | S | R | R | S | S | R[a] | R[a] | R | R[a] | S | S | S | R | S | S | S |
| | 17 | S | S | S | S | R | R | S | R | R | R | S | R[a] | R[a] | I | R[a] | S | S | S | R | R | I | R |
| | 19 | R | R | R | R | R | S | R | R | R | R | R | R[a] | R[a] | R | R[a] | S | R | R | R | R | I | R |
| | 20 | S | S | S | S | R | S | S | R | R | R | S | R[a] | R[a] | S | R[a] | S | S | R | R | R | I | S |
| | 22 | R | R | R | R | R | I | R | R | R | R | S | R[a] | R[a] | R | R[a] | S | R | R | R | R | I | S |
| | 23 | S | S | R | R | R | S | S | R | R | R | S | R[a] | R[a] | R | R[a] | S | S | S | R | S | I | R |
| Klebsiella pneumoniae (n = 4) | 6 | S | R[a] | R | R | R | S | S | R | R | S | S | R[a] | R[a] | S | R[a] | S | S | S | R | S | S | R |
| | 10 | I | R[a] | R | R | R | R | S | R | R | S | S | R[a] | R[a] | R | R[a] | S | I | S | R | S | S | S |
| | 12 | I | R[a] | R | R | R | R | S | R | R | R | S | R[a] | R[a] | R | R[a] | S | I | I | R | S | S | R |
| | 22 | R | R[a] | R | R | R | R | R | R | R | R | S | R[a] | R[a] | S | R[a] | S | R | R | R | S | S | R |
| Enterobacter cloacae (n = 2) | 2 | R | R[a] | R | S | R | R | R | R | R | S | S | R[a] | R[a] | S | R[a] | S | I | S | R | S | S | R |
| | 13 | S | S[a] | S | S | R | I | S | R | R | I | I | R[a] | R[a] | I | R[a] | S | S | R | R | S | I | S |
| Enterobacter gergoviae (n = 2) | 5 | S | R[a] | R | R | R | I | S | R | R | S | S | R[a] | R[a] | S | R[a] | S | I | S | R | S | I | S |
| | 9 | S | R[a] | R | S | R | S | S | R | R | S | S | R[a] | R[a] | S | R[a] | S | S | S | R | S | S | S |
| Escherichia fergusoni (n = 1) | 21 | S | S | S | S | R | S | S | R | R | S | S | R[a] | R[a] | S | R[a] | R | S | S | R | S | R | S |
| Proteus mirabilis (n = 1) | 20 | S | S | S | S | R | S | S | R | R | S | S | R[a] | R[a] | S | R[a] | S | S | S | R | S | R[a] | S |
| Salmonella enterica (n = 1) | 3 | S | R | R | R | R | I | S | R | R | I | S | R[a] | R[a] | R | R[a] | I | S | S | R | S | S | S |
| Pseudomonas aeruginosa (n = 1) | 12 | R[a] | R[a] | R[a] | R[a] | R[a] | R | S | R | R | S | I | R[a] | R[a] | S | R[a] | S | S | S | R | S[a] | S[a] | R |

Amoxicillin–clavulanic acid (AMC); ampicillin (AMP); cefadroxil (CFR); cephalexin (CL); cefuroxime (CXM); cefovecin (CVN); ceftriaxone (CRO); cefquinome (CEQ); methicillin (MET); aztreonam (ATM); imipenem (IPM); spiramycin (SP); clindamycin (DA); gentamicin (CN); vancomycin (VA); colistin sulfate (CT); enrofloxacin (ENR); marbofloxacin (MAR); metronidazole (MPZ); chloramphenicol (C); doxycycline (DO); sulfamethoxazole + trimethoprim (SXT). S: sensible; R: resistant; I: intermediate; [a] Intrinsic resistance.

**Table 3.** Antibiotic sensitivity results derived with Kirby–Bauer method for the Gram-positive strains (n = 12).

| Bacterial Isolates | Dog ID. | AMC | AMP | CFR | CL | CXM | CVN | CRO | CEQ | MET | ATM | IPM | SP | DA | CN | VA | CT | ENR | MAR | MPZ | C | DO | SXT |
|---|---|---|---|---|---|---|---|---|---|---|---|---|---|---|---|---|---|---|---|---|---|---|---|
| *Clostridium perfringens* (n = 3) | 2 | S | R | R | R | R | R | R | R | R | R[a] | S | R | R | R | S | R[a] | I | S | R | S | I | R |
|  | 3 | S | S | S | S | R | I | S | R | S | R[a] | S | I | S | R | S | R[a] | S | S | S | S | S | R |
|  | 20 | S | S | S | S | S | R | S | R | S | R[a] | S | S | S | R | S | R[a] | S | S | S | S | S | S |
| *Enterococcus faecium* (n = 2) | 4 | I | R | R[a] | R[a] | R[a] | R[a] | R[a] | R[a] | R | R[a] | R | I[a] | R | R | S | R[a] | R | R | R | S | I | I[a] |
|  | 12 | I | R | R[a] | R[a] | R[a] | R[a] | R[a] | R[a] | R | R[a] | R | I[a] | I | R | S | R[a] | R | R | R | S | I | R[a] |
| *Enterococcus faecalis* (n = 1) | 9 | S | S | S[a] | R[a] | R[a] | R[a] | I[a] | R[a] | R | R[a] | S | R[a] | R[a] | S | S | R[a] | R | R | R | S | R | R[a] |
| *Staphylococcus lentus* (n = 1) | 20 | S | S | S | S | S | S | S | R | S[a] | R[a] | S | I | I | S | S | R[a] | S | S | R | S | S | S |
| *Staphylococcus sciuri* (n = 1) | 10 | S | S | S | S | R | S | S | R | S[a] | R[a] | S | I | I | S | S | R[a] | S | S | R | S | S | S |
| *Staphylococcus xylosus* (n = 1) | 4 | S | R | R | R | R | R | I | R | R[a] | R[a] | S | R | R | S | S | R[a] | R | S | R | S | S | S |
| *Streptococcus canis* (n = 2) | 1 | S | I | I | S | S | S | S | R | S | R[a] | S | I | R | R | S | R[a] | I | S | R | S | S | S |
|  | 5 | S | S | S | S | R | R | S | R | S | R[a] | S | I | S | I | S | R[a] | I | S | R | S | R | S |
| *Streptococcus pseudoporcinus* (n = 1) | 18 | S | S | S | S | R | I | S | R | S | R[a] | S | I | I | I | S | R[a] | I | I | R | S | S | S |

Amoxicillin-clavulanic acid (AMC); ampicillin (AMP); cefadroxil (CFR); cephalexin (CL); cefuroxime (CXM); cefovecin (CVN); ceftriaxone (CRO); cefquinome (CEQ); methicillin (MET); aztreonam (ATM); imipenem (IPM); spiramycin (SP); clindamycin (DA); gentamicin (CN); vancomycin (VA); colistin sulfate (CT); enrofloxacin (ENR); marbofloxacin (MAR); metronidazole (MPZ); chloramphenicol (C); doxycycline (DO); sulfamethoxazole + trimethoprim (SXT). S: sensible; R: resistant; I: intermediate; [a] Intrinsic resistance.

## 2.6. Molecular Analysis of β-Lactamase Genes

All the *Enterobacteriaceae* (30 isolates in Table 4) from the dogs were further analyzed for the presence of β-lactamase genes. The results show that almost 50% (15/32) of the isolates were positive, according to PCR, for at least one β-lactamase gene, with the majority also carrying more genes simultaneously. Of the 15 β-lactamase-positive strains, 11 isolates carried the $bla_{TEM}$ gene and nine the $bla_{CTXM-II}$ gene.

Some isolates of *E. coli* tested positive for at least one β-lactamase gene (8/19). All but one carried the $bla_{TEM}$ gene, mostly associated with other genes. Only one carried just $bla_{OXA}$ and $bla_{CTX-M-II}$, and one, only $bla_{TEM}$ (Table 4). *Klebsiella pneumonia* was also isolated from four mixed breed dogs (three strays and one owned). Of these isolates, two carried four β-lactamase genes simultaneously ($bla_{SHV}$, $bla_{OXA}$, $bla_{TEM}$, and $bla_{CTXM-II}$), one carried three genes ($bla_{SHV}$, $bla_{TEM}$, and $bla_{CTXM-II}$), and one carried only the $bla_{SHV}$ gene, normally present in all *K. pneumonia* strains.

The unique isolate of *Salmonella enterica* tested negative for the presence of the β-lactamase gene, confirming the sensitivity of this strain in the MIC assay, in contrast to its ampicillin resistance as determined by the KB method. The unique isolate *E. fergusonii* was sensitive to all the antibiotics, although the $bla_{CTX-M-II}$ gene was present according to PCR. Of the *Enterobacter* spp., represented by two *gergoviae* and two *cloacae*, one *E. gergoviae* was positive for $bla_{SHV}$ only, and one *E. cloacae*, for the $bla_{TEM}$ and $bla_{DHA}$ genes (Table 4).

## 2.7. Molecular Analysis for Virulence Factors in Enterobacteriaceae, Staphylococcus spp. and Clostridium perfringens (A to E)

All the *E. coli* (19 isolates) were analyzed for the presence of genes that code for serogroup-specific O-antigens and four major virulence factors (intimin, enterohemorrhagic hemolysin, and Shiga toxins [Stx] 1 and 2), to detect O157, O26, O45, O103, O111, O121, and O145. The four virulence factors were also studied for all the other strains of *Enterobacteriaceae* (11 isolates). All the strains tested negative for the four virulent genes, except for one *E. coli* strain from dog id. 9, which carried the eae and the serogroup O111 genes (Table 4).

The *Staphylococcus* spp. strains showed negativity for the mecA and enterotoxin genes, except for *S. xilosus* (dog id. 4), which carried the enterotoxin D gene. One *Clostridium perfringens* strain (dog id. 3) showed the presence of the cpa gene, encoding the alpha-toxin.

## 2.8. Multidrug-Resistance Evaluation

To better assess the presence of multidrug-resistant strains among the 36 isolates tested using both methods (Kirby–Bauer and MIC), the results obtained with the two methods for the different antibiotic classes were compared. However, since the cards used to determine the MIC with VITEK® contain predetermined antibiotics, it was not possible to test the same molecules with both methods. For this reason, for the beta-lactam and tetracycline classes only, the comparison was based on different molecules of the same class, and for some other molecules (i.e., metronidazole), the comparison was not possible.

Among the Gram-negative strains, for the 27 *Enterobacteriaceae*, both methods confirmed sensitivity to the chloramphenicol class. Few variations were found between the two methods for penicillin and sulfonamides, while clearer differences emerged for cephalosporins, beta-lactams, aminoglycosides, fluoroquinolones, and tetracyclines (Table 5). The *Pseudomonas aeruginosa* strain was proven sensitive to all the antibiotic classes.

Table 4. β-lactamase genes, and antibiotic sensitivity results derived with the Kirby–Bauer method for the Enterobacteriaceae isolates.

| Dog ID. | Bacterial Isolates | Source | β-Lactamase Genes | AMC | AMP | CFR | CL | CXM | CVN | CRO | CEQ | MET | ATM | IPM |
|---|---|---|---|---|---|---|---|---|---|---|---|---|---|---|
| 1 | E. coli | Intestine | bla$_{TEM}$, bla$_{CMY-II}$, bla$_{CTX-M-I}$ | I | R | R | R | R | R | I | R | R | S | S |
| 2 | E. cloacae | Intestine | bla$_{TEM}$, bla$_{DHA}$ | R | R$^a$ | R | R | R | R | R | R | R | R | S |
| 3 | S. enterica | Intestine | negative | S | R | R | R | R | I | S | R | R | I | S |
| 4 | E. coli | Intestine | negative | I | R | R | R | R | R | S | R | R | S | I |
| 5 | E. coli | Intestine | bla$_{TEM}$, bla$_{CTX-M-II}$ | I | R | R | R | R | R | R | R | R | R | I |
| 5 | E. gergoviae | Brain | negative | S | R$^a$ | R | R | R | I | S | R | R | I | S |
| 5 | E. coli | Intestine | negative | S | S | R | R | R | I | S | R | R | I | S |
| 6 | E. coli | Intestine | negative | S | S | R | R | R | I | S | R | R | I | S |
| 6 | K. pneumoniae | Brain | bla$_{TEM}$, bla$_{SHV}$, bla$_{CTX-M-II}$ | S | R$^a$ | R | R | R | I | S | R | R | S | S |
| 7 | E. coli | Intestine | negative | S | R | R | R | R | S | S | R | R | S | S |
| 8 | E. coli | Intestine | bla$_{TEM}$ | S | R | R | R | R | I | S | R | R | I | S |
| 9 | E. coli (O111, eae) | Intestine | bla$_{TEM}$, bla$_{CTX-M-II}$ | I | R | R | R | R | I | S | R | R | I | S |
| 9 | E. gergoviae | Intestine | bla$_{SHV}$ | S | R$^a$ | R | S | R | R | S | R | R | S | S |
| 9 | E. coli | Intestine | negative | R | R$^a$ | R | R | R | S | S | R | R | S | S |
| 10 | K. pneumoniae | Brain | bla$_{SHV}$ | I | R$^a$ | R | R | R | R | S | R | R | S | S |
| 11 | E. coli | Intestine | bla$_{TEM}$, bla$_{OXA}$ | I | R | R | R | R | I | S | R | R | I | S |
| 12 | K. pneumoniae | Intestine | bla$_{TEM}$, bla$_{OXA}$, bla$_{SHV}$ bla$_{CTX-M-II}$ | I | R$^a$ | R | R | R | R | R | R | R | R | S |
| 13 | E. coli | Intestine | negative | S | I | R | R | R | R | R | R | R | R | S |
| 13 | E. cloacae | Brain | negative | S | S$^a$ | S | R | R | I | S | R | R | I | S |
| 14 | E. coli | Intestine | bla$_{TEM}$, bla$_{CTX-M-II}$ | S | R | S | R | R | S | S | R | R | S | S |
| 15 | E. coli | Intestine | negative | S | S | R | R | R | S | S | R | R | S | S |
| 16 | E. coli | Intestine | negative | S | S | S | S | R | S | S | R | R | R | I |
| 17 | E. coli | Intestine | negative | S | S | S | S | R | S | S | R | R | S | S |
| 19 | E. coli | Intestine | bla$_{OXA}$, bla$_{CTX-M-II}$ | R | R | R | R | R | S | R | R | R | R | S |
| 20 | P. mirabilis | Intestine | negative | S | S | S | R | R | S | S | R | R | S | S |
| 21 | E. fergusonii | Intestine | bla$_{CTX-M-II}$ | S | S | S | S | R | I | S | R | R | S | S |
| 22 | E. coli | Intestine | bla$_{TEM}$, bla$_{OXA}$, bla$_{SHV}$, bla$_{CTX-M-II}$ | R | R | R | R | R | R | S | R | R | R | R |
| 22 | K. pneumoniae | Intestine | bla$_{TEM}$, bla$_{OXA}$, bla$_{SHV}$, bla$_{CTX-M-II}$ | R | R$^a$ | R | R | R | R | R | R | R | R | S |
| 23 | E. coli | Intestine | negative | S | S | S | S | R | S | S | R | R | R | S |

Amoxicillin–clavulanic acid (AMC); ampicillin (AMP); cefadroxil (CFR); cephalexin (CL); cefuroxime (CXM); cefovecin (CVN); ceftriaxone (CRO); cefquinome (CEQ); methicillin (MET); aztreonam (ATM); imipenem (IPM); $^a$ Intrinsic resistance.

**Table 5.** Multidrug-resistance evaluation of 27 strains of the *Enterobacteriaceae* family.

| Bacterial Isolates | Dog Id | Penicillins | | | | | Cephalosporins | | | | | Carbapenem | | Aminoglycosides | | Fluoroquinolones | | | | Chloramphenicol | | Sulfonamides | | Beta Lactams | | Tetracycline | |
|---|---|---|---|---|---|---|---|---|---|---|---|---|---|---|---|---|---|---|---|---|---|---|---|---|---|---|---|
| | | AMC | | AMP | | CL | | CVN | | IPM | | CN | | ENR | | MAR | | C | | SXT | | MET | PIP | DO | TE |
| | | KB | MIC | KB | MIC | KB | MIC | KB | MIC | KB | MIC | KB | MIC | KB | MIC | KB | MIC | KB | MIC | KB | MIC | KB | KB | MIC | KB | MIC |
| *E. coli* (n = 16) | 1 | I | R | R | R | R | R | R | R | S | S | R | S | S | S | S | S | S | S | R | R | R | R | I | R |
| | 3 | I | S | R | S | R | R | R | S | I | S | R | R | S | S | S | S | S | S | S | S | R | S | S | S |
| | 4 | I | R | R | S | R | R | R | R | I | S | I | R | I | S | S | S | S | S | R | R | R | R | S | S |
| | 5 | S | S | S | S | R | R | R | I | S | S | I | I | S | S | S | S | S | S | S | S | R | S | S | S |
| | 6 | S | S | S | S | R | R | I | S | S | S | I | R | S | S | S | S | S | S | R | R | R | R | S | R |
| | 7 | S | S | R | R | R | R | I | S | S | S | R | R | S | S | S | S | S | S | R | R | R | R | R | S |
| | 8 | S | S | R | R | R | R | I | S | S | S | R | S | S | S | S | S | S | S | R | R | R | R | S | R |
| | 9 | I | S | R | R | R | R | R | S | S | S | I | R | S | S | S | S | S | S | S | S | R | R | S | S |
| | 10 | R | R | R | R | R | R | R | R | S | S | R | R | R | R | R | R | S | S | R | R | R | R | R | R |
| | 11 | I | R | S | S | R | R | I | S | S | S | R | R | R | R | R | R | S | S | R | R | R | R | R | S |
| | 13 | S | S | I | S | R | R | R | S | S | S | I | S | S | S | S | S | I | S | S | S | R | S | S | S |
| | 14 | S | S | R | R | R | R | R | S | S | S | S | S | S | S | S | S | I | I | S | S | R | R | R | S |
| | 15 | S | S | S | S | R | R | S | S | I | S | R | R | R | R | R | R | S | S | R | R | R | S | R | S |
| | 16 | S | S | S | S | S | R | S | S | S | S | R | R | S | S | S | S | S | S | S | S | R | S | S | S |
| | 17 | R | R | R | R | R | R | R | R | S | S | I | R | R | R | R | R | R | S | R | R | R | R | I | R |
| | 19 | R | R | R | R | R | R | R | R | S | S | R | R | R | R | R | R | S | S | S | S | R | R | I | R |
| | 20 | S | S | S | R | R | R | S | S | R | S | R | R | S | S | S | S | S | S | R | R | R | R | I | R |
| *Klebsiella pneumoniae* (n = 4) | 6 | S | R | R[a] | R[a] | R | R | S | S | S | S | S | S | S | S | S | S | S | S | S | S | R | R | R | R |
| | 10 | S | I | I | R[a] | S | I | R | R | S | S | S | S | I | S | I | S | S | S | R | R | R | R | R | S |
| | 12 | I | I | I | R[a] | R | R | R | R | S | S | R | R | I | I | I | I | S | S | R | R | R | R | I | S |
| | 20 | R | R | R | R[a] | R | R | R | R | S | S | R | R | R | R | R | R | S | S | R | R | R | R | R | R |
| *Enterobacter cloacae* (n = 2) | 2 | R | R | R | nd | R | R | R | S | S | S | S | S | I | I | S | S | S | S | S | S | R | R | I | S |
| | 13 | S | S | S[a] | nd | R | R | I | S | S | S | S | S | I | S | S | S | S | S | S | S | R | S | R | S |
| *Enterobacter gergoviae* (n = 2) | 5 | S | R | R[a] | nd | R | R | S | S | S | S | S | S | S | S | S | S | S | S | S | S | R | S | R | S |
| | 9 | S | S | R[a] | nd | S | R | S | S | S | S | S | S | S | S | S | S | S | S | S | S | R | I | S | S |
| *Escherichia fergusoni* (n = 1) | 23 | S | S | S | S | S | S | S | S | S | S | S | S | S | S | S | S | S | S | S | S | R | S | R | S |
| *Proteus mirabilis* (n = 1) | 22 | S | S | S | S | S | I | S | S | S | S | S | S | S | S | S | S | S | S | S | S | R | S | R[a] | R |
| *Salmonella enterica* (n = 1) | 3 | S | S | R | R | R | S | I | S | S | S | R | S | S | S | S | S | S | S | S | S | R | S | S | S |

Amoxicillin + clavulanic acid (AMC); ampicillin (AMP); cephalexin (CL); cefovecin (CVN); imipenem (IPM); gentamicin (CN); enrofloxacin (ENR); marbofloxacin (MAR); chloramphenicol (C); sulfamethoxazole + trimethoprim (SXT); methicillin (MET); piperacillin (PIP); doxycycline (DO); tetracycline (TE); [a] Intrinsic resistance; nd: not determined.

For the Gram-positives, no differences were found between the two methods for two of the eight *Streptococcus* spp., and the resistance of one strain to the tetracycline class was confirmed. For three of the eight *Enterococcus* spp., sensitivity to the chloramphenicol class was confirmed, but differences were evidenced for the fluoroquinolones and tetracyclines. For three of the eight *Staphylococcus* spp., both methods confirmed sensitivity to the aminoglycosides, chloramphenicol, and sulfonamides classes, and the resistance of only one strain to the lincosamides and fluoroquinolones. With MIC evaluation, the resistance of one strain of *Staphylococcus* spp. to macrolides was not confirmed, whereas resistance to the tetracycline class in one strain was observed.

Due to the variations among the methods, the results of the MIC method were considered to limit the overestimation of antimicrobial resistance. Bacterial strains showing resistance toward three or more antimicrobial classes were considered multidrug-resistant (MDR).

As a result of this comparison, 17 (47.2%) of the strains tested with both methods (15/27 *Enterobacteriaceae*, 1/2 *Enterococcus faecium*, and 1/1 *Staphylococcus xylosus*) were considered multidrug-resistant (Supplementary Material Tables S4 and S5). In particular, five strains of different bacterial species (1/16 *E. coli*, 1/4 *Klebsiella pneumoniae*, 1/2 *Enterobacter cloacae*, 1/2 *Enterococcus faecium*, and 1/1 *Staphylococcus xylosus*) showed resistance to three antibiotic classes; 1/16 strain of *E. coli* showed resistance to four antibiotics classes; seven strains (4/16 *E. coli*, 2/4 *Klebsiella pneumoniae*, and 1/2 *Enterobacter cloacae*), to five antibiotics classes; 2/16 strains of *E. coli*, to six antibiotics classes; and two strains (1/4 *Klebsiella pneumoniae* and 1/16 *E. coli*) showed resistance to seven and eight classes, respectively.

The multidrug-resistant strains were isolated from 13 dogs, and in one case, the presence of MDR was shown in all the strains isolated from the same dog. Indeed, the two strains, *Klebsiella pneumoniae* and *E. coli*, isolated from the stray dog id. 22 were resistant to seven (penicillin, cephalosporins, beta lactams, sulfonamides, fluoroquinolones, aminoglycosides, and tetracyclines) and five (penicillin, fluoroquinolones, aminoglycosides, chloramphenicol, and tetracyclines) classes, respectively. The same two bacterial species from dog id. 22 tested positive for the presence of the same four β-lactamase genes (Table 4). *E. coli* from dog id. 4 was resistant to five classes (penicillin, cephalosporins, beta lactams, sulfonamides, and tetracyclines), while *Staphylococcus xylosus* was resistant to three classes (tetracyclines, fluoroquinolones, and lincosamides); in the molecular analysis for the β-lactamase gene, the *E. coli* strain from dog 4 showed the presence of $bla_{TEM}$ and $bla_{CTX-M-II}$ genes (Table 4). In dog id. 10, the *E. coli* strain was resistant to eight antibiotic classes (penicillin, cephalosporins, beta lactams, sulfonamides, fluoroquinolones, aminoglycosides, tetracyclines, and chloramphenicol), although it was negative for the presence of β-lactamase genes when assessed by PCR, in contrast to the *Klebsiella pneumoniae* isolate, which was shown to be positive for the $bla_{SHV}$ gene and was resistant to three classes (penicillin, beta lactams, and tetracyclines). Multidrug-resistant strains of *E. coli* (the species isolated with the higher rate) were isolated from the intestines of three dogs and from the intestines and other organs of another five dogs.

## 3. Discussion

Despite the fact that vaccination has considerably reduced the occurrence, canine parvovirus infection remains a global threat to domestic and wild carnivores. Until now, studies have been focused on CPV infection and global spread, with limited studies on co-infections with bacteria or other viruses [17,20,33,34]. In this study, samples collected from dog carcasses with CPV infection were analyzed to evaluate the impact of the bacterial species, their susceptibility to antibiotics, and their multidrug resistance, along with other viral co-infections. In total, 18 dogs were strays, three were owned, one was housed in a city shelter, and one was just imported from an Eastern European country. The lack of any specific therapeutic treatment or previous vaccination for stray dogs and the potential stressful conditions for the others could have contributed to the fatal infection outcome.

The occurrence of CPV infection has been mainly reported in young dogs, probably related to the lack of specific and protective immunization or stressful conditions [5,35]. The vaccines currently used for CPV are safe and effective and cross-protect against all three variants [3,36,37]. Their rational use [38], together with appropriate sanitation procedures [39], still represents the most effective protective approach to preventing viral infection [40]. Moreover, vaccines could also reduce the unnecessary use of antimicrobials, as recently suggested [41,42].

The most commonly described pathological findings for CPV infection [5] were observed in all the carcasses during the anatomopathological examinations. However, other lesions not specifically associated with CPV were also observed. These anatomopathological observations might suggest a mixed pathological pattern, potentially due to bacterial co-infections, the effect of the bacterial toxins, or the systemic inflammatory response (SIRS) [14,43,44]. The data in this study suggest the need for more specific assays, particularly in the extra-intestinal organs from which bacteria were isolated, to assess their role and/or the roles of their toxins in determining pathological lesions. Additional studies are also necessary to evaluate CPV's action in extra-intestinal sites, such as the central nervous system (CNS) or bone marrow.

Although in a few dogs (id. 6, 7, 11, 21, 22, 19) co-infections with other viruses (CCoV and CAdV-1) were assessed, the results confirm that CPV infection remained the main cause of viral enteritis and acute hemorrhagic diarrhea syndrome (AHDS) in young dogs [33,34]. Therefore, a diagnostic panel for the main pathogenic bacteria and multiple viral agents should be considered in dogs with suspected infectious gastrointestinal disease [21,34].

From all the samples, forty-three bacterial strains were isolated, with a prevalence of Gram-negative groups and, particularly, *E. coli* species, isolated mainly from the organs of the gastrointestinal tract (liver, spleen, and intestine) and, less frequently, from extraintestinal organs. Furthermore, few species belonging to the Gram-positive group were isolated. Bacterial isolation from intestinal tissues was performed in five dogs only, while, in the others, bacteria were isolated mainly from the brain but also other tissues, suggesting a systemic or multi-organ infection. The evidence in this study of toxin-producing bacteria, such as *Clostridium perfringens*, and of other pathogenic bacterial strains in the brain suggests their role in the development of the neurological clinical signs, such as depression, commonly observed in live dogs with CPV infection [5,14,45]. However, further studies on the potential association of CPV with neurological lesions, as suggested in other reports [34,46–49], are necessary.

According to the results, the risk some bacteria pose of fatal outcomes in dogs with CPV infection appears to be partially limited. Indeed, most of the isolated bacteria (*E. coli* strains) represented normal intestinal flora and the fact that their presence was restricted to the enteric tract confirms their limited role in the pathogenesis of the dogs. Therefore, antibiotic therapy would most likely not have been necessary in these cases. Conversely, in eleven dogs, *E. coli* was isolated from extra-enteric organs, and in two dogs, bacteria harboring toxin genes (*Clostridium perfringens* and *Staphylococcus xylosus*) were also evidenced. In almost half of the analyzed canine carcasses, two or three different bacterial species were isolated, suggesting their potential role in developing the clinical signs and contributing to the *exitus*, or the observed pathological findings, as previously suggested [21,50]. In these cases, antimicrobial therapy in vivo might have been suggested and could have been effective. However, the accurate evaluation of the clinical evidence of sepsis status and antimicrobial resistance is important before considering any empirical therapy in order to avoid unnecessary treatment which could favor the spread of antimicrobial-resistant strains.

Despite the potential marginal role of the bacteria in the clinical outcome, this study evidenced the presence of multidrug-resistant bacteria in dogs with parvovirosis. In some cases, the isolates showed resistance to the most important antimicrobial drugs in human medicine, such as second- and fourth-generation cephalosporins, macrolides, lincosamides, nitroimidazoles, and glycopeptides while all the Gram-positive bacteria were resistant to fourth-generation cephalosporins and, with the exception of two *Clostridium perfringens* strains, also to nitroimidazoles. A slightly higher sensitivity to the ceftriaxone over cefovecin (third gen. cephalosporins) was also observed.

The analysis of the β-lactamase genes of *Enterobacteriaceae* showed that 15/30 of the strains harbored one to four genes of resistance. In one *E. coli* and one *Klebsiella pneumoniae* from dog id. 22, four genes of resistance ($bla_{TEM}$, $bla_{SHV}$, $bla_{OXA}$, and $bla_{CTX-M-II}$) were detected. Although the gene $bla_{SHV}$ is commonly present in most *K. pneumoniae* strains at chromosomal locations, the same combination of different genes present in different bacterial strains in the same dog suggests acquisition through genetic horizontal transfer. Another *K. pneumoniae* derived from dog id. 12 carried the same four genes. The evidence of these bacteria in the enteric tract suggests their potential shedding via feces, and this deserves attention considering their potential zoonotic role and the possibility of spreading to humans. These strains also showed the highest resistance in both the Kirby–Bauer and MIC assays.

In the treatment of dogs with parvoviral enteritis there is no specific therapy, only supportive care approaches. Although some reports warn about the potential risks connected to the use of antibiotics [14,43], an intravenous or subcutaneous broad spectrum of bactericidal antibiotics is commonly used in addition to therapy. Penicillin, alone or in combination with beta-lactamase inhibitors, cephalosporins, fluoroquinolones, metronidazole, and aminoglycosides, is the most commonly used antibiotics that have been reported [15,51,52]. To date, official data on the use or sale of antimicrobials in Italy for the treatment of gastrointestinal infections in dogs are not available. Nonetheless, a guideline for the prudent use of antibiotics in companion animals has been provided [53] along with surveys and cross-sectional studies describing the use of antimicrobials for companion animals [54–56]. Similar studies involving other European countries, including Italy, have recently been published [57,58]. Moreover, most recent updates of canine parvoviral enteritis recommend the use of broad-spectrum antibiotics such as ampicillins, cephalosporins, nitroimidazoles, or fluoroquinolones [59]. Although a national survey specifically on the use of antimicrobials in dogs with CPV infection is not available, all of these studies, as well as the guidelines, cite specific antibiotics (i.e., nitroimidazoles such as metronidazole, alone or in addition with spiramycin or cephalosporins) and CIAs (i.e., fluoroquinolones or third-generation cephalosporins) for common use in the generically defined gastrointestinal disease. Since 2017, computerized prescriptions for veterinary medical products (defined as Ricetta Elettronica Veterinaria, REV) have been available in Italy, replacing paper prescriptions for antimicrobials under the direct control of the Ministry of Health. Data analysis could contribute to the categorization of the antimicrobials used for companion animals, supporting future strategies to combat AMR, along with the increasing attention being paid to multi-resistant pathogens found in companion animals that are harmful for humans.

This study outlines the high bacterial resistance to some of the antibiotics commonly used in the treatment of parvoviral enteritis, such as third- and fourth-generation cephalosporins and metronidazole, which pose a high risk of the spread of resistance to antibiotics that are very important for human health. Moreover, inappropriate and ineffective empirical treatments of CPV infection, such as intravenous therapy with narrow-spectrum antimicrobials, potentially contribute to the occurrence of other short- or long-term effects, such as damage to fecal microbiota, neurotoxicity, and chronic gastrointestinal disease [60–62]. Given this evidence, the real need for antibiotic therapy and its benefits should be assessed.

The rational rather than empirical use of antibiotics could contribute to the effective control of antimicrobial resistance. The concerns related to AMR are increasing, especially for those involving important antimicrobial classes, such as the third- or higher-generation cephalosporins, glycopeptides, macrolides, ketolides, polymyxins, and quinolones included in the lists of international health institutions [24]. Due to the threat posed to human health, the guidelines on the rational use of antibiotics mainly refer to food-producing animals or animal production practices and the role of companion animals is neglected [63,64]. Moreover, the need to elucidate the role of companion animals in the spread of antibiotic resistance is highlighted by the fact that some of the microorganisms included in the WHO's list of globally prioritized antibiotic-resistant bacteria [65] are often isolated from companion animals. In our study, four strains of *Klebsiella pneumoniae*, representing a threat to human health in hospital settings [66], showed more than one β-lactamase gene and multidrug resistance. An *E. coli* strain isolated from a young stray dog showed the O111 serogroup and eae genes. The O111 serotype and enteroaggregative intimin (eae) genes related to *E. coli* strains are responsible for diarrhea problems in children [67]. Moreover, four *E. coli*, one *Escherichia fergusonii*, two *Klebsiella pneumoniae*, and one *Enterobacter cloacae* were shown to be resistant to antibiotics considered a last line of defense against resistant infections such as colistin sulphate, imipenem, chloramphenicol, and ceftriaxone. We cannot rule out the possibility that resistant bacterial strains were transferred from humans to animals, since some of the tested puppies might have been abandoned by owners that could not keep the newborn animals. The presence of multidrug resistance could be related to the household environment and it is possible that, for pets with close relations to humans, AMR originates from human sources thus confirming the importance of the One Health approach. Moreover, less common bacteria indicated as potential agents of zoonoses were also isolated: *Salmonella enterica* subsp. *enterica* serovar Schleissheim [68], *E. fergusonii* [69], *Str. pseudoporcinus* [70], and *Str. canis* [71]. This evidence suggests a potential risk for humans connected to the shedding of zoonotic bacteria species carrying drug resistance. Due to this evidence being found in stray and shelter-housed dogs, the roles of these species should be assessed and considered as part of sanitation protocols to limit the contamination of shelters and veterinary clinics, thus limiting the risks posed to the personnel of shelters and veterinarians.

Some limitations—particularly the low availability of tissue samples from dead dogs naturally infected with canine parvovirus—prevent in-depth data analysis. First, the lack of negative controls is a potential limitation: since this was a descriptive study, intended only to evaluate the antimicrobial susceptibility and multidrug-resistance profiles of bacterial species derived from tissue samples of dogs with canine parvovirus infection, samples from CPV-negative dogs were considered non-ideal as negative controls.

As this observational study was based only on samples collected for routine diagnostic purposes, aiming to describe and highlight the presence of multi-resistant bacteria in these targeted individuals, no negative controls were defined.

Another limit was related to the lack of specific anamnestic and clinical information, particularly on the use of antimicrobials for therapies, which prevents speculation on the meaning of the resistance found in the analyzed strains. Therefore, in light of these limitations, further studies are necessary in order to derive in-depth deductions.

Antibiotic treatment is sometimes used in canine parvoviral infection but, as shown in this study, the evidence of multi-resistant bacteria with potential for intra- or cross-species transmission should be carefully considered before unnecessary antimicrobial treatments are undertaken. Dogs, as companion animals, are usually reared and housed in close contact with humans [72,73] and, therefore, a One Health perspective is imperative for global public health.

## 4. Materials and Methods

### 4.1. Clinical Samples

Tissue samples from 23 dead dogs suspected of having parvovirosis were analyzed. Samples were collected from May 2018 to October 2019 and analyzed for diagnostic purposes. Carcasses had already been submitted by public and private veterinary practitioners to ascertain the causa mortis. Most of these subjects were stray dogs (n = 18) and the others were owned dogs (n = 3), shelter dogs (n = 1) and imported dogs (n = 1). The veterinary public services recovered all but one of the roaming strays showing clinical gastroenteric signs, all of which died just after admittance; the other died just before it could be recovered. Other carcasses were submitted by private or public veterinary practitioners with clinical suspicion of infectious gastrointestinal disease in almost all of them. No other anamnestic or clinical information was provided, including vaccination statuses or therapies. The carcasses were subjected to necropsy after admittance or storage at $-20\ °C$. During necropsy, tissue samples (brain, lungs, heart, spleen, liver, intestine, mesenteric lymph nodes, and kidneys) were collected, stored at $-20\ °C$, and subjected to virological and bacteriological assays. The details are summarized in Supplementary Materials Table S1.

*4.2. Parvovirus PCR and Molecular Characterization of CPV Strains*

Organ homogenates were obtained as previously described [74]. DNA was extracted from homogenates using the DNeasy Blood & Tissue Kit (Qiagen S.p.A., Hilden, Germany), according to the manufacturer's instructions. The presence of CPV DNA was confirmed using a primer pair [75] in a PCR protocol amplifying a 700 bp fragment of the VP2 gene, as previously described [28]. Briefly, PCR was carried out using the GoTaq G2 DNA Polymerase (Promega Italia s.r.l., Milan, Italy) in a 50 μL reaction mix consisting of 10 μL of 5× GoTaq® Reaction Buffer, 1 μL of $MgCl_2$ (25 mM), 1 μL of dNTP mix (10 mM), 0.5 μL of each primer VP2-850-Forward and VP2-1550-Reverse (0.5 μM), 0.25 μL of GoTaq® G2 DNA Polymerase, 31.75 μL of nuclease-free water, and 5 μL of DNA extract. Amplification was conducted under the following thermal conditions: 94 °C for 2 min to activate TaqPol followed by 40 cycles of 94 °C for 30 s, 55 °C for 1 min, and 72 °C for 1 min as well as a final extension of 72 °C for 10 min.

The nearly complete VP2 gene sequence (a 1745-bp fragment) was assessed using a primer pair [76] and direct sequencing [77].

Sequencing encompassing both CPV ORFs (including NS and VP genes) was carried out using the primer pairs developed by Pérez et al. [78], as previously described, and the amplicons were directly sequenced using forward, reverse, and internal primers [29].

The nucleotide VP2 coding sequences were obtained using the ClustalW program and analyzed using the BioEdit software. The sequences were submitted to nBLAST to search related sequences in public domain databases. The CPV antigenic variants (CPV-2a, 2b and 2c) were deduced based on the 426-VP2 amino acid residue [79].

To elucidate the genetic relationships between the obtained CPV strains and the dataset of sequences obtained from the NCBI database, a phylogenetic tree was constructed with the MEGA-X software, using the maximum-likelihood (ML) method according to the Tamura 3-parameter (T92) model with discrete Gamma distribution (+G) employing five rate categories, assuming that a certain fraction of the sites were evolutionarily invariable (+I), and employing bootstrap analyses with 1000 replicates. The phylogeny is depicted in Supplementary Materials Figure S2, showing a representative CPV strain for each genetic and antigenic variant.

These sequence data have been previously or newly submitted to the DDBJ/EMBL/GenBank databases under accession numbers reported in Supplementary Materials Table S1.

*4.3. Additional Virologic Tests*

RNA was extracted from samples using the QIAamp Viral RNA Mini Kit (Qiagen S.p.A., Hilden, Germany), according to the manufacturer's instructions. The extracted DNA and RNA were amplified using a set of gel-based or real-time (RT) PCR assays useful for the detection of CDV [80], CAdVs types 1 and 2 [81], CCoV [82], and CRoV [83]. The details are summarized in Supplementary Materials Table S6.

*4.4. Bacterial Isolation*

For the tissue samples collected from all the dogs, bacterial isolation was performed using selective and differential agar (MacConkey agar, Columbia blood agar and Mannitol Salt agar) incubated at 37 °C for 24 h. Moreover, Columbia blood agar plates were anaerobically incubated with the AnaeroGen™ Anaerobic System (Oxoid, Milano, Italy) to isolate anaerobic bacteria.

For the *Salmonella* spp. culture, pre-enrichment in Buffered Peptone water was performed, followed by two enrichments in Selenite Cystine (SC) and Rappaport-Vassiliadis (RV) broths, and incubated, respectively, at 37 °C and 42 °C for 24 h. The enrichment broths were then plated on Xylose–Lysine Deoxycholate Agar (XLD) and Brilliant Green Agar (BGA).

The identification of the isolated strains was carried out with the biochemical API® system and Vitek® 2 system (bioMérieux, Craponne, France). For the *Salmonella* spp. strains, after identification by API20E®, serological typing was performed.

### 4.5. Disk Diffusion Method

The antimicrobial susceptibility of the bacterial strains isolated (n = 43) was evaluated by the disk diffusion method (Kirby-Bauer) on Mueller-Hinton agar, according to the guidelines of the Clinical and Laboratory Standards Institute [84]. A standard panel of 22 antibiotics was used: amoxicillin-clavulanic acid (AMC), 30 µg; ampicillin (AMP), 10 µg; aztreonam (ATM), 30 µg; cefadroxil (CFR), 30 µg; cephalexin (CL), 30 µg; cefovecin (CVN), 30 µg; ceftriaxone (CRO), 30 µg; cefquinome (CEQ), 30 µg; cefuroxime (CXM), 30 µg; clindamycin (DA), 2 µg; chloramphenicol (C), 30 µg; colistin sulfate (CT), 10 µg; doxycycline (DO), 30 µg; enrofloxacin (ENR), 5 µg; gentamicin (CN), 10 µg; imipenem (IPM), 10 µg; marbofloxacin (MAR), 5 µg; methicillin (MET), 5 µg; metronidazole (MPZ), 4 µg; spiramycin (SP), 100 µg; sulfamethoxazole/trimethoprim (SXT), 23.75 µg/1.25 µg; vancomycin (VA), 30 µg. The sensitivity model was evaluated by measuring the diameter of the inhibition zone, and isolates were considered resistant, intermediate, or susceptible according to the CLSI ranges [84].

### 4.6. Determination of Minimum Inhibitory Concentration (MIC)

The minimum inhibitory concentrations (MICs) of 36 of the isolated strains were determined with the Vitek® 2 system (bioMérieux, Craponne, France), with specific panels of antibiotics selected according to the identified species. The VITEK® AST-GN65 card was used to determine the susceptibility of 28 strains of isolated Gram-negative aerobic bacilli, while the VITEK® AST-GP81 card was used to determine the susceptibility of three *Enterococcus* spp. And three Staphylococcus spp. The VITEK® AST-ST03 card was used for the two *Streptococcus* spp., whose MIC values were expressed in µg/mL. According to the breakpoints expressed in vet CLSI 2017 v8.02 and CLSI M100-S25 (2015) [84,85], the isolates were categorized as resistant, intermediate, or susceptible.

### 4.7. Detection of β-Lactamase Genes

Two multiplex PCRs were performed to amplify the β-lactamase genes in the Enterobacteriaceae isolates as described by Kim et al. [86]. The first multiplex assay (named Set I) was designed to detect the $bla_{TEM}$, $bla_{SHV}$, and $bla_{CTX-M-IV}$ group- (8–10) and $bla_{OXA}$ β-lactamase-encoding genes, and the second assay (named Set II) was designed to detect $bla_{CTX-M-I}$ group-, $bla_{CTX-M-II}$ group-, $bla_{CMY-II}$-, and $bla_{DHA}$-encoding genes. The DNA amplifications were carried out in the GeneAmp™ PCR System 2700 thermal cycle (Applied Biosystems, Foster City, CA, USA). Both assays used identical cycling conditions: the thermal cycling profile consisted of an initial denaturation at 95 °C for 15 min, followed by 30 cycles of 94 °C for 30 s, 61 °C for 90 s, and 72 °C for 90 s and a final extension at 72 °C for 10 min. The sizes of the PCR products were analyzed by electrophoresis on a 2% agarose gel containing GelRed® (Biotium, San Francisco, CA, USA) (4 µL per 100 mL) in 0.5× TBE at 100 V for 1 h, and visualized using GeneSys (Syngene, Cambridge, UK).

### 4.8. Detection of Genes for Toxins of Staphylococcus spp. and of Clostridium perfringens (A to E)

Two multiplex PCR assays were used to amplify the sea-see and tsst-1, eta, etb, mecA (Set I), and seg, seh, sei, sej, and sep (Set II) genes for toxins of *Staphylococcus* spp. as described by Vitale et al. [87].

A multiplex PCR assay was used to detect the toxin genes cpa, cpb, etx, iap, cpe, and cpb2 of *Clostridium perfringens*, according to the method described by Baums et al. [88]. The PCR results were visualized by electrophoresis on a 1.5% agarose gel containing GelRed® (Biotium, San Francisco, CA, USA) (4 µL per 100 mL) in 0.5× TBE at 100 V for 1 h and visualized using GeneSys (Syngene, Cambridge, UK).

*4.9. Serogroup Identification in E. coli and Virulent Genes' Identification in Enterobacteriaceae*

A multiplex polymerase chain reaction (mPCR) was used to detect the 11 genes that encode serogroup-specific O-antigens and four major virulence factors (eae–intimin adherence protein, enterohemorrhagic hemolysin A (EHEC hlyA), and Shiga toxins [Stx] 1 and 2) so as to detect O157 and the "top six" non-O157 (O26, O45, O103, O111, O121, and O145) Shiga toxin-producing Escherichia coli (STEC) as described by Bai et al. [89]. The search for genes coding for the four virulence factors mentioned above was conducted on all the strains of *Enterobacteriaceae* isolated.

**Supplementary Materials:** The following are available online at https://www.mdpi.com/article/10.3390/antibiotics11020142/s1. Figure S1: Gross lesions observed at necropsy, Figure S2: Maximum likelihood tree based on 158 full-length VP2 gene sequences of canine parvovirus type 2 strains, Table S1: Details of collected and tested samples, Table S2: Antibiotic sensitivity results according to minimum inhibitory concentration (MIC) method for the Gram-negative strains (n = 28), Table S3: Antibiotic sensitivity results with minimum inhibitory concentration (MIC) method for the Gram-positive strains (n = 8), Table S4: Comparison of the results obtained with the two methods for MDR Enterobacteriaceae strains (n = 15), Table S5: Comparison of the results obtained with the two methods for MDR Gram-positive strains (n = 2), Table S6: Details on additional virologic tests.

**Author Contributions:** Conceptualization, G.S., D.G. and F.M.; methodology, G.S., D.G., M.V. and F.A.; formal analysis, G.S., D.G., F.M., M.V. and F.A.; investigation, G.S., D.G., F.L., G.C., M.L.G. and V.R.; resources, G.P., M.V., F.A. and D.V.; data curation, G.S., D.G., F.M. and M.V.; writing—original draft preparation, G.S., D.G., F.M. and M.V.; writing—review and editing, G.S., D.G., F.M., M.V. and D.V.; visualization, G.S. and F.M.; supervision, M.V., A.G., G.P., F.A. and D.V.; project administration, F.M., A.G. and D.V.; funding acquisition, A.G. All authors have read and agreed to the published version of the manuscript.

**Funding:** This research was funded by the Ministero della Salute (Italy), Ricerca Corrente IZS SI 03/18 RC "Studio del potenziale zoonosico e caratterizzazione genomica dei virus enterici del cane".

**Institutional Review Board Statement:** Ethical review and approval were not required for this study since no experiment on live animals was performed; the study was carried out using tissue samples collected from dead animals submitted at the Istituto Zooprofilattico Sperimentale della Sicilia "A. Mirri" for diagnostic purposes.

**Informed Consent Statement:** Not applicable.

**Data Availability Statement:** Sequence data were submitted to the DDBJ/EMBL/GenBank databases under accession numbers MT981020–MT981039.

**Conflicts of Interest:** The authors declare no conflict of interest. The funders had no role in the design of the study; in the collection, analyses, or interpretation of data; in the writing of the manuscript; or in the decision to publish the results.

# References

1. Carmichael, L.E. An annotated historical account of canine parvovirus. *J. Vet. Med. B Infect. Dis. Vet. Public Health* **2005**, *52*, 303–311. [CrossRef] [PubMed]
2. Fratelli, A.; Cavalli, A.; Martella, V.; Tempesta, M.; Decaro, N.; Carmichael, L.E.; Buonavoglia, C. Canine parvovirus (CPV) vaccination: Comparison of neutralizing antibody responses in pups after inoculation with CPV2 or CPV2b modified live virus vaccine. *Clin. Diagn. Lab. Immunol.* **2001**, *8*, 612–615. [CrossRef] [PubMed]
3. Spibey, N.; Greenwood, N.M.; Sutton, D.; Chalmers, W.S.K.; Tarpey, I. Canine parvovirus type 2 vaccine protects against virulent challenge with type 2c virus. *Vet. Microbiol.* **2008**, *128*, 48–55. [CrossRef] [PubMed]

4. Voorhees, I.E.H.; Lee, H.; Allison, A.B.; Lopez-Astacio, R.; Goodman, L.B.; Oyesola, O.O.; Omobowale, O.; Fagbohun, O.; Dubovi, E.J.; Hafenstein, S.L.; et al. Limited Intrahost Diversity and Background Evolution Accompany 40 Years of Canine parvovirus Host Adaptation and Spread. *J. Virol.* **2019**, *94*, e01162-19. [CrossRef]
5. Decaro, N.; Buonavoglia, C. Canine parvovirus—A review of epidemiological and diagnostic aspects, with emphasis on type 2c. *Vet. Microbiol.* **2012**, *155*, 1–12. [CrossRef]
6. Cotmore, S.F.; Agbandje-McKenna, M.; Canuti, M.; Chiorini, J.A.; Eis-Hubinger, A.-M.; Hughes, J.; Mietzsch, M.; Modha, S.; Ogliastro, M.; Pénzes, J.J.; et al. ICTV Virus Taxonomy Profile: Parvoviridae. *J. Gen. Virol.* **2019**, *100*, 367–368. [CrossRef]
7. Cotmore, S.F.; Agbandje-McKenna, M.; Chiorini, J.A.; Mukha, D.V.; Pintel, D.J.; Qiu, J.; Soderlund-Venermo, M.; Tattersall, P.; Tijssen, P.; Gatherer, D.; et al. The family Parvoviridae. *Arch. Virol.* **2014**, *159*, 1239–1247. [CrossRef]
8. Parrish, C.R.; O'Connell, P.H.; Evermann, J.F.; Carmichael, L.E. Natural variation of canine parvovirus. *Science* **1985**, *230*, 1046–1048. [CrossRef]
9. Parrish, C.R.; Aquadro, C.F.; Strassheim, M.L.; Evermann, J.F.; Sgro, J.Y.; Mohammed, H.O. Rapid antigenic-type replacement and DNA sequence evolution of canine parvovirus. *J. Virol.* **1991**, *65*, 6544–6552. [CrossRef]
10. Buonavoglia, C.; Martella, V.; Pratelli, A.; Tempesta, M.; Cavalli, A.; Buonavoglia, D.; Bozzo, G.; Elia, G.; Decaro, N.; Carmichael, L. Evidence for evolution of Canine parvovirus type 2 in Italy. *J. Gen. Virol.* **2001**, *82*, 3021–3025. [CrossRef]
11. Mohr, A.J.; Leisewitz, A.L.; Jacobson, L.S.; Steiner, J.M.; Ruaux, C.G.; Williams, D.A. Effect of early enteral nutrition on intestinal permeability, intestinal protein loss, and outcome in dogs with severe parvoviral enteritis. *J. Vet. Intern. Med.* **2003**, *17*, 791–798. [CrossRef] [PubMed]
12. Armenise, A.; Trerotoli, P.; Cirone, F.; De Nitto, A.; De Sario, C.; Bertazzolo, W.; Pratelli, A.; Decaro, N. Use of recombinant canine granulocyte-colony stimulating factor to increase leukocyte count in dogs naturally infected by canine parvovirus. *Vet. Microbiol.* **2019**, *231*, 177–182. [CrossRef] [PubMed]
13. Gerlach, M.; Proksch, A.-L.; Dörfelt, R.; Unterer, S.; Hartmann, K. Therapy of Canine parvovirus infection—Review and current insights. *Tierarztl. Prax. Ausg. K Kleintiere Heimtiere* **2020**, *48*, 26–37. [CrossRef] [PubMed]
14. Goddard, A.; Leisewitz, A.L. Canine parvovirus. *Vet. Clin. N. Am. Small Anim. Pract.* **2010**, *40*, 1041–1053. [CrossRef] [PubMed]
15. Pereira, G.Q.; Gomes, L.A.; Santos, I.S.; Alfieri, A.F.; Weese, J.S.; Costa, M.C. Fecal microbiota transplantation in puppies with Canine parvovirus infection. *J. Vet. Intern. Med.* **2018**, *32*, 707–711. [CrossRef] [PubMed]
16. Park, J.S.; Guevarra, R.B.; Kim, B.-R.; Lee, J.H.; Lee, S.H.; Cho, J.H.; Kim, H.; Cho, J.H.; Song, M.; Lee, J.-H.; et al. Intestinal Microbial Dysbiosis in Beagles Naturally Infected with Canine Parvovirus. *J. Microbiol. Biotechnol.* **2019**, *29*, 1391–1400. [CrossRef] [PubMed]
17. Zheng, Y.; Hao, X.; Lin, X.; Zheng, Q.; Zhang, W.; Zhou, P.; Li, S. Bacterial diversity in the feces of dogs with CPV infection. *Microb. Pathog.* **2018**, *121*, 70–76. [CrossRef]
18. Otto, C.M.; Drobatz, K.J.; Soter, C. Endotoxemia and tumor necrosis factor activity in dogs with naturally occurring parvoviral enteritis. *J. Vet. Intern. Med.* **1997**, *11*, 65–70. [CrossRef]
19. Botha, W.J.; Schoeman, J.P.; Marks, S.L.; Whitehead, Z.; Annandale, C.H. Prevalence of Salmonella in juvenile dogs affected with parvoviral enteritis. *J. S. Afr. Vet. Assoc.* **2018**, *89*, e1–e6. [CrossRef]
20. Silva, R.O.S.; Dorella, F.A.; Figueiredo, H.C.P.; Costa, É.A.; Pelicia, V.; Ribeiro, B.L.D.; Ribeiro, M.G.; Paes, A.C.; Megid, J.; Lobato, F.C.F. Clostridium perfringens and C. difficile in parvovirus-positive dogs. *Anaerobe* **2017**, *48*, 66–69. [CrossRef]
21. Duijvestijn, M.; Mughini-Gras, L.; Schuurman, N.; Schijf, W.; Wagenaar, J.A.; Egberink, H. Enteropathogen infections in canine puppies: (Co-)occurrence, clinical relevance and risk factors. *Vet. Microbiol.* **2016**, *195*, 115–122. [CrossRef] [PubMed]
22. Da Rocha Gizzi, A.B.; Oliveira, S.T.; Leutenegger, C.M.; Estrada, M.; Kozemjakin, D.A.; Stedile, R.; Marcondes, M.; Biondo, A.W. Presence of infectious agents and co-infections in diarrheic dogs determined with a real-time polymerase chain reaction-based panel. *BMC Vet. Res.* **2014**, *10*, 23. [CrossRef]
23. McEwen, S.A.; Collignon, P.J. Antimicrobial Resistance: A One Health Perspective. *Microbiol. Spectr.* **2018**, *6*, ARBA-0009-2017. [CrossRef] [PubMed]
24. WHO (World Health Organization). *Critically Important Antimicrobials for Human Medicine*, 6th ed.; WHO Press: Geneva, Switzerland, 2019; Available online: https://apps.who.int/iris/bitstream/handle/10665/312266/9789241515528-eng.pdf?ua=1 (accessed on 7 October 2020).
25. Collignon, P.J.; McEwen, S.A. One Health-Its Importance in Helping to Better Control Antimicrobial Resistance. *Trop. Med. Infect. Dis.* **2019**, *4*, 22. [CrossRef] [PubMed]
26. Guardabassi, L.; Schwarz, S.; Lloyd, D.H. Pet animals as reservoirs of antimicrobial-resistant bacteria. *J. Antimicrob. Chemother.* **2004**, *54*, 321–332. [CrossRef]
27. Decaro, N.; Martella, V.; Elia, G.; Desario, C.; Campolo, M.; Lorusso, E.; Colaianni, M.L.; Lorusso, A.; Buonavoglia, C. Tissue distribution of the antigenic variants of Canine parvovirus type 2 in dogs. *Vet. Microbiol.* **2007**, *121*, 39–44. [CrossRef]
28. Mira, F.; Dowgier, G.; Purpari, G.; Vicari, D.; Di Bella, S.; Macaluso, G.; Gucciardi, F.; Randazzo, V.; Decaro, N.; Guercio, A. Molecular typing of a novel Canine parvovirus type 2a mutant circulating in Italy. *Infect. Genet. Evol.* **2018**, *61*, 67–73. [CrossRef]
29. Mira, F.; Canuti, M.; Purpari, G.; Cannella, V.; Di Bella, S.; Occhiogrosso, L.; Schirò, G.; Chiaramonte, G.; Barreca, S.; Pisano, P.; et al. Molecular Characterization and Evolutionary Analyses of Carnivore Protoparvovirus 1 NS1 Gene. *Viruses* **2019**, *11*, 308. [CrossRef]

30. Mira, F.; Purpari, G.; Lorusso, E.; Di Bella, S.; Gucciardi, F.; Desario, C.; Macaluso, G.; Decaro, N.; Guercio, A. Introduction of Asian *Canine parvovirus* in Europe through dog importation. *Transbound. Emerg. Dis.* 2018, 65, 16–21. [CrossRef]
31. Mira, F.; Purpari, G.; Di Bella, S.; Colaianni, M.L.; Schirò, G.; Chiaramonte, G.; Gucciardi, F.; Pisano, P.; Lastra, A.; Decaro, N.; et al. Spreading of *Canine parvovirus* type 2c mutants of Asian origin in southern Italy. *Transbound. Emerg. Dis.* 2019, 66, 2297–2304. [CrossRef]
32. Leclercq, R.; Cantón, R.; Brown, D.F.J.; Giske, C.G.; Heisig, P.; MacGowan, A.P.; Mouton, J.W.; Nordmann, P.; Rodloff, A.C.; Rossolini, G.M.; et al. EUCAST expert rules in antimicrobial susceptibility testing. *Clin. Microbiol. Infect.* 2013, 19, 141–160. [CrossRef] [PubMed]
33. Cardillo, L.; Piegari, G.; Iovane, V.; Viscardi, M.; Alfano, F.; Cerrone, A.; Pagnini, U.; Montagnaro, S.; Galiero, G.; Pisanelli, G.; et al. Lifestyle as Risk Factor for Infectious Causes of Death in Young Dogs: A Retrospective Study in Southern Italy (2015–2017). *Vet. Med. Int.* 2020, 2020, 6207297. [CrossRef] [PubMed]
34. Dowgier, G.; Lorusso, E.; Decaro, N.; Desario, C.; Mari, V.; Lucente, M.S.; Lanave, G.; Buonavoglia, C.; Elia, G. A molecular survey for selected viral enteropathogens revealed a limited role of Canine circovirus in the development of canine acute gastroenteritis. *Vet. Microbiol.* 2017, 204, 54–58. [CrossRef] [PubMed]
35. Greene, C.E.; Decaro, N. Canine Viral Enteritis. In *Infectious Diseases of Dog and Cat*, 4th ed.; Greene, C.E., Ed.; Elsevier Saunders: Philadelphia, PA, USA, 2012; pp. 67–80.
36. Wilson, S.; Illambas, J.; Siedek, E.; Stirling, C.; Thomas, A.; Plevová, E.; Sture, G.; Salt, J. Vaccination of dogs with *canine parvovirus* type 2b (CPV-2b) induces neutralising antibody responses to CPV-2a and CPV-2c. *Vaccine* 2014, 32, 5420–5424. [CrossRef] [PubMed]
37. Larson, L.J.; Schultz, R.D. Do two current *Canine parvovirus* type 2 and 2b vaccines provide protection against the new type 2c variant? *Vet. Ther.* 2008, 9, 94–101. [PubMed]
38. Day, M.J.; Horzinek, M.C.; Schultz, R.D.; Squires, R.A.; Vaccination Guidelines Group (VGG) of the World Small Animal Veterinary Association (WSAVA). WSAVA Guidelines for the vaccination of dogs and cats. *J. Small Anim. Pract.* 2016, 57, E1–E45. [CrossRef] [PubMed]
39. Cavalli, A.; Marinaro, M.; Desario, C.; Corrente, M.; Camero, M.; Buonavoglia, C. In vitro virucidal activity of sodium hypochlorite against *Canine parvovirus* type 2. *Epidemiol. Infect.* 2018, 146, 2010–2013. [CrossRef]
40. Decaro, N.; Buonavoglia, C.; Barrs, V.R. *Canine parvovirus* vaccination and immunisation failures: Are we far from disease eradication? *Vet. Microbiol.* 2020, 247, 108760. [CrossRef]
41. Buchy, P.; Ascioglu, S.; Buisson, Y.; Datta, S.; Nissen, M.; Tambyah, P.A.; Vong, S. Impact of vaccines on antimicrobial resistance. *Int. J. Infect. Dis.* 2020, 90, 188–196. [CrossRef]
42. Bloom, D.E.; Black, S.; Salisbury, D.; Rappuoli, R. Antimicrobial resistance and the role of vaccines. *Proc. Natl. Acad. Sci. USA* 2018, 115, 12868–12871. [CrossRef]
43. Prittie, J. Canine parvoviral enteritis: A review of diagnosis, management, and prevention. *J. Vet. Emerg. Crit. Car.* 2004, 14, 167–176. [CrossRef]
44. Alves, F.; Prata, S.; Nunes, T.; Gomes, J.; Aguiar, S.; Aires da Silva, F.; Tavares, L.; Almeida, V.; Gil, S. Canine parvovirus: A predicting canine model for sepsis. *BMC Vet. Res.* 2020, 16, 199. [CrossRef] [PubMed]
45. Miranda, C.; Carvalheira, J.; Parrish, C.R.; Thompson, G. Factors affecting the occurrence of *Canine parvovirus* in dogs. *Vet. Microbiol.* 2015, 180, 59–64. [CrossRef] [PubMed]
46. Marenzoni, M.L.; Calò, P.; Foiani, G.; Tossici, S.; Passantino, G.; Decaro, N.; Mandara, M.T. Porencephaly and Periventricular Encephalitis in a 4-month-old Puppy: Detection of *Canine parvovirus* Type 2 and Potential Role in Brain Lesions. *J. Comp. Pathol.* 2019, 169, 20–24. [CrossRef]
47. Zhao, Y.; Lin, Y.; Zeng, X.; Lu, C.; Hou, J. Genotyping and pathobiologic characterization of *Canine parvovirus* circulating in Nanjing, China. *Virol. J.* 2013, 10, 272. [CrossRef]
48. Schaudien, D.; Polizopoulou, Z.; Koutinas, A.; Schwab, S.; Porombka, D.; Baumgärtner, W.; Herden, C. Leukoencephalopathy associated with parvovirus infection in Cretan hound puppies. *J. Clin. Microbiol.* 2010, 48, 3169–3175. [CrossRef]
49. Schwab, S.; Herden, C.; Seeliger, F.; Papaioannou, N.; Psalla, D.; Polizopoulou, Z.; Baumgärtner, W. Non-suppurative meningoencephalitis of unknown origin in cats and dogs: An immunohistochemical study. *J. Comp. Pathol.* 2007, 136, 96–110. [CrossRef]
50. Schoeman, J.P.; Goddard, A.; Leisewitz, A.L. Biomarkers in *Canine parvovirus* enteritis. *N. Z. Vet. J.* 2013, 61, 217–222. [CrossRef]
51. Venn, E.C.; Preisner, K.; Boscan, P.L.; Twedt, D.C.; Sullivan, L.A. Evaluation of an outpatient protocol in the treatment of canine parvoviral enteritis. *J. Vet. Emerg. Crit. Care* 2017, 27, 52–65. [CrossRef]
52. Mylonakis, M.E.; Kalli, I.; Rallis, T.S. Canine parvoviral enteritis: An update on the clinical diagnosis, treatment, and prevention. *Vet. Med. Auckl* 2016, 7, 91–100. [CrossRef]
53. Barbarossa, A.; Casadio, C.; Diegoli, G.; Fontana, M.C.; Giunti, M.; Miraglia, V.; Rambaldi, J.; Rubini, M.; Torresani, G.; Trambajolo, G.; et al. LINEE GUIDA Uso Prudente Dell'antibiotico Negli Animali da Compagnia. 2018. Available online: https://www.alimenti-salute.it/sites/default/files/Linee%20Guida%20PETs%202018.pdf (accessed on 22 November 2021).
54. Escher, M.; Vanni, M.; Intorre, L.; Caprioli, A.; Tognetti, R.; Scavia, G. Use of antimicrobials in companion animal practice: A retrospective study in a veterinary teaching hospital in Italy. *J. Antimicrob. Chemoter.* 2011, 66, 920–927. [CrossRef] [PubMed]
55. Barbarossa, A.; Rambaldi, J.; Miraglia, V.; Giunti, M.; Diegoli, G.; Zaghini, A. Survey on antimicrobial prescribing patterns in small animal veterinary practice in Emilia Romagna, Italy. *Vet. Rec.* 2017, 181, 69. [CrossRef] [PubMed]

56. Chirollo, C.; Nocera, F.P.; Piantedosi, D.; Fatone, G.; Della Valle, G.; De Martino, L.; Cortese, L. Data on before and after the Traceability System of Veterinary Antimicrobial Prescriptions in Small Animals at the University Veterinary Teaching Hospital of Naples. *Animals* **2021**, *11*, 913. [CrossRef] [PubMed]
57. De Briyne, N.; Atkinson, J.; Pokludová, L.; Borriello, S.P. Antibiotics used most commonly to treat animals in Europe. *Vet. Rec.* **2014**, *175*, 325. [CrossRef] [PubMed]
58. Joosten, P.; Ceccarelli, D.; Odent, E.; Sarrazin, S.; Graveland, H.; Van Gompel, L.; Battisti, A.; Caprioli, A.; Franco, A.; Wagenaar, J.A.; et al. Antimicrobial Usage and Resistance in Companion Animals: A Cross-Sectional Study in Three European Countries. *Antibiotics* **2020**, *9*, 87. [CrossRef]
59. Mazzaferro, E.M. Update on Canine Parvoviral Enteritis. *Vet. Clin. N. Am. Small Anim. Pract.* **2020**, *50*, 1307–1325. [CrossRef] [PubMed]
60. Chaitman, J.; Ziese, A.-L.; Pilla, R.; Minamoto, Y.; Blake, A.B.; Guard, B.C.; Isaiah, A.; Lidbury, J.A.; Steiner, J.M.; Unterer, S.; et al. Fecal Microbial and Metabolic Profiles in Dogs with Acute Diarrhea Receiving Either Fecal Microbiota Transplantation or Oral Metronidazole. *Front. Vet. Sci.* **2020**, *7*, 192. [CrossRef] [PubMed]
61. Tauro, A.; Beltran, E.; Cherubini, G.B.; Coelho, A.T.; Wessmann, A.; Driver, C.J.; Rusbridge, C.J. Metronidazole-induced neurotoxicity in 26 dogs. *Aust. Vet. J.* **2018**, *96*, 495–501. [CrossRef]
62. Kilian, E.; Suchodolski, J.S.; Hartmann, K.; Mueller, R.S.; Wess, G.; Unterer, S. Long-term effects of *Canine parvovirus* infection in dogs. *PLoS ONE* **2018**, *13*, e0192198. [CrossRef]
63. WHO (World Health Organization). Antimicrobial Resistance: Global Report on Surveillance 2014. 2014. Available online: https://www.who.int/antimicrobial-resistance/publications/surveillancereport/en/ (accessed on 7 October 2020).
64. WHO (World Health Organization). WHO Guidelines on Use of Medically Important Antimicrobials in Food-Producing Animals. 2017. Available online: https://www.who.int/foodsafety/areas_work/antimicrobial-resistance/cia_guidelines/en/ (accessed on 7 October 2020).
65. WHO (World Health Organization). Global Priority List of Antibiotic-Resistant Bacteria to Guide Research, Discovery, and Development of New Antibiotics. 2017. Available online: https://www.who.int/medicines/publications/global-priority-list-antibiotic-resistant-bacteria/en/ (accessed on 7 October 2020).
66. Effah, C.Y.; Sun, T.; Liu, S.; Wu, Y. Klebsiella pneumoniae: An increasing threat to public health. *Ann. Clin. Microbiol. Antimicrob.* **2020**, *19*, 1. [CrossRef]
67. Alikhani, M.Y.; Asl, H.M.; Khairkhah, M.; Farajnia, S.; Aslani, M.M. Phenotypic and genotypic characterization of Escherichia Coli O111 serotypes. *Gastroenterol. Hepatol. Bed Bench* **2011**, *4*, 147–152. [PubMed]
68. Kim, S.; Kim, S.-H.; Kim, J.; Shin, J.-H.; Lee, B.-K.; Park, M.-S. Occurrence and distribution of various genetic structures of class 1 and class 2 integrons in Salmonella enterica isolates from foodborne disease patients in Korea for 16 years. *Foodborne Pathog. Dis.* **2011**, *8*, 319–324. [CrossRef] [PubMed]
69. Gaastra, W.; Kusters, J.G.; van Duijkeren, E.; Lipman, L.J.A. Escherichia fergusonii. *Vet. Microbiol.* **2014**, *172*, 7–12. [CrossRef] [PubMed]
70. Gullett, J.C.; Westblade, L.F.; Green, D.A.; Whittier, S.; Burd, E.M. The Brief Case: Too beta to be a "B". *J. Clin. Microbiol.* **2017**, *55*, 1604–1607. [CrossRef] [PubMed]
71. Pinho, M.D.; Matos, S.C.; Pomba, C.; Lübke-Becker, A.; Wieler, L.H.; Preziuso, S.; Melo-Cristino, J.; Ramirez, M. Multilocus sequence analysis of Streptococcus canis confirms the zoonotic origin of human infections and reveals genetic exchange with Streptococcus dysgalactiae subsp. equisimilis. *J. Clin. Microbiol.* **2013**, *51*, 1099–1109. [CrossRef]
72. Sato, Y.; Kuwamoto, R. A case of canine salmonellosis due to Salmonella infantis. *J. Vet. Med. Sci.* **1999**, *61*, 71–72. [CrossRef]
73. Chomel, B.B. Emerging and Re-Emerging Zoonoses of Dogs and Cats. *Animals* **2014**, *4*, 434–445. [CrossRef]
74. Purpari, G.; Mira, F.; Di Bella, S.; Di Pietro, S.; Giudice, E.; Guercio, A. Investigation on *Canine parvovirus* circulation in dogs from Sicily (Italy) by biomolecular assay. *Acta Vet. Beogr.* **2018**, *68*, 80–94.
75. Touihri, L.; Bouzid, I.; Daoud, R.; Desario, C.; El Goulli, A.F.; Decaro, N.; Ghorbel, A.; Buonavoglia, C.; Bahloul, C. Molecular characterization of canine parvovirus-2 variants circulating in Tunisia. *Virus Genes* **2009**, *38*, 249–258. [CrossRef]
76. Battilani, M.; Modugno, F.; Mira, F.; Purpari, G.; Di Bella, S.; Guercio, A.; Balboni, A. Molecular epidemiology of *Canine parvovirus* type 2 in Italy from 1994 to 2017: Recurrence of the CPV-2b variant. *BMC Vet. Res.* **2019**, *15*, 393. [CrossRef]
77. Ogbu, K.I.; Mira, F.; Purpari, G.; Nwosuh, C.; Loria, G.R.; Schirò, G.; Chiaramonte, G.; Tion, M.T.; Di Bella, S.; Ventriglia, G.; et al. Nearly full-length genome characterization of *Canine parvovirus* strains circulating in Nigeria. *Transbound. Emerg. Dis.* **2020**, *67*, 635–647. [CrossRef]
78. Pérez, R.; Calleros, L.; Marandino, A.; Sarute, N.; Iraola, G.; Grecco, S.; Blanc, H.; Vignuzzi, M.; Isakov, O.; Shomron, N.; et al. Phylogenetic and genome-wide deep-sequencing analyses of *Canine parvovirus* reveal co-infection with field variants and emergence of a recent recombinant strain. *PLoS ONE* **2014**, *9*, e111779. [CrossRef] [PubMed]
79. Martella, V.; Decaro, N.; Elia, G.; Buonavoglia, C. Surveillance activity for *Canine parvovirus* in Italy. *J. Vet. Med. B Infect. Dis. Vet. Public Health* **2005**, *52*, 312–315. [CrossRef] [PubMed]
80. Barrett, T.; Visser, I.K.; Mamaev, L.; Goatley, L.; van Bressem, M.F.; Osterhaust, A.D. Dolphin and porpoise morbilliviruses are genetically distinct from phocine distemper virus. *Virology* **1993**, *193*, 1010–1012. [CrossRef] [PubMed]
81. Hu, R.L.; Huang, G.; Qiu, W.; Zhong, Z.H.; Xia, X.Z.; Yin, Z. Detection and differentiation of CAV-1 and CAV-2 by polymerase chain reaction. *Vet. Res. Commun.* **2001**, *25*, 77–84. [CrossRef] [PubMed]

82. Pratelli, A.; Martella, V.; Decaro, N.; Tinelli, A.; Camero, M.; Cirone, F.; Elia, G.; Cavalli, A.; Corrente, M.; Greco, G.; et al. Genetic diversity of a canine coronavirus detected in pups with diarrhoea in Italy. *J. Virol. Methods* **2003**, *110*, 9–17. [CrossRef]
83. Freeman, M.M.; Kerin, T.; Hull, J.; McCaustland, K.; Gentsch, J. Enhancement of detection and quantification of rotavirus in stool using a modified real-time RT-PCR assay. *J. Med. Virol.* **2008**, *80*, 1489–1496. [CrossRef]
84. CLSI. *Performance Standards for Antimicrobial Disk and Dilution Susceptibility Tests for Bacteria Isolated from Animals*, 4th ed.; CLSI Supplement VET08; Clinical and Laboratory Standards Institute: Wayne, PA, USA, 2018; ISBN 978-1-68440-010-2.
85. CLSI. *Performance Standards for Antimicrobial Susceptibility Testing*, 25th ed.; CLSI supplement M100-S25; Clinical and Laboratory Standards Institute: Wayne, PA, USA, 2015; ISBN 978-1-56238-989-5/978-1-56238-990-1.
86. Kim, J.; Jeon, S.; Rhie, H.; Lee, B.; Park, M.; Lee, H.; Lee, J.; Kim, S. Rapid Detection of Extended Spectrum β-Lactamase (ESBL) for Enterobacteriaceae by use of a Multiplex PCR-based Method. *Infect. Chemother.* **2009**, *41*, 181–184. [CrossRef]
87. Vitale, M.; Gaglio, S.; Galluzzo, P.; Cascone, G.; Piraino, C.; Di Marco Lo Presti, V.; Alduina, R. Antibiotic Resistance Profiling, Analysis of Virulence Aspects and Molecular Genotyping of Staphylococcus aureus Isolated in Sicily, Italy. *Foodborne Pathog. Dis.* **2018**, *15*, 177–185. [CrossRef]
88. Baums, C.G.; Schotte, U.; Amtsberg, G.; Goethe, R. Diagnostic multiplex PCR for toxin genotyping of Clostridium perfringens isolates. *Vet. Microbiol.* **2004**, *100*, 11–16. [CrossRef]
89. Bai, J.; Paddock, Z.D.; Shi, X.; Li, S.; An, B.; Nagaraja, T.G. Applicability of a multiplex PCR to detect the seven major Shiga toxin-producing Escherichia coli based on genes that code for serogroup-specific O-antigens and major virulence factors in cattle feces. *Foodborne Pathog. Dis.* **2012**, *9*, 541–548. [CrossRef] [PubMed]

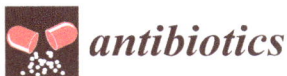 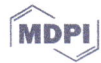

*Article*

# Knowledge, Attitude, and Practices (KAP) Survey among Veterinarians, and Risk Factors Relating to Antimicrobial Use and Treatment Failure in Dairy Herds of India

Deepthi Vijay [1], Jasbir Singh Bedi [1,*], Pankaj Dhaka [1], Randhir Singh [1], Jaswinder Singh [2], Anil Kumar Arora [3] and Jatinder Paul Singh Gill [1]

[1] School of Public Health and Zoonoses, College of Veterinary Science, Guru Angad Dev Veterinary and Animal Sciences University, Ludhiana 141004, India; deepthivijay@kvasu.ac.in (D.V.); pankaj.dhaka2@gmail.com (P.D.); sainirandhir74@gmail.com (R.S.); gilljps@gmail.com (J.P.S.G.)

[2] Department of Veterinary and Animal Husbandry Extension Education, College of Veterinary Science, Guru Angad Dev Veterinary and Animal Sciences University, Ludhiana 141004, India; jaswindervet@rediffmail.com

[3] Department of Veterinary Microbiology, College of Veterinary Science, Guru Angad Dev Veterinary and Animal Sciences University, Ludhiana 141004, India; aroraak65@gmail.com

\* Correspondence: bedijasbir78@gmail.com; Tel.: +91-9855425578

**Abstract:** The indiscriminate usage of antimicrobials in the animal health sector contributes immensely to antimicrobial resistance (AMR). The present study aims to assess the antimicrobial usage pattern and risk factors for AMR in animal husbandry sector of India. A cross-sectional survey about Knowledge, Attitude, and Practices (KAP) among veterinarians was carried out using a questionnaire comprising of 52 parameters associated with antibiotic use and the emergence of AMR in dairy herds. Respondents' KAP scores were estimated to rank their level of knowledge, attitude, and practice. Furthermore, risk factors associated with treatment failure were analyzed by univariable and multivariable analyses. Out of a total of 466 respondents, the majority had average knowledge (69.5%), neutral attitude (93.2%), and moderate practice (51.3%) scores toward judicious antibiotic usage. Veterinarians reported mastitis (88.0%), reproductive disorders (76.6%), and hemoprotozoan infections (49.6%) as the top three disease conditions that require antibiotic usage. Most of the veterinarians (90.6%) resorted to their "own experience" as the main criteria for antibiotic choice. The use of the highest priority critically important antimicrobials (HPCIA) listed by the World Health Organization (WHO) in animals, particularly quinolones (76.8%) and third-generation cephalosporins (47.8%), has been reported. On multivariable regression analysis of the risk factors, the lack of cooperation of the dairy farmers in the completion of a prescribed antibiotic course by the veterinarian and the demand for antibiotic use even in conditions not requiring antibiotic use were found to be significantly associated with the outcome variable "treatment failure" having respective odds of 1.8 (95%CI: 1.1–3.0) and 3.6 (95%CI: 2.3–5.8) ($p < 0.05$). The average KAP score of veterinarians, poor farm management practices, lack of awareness among farmers on prudent antibiotic use, and lack of antibiotic stewardship are the significant factors that need attention to combat the rising AMR in veterinary sector in India.

**Keywords:** antimicrobial resistance; antimicrobial usage; bovine; India; KAP survey; veterinarians

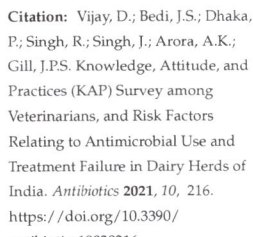

Citation: Vijay, D.; Bedi, J.S.; Dhaka, P.; Singh, R.; Singh, J.; Arora, A.K.; Gill, J.P.S. Knowledge, Attitude, and Practices (KAP) Survey among Veterinarians, and Risk Factors Relating to Antimicrobial Use and Treatment Failure in Dairy Herds of India. *Antibiotics* **2021**, *10*, 216. https://doi.org/10.3390/antibiotics10020216

Academic Editor: Jeroen Dewulf

Received: 13 November 2020
Accepted: 15 January 2021
Published: 22 February 2021

**Publisher's Note:** MDPI stays neutral with regard to jurisdictional claims in published maps and institutional affiliations.

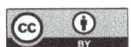

**Copyright:** © 2021 by the authors. Licensee MDPI, Basel, Switzerland. This article is an open access article distributed under the terms and conditions of the Creative Commons Attribution (CC BY) license (https://creativecommons.org/licenses/by/4.0/).

## 1. Introduction

Antimicrobial resistance is one of the greatest public health threats that has been projected to cause globally 10 million deaths and US$100 trillion economic loss by 2050 [1]. In order to meet the food security of burgeoning human population, the economic scale production of food animals favor the high-density farming operations, which could double the antibiotic consumption by livestock in developing countries by 2030 [2,3]. The widespread application of antibiotics to food animal populations imposes strong selection pressure, which contributes to the emergence, spread, and persistence of resistant pathogens to other animals, humans, and the environment [4]. The awareness on antibiotic resistance in human medicine has gained momentum; however, the role of animal husbandry practices in tackling antibiotic resistance are still being discussed with limited awareness among stakeholders, especially in developing countries [5].

India is bestowed with huge livestock wealth comprising of 193.5 million cattle and 109.9 million buffaloes [6]. The emerging intensive farming practices of the country has been posited as the hotspots of antibiotic resistance, and by 2030, the use of antibiotics in food animals has been projected to increase by 82% [2]. The threat of antibiotic resistance from the foods of animal origin has been discussed in many recent studies in India, highlighting the need for the judicious use of antibiotics in the animal health sector of the country [7–9]. Albeit, a "National Action Plan on Antimicrobial Resistance" has been enforced for optimizing antibiotic use in the country, strict enforcement still needs to be executed at the ground level [10–12].

While the reliability of data on the usage of antibiotics in the animal husbandry sector is questioned in general, some developing countries including India have a negligible amount of data [2,13]. In the midst of antimicrobial resistance crises with limited existing treatment options, mitigation strategies mainly revolve around awareness and proper stewardship for antibiotic usage among the key stakeholders. Thereby, understanding of knowledge, attitude, and practices (KAP) among the main stakeholders (e.g., veterinarians) with regard to antimicrobial use and resistance can help in the development of tailored intervention strategies to address poor practices, lack of knowledge, and negative attitude. Keeping in view the fact that there is no systematic KAP study along with prevailing antibiotic usage patterns and resistance in animal husbandry sector in Indian settings, the objectives of the present study were to assess Knowledge, Attitude, and Practices (KAP) among veterinarians in relevant to antimicrobial usage in animal husbandry sector through cross-sectional surveys, and identify the risk factors for the development of antimicrobial resistance (AMR) in India.

## 2. Material and Methods

### 2.1. Study Design and Questionnaire Development

The descriptive study was designed as a questionnaire-based cross-sectional analysis among the veterinarians of India during February 2020 to June 2020. A comprehensive review of the literature has been conducted to identify the factors influencing knowledge, attitude, and practices (KAP) on antimicrobial usage and resistance among veterinarians [14–16]. The questionnaire design was guided by the results from qualitative interviews and focus group discussions with veterinary academicians and farm animal practitioners of the Guru Angad Dev Veterinary and Animal Sciences University, Ludhiana, India. The questionnaire consisted of close-end questions, Likert scale statements, and open-ended questions exploring the existing knowledge, antimicrobial prescribing behaviors, perceptions on antimicrobial usage, and field practices associated with antimicrobial resistance. In addition, the veterinarian's recommendations were also requested for suggesting the interventions to combat antimicrobial resistance in the animal husbandry sector.

The questionnaire was divided into five sections: (1) Personal information; (2) Health services; (3) Knowledge, attitude, and practices toward antibiotic use; (4) Knowledge, attitude, and practices toward antimicrobial resistance; and (5) Miscellaneous section covering practices and recommendations for combating antimicrobial resistance.

The preliminary draft of the questionnaire having 58 questions was reviewed by five expert researchers to identify ambiguity and content validity. Later, the questionnaire was piloted among 20 veterinarians to assess its duration, clarity, and sequence. During the processing, six questions were omitted that were inappropriate, resulting in a total of 52 questions in the final questionnaire (Supplementary Material File S1).

## 2.2. Sampling Procedure

The source population of the present study comprised of registered veterinarians (Veterinary Council of India and/or State Veterinary Council) of India, and the study population included veterinarians who fulfilled the inclusion criteria of being farm animal practitioners. The sample size was calculated using the 'Raosoft calculator' (Raosoft: http://www.raosoft.com/samplesize.html?nosurvey). The sample size of 377 was estimated based on 50% response distribution, a 5% margin of error, and a 95% confidence interval. The expected response proportion of 50% was assumed based on the fact that both responses and response rates were completely unknown, since there are no previously published similar studies from India. Thereby, a total of 800 questionnaires were sent to the veterinarians selected through registered emails and/or personal contacts from professional societies and social media groups. The questionnaire was administrated by using the online interface of Google Forms (Google LLC, Mountain View, CA, USA) to the target population, and the survey remained open from May 2020 to June 2020.

## 2.3. Ethical Statement

The research was conducted in accordance with the Declaration of Helsinki and national standards. All the required ethical considerations have been taken into account. The nature of the study was completely voluntary, and informed consent was obtained from study participants. The details of the participants were anonymous, and data confidentiality was properly maintained.

## 2.4. Statistical Analysis

The completed questionnaires were manually checked for data quality before coding on Microsoft® Office Excel 2010. The study variables were summarized using proportions for qualitative variables and median and median absolute deviation for quantitative variables. The Likert-scale questions were condensed into two categories for analysis. A scoring system was generated by the subject experts of the University, in which the participants were given a score for knowledge, attitude, and practices based on the number of correct or appropriate responses. The overall score was determined based on the sum of correct answers to the eleven knowledge-based questions, four attitude-based questions, and thirteen practice-based questions. The respondent's level of knowledge/attitude/practices were categorized as "high/positive/good", "average/neutral/moderate", or "low/negative/poor" using the $\geq$75th percentile, <75th to 25th percentile, and <25th percentile of the individual scores, respectively. The Mann–Whitney U test/Kruskal–Wallis H test were used to determine the relationship between demographic characteristics of the veterinarians and their KAP scores. The correlation among the knowledge, attitude, and practice scores were assessed by the Spearman correlation. A $p$-value of $\leq 0.05$ was interpreted as significant. The logistic regression analysis was performed to estimate predictors for the outcome variable, "frequent treatment failure". The outcome variable "frequent treatment failure" depicting the failure of response of the animal to the first line of antibiotic treatment by the veterinarians was ascertained from the questionnaire. Various risk factors associated with "frequent treatment failure" were used as predictors determined by univariate odds ratio. The multicollinearity was checked to rule out the relationship amongst the independent variables based on the Variable Inflation Factor value (VIF) calculated in an iterative manner. The associations between the selected variables for multivariable analysis had a VIF of less than 2. The interactions between the predictors were checked and were found to be non-significant. The model was constructed by considering all these explanatory variables using the backward stepwise approach using the Likelihood Ratio Test (LRT). The analyses were conducted using SPSS version 24.0 (SPSS Inc., IBM, Armonk, NY, USA).

## 3. Results

A total of 478 (59.7%) responses were received out a total of 800 questionnaires, of which 466 were with complete information. The questionnaires that contained incomplete ($n = 7$) and vague information ($n = 5$) were excluded from the study.

### 3.1. Demographic Information

The demographic profile of the participants belonged to twenty-five states of India, which were grouped into six geographical regions (Table 1). Out of 466 participants with a median age of 32 years, 70.0% were males and 30.0% were females. The highest number of respondents belonged to the 30–40 age group (37.5%). It was observed that 48.1% of veterinarians had post-graduate qualifications. Most of the veterinarians (62.9%) had less than 10 years of field experience. The majority of the respondents were working in veterinary hospitals (85.6%), while 14.4% were in veterinary polyclinics that had established laboratory facilities.

Table 1. Demographic information of respondents.

| Characteristics | n | (%) |
|---|---|---|
| **Age (years)** | | |
| <30 | 148 | 31.8 |
| 30–40 | 175 | 37.5 |
| 40–50 | 103 | 22.1 |
| 50–60 | 32 | 6.9 |
| 60–70 | 8 | 1.7 |
| **Sex** | | |
| Male | 326 | 70.0 |
| Female | 140 | 30.0 |
| **Level of education** | | |
| Bachelor of Veterinary Sciences and Animal husbandry (B.V.Sc and A.H) | 208 | 44.6 |
| Master of Veterinary Sciences (M.V.Sc) | 224 | 48.1 |
| Ph.D. | 34 | 7.3 |
| **Field Experience (years)** | | |
| <10 | 293 | 62.9 |
| 10–20 | 105 | 22.5 |
| 20–30 | 50 | 10.7 |
| 30–40 | 17 | 3.6 |
| 40–50 | 1 | 0.2 |
| **Regional distribution (6 regions: 25 States)** | | |
| Northern Region (Jammu and Kashmir, Haryana, Himachal Pradesh, Punjab, Delhi, Uttarakhand, Uttar Pradesh) | 181 | 38.8 |
| Southern Region (Andhra Pradesh, Telangana, Karnataka, Kerala, Tamil Nadu) | 158 | 33.9 |
| Western Region (Rajasthan, Gujarat, Maharashtra) | 55 | 11.8 |
| Eastern Region (Bihar, Orissa, West Bengal) | 38 | 8.1 |
| Central Region (Madhya Pradesh, Chhattisgarh) | 22 | 4.7 |
| North-East Region (Assam, Sikkim, Nagaland, Meghalaya, Mizoram) | 12 | 2.6 |

Table 1. Cont.

| Characteristics | n | (%) |
|---|---|---|
| **Type of Hospital** | | |
| Veterinary Hospital (Institutes with basic facilities for day-to-day treatment and care of livestock) | 399 | 85.6% |
| Veterinary Polyclinic (Institutes with specialized facilities including diagnostic laboratories) | 67 | 14.4% |

### 3.2. Common Diseases Requiring Antibiotic Usage in Bovines

Major disease conditions found in bovines requiring antibiotic usage are listed in Figure 1. The veterinarians reported mastitis ($n = 410$), reproductive disorders ($n = 343$), and hemoprotozoan infections ($n = 231$) as the top three disease conditions in bovines where antibiotics are widely used.

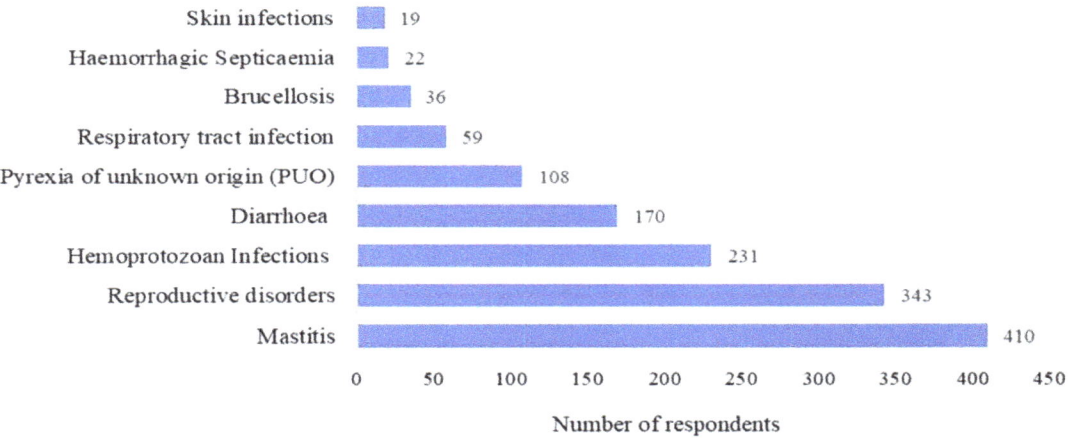

**Figure 1.** Major disease conditions requiring antibiotic use in bovines in India * (* Question: Top 03 disease conditions that require antibiotic use in bovines. Each veterinarian was asked to choose up to three disease conditions).

### 3.3. Antibiotic Prescribing Decisions

The decision over the choice of antibiotics in various diseases/conditions in bovines was influenced by different factors (Figure 2). The majority of the veterinarians (90.6%) depended on their own experience as the top criteria for choosing antibiotics followed by the availability (63.3%) and cost (59.0%) of the antibiotic. Recommendations from other veterinarians (31.8%) and pharmaceutical companies (7.1%) also influenced their decision regarding antibiotic use. Around 28% of the veterinarians took into account positive culture and sensitivity test results, whereas the withdrawal period of the drug influenced only 15% of veterinarians in prescribing the antibiotics. In addition, 24.9% veterinarians reported that the demand and expectation of farmers influences the prescription behaviors of antibiotics, even for conditions that do not require their use.

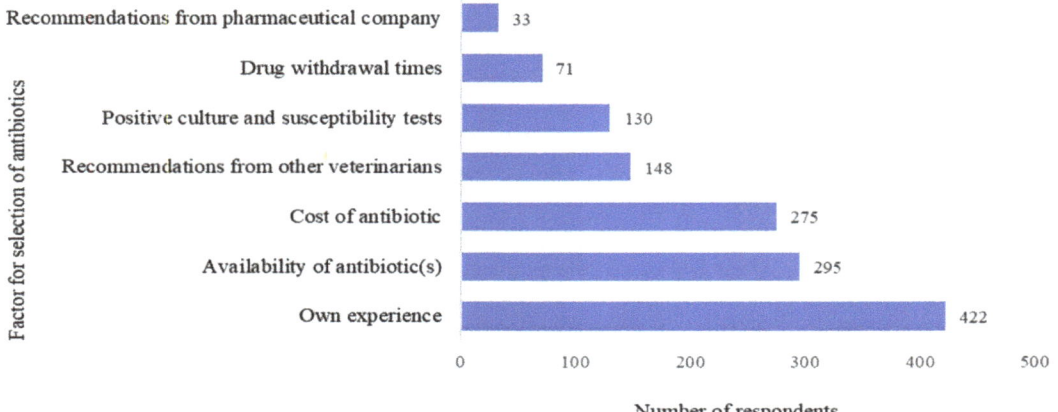

**Figure 2.** Factors determining the choice of antimicrobial use by veterinarians * (* Question: What are the top three factors in determining the choice of antibiotics use in your treatment? Choose among the following (Own experience/Availability of antibiotic(s)/Recommendations from other veterinarians/Cost of antibiotic/Positive culture and susceptibility tests/Drug withdrawal times/Recommendations from pharmaceutical company). Each veterinarian was asked to choose up to three top factors determining the choice of antimicrobials).

The veterinarians reported the use of "highest priority critically important antimicrobials" (HPCIA) mentioned by World Health Organization (WHO) [17] in their choices for treatment, *viz.*, quinolones (76.8%; $n = 358$), third-generation cephalosporins (47.8%; $n = 223$), and fourth-generation cephalosporins (6.0%; $n = 28$) (Figure 3a). The quinolones (71.9%, $n = 335$) were the most commonly prescribed antibiotic for mastitis followed by third-generation cephalosporins (64.2%; $n = 299$) (Figure 3b). In case of metritis, third-generation cephalosporins (55.6%; $n = 259$) followed by tetracycline (50.6%; $n = 236$) and quinolones (50.0%; $n = 233$) were the top three commonly used antibiotics (Figure 3c).

However, 45.5% of the veterinarians were aware of the 'critically important list of antimicrobials' of the WHO [17], while 59.2% opined that restriction on the WHO suggested 'priority antibiotics for human-use only' is not possible in veterinary therapeutics. The antibiotics in the 'reserve group' as proposed by the WHO [18], particularly fourth-generation cephalosporins, were used by 13.5% of the veterinarians in mastitis and by 6.9% of veterinarians in metritis. Moreover, 1.9% of the veterinarians reported the use of fifth-generation cephalosporins in mastitis. In addition, uses of alternate therapies such as herbal medicines were reported by 74.0% veterinarians, whereas 67.2% used probiotics, 43.8% used homeopathic medicine, and 2.4% used indigenous remedies for different disease conditions.

### 3.4. Knowledge, Attitude, and Practice (KAP) Analysis

The knowledge of the respondents on antimicrobial use and resistance was assessed by scoring eleven questions, with the score 1 given to correct answer while 0 was given to incorrect or not sure response (Table 2; Supplementary Material Table S1). The knowledge was scaled as high with a score $\geq 9$, average with a score 6–9, and low with a score < 6. The median knowledge score of the respondents was $8.0 \pm 1.0$. Only 14.2% of the respondents had a high knowledge score, whereas most respondents (69.5%) had an average knowledge score. The majority of the respondents (73%) were regularly updating themselves on antimicrobial resistance, where the internet was the most common information source (Figure 4). A significantly higher knowledge score was observed among the veterinarians who regularly updated themselves compared with those who did not (U statistic: 4.6, *p*-value: 0.00).

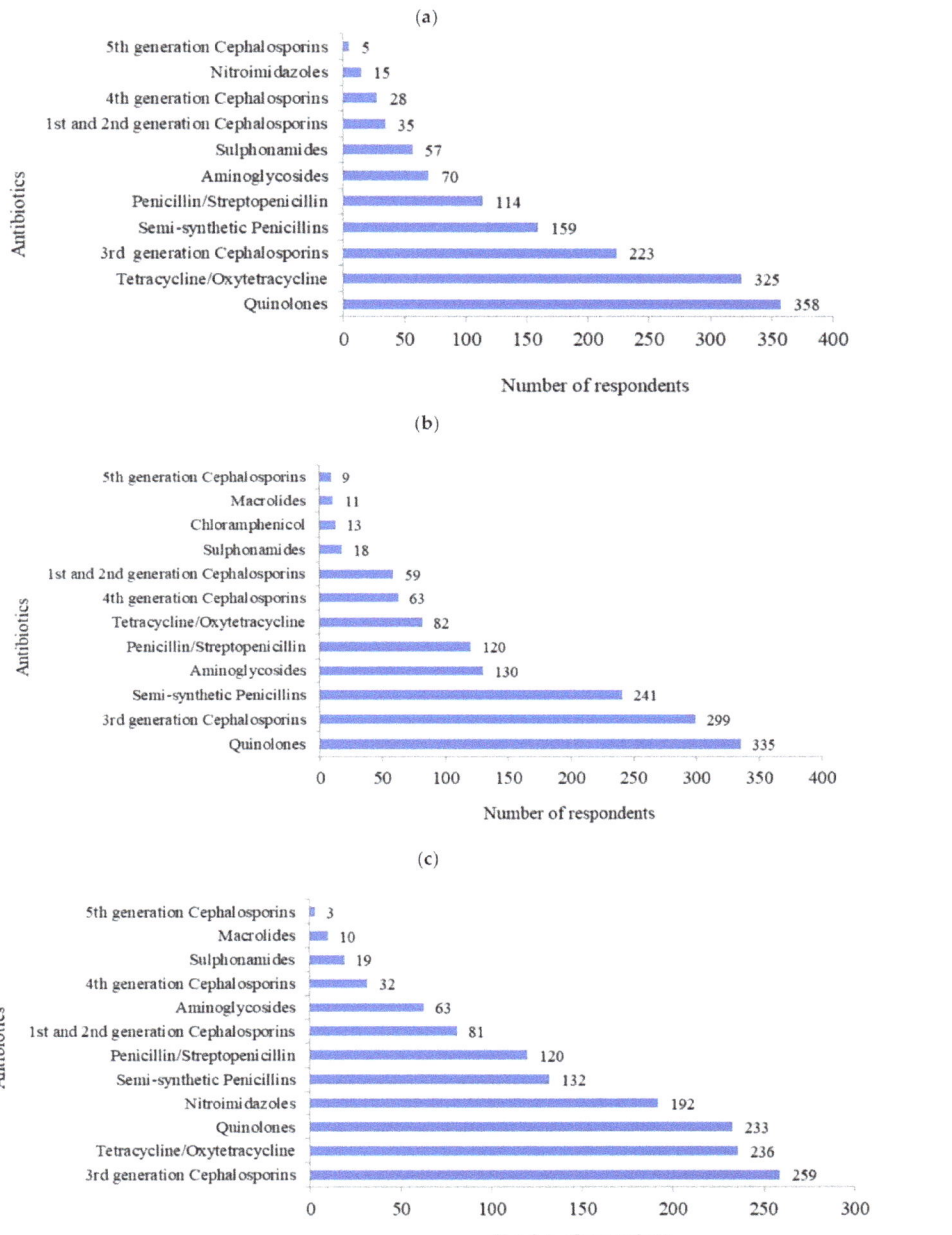

**Figure 3.** Commonly used antibiotics in bovines ((**a**) overall use; (**b**) use in mastitis; (**c**) use in metritis)* (* Questions: (**a**) Top three frequently used antibiotics in the treatment of bovines; (**b**) Top three frequently used antibiotics for the treatment of mastitis in bovines; (**c**) Top three frequently used antibiotics for the treatment of metritis in bovines. Each veterinarian was asked to choose up to three most commonly used antibiotics).

Table 2. Knowledge, attitude, and practices (KAP) of veterinarians regarding antibiotic use and resistance.

| KAP Parameters ¶ | Correct Answer | Percentage (%) |
|---|---|---|
| **Knowledge parameters** | | |
| Is there an ongoing antibiotic abuse in therapeutics in the veterinary sector? | 401 | 86.0 |
| Do you know about the critically important list of antimicrobials specified by the World Health Organization (WHO)? | 212 | 45.5 |
| Is antibiotic resistance a serious public health issue? | 460 | 98.7 |
| Is antibiotic resistance a natural as well as anthropogenic phenomenon? | 268 | 57.5 |
| Does irrational antibiotics use in animals lead to resistance in humans? | 409 | 87.8 |
| Are you familiar with superbug New Delhi metallo-beta-lactamase 1? | 233 | 50.0 |
| Are you familiar with Livestock-associated methicillin-resistant *Staphylococcus aureus* (LA-MRSA)? | 297 | 63.7 |
| Does the use of expired antibiotics lead to emergence of resistance? | 195 | 41.8 |
| Does injudicious use of antibiotics lead to antibiotic residues in milk and meat? | 450 | 96.6 |
| Does antibiotic residues in milk/meat lead to emergence of resistance? | 427 | 91.6 |
| Are you aware about recommendations of National Antimicrobial Resistance Plan 2017 of India? | 97 | 20.8 |
| **Attitude parameters** | | |
| I believe the use of two or more classes of antibiotics in combination is always a better choice to control infections | 18 / 387 * | 3.9 / 83.0 |
| I believe a broad spectrum antibiotics is a better choice than using highly selective antibiotics, even when narrow-spectrum drugs are available | 24 | 5.1 |
| I believe priority antibiotics must be restricted for human-use only | 190 | 40.8 |
| I believe that skipping 1 or 2 doses of antibiotics contributes to the development of resistance | 269 | 57.7 |
| **Practice parameters** | | |
| What is your first line of treatment for pyrexia of unknown origin (PUO)? | 138 | 29.6 |
| How often do you use bacterial culture and susceptibility testing to select the appropriate antibiotics during your treatment? | 15 / 161 * | 3.2 / 34.5 |
| Illegitimate demands of farmers lead to use of antibiotics in conditions which do not require their use | 163 | 35.0 |
| How often do you advise the farmer to administer antibiotics through a telephonic conversation (vocal prescription)? | 284 | 60.9 |
| Do you write a prescription of antibiotics to farmers who come to you at the hospital without presenting their animals? | 253 | 54.3 |
| How often do you give free samples of antibiotics to farmers? | 189 | 40.6 |
| Do you use antibiotics for prophylaxis? | 284 | 60.9 |
| Do you check the expiry date of the antibiotics before use? | 439 | 94.2 |
| Do you allow the farmer to inject the subsequent doses of antibiotics after you have administered the first dose of the treatment? | 292 | 62.7 |
| After antibiotic treatment, do you advise farmers about not to use or sell milk up to recommended withdrawal period? | 233 / 197 * | 50.0 / 42.3 |
| Do you adhere to the recommendations of the National Antimicrobial Resistance Plan of India? | 48 / 180 * | 10.3 / 38.6 |
| Have you attended any trainings/conferences to update your knowledge on antibiotic usage and antimicrobial resistance? | 127 | 27.2 |
| Have you conducted/organized any training to improve the knowledge of farmers on antibiotic usage and antimicrobial resistance emergence? | 148 | 31.8 |

* Partially correct answers. ¶ Each question was scored with score of 1 for correct, 0.5 for partially correct, and 0 for incorrect or not sure responses.

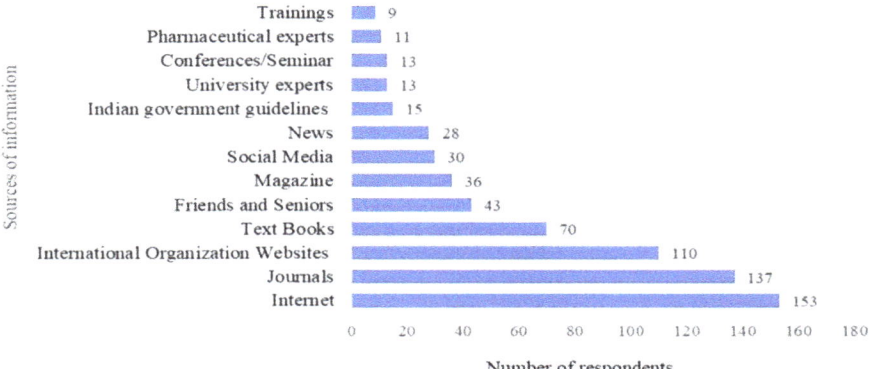

**Figure 4.** Information sources referred by veterinarians on antibiotic use and resistance * (* Question: What are the major information sources that you refer regularly to for knowledge on antibiotic use and resistance? (The question was open-ended with the provision to answer more than one source of information)).

Attitude toward antibiotic use and associated resistance was assessed by four questions (Table 2, Supplementary Material Table S1) with score of 1 for correct, 0.5 for partially correct, and 0 for incorrect or not sure response. The attitude score of ≥2.5 was classified as positive, 0.5–2.5 was classified as neutral and < 0.5 was classified as negative. The majority of the respondents (93.3%) had attitude score in the neutral range, with an overall median of $1.5 \pm 0.5$.

The practice scores were assessed for thirteen questions (Table 2; Supplementary Material Table S1) with a score of 1 for correct, 0.5 for partially correct and 0 for incorrect practice. The practice scale with a score of ≥7.5 was classified as good, 4.5–7.5 was classified as moderate and <4.5 was classified as poor. The respondents had a median practice score of $6.0 \pm 1.5$. The majority of the respondents (51.3%) had a moderate practice score and 27.7% stated poor practice toward antimicrobial usage. In addition, 27.2% of veterinarians had attended training programs on antibiotic usage and resistance. The veterinarians who attended the training program had significantly higher practice scores (U statistic: 5.3, $p$-value: 0.00) and knowledge scores (U statistic: 3.8, $p$-value: 0.00).

### 3.5. Association of KAP Scores with Demographic Characteristics

The association of demographic characteristics and KAP scores were analyzed using the Mann–Whitney U test/Kruskal–Wallis H test (Table 3). A significant difference was observed among the age groups, with higher knowledge (H statistic: 10.9, df: 4, $p$-value: 0.03) score in the <30-year age group. Post hoc analysis revealed that the knowledge scores of veterinarians having age <30 differed significantly from the other age groups. The veterinarians with PhD degrees had significantly higher knowledge scores (H statistic: 37.8, df: 2, $p$-value: 0.00), and on post hoc analysis, the knowledge scores of all the groups having different educational qualifications differed significantly from each other. Moreover, a higher knowledge (H statistic: 19.1, df: 3, $p$-value: 0.00) score was observed among veterinarians having less than 10 years of experience, and post hoc analysis revealed that the knowledge score of veterinarians having less than 10 years of experience and veterinarians with 20–30 years of experience differed significantly from the knowledge score of veterinarians with 30–40 years of experience. The knowledge and attitude scores had no significant difference between the regions, while a higher practice score was observed amongst the veterinarians from the Western region (H statistic: 13.7, df: 5, $p$-value: 0.02), and post hoc analysis revealed that the practice score of veterinarians of the Western region differed significantly from that of respondents of the Northern and Eastern region. The veterinarians working in veterinary polyclinics had higher knowledge scores than those working in veterinary hospitals (U statistic: 2.2, p-value: 0.03).

Table 3. Demographic characteristics and associated KAP scores.

| Variables | Median Knowledge Score | p-Value * | Median Attitude Score | p-Value * | Median Practice Score | p-Value * |
|---|---|---|---|---|---|---|
| Age group (years) ¶ | | | | | | |
| <30 | 8.0 | | 1.5 | | 6.0 | |
| 30–40 | 7.0 | | 1.0 | | 6.0 | |
| 40–50 | 7.0 | 0.03 | 1.0 | 0.08 | 5.5 | 0.73 |
| 50–60 | 7.0 | | 0.8 | | 5.8 | |
| 60–70 | 5.5 | | 1.3 | | 6.8 | |
| Educational qualification ¶ | | | | | | |
| B.V.Sc and A.H | 7.0 | | 1.0 | | 6.0 | |
| M.V.Sc | 8.0 | 0.00 | 1.5 | 0.19 | 6.0 | 0.19 |
| PhD | 9.0 | | 1.3 | | 7.0 | |
| Years of Experience ¶ | | | | | | |
| <10 | 8.0 | | 1.5 | | 6.0 | |
| 10–20 | 7.0 | 0.00 | 1.0 | 0.24 | 5.5 | 0.33 |
| 20–30 | 7.0 | | 1.3 | | 6.5 | |
| 30–40 | 5.0 | | 0.5 | | 5.5 | |
| Gender # | | | | | | |
| Male | 7.5 | 0.44 | 1.0 | 0.37 | 6.0 | 0.50 |
| Female | 8.0 | | 1.5 | | 6.0 | |
| Region ¶ | | | | | | |
| Northern | 8.0 | | 1.5 | | 5.5 | |
| Southern | 7.0 | | 1.5 | | 6.3 | |
| Central | 8.0 | 0.12 | 0.5 | 0.09 | 5.5 | 0.02 |
| Western | 8.0 | | 1.0 | | 7.0 | |
| Eastern | 8.0 | | 1.5 | | 5.5 | |
| North Eastern | 8.5 | | 1.5 | | 6.3 | |
| Type of hospital # | | | | | | |
| Veterinary hospital | 7.0 | 0.03 | 1.5 | 0.63 | 6.0 | 0.40 |
| Veterinary polyclinic | 8.0 | | 1.5 | | 6.0 | |

* Significant p-values are presented in bold characters. ¶ Kruskal–Wallis H test; # Mann–Whitney U test.

### 3.6. Correlation between Knowledge, Attitude and Practice Scores

The present study revealed weak linear correlations between knowledge–attitude ($r = 0.23$, $p < 0.000$), knowledge–practice ($r = 0.20$, $p < 0.000$), and attitude–practice ($r = 0.18$, $p < 0.001$) as per the criteria by Cohen (2013) (0–0.25 = weak correlation, 0.25–0.5 = fair correlation, 0.5–0.75 = good correlation, and >0.75 = excellent correlation) [19].

### 3.7. Risk Factors Associated with Treatment Failure

Most of the veterinarians (86.0%) admitted about ongoing antibiotic abuse in therapeutics, and 98.7% considered antimicrobial resistance as a serious public health issue. Frequent treatment failure has been reported by 21.7% of veterinarians, and therapeutic failure has been observed in mastitis treatment against HPCIA such as quinolones (13.5%), third-generation cephalosporins (11.4%), and high-priority antimicrobials such as synthetic penicillin (11.6%), penicillin (11.4%), and aminoglycosides (9.2%). For metritis treatment, veterinarians reported therapeutic failure against quinolones (2.4%), tetracyclines (2.1%), synthetic penicillins (1.9%), and third-generation cephalosporins (1.7%). The failure of effective therapeutic response to antimicrobials other than antibiotics was reported by 66.1% of veterinarians for antiparasitic drugs and 9.4% for antifungal drugs.

The majority of the veterinarians (86.5%) attributed unauthorized practitioners (commonly called "quacks") followed by farmers and para-vets (43.6% each) as responsible for irrational use of antimicrobials in livestock (Figure 5). The practice of farmers directly acquiring antibiotics from a pharmacy without prescription was reported by 82.8% of the veterinarians, whereas 39.5% of the veterinarians reported non-cooperation of the farmers in the completion of the antibiotic course prescribed by them. However, 31.8% veterinarians organized awareness camps on antibiotic usage and resistance for farmers.

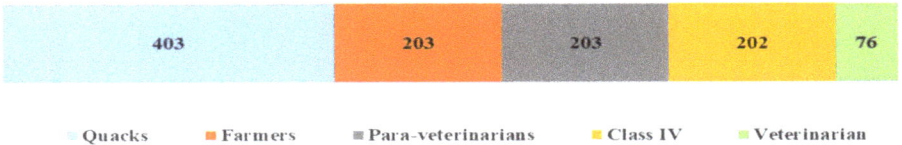

**Figure 5.** Personnel responsible for irrational use of antibiotics in field *. (Quacks: unauthorized practitioners; Para-veterinarians: diploma holders in Veterinary Science, Class IV: helping staff in veterinary hospitals) (* Question: Whom do you think as responsible for the irrational use of antibiotic in bovines at the field level (select all that apply)? (The question was having the provision to select more than one option)).

Around 16.3% of veterinarians considered themselves responsible for the injudicious use of antimicrobials, and 39.1% of veterinarians used antibiotics for prophylaxis, especially to prevent outbreaks. The majority of the veterinarians (62.2%) rarely performed antibiotic susceptibility testing to complement their treatment, while 70.6% of veterinarians reported lack of laboratory facilities for performing antibiotic sensitivity testing in/near their hospital. Moreover, only 20.8% veterinarians were aware about the recommendations of the National Antimicrobial Resistance Plan of 2017, India [20].

### 3.8. Univariable and Multivariable Analysis

The univariable analysis for frequent treatment failure associated risk factors pertaining to veterinarian's and farmer's practices was carried out by calculating the odds ratio (Table 4). All the variables of univariable analysis were used for building logistic regression models using independent predictors of practices associated with veterinarians and farmers in respect to frequent treatment failure.

On multivariable logistic regression analysis with a backward stepwise approach using the Likelihood Ratio Test (LRT), the final model contained two variables as depicted in Table 5. With respect to the risk factors associated with veterinarians, "skipping doses of antibiotics" and "allowing farmer to inject subsequent doses of antibiotics after administering first dose of the treatment" were significantly found to be associated with frequent treatment failure, with respective odds ratios of 1.7 (95%CI: 1.1–2.6) and 1.8 (95%CI: 1.1–2.8) ($p$-value: <0.05) (Table 5a). The adjusted odds ratio of "illegitimate demands of farmers for antibiotic use" and "farmer's non-cooperation in completion of antibiotic course" were found to be significantly associated with "frequent treatment failure", with respective odds ratios of 3.6 (95%CI: 2.3–5.8) and 1.8 (95%CI: 1.1–3.0) ($p$-value: <0.05) (Table 5b). The Hosmer–Lemeshow test for goodness of fit was found to be non-significant for both the models of veterinarians and farmers (Table 5).

Table 4. Univariable analysis: (a) Veterinarians; (b) Farmers.

| Variables | Odds Ratio (95% C.I.) | $p$-Value |
|---|---|---|
| (a) | | |
| Use of antibiotics for prophylaxis | 1.6 (1.0–2.4) | 0.05 |
| Allowing farmer to inject the subsequent doses of antibiotics after administering the first dose of treatment | 1.8 (1.2–2.8) | 0.009 |
| After antibiotic treatment, advising farmers not to use or sell milk up to the recommended withdrawal period | 1.1 (0.7–1.7) | 0.74 |
| Checking of expiry date of the antibiotics before use | 1.9 (0.8–4.3) | 0.14 |
| Vocal prescription of antibiotics to farmers | 1.5 (0.8–2.6) | 0.20 |
| Giving free samples of antibiotic to farmers | 1.3 (0.7–2.2) | 0.39 |
| Skipping of 1 or 2 doses of antibiotics in the course | 1.7 (1.1–2.6) | 0.02 |
| (b) | | |
| Illegitimate demand of farmers for antibiotics in conditions that do not require their use | 3.7 (2.3–6.0) | 0.00 |
| Farmer's non-cooperation in completion of the antibiotic course specified by the veterinarians | 1.9 (1.2–3.1) | 0.007 |
| Farmers acquiring antibiotics directly from a pharmacy without prescription | 2.2 (1.1–4.4) | 0.03 |

Table 5. Multivariable logistic regression analysis: (a) Veterinarians; (b) Farmers.

| Variable | B | S.E | Odds Ratio (95% C.I.) | $p$-Value |
|---|---|---|---|---|
| (a) | | | | |
| Skipping of 1 or 2 doses of antibiotics in the course | 0.5 | 0.2 | 1.7 (1.1–2.6) | 0.02 |
| Allowing the farmer to inject the subsequent doses of antibiotics after administering the first dose of treatment | 0.6 | 0.2 | 1.8 (1.1–2.8) | 0.01 |
| Constant | −1.8 | 0.2 | 0.2 | 0.00 |
| Hosmer–Lemeshow test for Goodness of Fit: $p$-value = 0.93 | | | | |
| (b) | | | | |
| Illegitimate demand of farmers for antibiotics in conditions that do not require their use | 1.3 | 0.2 | 3.6 (2.3–5.8) | 0.00 |
| Farmer's non-cooperation in completion of antibiotic course specified by the veterinarians | 0.6 | 0.2 | 1.8 (1.1–3.0) | 0.02 |
| Constant | −2.1 | 0.2 | 0.1 | 0.00 |
| Hosmer–Lemeshow test for Goodness of Fit: $p$-value = 0.55 | | | | |

### 3.9. Veterinarian's Recommendations

The respondents were asked to provide a single best suggestion to combat antimicrobial resistance. The suggestions overlapped in many cases, and the duplicate suggestions were removed and are categorized into field level, policy level, and research level suggestions in Supplementary Material Table S2.

### 4. Discussion

In developing countries, possible factors for antibiotic resistance include increased and indiscriminate use of antibiotics in animal production, poor farm biosecurity, inadequate infection control practices in consort with lack of compliance with regulatory frameworks [21]. In Indian dairy herds, more than 70% of production losses have been incurred by mastitis, which remains the condition requiring the most antibiotic use [22]. Similarly, in the present study, veterinarians reported mastitis as the most common condition in bovines requiring antibiotic use followed by reproductive disorders and hemoprotozoan infections.

There are limited studies from India on antibiotic usage patterns for various conditions in animal husbandry [12]. The present study listed major disease conditions of bovines requiring antibiotic usage. Our study reports the use of HPCIA in animal therapeutics, with quinolones and third-generation cephalosporins as prime antibiotics used for mastitis and metritis. However, studies from western countries reported the use of non-HPCIA predominating in animal agriculture, while the use of critically important antimicrobials was limited to the treatment of diarrhea and respiratory diseases in bovines [23]. Similarly, in Australia, the major antibiotics in bovine therapeutics were tetracycline/doxycycline, penicillin, synthetic penicillin, and trimethoprim–sulfamethoxazole [16]. In addition, the alternate systems of medicine are prevalent both in the human and veterinary sector in India [24–26], and the veterinarians in the study also reported the widespread usage of herbal medicines and homeopathy in bovine therapeutics.

While choosing the antibiotics, previous experience of veterinarians remained the topmost criteria, which is in accordance with previous studies where veterinarian's prior experience of a drug was decisive for antibiotic selection [27]. Moreover, the cost of antibiotics had a moderate influence on antibiotic choice, as also reported by Australian veterinarians [16]. The lower use of antimicrobial culture and susceptibility testing in choosing antibiotics was in accordance with the study on New Zealand veterinarians [28]. The recommendations from the pharmaceutical company were a minor factor in the choice of antibiotics in contrary to the previous reports, where half of the veterinarians were influenced by the pharmaceutical companies [29].

In the present study, 69.5% of veterinarians had average knowledge score similar to earlier regional study from India, where 58.3% of veterinarians had a medium level of awareness on antibiotic resistance [30]. The majority of veterinarians had attitude in the neutral range and moderate practice scores, suggesting the need for more directed efforts on improving attitude and practices toward judicious antibiotic use. The highest knowledge and attitude scores were in the age group of <30 years and in veterinarians with <10 years of experience, which is in similar to earlier studies, where Dutch veterinarians with more years of experience were found to be less concerned about the possible contribution of veterinary antibiotic use to antimicrobial resistance [14]. The higher knowledge score among veterinarians working in veterinary polyclinics with established facilities is in accordance with reported higher social responsibility among veterinarians working in referral clinics [31]. The regional differences noted in the present study with a higher practice score for the Western region is in accordance with earlier studies where regional differences were observed [32], which might be due to the higher awareness of activities on animal husbandry practices, including farm biosecurity.

The highest consumption of antimicrobials in livestock has been reported in low- and middle-income countries where antibiotics are used for therapeutics, growth promotion, and prophylaxis [2]. In the present study, 39.0% of veterinarians reported the use of antibiotics for prophylaxis, mainly to prevent disease outbreaks, on contrary with developed nations where most veterinarians had abandoned the practice of using antibiotics for prophylaxis [33].

The reliability on diagnostic and antibiotic sensitivity testing is posited to be crucial for responsible antimicrobial use, while in the present study, 37.8% of veterinarians resorted to bacterial culture and susceptibility test results for choosing antibiotics. In addition, 70% veterinarians were not having access to well-equipped laboratory facilities for antibiotic susceptibility testing. This is in accordance with previous studies where in both veterinary [23,33] and human medicine [34], the use of antibiotic susceptibility testing for choosing antibiotics was less frequent. The lack of access to laboratory facilities for the majority of the veterinarians for confirming the root cause of treatment failure might have led to the assumption that treatment failure was due to antimicrobial resistance. Even though treatment failure may also arise due to other causes, such as the inadequate antimicrobial spectrum of the prescribed antibiotics due to the use of ineffective drugs or incorrect dosage or incorrect diagnosis, in the present study, more emphasis has been laid on antimicrobial resistance as leading causes of treatment failure, which might pose a limitation to the study.

The majority of veterinarians (87%) believed there is an ongoing antibiotic abuse in therapeutics in India, while a lower proportion of Australian livestock veterinarians opined the current usage of antibiotics as "significant" for antibiotic resistance [16]. Moreover, 98.7% veterinarians believed that antibiotic resistance was a serious public health issue, in similar line with the previous studies [35,36]. In addition, earlier studies also have reported a large number of untrained personnel (quacks) in veterinary practice in India, which might be due to unaffordable professional veterinary services for marginalized farmers [12,30,37].

The present study analyzed the possible risk factors of farmers and veterinarians for the development of treatment failure. The "illegitimate demands of farmers for antibiotic use" was significantly associated with treatment failure in accordance with the earlier studies, where around 33% veterinarians reported explicit demand of farmers for antibiotics [30]. On contrary, other study from Australia reported that the expectations of the client had a minimal influence on antibiotic prescription [16].

The majority of the veterinarians (82.8%) reported the purchase of antibiotics without prescription by farmers in accordance with earlier studies from India, where the lack of adequate knowledge among farmers and easy access to antibiotics without prescriptions were considered as possible drivers of this risk practice [38]. Around 31.8% of veterinarians have conducted training programs to improve knowledge of farmers on antibiotic usage. Earlier studies also reported that the majority of veterinarians believed in educating farmers on good management practices for reducing antimicrobial use [15,39].

In accordance with earlier studies where the Australian veterinarians have highlighted the need for cost-effective culture and susceptibility testing as well as rapid and affordable diagnostic tests for facilitating judicious antibiotic use [16], the present study has also put forward similar suggestions at the field level, regulatory level, and research level. The participating veterinarians of the present study have also emphasized the need for a data-driven interdisciplinary approach that is crucial for combating antimicrobial resistance. The present study could not have the exact proportional number of respondents from different regions of the country, which might pose a limitation. However, the study is the first of its kind to have a comprehensive approach on the existing antibiotic usage practices, KAP survey, and veterinarian's recommendations to address antimicrobial resistance.

## 5. Conclusions

To conclude, the facilitating changes in the attitude and practices of veterinarians can be augmented by the implementation of continuing veterinary education programs. The effective flow of information from veterinarians to farmers can create a paradigm shift in the perceptions of the farmers for judicious antibiotic use as well as less reliability on quacks. There is need to strengthen the laboratory surveillance networks, research and diagnostics, and judicious antimicrobial stewardship. More stringent guidelines on the use of HPCIA in the animal sector and the compliance with responsible antimicrobial prescription behaviors by veterinarians need to be implemented. A "One Health" framework facilitating behavioural change interventions in farmers and veterinarians by bringing all the stakeholders together and promoting prudent antimicrobial use and judicious antimicrobial stewardship is the need of the hour.

**Supplementary Materials:** The following are available online at https://www.mdpi.com/2079-6382/10/2/216/s1, File S1: Questionnaire for veterinarians, Table S1: List of KAP parameters and their correct responses in questionnaire, Table S2: Recommendations at various levels from the study.

**Author Contributions:** Conceptualization, D.V., J.S.B, P.D., A.K.A. and J.P.S.G.; Methodology, D.V., J.S.B., P.D., J.S. and R.S.; Software, D.V., P.D. and J.S.B.; Formal Analysis, D.V., J.S.B., P.D. and J.S.; Investigation, D.V., P.D., J.S. and J.S.B.; Validation, R.S., A.K.A., J.S.B. and J.P.S.G.; Writing—Original Draft Preparation: D.V., J.S.B., and P.D.; Writing—Review and Editing: R.S., J.S., A.K.A., J.S.B. and J.P.S.G.; Supervision, A.K.A. and J.P.S.G.; and Project Administration, A.K.A. and J.P.S.G. All authors have read and agreed to the published version of the manuscript.

**Funding:** The research was supported by grants from the Indian Council of Agricultural Research, Niche Area of Excellence project on 'Antibiotic Resistance: Animal Human Interface' (ICAR/Edn.10(8)/2016-EP&HS).

**Institutional Review Board Statement:** The study was conducted according to the guidelines of the Declaration of Helsinki, and approved by the Institutional Advisory Committee of Guru Angad Dev Veterinary and Animal Sciences University, Ludhiana. The study was survey based and there was no involvement of any invasive procedures or experimental protocols on the study subjects.

**Informed Consent Statement:** The study was completely voluntary and proper consent of the participants were obtained before enrollment in the study.

**Data Availability Statement:** The data presented in this study are available on request from the corresponding author. The data are not publicly available due to privacy and confidentiality agreements to the participants.

**Acknowledgments:** Authors are thankful to Guru Angad Dev Veterinary and Animal Sciences University, Ludhiana for providing necessary support for the study.

**Conflicts of Interest:** The authors declare no conflict of interest.

# References

1. O'Neill, J. Review on Antimicrobial Resistance. Tackling Drug-Resistant Infections Globally: Final Report and Recommendations. 2016. Available online: https://amr-review.org/sites/default/files/160518_Final%20paper_with%20cover.pdf (accessed on 8 April 2020).
2. Van Boeckel, T.P.; Brower, C.; Gilbert, M.; Grenfell, B.T.; Levin, S.A.; Robinson, T.P.; Teillant, A.; Laxminarayan, R. Global trends in antimicrobial use in food animals. *Proc. Natl. Acad. Sci. USA* **2015**, *112*, 5649–5654. [CrossRef] [PubMed]
3. Bellet, C.; Rushton, J. World food security, globalisation and animal farming: Unlocking dominant paradigms of animal health science. *Rev. Sci. Tech.* **2019**, *38*, 383–393. [CrossRef] [PubMed]
4. Economou, V.; Gousia, P. Agriculture and food animals as a source of antimicrobial-resistant bacteria. *Infect. Drug Resist.* **2015**, *8*, 49–61. [CrossRef] [PubMed]
5. Founou, L.L.; Founou, R.C.; Essack, S.Y. Antibiotic resistance in the food chain: A developing country-perspective. *Front. Microbiol.* **2016**, *7*, 1–19. [CrossRef]
6. 20th Livestock Census 2019—All India Report. Department of Animal Husbandry and Dairying (AH&D). Available online: http://dadf.gov.in/sites/default/filess/20th%20Livestock%20census-2019%20All%20India%20Report.pdf (accessed on 6 July 2020).
7. Mahato, S.; Mistry, H.U.; Chakraborty, S.; Sharma, P.; Saravanan, R.; Bhandari, V. Identification of variable traits among the methicillin resistant and sensitive coagulase negative staphylococci in milk samples from mastitic cows in India. *Front. Microbiol.* **2017**, *8*, 1446. [CrossRef]
8. Khan, J.A.; Rathore, R.S.; Abulreesh, H.H.; Al-Thubiani, A.S.; Khan, S.; Ahmad, I. Diversity of antibiotic-resistant Shiga toxin-producing Escherichia coli serogroups in foodstuffs of animal origin in northern India. *J. Food Saf.* **2018**, *38*, 12566. [CrossRef]
9. Moudgil, P.; Bedi, J.S.; Moudgil, A.D.; Gill, J.P.S.; Aulakh, R.S. Emerging issue of antibiotic resistance from food producing animals in India: Perspective and legal framework. *Food Rev. Int.* **2018**, *34*, 447–462. [CrossRef]
10. Sharma, C.; Rokana, N.; Chandra, M.; Singh, B.P.; Gulhane, R.D.; Gill, J.P.S.; Ray, P.; Puniya, A.K.; Panwar, H. Antimicrobial resistance: Its surveillance, impact, and alternative management strategies in dairy animals. *Front. Vet. Sci.* **2018**, *4*, 237. [CrossRef]
11. Walia, K.; Madhumathi, J.; Veeraraghavan, B.; Chakrabarti, A.; Kapil, A.; Ray, P.; Singh, H.; Sistla, S.; Ohri, V. Establishing antimicrobial resistance surveillance & research network in India: Journey so far. *Indian J. Med. Res.* **2019**, *149*, 164–179.
12. Mutua, F.; Sharma, G.; Grace, D.; Bandyopadhyay, S.; Shome, B.; Lindahl, J. A review of animal health and drug use practices in India, and their possible link to antimicrobial resistance. *Antimicrob. Resist. Infect. Control* **2020**, *9*, 103. [CrossRef]
13. Kirchhelle, C. Pharming animals: A global history of antibiotics in food production (1935–2017). *Palgrave Commun.* **2018**, *4*, 1–13. [CrossRef]
14. Speksnijder, D.C.; Jaarsma, D.A.C.; Verheij, T.J.M.; Wagenaar, J.A. Attitudes and perceptions of Dutch veterinarians on their role in the reduction of antimicrobial use in farm animals. *Prev. Vet. Med.* **2015**, *121*, 365–373. [CrossRef] [PubMed]
15. Coyne, L.A.; Latham, S.M.; Dawson, S.; Donald, I.J.; Pearson, R.B.; Smith, R.F.; Williams, N.J.; Pinchbeck, G.L. Antimicrobial use practices, attitudes and responsibilities in UK farm animal veterinary surgeons. *Prev. Vet. Med.* **2018**, *161*, 115–126. [CrossRef]
16. Norris, J.M.; Zhuo, A.; Govendir, M.; Rowbotham, S.J.; Labbate, M.; Degeling, C.; Gilbert, G.L.; Dominey-Howes, D.; Ward, M.P. Factors influencing the behaviour and perceptions of Australian veterinarians towards antibiotic use and antimicrobial resistance. *PLoS ONE* **2019**, *14*, e0223534.
17. World Health Organization. WHO List of Critically Important Antimicrobials. 2019. Available online: https://www.who.int/foodsafety/areas_work/antimicrobial-resistance/cia/en (accessed on 26 February 2020).

18. World Health Organization. WHO AWaRe Classification Antibiotics. 2019. Available online: https://www.who.int/medicines/news/2019/WHO_releases2019AWaRe_classification_antibiotics/en/#:~{}:text=RESERVE%20GROUP%20ANTIBIOTICS&text=22%20antibiotics%20have%20been%20classified,Model%20List%20of%20Essential%20Medicines (accessed on 26 February 2020).
19. Cohen, J. *Statistical Power Analysis for the Behavioral Sciences*; Academic Press: Cambridge, MA, USA, 2013.
20. National Action Plan on Antimicrobial Resistance. India. 2017. Available online: https://www.ncdc.gov.in/WriteReadData/linkimages/AMR/File645.pdf (accessed on 3 March 2020).
21. Ayukekbong, J.A.; Ntemgwa, M.; Atabe, A.N. The threat of antimicrobial resistance in developing countries: Causes and control strategies. *Antimicrob. Resist. Infect. Control* 2017, *6*, 47. [CrossRef]
22. Verma, H.; Rawat, S.; Sharma, N.; Jaiswal, V.; Singh, R.; Harshit, V. Prevalence, bacterial etiology and antibiotic susceptibility pattern of bovine mastitis in Meerut. *J. Entomol. Zool. Stud.* 2018, *6*, 706–709.
23. De Briyne, N.; Atkinson, J.; Pokludová, L.; Borriello, S.P.; Price, S. Factors influencing antibiotic prescribing habits and use of sensitivity testing amongst veterinarians in Europe. *Vet. Rec.* 2013, *173*, 475. [CrossRef]
24. Varshney, J.P.; Naresh, R. Comparative efficacy of homeopathic and allopathic systems of medicine in the management of clinical mastitis of Indian dairy cows. *Homeopathy* 2005, *94*, 81–85. [CrossRef]
25. Mishra, S.; Sharma, S.; Vasudevan, P.; Bhatt, R.K.; Pandey, S.; Singh, M.; Meena, B.S.; Pandey, S.N. Livestock feeding and traditional healthcare practices in Bundelkhand region of Central India. *Indian J. Tradit. Knowl.* 2010, *9*, 333–337.
26. Sen, S.; Chakraborty, R.; De, B. Challenges and opportunities in the advancement of herbal medicine: India's position and role in a global context. *J. Herb. Med.* 2011, *1*, 67–75. [CrossRef]
27. Gibbons, J.F.; Boland, F.; Buckley, J.F.; Butler, F.; Egan, J.; Fanning, S.; Markey, B.K.; Leonard, F.C. Influences on antimicrobial prescribing behaviour of veterinary practitioners in cattle practice in Ireland. *Vet. Rec.* 2013, *172*, 14. [CrossRef] [PubMed]
28. McDougall, S.; Compton, C.W.R.; Botha, N. Factors influencing antimicrobial prescribing by veterinarians and usage by dairy farmers in New Zealand. *N. Z. Vet. J.* 2017, *65*, 84–92. [CrossRef] [PubMed]
29. Postma, M.; Speksnijder, D.C.; Jaarsma, A.D.C. Opinions of veterinarians on antimicrobial use in farm animals in Flanders and the Netherlands. *Vet. Rec.* 2016, *179*, 68. [CrossRef] [PubMed]
30. Kumar, V.; Gupta, J.; Meena, H.R. Assessment of Awareness about Antibiotic Resistance and Practices Followed by Veterinarians for Judicious Prescription of Antibiotics: An Exploratory Study in Eastern Haryana Region of India. *Trop. Anim. Health Prod.* 2019, *51*, 677–687. [CrossRef] [PubMed]
31. Hopman, N.E.; Mughini-Gras, L.; Speksnijder, D.C.; Wagenaar, J.A.; Van Geijlswijk, I.M.; Broens, E.M. Attitudes and perceptions of Dutch companion animal veterinarians towards antimicrobial use and antimicrobial resistance. *Prev. Vet. Med.* 2019, *170*, 104717. [CrossRef] [PubMed]
32. De Briyne, N.; Atkinson, J.; Pokludová, L. Antibiotics used most commonly to treat animals in Europe. *Vet. Rec.* 2014, *175*, 325. [CrossRef]
33. Coyne, L.A.; Latham, S.M.; Williams, N.J.; Dawson, S.; Donald, I.J.; Pearson, R.B.; Smith, R.F.; Pinchbeck, G.L. Understanding the culture of antimicrobial prescribing in agriculture: A qualitative study of UK pig veterinary surgeons. *J. Antimicrob. Chemother.* 2016, *71*, 3300–3312. [CrossRef] [PubMed]
34. Peterson, L.R.; Dalhoff, A. Towards targeted prescribing: Will the cure for antimicrobial resistance be specific, directed therapy through improved diagnostic testing? *J. Antimicrob. Chemother.* 2014, *53*, 902–905. [CrossRef]
35. Rather, I.A.; Kim, B.C.; Bajpai, V.K. Self-medication and antibiotic resistance: Crisis, current challenges, and prevention. *Saudi J. Biol. Sci.* 2017, *24*, 808–812. [CrossRef]
36. Robinson, T.P.; Bu, D.P.; Carrique-Mas, J.; Fèvre, E.M.; Gilbert, M.; Grace, D.; Hay, S.I.; Jiwakanon, J.; Kakkar, M.; Kariuki, S.; et al. Antibiotic resistance is the quintessential One Health issue. *Trans. R. Soc. Trop. Med. Hyg.* 2016, *110*, 377–380. [CrossRef]
37. Sarita, S.; Gautam, S.P.; Ahuja, R. An analysis of constraints perceived by dairy farmers in Murrah tract of Haryana state. *Int. J. Pure App. Biosci.* 2017, *5*, 1048–1053.
38. Chauhan, A.S.; George, M.S.; Chatterjee, P.; Lindahl, J.F.; Grace, D.; Kakkar, M. The social biography of antibiotic use in smallholder dairy farms in India. *Antimicrob. Resist. Infect. Control* 2018, *7*, 60. [CrossRef] [PubMed]
39. Kramer, T.; Jansen, L.E.; Lipman, L.J.; Smit, L.A.; Heederik, D.J.; Dorado-García, A.; Dorado-García, A. Farmers' knowledge and expectations of antimicrobial use and resistance are strongly related to usage in Dutch livestock sectors. *Prev. Vet. Med.* 2017, *147*, 142–148. [CrossRef] [PubMed]

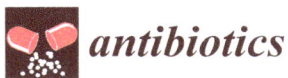 

*Article*

# Antimicrobial Use in Animals in Timor-Leste Based on Veterinary Antimicrobial Imports between 2016 and 2019

Shawn Ting [1,*], Abrao Pereira [1], Amalia de Jesus Alves [1], Salvador Fernandes [2], Cristina da Costa Soares [2], Felix Joanico Soares [2], Onofre da Costa Henrique [2], Steven Davis [1], Jennifer Yan [1,3], Joshua R. Francis [1,3], Tamsin S. Barnes [4] and Joanita Bendita da Costa Jong [2]

[1] Global and Tropical Health Division, Menzies School of Health Research, Charles Darwin University, Ellengowan Drive, Darwin, NT 0909, Australia; abrao.pereira@menzies.edu.au (A.P.); amalia.dejesusalves@menzies.edu.au (A.d.J.A.); steven.davis@menzies.edu.au (S.D.); jennifer.yan@menzies.edu.au (J.Y.); josh.francis@menzies.edu.au (J.R.F.)

[2] Ministry of Agriculture and Fisheries, Government of Timor-Leste, Av. Nicolao Lobato, Comoro, Dili 0332, Timor-Leste; baduhlareanatena@gmail.com (S.F.); cristinasoares@gmail.com (C.d.C.S.); romakabureno@gmail.com (F.J.S.); henriqueonofre11@gmail.com (O.d.C.H.); katitadog_2001@yahoo.com (J.B.d.C.J.)

[3] Department of Paediatrics, Royal Darwin Hospital, Darwin, NT 0810, Australia

[4] Epivet Pty. Ltd., Withcott, QLD 4352, Australia; tamsin.barnes@gmail.com

* Correspondence: shawn.ting@menzies.edu.au; Tel.: +61-(08)-8946-8505

**Abstract:** Monitoring veterinary antimicrobial use is part of the global strategy to tackle antimicrobial resistance. The purpose of this study was to quantify veterinary antimicrobials imported into Timor-Leste between 2016 and 2019 and describe the antimicrobial import profile of importers. Data were obtained from import applications received by the Ministry of Agriculture and Fisheries (MAF) of Timor-Leste. Import quantities were analysed by antimicrobial class, importance for human medicine, recommended route of administration and type of importer. An average of 57.4 kg (s.d. 31.0 kg) and 0.55 mg/kg (s.d. 0.27 mg/kg) animal biomass of antimicrobials was imported per year. Tetracyclines (35.5%), penicillins (23.7%), and macrolides (15.9%) were the commonly imported antimicrobial classes. Antimicrobials imported for parenteral administration were most common (60.1%). MAF was the largest importer (52.4%). Most of the critically important antimicrobials for human medicine were imported by poultry farms for oral administration and use for growth promotion could not be ruled out. In conclusion, the use of antimicrobials in animals in Timor-Leste is very low, in keeping with its predominantly subsistence agriculture system. Farmer education, development of treatment guidelines, and strengthening of the veterinary service is important for addressing the potential future misuse of antimicrobials especially in the commercial poultry industry.

**Keywords:** antimicrobial use; antimicrobial resistance (AMR); Timor-Leste; antibiotic; antimicrobial; veterinary; prudent use; critically important antimicrobials; growth promotion; poultry

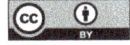

## 1. Introduction

The emergence of antimicrobial resistance is a major global health threat for the 21st century [1]. It is also a One Health challenge that requires coordinated action as transmission of resistant bacteria can occur between humans, animals, plants and the environment [2–4]. This emergence has been rapid and is linked to the overuse and misuse of antimicrobials in humans and animals [5,6]. Despite this, it is projected that the use of antimicrobials in humans and animals will continue to rise over the next decade [7,8]. In particular, the use of antimicrobials in food producing animals has received attention due to high levels of use globally for disease prevention and growth promotion [9,10]. While some developed countries have demonstrated a reduction in usage levels [11–15], usage in many developing countries have risen due to farm intensification and demand for animal-based protein associated with rising incomes [16–18]. This puts low- and middle-income countries at a higher risk for emergence of resistance.

Antimicrobial resistance limits the effectiveness of antimicrobial therapy which has a greater impact in low and middle-income countries due to their weaker health systems, higher prevalence of infectious diseases and limited access to more expensive treatment alternatives [19,20]. To preserve the effectiveness of antimicrobials, a global strategy has been developed to tackle antimicrobial resistance [21]. This strategy is wide-ranging and multi-sectoral and includes initiatives to strengthen monitoring of antimicrobial use in animals [21].

Monitoring of antimicrobial use in animals at the national level enables a country to identify trends of use over time and assess the impact of policy measures to promote prudent use in animals [22]. When analysed in conjunction with data on antimicrobial resistance in animal and humans, it can also identify potential associations between antimicrobial use and resistance patterns [23,24]. To harmonize antimicrobial use data collection, the World Organisation for Animal Health (OIE) has published guidelines for monitoring the use of antimicrobials in food producing animals [25]. The guidelines acknowledge that antimicrobial use data can be obtained from different levels such as import, manufacturing, sales, dispensing records or from end-use sources [25]. While many higher income countries have been collecting data for many years [26,27], some low to middle income countries in Africa and Asia-Pacific are still facing challenges such as a lack of regulation, under-reporting and unreliable data when monitoring antimicrobial use in animals [10,28,29].

Timor-Leste is a lower-middle income country [30] located in the south-east portion of the Malay Archipelago with a population of 1.3 million [31]. Subsistence farming is the main livelihood for most of the rural population [32,33], with a high proportion of households owning livestock [34]. Chicken and pigs are the two most commonly reared species in the country [35]. Commercial animal farming is uncommon [36,37] but may increase with rising income levels [33]. Currently, there are two large commercial layer farms [38] and a growing number of commercial broiler farms. There are no major commercial livestock farms for other species. There is no local manufacture of antimicrobials, and all antimicrobials are imported into the country. All applications to import veterinary medicines into the country must be submitted to the Ministry of Agriculture and Fisheries (MAF) and there is no re-export of veterinary antimicrobials.

The aims of this study were to quantify veterinary antimicrobial imports into Timor-Leste between 2016 to 2019; and to describe these imports based on antimicrobial class, importance for human medicine, recommended route of administration and type of importer. The findings can help improve monitoring and control of veterinary antimicrobial use in Timor-Leste.

## 2. Materials and Methods

### 2.1. Data Collection for Antimicrobial Imports

All applications to import veterinary medicines into Timor-Leste submitted to MAF between January 2016 to December 2019 were screened to identify veterinary antimicrobials using OIE's list of antimicrobials of veterinary importance [39]. Data on the date of application, name of importer, brand name, quantity imported, name of active ingredient, concentration of active ingredient, route of administration and target species was extracted for each veterinary antimicrobial. Any missing details on the name of active ingredient, concentration of active ingredient and route of administration was obtained from the technical product sheets. Data collection was performed by two MAF staff who received training on recording antimicrobial import data from received import applications through three workshops and ongoing side-by-side mentorship [40]. The data was stored on an Excel spreadsheet (Microsoft Corporation, Redmond, WA, USA). Data accuracy was checked independently by three researchers from Menzies School of Health Research between November and December 2020.

## 2.2. Data Categorisation for Antimicrobial Imports

Using the name of the active ingredient, each antimicrobial was classified into an antimicrobial class/subclass based on OIE guidelines [41]. The name of the active ingredient was also used to classify antimicrobials as a critically important antimicrobial (CIA), highly important antimicrobial (HIA) or an important antimicrobial (IA) using the World Health Organization (WHO) List of Critically Important Antimicrobials for Human Medicine [42]. The importer name was used to classify importers into 6 types to understand their individual import patterns: "MAF", "agriculture shops", "veterinary clinics", "layer farms", "broiler farms", and "education institutions". Layer and broiler farms were placed in separate categories because they may have different antimicrobial use patterns. In Timor-Leste, agriculture shops are enterprises where veterinary medicines can be procured without a prescription.

## 2.3. Animal Biomass Calculation

Data for biomass calculation (i.e., number of live animals, number of animals slaughtered and meat product quantity) were obtained from the Food and Agricultural Organization Global Statistical Database (FAOSTAT) [43,44]. Common animal species in Timor-Leste (buffalo, cattle, chicken, goats, horse, pigs, and sheep) [34] were included in the biomass calculation. Ducks, rabbits, dogs, and cats were excluded because data were not available. Total animal biomass was calculated for each year between 2016 and 2019 using an OIE method [25] except for bovine biomass because the proportion of animals in different age groups are not known. The data for total animal biomass calculation and estimates for annual biomass can be found in Supplementary Table S1.

## 2.4. Data Analysis

The weight of active ingredient in one unit of imported product per pharmaceutical form (e.g., bottle, bag, or tube) was estimated by multiplying the strength of the antimicrobial active ingredient by the volume or weight. All weights were expressed in kilograms (kg). Conversion factors based on OIE guidelines was used to mathematically convert international units (IU) into kilograms [29].

The weight of each active ingredient imported between 2016 to 2019 was calculated by multiplying the weight of active ingredient in one unit of product by the quantity imported. Adjustment for animal biomass was achieved by dividing the total weight of active ingredient by the total animal biomass. The result was expressed in milligram (mg) of active ingredient per kilogram (kg) of animal biomass.

Annual and total imports were calculated for each active ingredient, antimicrobial class, WHO class of importance in human medicine, route of administration and type of importer. Total annual imports of all antimicrobials by weight and weight adjusted for biomass were summarized as mean $\pm$ s.d. Spearman's rank correlation coefficient ($r_s$) was used to test the hypothesis of a monotonic (increasing or decreasing) trend in imports by total weight, total weight adjusted for biomass, individual active ingredient and type of importer. Data analysis was performed using Stata 15 software (StataCorp, College Station, TX, USA)

## 2.5. Ethical Approval

The study was conducted in accordance with the Declaration of Helsinki, and the protocol was approved by Human Research Ethics Committee of the Northern Territory (NT) Department of Health and Menzies School of Health Research (2020-3841) and Institute Nacional de Saude in Timor-Leste (MS-INS/DE/IX/2020/1411).

## 3. Results

### 3.1. Import Quantities and Trends

Between 2016 to 2019, a total of 229.8 kg of active ingredients of veterinary antimicrobials were imported into Timor-Leste (mean: 57.4 $\pm$ 31.0 kg per year). Import quantities were lower in 2017 and 2018 compared to 2016 and 2019 (see Table 1). After adjusting for animal biomass, the average amount of imported antimicrobials was $0.55 \pm 0.27$ mg/kg biomass per year. There was no evidence of a significant monotonic trend in antimicrobial imports based on total weight ($r_s$: $-0.40$, $p$ value: 0.60) or weight adjusted by biomass ($r_s$: $-0.40$, $p$ value: 0.60) (see Figure 1).

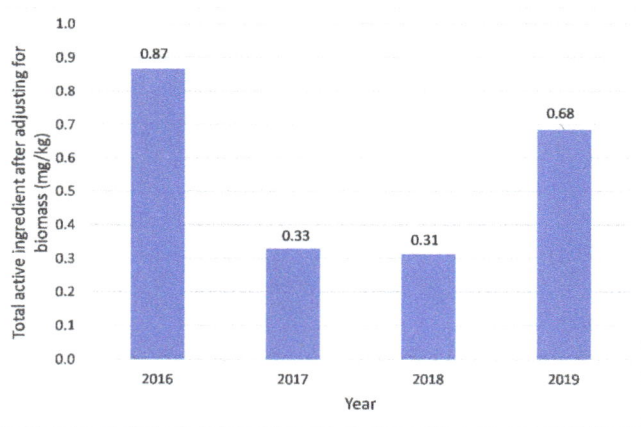

**Figure 1.** Antimicrobial import weight (mg) adjusted by animal biomass (kg) into Timor-Leste between 2016 and 2019.

A total of 21 antimicrobial active ingredients belonging to 8 classes of antimicrobials were imported during the study period. The import quantities of different antimicrobials between 2016 and 2019 can be found in Table 1. The active ingredients imported in the largest quantities were oxytetracyline (81.7 kg; 35.5%), amoxicillin (34.8 kg; 15.2%), tylosin (25.2 kg; 11.0%) and dihydrostreptomycin (25.8 kg; 11.2%). The classes of antimicrobials imported in the largest quantities were tetracyclines (81.7 kg; 35.5%), penicillins (54.4 kg; 23.7%), macrolides (36.5 kg; 15.9%) and aminoglycosides (25.8 kg; 11.3%). There was some evidence of monotonic increase in imports of neomycin ($r_s$: 0.95, $p$ value: 0.05) but quantities imported each year were extremely small. There was also some evidence of a monotonic decrease in imports of tylosin ($r_s$: $-0.95$, $p$ value: 0.05) driven by a relatively large import in 2016 and sulfamonomethoxine ($r_s$: $-0.95$, $p$ value: 0.05) although quantities imported each year were extremely small. There was no strong evidence of a monotonic trend in the import of any of the other individual antimicrobials (see Table 1). Based on WHO classification, most of the imported veterinary antimicrobials were CIAs (117.9 kg; 51.3%) followed by HIAs (111.8 kg; 48.7%).

Table 1. Weight of veterinary antimicrobials imported into Timor-Leste between 2016 and 2019, by year and overall for individual antimicrobial and antimicrobial class.

| Antimicrobial Class | Antimicrobial (WHO Classification [1]) | Kilogram of Active Ingredient (%) | | | | $r_s$ ($p$ Value) [2] | Kilogram for all Years (%) | Kilogram for all Years for Each Class (%) |
|---|---|---|---|---|---|---|---|---|
| | | 2016 | 2017 | 2018 | 2019 | | | |
| Aminoglycosides | Neomycin (CIA) | 0 | $2.5 \times 10^{-4}$ (<0.01) | 0.01 (0.05) | 0.01 (0.02) | 0.95 (0.05) | 0.03 (0.01) | 25.85 (11.25) |
| | Dihydrostreptomycin (CIA) | 4.64 (4.83) | 6.20 (18.56) | 5.80 (18.5) | 9.18 (13.32) | 0.80 (0.20) | 25.82 (11.24) | |
| Cephalosporins (3rd/4th gen) | Cefotaxime (CIA) | 0 | 0.01 (0.03) | 0 | 0 | −0.26 (0.74) | 0.01 (<0.00) | 0.01 (<0.00) |
| Fluroquinolones | Norfloxacin (CIA) | 0.20 (0.21) | 0.20 (0.60) | 0 | 0 | −0.89 (0.11) | 0.40 (0.17) | 6.01 (2.62) |
| | Enrofloxacin (CIA) | 3.61 (3.76) | 0 | 0 | 2.00 (2.90) | −0.32 (0.68) | 5.61 (2.44) | |
| Macrolides | Tylosin (CIA) | 25.10 (26.12) | 0.10 (0.30) | 0 | 0 | −0.95 (0.05) | 25.20 (10.97) | 36.45 (15.86) |
| | Tilmicosin (CIA) | 0 | 0 | 0 | 11.25 (16.33) | 0.77 (0.23) | 11.25 (4.9) | |
| | Ampicillin (CIA) | 0 | 0 | 3.27 (10.41) | 0.63 (0.91) | 0.74 (0.26) | 3.89 (1.69) | |
| Penicillins | Benzylpenicillin (HIA) | 2.78 (2.90) | 3.72 (11.13) | 3.48 (11.10) | 5.70 (8.28) | 0.80 (0.20) | 15.69 (6.83) | 54.39 (23.67) |
| | Amoxicillin (CIA) | 20.31 (21.13) | 0 | 0 | 14.51 (21.05) | −0.32 (0.68) | 34.82 (15.15) | |
| | Bacitracin (IA) | 0 | 0 | 0.02 (0.06) | 0 | 0.26 (0.74) | 0.02 (0.01) | |
| Polypeptides | Colistin (CIA) | 10.04 (10.45) | 0 | 0.31 (0.98) | 0.57 (0.82) | −0.20 (0.80) | 10.91 (4.75) | 10.93 (4.76) |
| | Polymyxin B (CIA) | 0 | $9.5 \times 10^{-5}$ (<0.01) | 0 | 0 | −0.26 (0.74) | $9.5 \times 10^{-5}$ (<0.01) | |
| Sulfonamides | Sulfamonomethoxine (HIA) | 0.40 (0.42) | 0.20 (0.60) | 0 | 0 | −0.95 (0.05) | 0.60 (0.26) | 14.46 (6.29) |
| | Sulfaquinoxaline (HIA) | 0.33 (0.34) | 0 | 0 | 0 | −0.77 (0.23) | 0.33 (0.14) | |
| | Sulfadoxine (HIA) | 0 | 0 | 0 | 0.04 (0.06) | 0.77 (0.23) | 0.04 (0.02) | |
| | Sulfamerazine (HIA) | 0 | 0.08 (0.23) | 0.02 (0.06) | 0.78 (1.14) | 0.80 (0.20) | 0.88 (0.38) | |
| | Sulfadiazine (HIA) | 2.09 (2.17) | 1.48 (4.42) | 1.59 (5.06) | 1.57 (2.27) | −0.40 (0.60) | 6.72 (2.92) | |
| | Sulfadimidine (HIA) | 1.67 (1.74) | 0.58 (1.73) | 0.80 (2.56) | 2.35 (3.41) | 0.40 (0.60) | 5.40 (2.35) | |
| | Trimethoprim (HIA) | 0.20 (0.21) | 0.28 (0.84) | 0 | 0.01 (0.01) | −0.06 (0.40) | 0.49 (0.21) | |
| Tetracyclines | Oxytetracycline (HIA) | 24.73 (25.73) | 20.56 (61.55) | 16.07 (51.23) | 20.32 (29.48) | −0.80 (0.20) | 81.67 (35.54) | 81.67 (35.54) |
| Overall | | 96.1 (100) | 33.41 (100) | 31.36 (100) | 68.91 (100) | −0.40 (0.60) | 229.77 (100) | 229.77 (100) |

[1] CIA refers to critically important antimicrobials; HIA refers to highly important antimicrobials; IA refers to important antimicrobials. [2] Spearman rank-order correlation coefficient ($r_s$) and $p$-value assessing the strength and direction of possible monotonic trends in the quantities of antimicrobials imported over time.

## 3.2. Import Pattern by Recommended Route of Administration

Recommended routes of administration for imported veterinary antimicrobials during the study period were parenteral (138.0 kg; 60.1%), oral (91.5 kg; 39.8%), and topical (0.3 kg; 0.1%). The majority of tetracyclines (81.3 kg; 99.6%), aminoglycosides (25.8 kg; 99.9%), sulphonamides (13.4 kg; 96.2%), and cephalosporins (0.01 kg; 100%) were for parenteral administration, while the majority of penicillins (37.6 kg; 69.2%), macrolides (36.3 kg; 99.5%), polypeptides (10.9 kg; 100%), and fluoroquinolones (6.0 kg; 100%) were for oral administration. The quantities of different antimicrobial classes for parenteral, oral and topical administration are shown in Figure 2. The weight of antimicrobial classes recommended for administration through different routes for each year over the study period can be found in Supplementary Table S2.

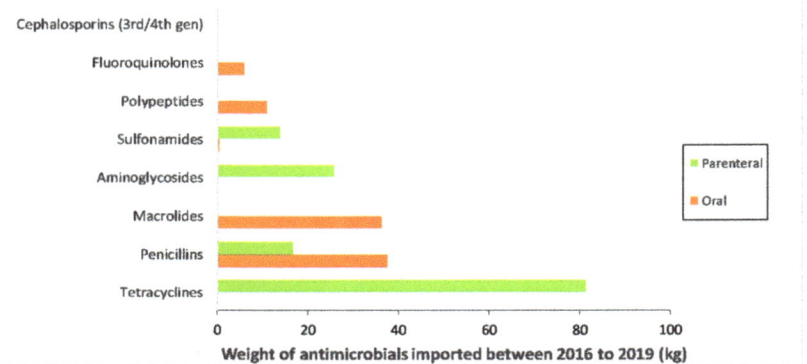

**Figure 2.** Total weight of veterinary antimicrobials imported into Timor-Leste between 2016 and 2019, by route of administration and antimicrobial class. Antimicrobials for administration via the topical route represented less than 0.3 kg (0.1%) of total imports and were therefore not included in the diagram.

## 3.3. Import Pattern by Importer Type

Between 2016 and 2019, the biggest importers of antimicrobials were MAF (120.4 kg; 52.4%), followed by layers farms (81.1 kg; 35.3%) and agriculture shops (15.9 kg; 6.9%) (See Figure 3). There was very strong evidence of a monotonic increase in antimicrobial imports by MAF ($r_s$: 1.0, $p$ value: <0.001) and evidence of a monotonic increase in antimicrobial imports by broiler farms ($r_s$: 0.95, $p$ value: 0.05) but no evidence of a monotonic trend in antimicrobial import patterns for other types of importers (see Figure 4A,B). The pattern of imports by layer farms was unique as imports were high in 2016 (58.6 kg) and 2019 (22.5 kg) but negligible between those years (see Figure 4A). Educational institutions imported a relatively small amount (0.6 kg) of antimicrobials once in 2016. Colistin, neomycin and enrofloxacin were only imported by layer or broiler farms. Cephalosporins were only imported by veterinary clinics. The weights of individual antimicrobials and antimicrobial classes imported by different type of importers for each year during the study period can be found in Supplementary Table S3.

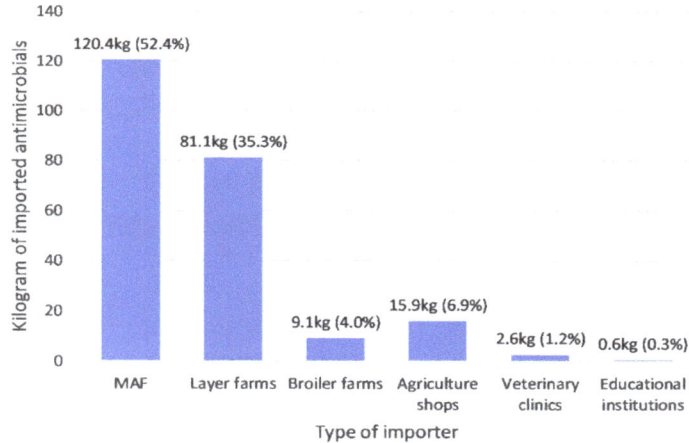

**Figure 3.** Total active ingredients imported between 2016 and 2019, by type of importer.

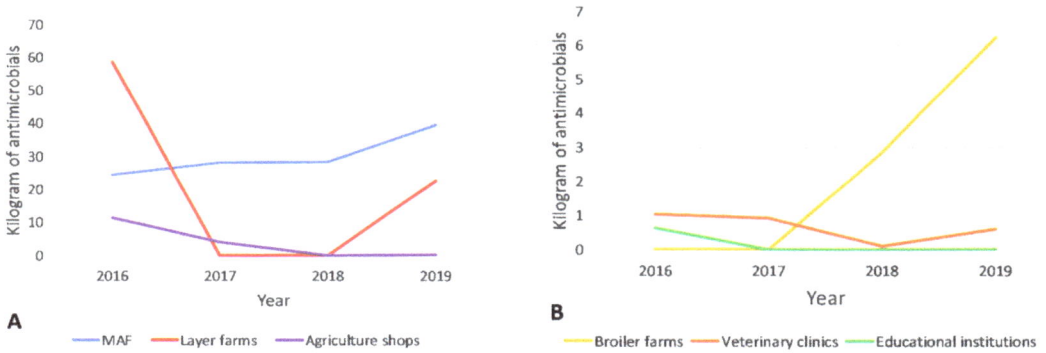

**Figure 4.** (**A**,**B**): Trend of antimicrobials imported by different importers between 2016 and 2019. Bigger importers are represented in (**B**) and smaller importers in (**B**), thus *y*-axes differ between diagrams.

The biggest importers of CIAs were layer farms (81.1 kg), MAF (25.6 kg) and broiler farms (9.0 kg). Layer and broiler farms imported CIAs almost exclusively; while CIAs accounted for less than a quarter of imports by MAF, agriculture shops and veterinary clinics (see Figure 5). Almost all antimicrobial imports by layer and broiler farms were for oral administration; while almost all imports by MAF and agriculture shops were for parenteral administration (see Figure 6).

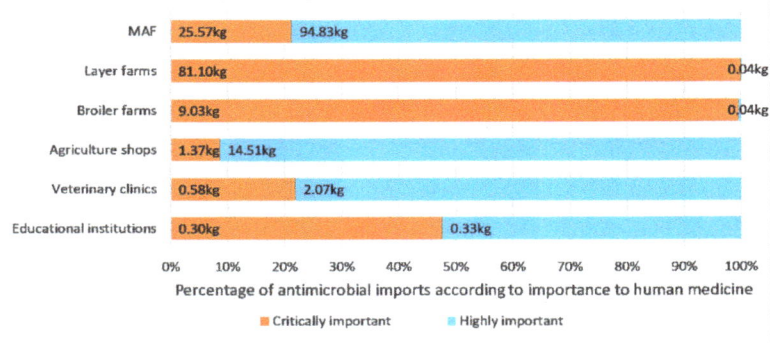

**Figure 5.** Profile of antimicrobial imports of different importer types by WHO classification of importance to human medicine. Important antimicrobials for human medicine represented less than 0.02 kg (0.01%) of total imports and were therefore not included in the diagram.

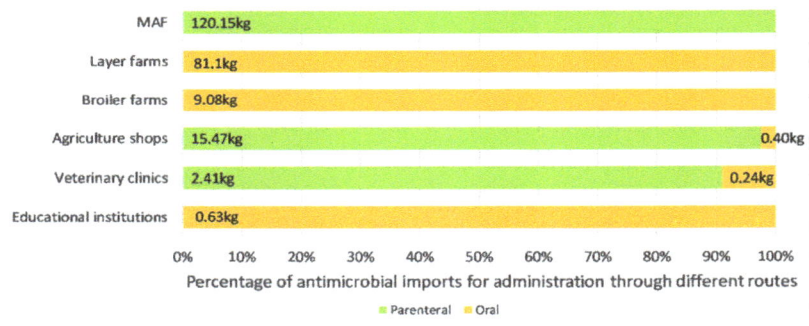

**Figure 6.** Profile of antimicrobial imports of different importer types, by recommended route of administration. Antimicrobials for administration via the topical route represented less than 0.3 kg (0.1%) of total imports and were therefore not included in the diagram.

## 4. Discussion

### 4.1. Strengths of the Study

This is the first study to describe veterinary antimicrobial imports into Timor-Leste. It showed a very low level of antimicrobial use in animals. Future studies of a similar nature will enable analysis of long-term trends and identification of changes in import patterns arising from interventions. Import data is a reasonable proxy for actual antimicrobial use for Timor-Leste since there is no local manufacture of veterinary antimicrobials and no re-export of antimicrobials. The data collection method was implemented consistently as it was performed by trained personnel using a written protocol. The accuracy of data was checked rigorously by authors to minimise data entry errors, and calculations were done with methods aligned with international guidelines. The training during data collection strengthened the capacity of MAF personnel to record antimicrobial import data and facilitated the timely reporting of results to the OIE, which is often a challenge in developing countries.

### 4.2. Quantity of Antimicrobial Import

The quantity of antimicrobials imported for use in animals in Timor-Leste after adjusting for biomass (0.55 mg/kg biomass) is very low compared to the global average of 144.39 mg/kg and regional average (Asia, Far East, and Oceania) of 237.72 mg/kg in 2016 [29]. The use of veterinary antimicrobials in Timor-Leste was even lower than countries such as New Zealand, Norway, and Iceland which are known to have some of the lowest use levels in the world [45,46]. The low level of use is likely due to the subsistence agriculture system in Timor-Leste [33,47] where there is poor access to veterinary services and medicines. The low level of use is also consistent with another study in Timor-Leste which showed that only 1% of backyard chicken farmers used commercial medicines in their animals [48]. It would be interesting to compare the results from Timor-Leste to other countries with a similar agriculture background but similar studies from such countries could not be found [10]. Although antimicrobial use levels are currently low, use may increase in the future with farming intensification, as seen in other developing countries [49,50]. In this study, there is already evidence of increasing use in the broiler industry, with import levels rising by 119% between 2018 and 2019.

### 4.3. Trend of Antimicrobial Import

Trends in antimicrobial imports over the study period can be explained by looking individually at each importer. For MAF, the rise in antimicrobial imports during the study period represented increased procurement following annual feedback that government employed animal health professionals (e.g., veterinary and livestock technicians) faced shortages for field use [51].

For layer farms, it is likely that the import quantities were inconsistent between years because this group included only two large commercial layer farms that import antimicrobials in bulk quantities for use over a few years. For broiler farms, antimicrobial imports occurred only after 2018 following the import of day-old chicks from Indonesia after the lifting of avian-influenza related import restrictions [52]. The easing of restrictions was followed by a government effort to promote the growth of the broiler industry. The use of antimicrobials may also reflect the lack of resources to implement farm biosecurity and vaccination programmes on these farms [53,54]. Use of antimicrobials on broiler farms could be expected to rise in the future, mimicking the trends seen in neighbouring Indonesia where there was a rise of antimicrobial use due to industry growth, lack of alternative disease control options and a relatively low cost of antibiotics [55]. Therefore, farmer education programmes to improve knowledge on good animal husbandry practices and biosecurity could be useful [56]. The availability of quality vaccines would provide further options for disease prevention and control [57].

For agriculture shops, the reason for a decrease in imports during the study period was unclear but could be partially attributed to non-adherence to the MAF import application process resulting in data not being captured. For veterinary clinics, the low quantities imported reflect the small size of the industry—there were only four veterinary practices operating in Timor-Leste during the study period. The closure of one veterinary clinic in 2018 coincided with a drop in antimicrobial imports by veterinary clinics that year. For education institutions, there was only a once off import of antimicrobials by an agriculture school in 2016. There were no direct imports of antimicrobials by other types of commercial livestock farms apart from poultry, but animals on these farms could still receive antimicrobials imported by MAF or agriculture shops.

### 4.4. Antimicrobial Class and Importance for Human Medicine

The common antimicrobial classes in Timor-Leste (tetracycline, penicillin, and macrolide) are consistent with global and regional (Asia, Far East, and Oceania) usage patterns [29]. The most imported antimicrobials in Timor-Leste (oxytetracycline, amoxicillin, tylosin, and dihydrostreptomycin) were consistent with antimicrobials used in poultry and pig production in developing countries in Asia and Africa [18,50,58,59]. Oxytetracycline is popular because of its broad-spectrum action, low cost, and availability in long-acting formulations [60,61] and it is likely that similar reasons underpin its popularity in Timor-Leste. Amoxicillin and tylosin were imported almost exclusively in oral formulation by commercial poultry farms, and the popularity of these antimicrobials in small scale poultry farms were also reported in other studies in other countries [50,62]. Dihydrostreptomycin was commonly imported in formulations with benzylpenicillin by MAF due to the combination's broad-spectrum action across a wide range of livestock species. It was positive that colistin, which is an antibiotic of last resort for human medicine that is commonly used in developing countries [63,64] contributed to less than 5% of imports to Timor-Leste with the majority imported in 2016. However, the broiler industry has been importing colistin albeit in small quantities in recent years and this should be closely monitored.

There has been a strong push towards reducing the use of medically important antimicrobials in livestock globally [65]. The almost exclusive imports of CIAs by commercial poultry farms could be attributed to the lack of awareness on antimicrobial resistance and its impact on public health, which has been observed in studies elsewhere [66,67]. On the other hand, the low proportion of CIA imports by MAF (21.2%) and veterinary clinics (21.7%) puts the professional veterinary service in positive light in terms of preserving critically important antimicrobials for use in human health. Of important concern is the import of fluroquinolones, polymyxins, and 3rd and 4th generation cephalosporins which are highest priority critically important antimicrobials for human medicine. Although the combined quantity of these classes contributed to less than 8% of total imports, future import and distribution of these antimicrobials should be closely monitored because of the potential risk of the development and transmission of antimicrobial resistance from livestock to humans [68,69]. To address the high proportion of CIA usage in the commercial poultry sector, a jointly developed antimicrobial treatment guideline between government and industry preferencing the use of non-CIA antibiotics may be effective [70].

### 4.5. Route of Administration

In this study, antimicrobials recommended for oral administration (39.8%) were less common than reported in some countries [12,14,71]. Antimicrobials imported by MAF and agriculture shops were mostly for parenteral administration. This is likely to be because they were mainly for use in species such as pigs and cattle that are reared extensively on small-holder livestock farms. On the other hand, commercial poultry farms probably imported mainly antimicrobials for oral administration because they are convenient for mass administration in poultry reared in semi-intensive or intensive production environments. The use of orally administered antimicrobials should be monitored in Timor-Leste as it has been demonstrated elsewhere that this route is more prone to misuse from inappropriate dosing and promotes the development of antimicrobial resistance [72].

### 4.6. Use of Antimicrobials for Growth Promotion

The import of antimicrobials intended for oral administration raises the concern of use of antimicrobials for growth promotion. Ideally antimicrobials should not be used for growth promotion without a public health risk assessment and any use should be phased out especially for critically important antimicrobials [21,65]. According to MAF, antimicrobials are not known to be used for growth promotion in the country. However, oral bacitracin and tylosin that were imported by poultry farms have been used for growth promotion worldwide [28,73]. In addition, the technical fact sheet of some antimicrobials indicated that the products could be administered for growth promotion. Therefore, it is possible that commercial farmers are administering antimicrobials at low doses, as recommended for growth promotion, without being aware. This has also been reported in another study [49]. The possible use of antimicrobials for growth promotion in Timor-Leste should be further investigated.

### 4.7. Use of Antimicrobials in Aquaculture

Although antimicrobial use is common practice in aquaculture systems worldwide and regionally [74–76], there were no aquaculture importers in this study and no products were indicated for use in aquatic animals. The absence of antimicrobial use in this sector is likely due to the relatively small and underdeveloped aquaculture sector [77].

*4.8. Limitations*

Timor-Leste is not immune to the challenges and limitations of monitoring antimicrobial use. The study only included import data after 2016 because of the five-year holding limit of hardcopy applications in the MAF office and the lack of digital record keeping. Thus, only data from 2016 to 2020 were available. The study excluded data from 2020 because the calendar year of 2020 had not yet ended at the point of data collection. This short study period limited the power of the study to detect trends in import quantities. However, digital record keeping was initiated as part of the study which will enable future studies to cover a longer time period.

It is likely that the study provided an under-estimation of the total amount of antimicrobials used in Timor-Leste due to the non-submission of import applications by some importers as reported in another study [71]. The possible reasons for non-submission include an importer's desire to avoid waiting times for approval, a weak regulatory framework and the lack of enforcement. Antimicrobials intended for human use could have also been administered to animals although elsewhere this is usually limited to companion animals [78]. The authors predict that the underestimation would not result in more than a doubling in the total amount of imported antimicrobials during the study period. Even if this happened, Timor-Leste would still demonstrate one of the lowest use rates compared to other countries that have reported usage data.

There may be a small degree of inaccuracy for the animal biomass estimation because the data obtained from FAOSTAT was based on extrapolations. This source of data was used because annual census data was unavailable during the study period. The OIE method for biomass calculation involved the use of European conversion coefficients and breeding cycles that may be different to Timor-Leste. However, these default parameters were used as no suitable alternative for a Timor-Leste context was found. The exclusion of minor species such as ducks, rabbits, dogs, and cats from the biomass calculation is likely to have only a marginal impact on the result since the population is relatively small [25].

It was not possible to quantify the antimicrobials that were administered to different animal species based on the import data due to the multi-species indication for many of the antimicrobials. However, a rough estimation of the division of antimicrobial use between livestock and companion animals could be estimated by assuming that antimicrobials imported by veterinary clinics were administered exclusively to companion animals, and antimicrobials imported by all other importers were administered exclusively to livestock.

*4.9. Future Directions*

Although the use of antimicrobials in animals is Timor-Leste is very low, there is potential for future misuse and overuse with farming intensification. Future studies investigating the knowledge, attitudes and practices of animal health professionals and farmers on antimicrobial use would be useful for identify strategies for promoting prudent use of antimicrobials in animals as identified in other studies [79–81]. Even in the absence of such studies, early action can be informed by studies conducted in other developing countries [55,58,82]. In addition to farmer education, which was mentioned previously, improving farmers access to animal health professionals [64], and training of animal health professionals to engage with farmers on prudent antimicrobial use has been shown to be effective elsewhere [82]. The strengthening of laboratory capacity in bacterial culture and antimicrobial susceptibility testing will also facilitate better decision making on antimicrobial use [65].

To improve the quality of data collected, MAF is engaging with importers such as agriculture shops to understand their reservations on submitting import applications and exploring legislative tools to improve compliance on import application submission. Future monitoring could focus on collecting data more proximal to the site of usage such as at end-user level to elucidate species and production type usage patterns [83,84].

## 5. Conclusions

This baseline study demonstrated very low levels of antimicrobial use in animals in Timor-Leste consistent with its subsistence agriculture system. Antimicrobial classes imported in the largest quantities were tetracyclines, penicillins, and macrolides. This is very similar to usage patterns in other countries globally and regionally. Import of CIAs for administration via the oral route was high in the poultry industry, and antimicrobial use for growth promotion could not be ruled out. Antimicrobial use in the poultry industry is expected to rise due to industry growth and the limited alternative disease control strategies. Education of farmers, development of antimicrobial treatment guidelines and improving access to veterinary services can help to ensure good antimicrobial stewardship in the animal health sector. Through this study, in-country capacity to monitor antimicrobial imports according to OIE reporting requirements was developed.

**Supplementary Materials:** The following are available online at https://www.mdpi.com/article/10.3390/antibiotics10040426/s1, Table S1: Animal biomass for buffalo, cattle, chicken, goats, horses, pigs and sheep in Timor-Leste between 2016 and 2019. Table S2: Import weight of various veterinary antimicrobial classes by route of administration between 2016 and 2019. Table S3: Total weight of active ingredients of different classes of veterinary antimicrobials imported into Timor-Leste, by type of importer between 2016 and 2019.

**Author Contributions:** Conceptualization, S.T., J.Y., J.R.F. and J.B.d.C.J.; Methodology, S.T., A.P., A.d.J.A. and S.D.; Software, S.T.; Investigation and data curation, S.T., A.P., A.d.J.A., S.D., C.d.C.S., S.F., F.J.S., O.d.C.H. and J.B.d.C.J.; Formal analysis, S.T., A.P., A.d.J.A., S.D. and T.S.B.; Writing—original draft preparation, S.T., A.P., A.d.J.A. and S.D.; Writing—review and editing, S.T., A.P., A.d.J.A., S.D., C.d.C.S., S.F., F.J.S., O.d.C.H., J.Y., J.R.F., T.S.B. and J.B.d.C.J.; Visualization, S.T., A.P., A.d.J.A., S.D. and T.S.B.; Supervision, S.T.; J.Y. and J.R.F.; Project administration, S.T. All authors have read and agreed to the published version of the manuscript.

**Funding:** This study was supported by the Fleming Fund Country Grant for Timor-Leste (FF/17/233). The Fleming Fund is a UK aid investment programme to tackle antimicrobial resistance in low- and middle-income countries around the world and is managed by the UK Department of Health and Social Care.

**Institutional Review Board Statement:** The study was conducted in accordance with the Declaration of Helsinki, and the protocol was approved Human Research Ethics Committee of the Northern Territory (NT) Department of Health and Menzies School of Health Research (2020-3841) and Institute Nacional de Saude in Timor-Leste (MS-INS/DE/IX/2020/1411).

**Informed Consent Statement:** Not applicable.

**Data Availability Statement:** The data presented in this study are available in the Supplementary Materials.

**Acknowledgments:** We acknowledge the staff from the Ministry of Agriculture and Fisheries of Timor-Leste for their support in this study. We thank Winnie Chen (Menzies School of Health Research) and Agnes Agunos (Public Health Agency of Canada) for critically reviewing the manuscript.

**Conflicts of Interest:** The authors declare no conflict of interest. The funders had no role in the design of the study; in the collection, analyses, or interpretation of data; in the writing of the manuscript, or in the decision to publish the results.

## References

1. Robinson, T.P.; Bu, D.P.; Carrique-Mas, J.; Fèvre, E.M.; Gilbert, M.; Grace, D.; Hay, S.I.; Jiwakanon, J.; Kakkar, M.; Kariuki, S.; et al. Antibiotic resistance is the quintessential One Health issue. *Trans. R. Soc. Trop Med. Hyg.* **2016**, *110*, 377–380. [CrossRef]
2. Léger, A.; Lambraki, I.; Graells, T.; Cousins, M.; Henriksson, P.J.G.; Harbarth, S.; Carson, C.; Majowicz, S.; Troell, M.; Parmley, E.J.; et al. AMR-Intervene: A social–ecological framework to capture the diversity of actions to tackle antimicrobial resistance from a One Health perspective. *J. Antimicrob. Chemother.* **2021**, *76*, 1–21. [CrossRef]

3. Wall, B.A.; Mateus, A.L.P.; Marshall, L.; Pfeiffer, D.U.; Lubroth, J.; Ormel, H.J.; Otto, P.; Patriarchi, A. Drivers, Dynamics and Epidemiology of Antimicrobial Resistance in Animal Production. Available online: http://www.fao.org/feed-safety/resources/resources-details/en/c/452608/ (accessed on 16 February 2021).
4. Lim, K.; Chee, D.; Ting, S.; Choo, E.; Tan, W.L.; Lin, Y.N. Singapore's National Action Plan on Antimicrobial Resistance. *Asian Fish. Sci.* **2020**, *33*, 107–111. [CrossRef]
5. Tang, K.L.; Caffrey, N.P.; Nóbrega, D.B.; Cork, S.C.; Ronksley, P.E.; Barkema, H.W.; Polachek, A.J.; Ganshorn, H.; Sharma, N.; Kellner, J.D.; et al. Restricting the use of antibiotics in food-producing animals and its associations with antibiotic resistance in food-producing animals and human beings: A systematic review and meta-analysis. *Lancet Planet. Health* **2017**, *1*, e316–e327. [CrossRef]
6. Ventola, C.L. The antibiotic resistance crisis: Part 1: Causes and threats. *Pharm. Ther.* **2015**, *40*, 277–283.
7. Klein, E.; Boeckel, T.; Martinez, E.; Pant, S.; Gandra, S.; Levin, S.; Goossens, H.; Laxminarayan, R. Global increase and geographic convergence in antibiotic consumption between 2000 and 2015. *Proc. Natl. Acad. Sci. USA* **2018**, *115*, 201717295. [CrossRef]
8. Animal Production ScienceVan Boeckel, T.P.; Brower, C.; Gilbert, M.; Grenfell, B.T.; Levin, S.A.; Robinson, T.P.; Teillant, A.; Laxminarayan, R. Global trends in antimicrobial use in food animals. *Proc. Natl. Acad. Sci. USA* **2015**, *112*, 5649–5654. [CrossRef] [PubMed]
9. Van Boeckel, T.P.; Glennon, E.E.; Chen, D.; Gilbert, M.; Robinson, T.P.; Grenfell, B.T.; Levin, S.A.; Bonhoeffer, S.; Laxminarayan, R. Reducing antimicrobial use in food animals. *Science* **2017**, *357*, 1350. [CrossRef]
10. Tiseo, K.; Huber, L.; Gilbert, M.; Robinson, T.P.; Van Boeckel, T.P. Global Trends in Antimicrobial Use in Food Animals from 2017 to 2030. *Antibiotics (Basel)* **2020**, *9*, 918. [CrossRef] [PubMed]
11. BelVet-SAC. Belgium Veterinary Surveillance of Antimicrobial Consumption: National Consumption Report 2019. Available online: https://belvetsac.ugent.be/BelvetSac_report_2019.pdf (accessed on 21 February 2021).
12. ANSES-ANMV. Sales Survey of Veterinary Medicinal Products Containing Antimicrobials in France in 2019. Available online: https://www.anses.fr/en/system/files/ANMV-Ra-Antibiotiques2019EN.pdf (accessed on 21 February 2021).
13. Swedres-Svarm. Sales of Antibiotics and Occurrence of Resistance in Sweden 2019. Available online: https://www.folkhalsomyndigheten.se/contentassets/fb80663bc7c94d678be785e3360917d1/swedres-svarm-2019.pdf (accessed on 21 February 2021).
14. UK-VARSS. Veterinary Antibiotic Resistance and Sales Surveillance Report (UK-VARSS 2019). Available online: https://assets.publishing.service.gov.uk/government/uploads/system/uploads/attachment_data/file/950126/UK-VARSS_2019_Report__2020-TPaccessible.pdf (accessed on 20 February 2021).
15. National Food Institute; Statens Serum Institut. DANMAP 2019—Use of Antimicrobial Agents and Occurrence of Antimicrobial Resistance in Bacteria from Food Animals, Food and Humans in Denmark. Available online: https://www.danmap.org/-/media/Sites/danmap/Downloads/Reports/2019/DANMAP_2019.ashx?la=da&hash=AA1939EB449203EF0684440AC1477FFCE2156BA5 (accessed on 21 February 2021).
16. Van Boeckel, T.P.; Pires, J.; Silvester, R.; Zhao, C.; Song, J.; Criscuolo, N.G.; Gilbert, M.; Bonhoeffer, S.; Laxminarayan, R. Global trends in antimicrobial resistance in animals in low- and middle-income countries. *Science* **2019**, *365*, 1944. [CrossRef] [PubMed]
17. Goutard, F.L.; Bordier, M.; Calba, C.; Erlacher-Vindel, E.; Góchez, D.; de Balogh, K.; Benigno, C.; Kalpravidh, W.; Roger, F.; Vong, S. Antimicrobial policy interventions in food animal production in South East Asia. *BMJ* **2017**, *358*, j3544. [CrossRef]
18. Ström, G.; Halje, M.; Karlsson, D.; Jiwakanon, J.; Pringle, M.; Fernström, L.L.; Magnusson, U. Antimicrobial use and antimicrobial susceptibility in Escherichia coli on small- and medium-scale pig farms in north-eastern Thailand. *Antimicrob. Resist. Infect. Control* **2017**, *6*, 75. [CrossRef] [PubMed]
19. O'Neill, J. *Tackling Drug-Resistant Infections Globally: Final Report and Recommendations*; Government of the United Kingdom: London, UK, 2016.
20. Laxminarayan, R.P.; Duse, A.M.D.; Wattal, C.M.D.; Zaidi, A.K.M.M.D.; Wertheim, H.F.L.M.D.; Sumpradit, N.P.; Vlieghe, E.M.D.; Hara, G.L.P.; Gould, I.M.M.; Goossens, H.P.; et al. Antibiotic resistance—The need for global solutions. *Lancet Infect. Dis.* **2013**, *13*, 1057–1098. [CrossRef]
21. World Health Organization. *Global Action Plan on Antimicrobial Resistance*; World Health Organization: Geneva, Switzerland, 2015.
22. World Organisation for Animal Health (OIE). Terrestrial Animal Health Code: Chapter 6.9 Monitoring of the Quantities and Usage Patterns of Antimicrobial Agents Used in Food-Producing Animals. Available online: https://www.oie.int/index.php?id=169&L=0&htmfile=chapitre_antibio_monitoring.htm (accessed on 16 February 2021).
23. Chantziaras, I.; Boyen, F.; Callens, B.; Dewulf, J. Correlation between veterinary antimicrobial use and antimicrobial resistance in food-producing animals: A report on seven countries. *J. Antimicrob. Chemother.* **2014**, *69*, 827–834. [CrossRef]
24. Callens, B.; Cargnel, M.; Sarrazin, S.; Dewulf, J.; Hoet, B.; Vermeersch, K.; Wattiau, P.; Welby, S. Associations between a decreased veterinary antimicrobial use and resistance in commensal Escherichia coli from Belgian livestock species (2011–2015). *Prev. Vet. Med.* **2018**, *157*, 50–58. [CrossRef] [PubMed]
25. Góchez, D.; Raicek, M.; Pinto Ferreira, J.; Jeannin, M.; Moulin, G.; Erlacher-Vindel, E. OIE Annual Report on Antimicrobial Agents Intended for Use in Animals: Methods Used. *Front. Vet. Sci.* **2019**, *6*. [CrossRef]
26. Grave, K.; Torren-Edo, J.; Mackay, D. Comparison of the sales of veterinary antibacterial agents between 10 European countries. *J. Antimicrob. Chemother.* **2010**, *65*, 2037–2040. [CrossRef]

27. Hosoi, Y.; Asai, T.; Koike, R.; Tsuyuki, M.; Sugiura, K. Use of veterinary antimicrobial agents from 2005 to 2010 in Japan. *Int. J. Antimicrob. Agents* **2013**, *41*, 489–490. [CrossRef]
28. Page, S.W.; Gautier, P. Use of antimicrobial agents in livestock. *Rev. Sci. Tech. OIE* **2012**, *31*, 145–188. [CrossRef]
29. World Organisation for Animal Health (OIE). OIE Annual Report on Antimicrobial Agents Intended for Use in Animals. Fourth report. Available online: https://www.oie.int/fileadmin/Home/eng/Our_scientific_expertise/docs/pdf/AMR/A_Fourth_Annual_Report_AMR.pdf (accessed on 16 February 2021).
30. The World Bank. World Bank Country and Lending Groups. Available online: https://datahelpdesk.worldbank.org/knowledgebase/articles/906519 (accessed on 16 February 2021).
31. The World Bank. Population, Total—Timor-Leste. Available online: https://data.worldbank.org/indicator/SP.POP.TOTL?locations=TL (accessed on 16 February 2021).
32. General Directorate of Statistics—Ministry of Finance (Timor Leste) and ICF. *Timor-Leste Demographic and Health Survey 2016*; GDS and ICF: Dili, Timor-Leste, 2018.
33. Lundahl, M.; Sjöholm, F. Improving the Lot of the Farmer: Development Challenges in Timor-Leste during the Second Decade of Independence. *Asian Econ. Pap.* **2013**, *12*, 71–96. [CrossRef]
34. Bettencourt, E.; Tilman, M.; Narciso, V.; Da Silva Carvalho, M.L.; Henriques, P. The Livestock Roles in the Wellbeing of Rural Communities of Timor-Leste. *Revista de Economia e Sociologia Rural* **2015**, *53*, 63–80. [CrossRef]
35. General Directorate of Statistics—Ministry of Finance (Timor Leste); Food and Agriculture Organization of the United Nations (FAO); United Nations Population Fund (UNFPA). *Timor-Leste Population and Housing Census 2015: Thematic Report Volume 12*; Government of Timor-Leste: Canberra, Australia, 2018.
36. Spencer, P.R.; Sanders, K.A.; Judge, D.S. Rural Livelihood Variation and its Effects on Child Growth in Timor-Leste. *Hum. Ecol.* **2018**, *46*, 787–799. [CrossRef]
37. de Correia, V.P.; Rola-Rubzen, M.F. Breaking the poverty cycle through linking farmers to markets in Timor Leste: The World Vision income generation project. *Hum. Dev. Capacit. Build. Asia Pac. Trends Chall. Prospect. Future* **2016**. [CrossRef]
38. The Poultry Site. International Egg and Poultry Review: Timor-Leste. Available online: https://www.thepoultrysite.com/news/2011/06/international-egg-and-poultry-review-timorleste (accessed on 18 February 2021).
39. World Organisation for Animal Health (OIE). OIE List of Antimicrobial Agents of Veterinary Importance (July 2019). Available online: https://www.oie.int/fileadmin/Home/eng/Our_scientific_expertise/docs/pdf/AMR/A_OIE_List_antimicrobials_July2019.pdf (accessed on 19 February 2021).
40. Jong, J.B.D.C. Multi-Capacity Building for Antimicrobial Use (AMU) Data Collection: Improving the Recording of Antimicrobial Agents Intended for Use in Animals in Timor-Leste. Available online: https://rr-asia.oie.int/en/projects/antimicrobial-resistance/good-practices-addressing-amr-in-asia-and-the-pacific-region/multi-capacity-building-for-antimicrobial-use-amu-data-collection/ (accessed on 22 February 2021).
41. World Organisation for Animal Health (OIE). Guidance for completing the OIE Template for the Collection of Data on Antimicrobial Agents Intended for Use in Animals (Version 1_Sept 2020). Available online: https://www.oie.int/fileadmin/Home/eng/Our_scientific_expertise/docs/pdf/AMR/2020/ENG_AMUse_Guidance_Final_2020.pdf (accessed on 19 February 2021).
42. World Health Organization. *Critically Important Antimicrobials for Human Medicine 6th Revision*; World Health Organization: Geneva, Switzerland, 2019.
43. Food and Agriculture Organization of the United Nations. Live Animals in Timor-Leste: Stocks. Available online: http://www.fao.org/faostat/en/#data/QA (accessed on 10 January 2021).
44. Food and Agriculture Organization of the United Nations. Livestock Primary in Timor-Leste: Producing animals/slaughtered. Available online: http://www.fao.org/faostat/en/#data/QL (accessed on 10 January 2021).
45. Hillerton, J.E.; Irvine, C.R.; Bryan, M.A.; Scott, D.; Merchant, S.C. Use of antimicrobials for animals in New Zealand, and in comparison with other countries. *N. Z. Vet. J.* **2017**, *65*, 71–77. [CrossRef] [PubMed]
46. European Medicines Agency—European Surveillance of Veterinary Antimicrobial Consumption. Sales of Veterinary Antimicrobial Agents in 31 European Countries in 2018. Available online: https://www.ema.europa.eu/en/documents/report/sales-veterinary-antimicrobial-agents-31-european-countries-2018-trends-2010-2018-tenth-esvac-report_en.pdf (accessed on 16 February 2021).
47. Alders, R.G.; Ali, S.N.; Ameri, A.A.; Bagnol, B.; Cooper, T.L.; Gozali, A.; Hidayat, M.M.; Rukambile, E.; Wong, J.T.; Catley, A. Participatory Epidemiology: Principles, Practice, Utility, and Lessons Learnt. *Front. Vet. Sci.* **2020**, *7*, 532763. [CrossRef] [PubMed]
48. Serrao, E.A. Constraints to Production of Village Chickens in Timor-Leste. Ph.D. Thesis, University of Queensland, Queensland, Australia, 2012.
49. Om, C.; McLaws, M.-L. Antibiotics: Practice and opinions of Cambodian commercial farmers, animal feed retailers and veterinarians. *Antimicrob. Resist. Infect. Control* **2016**, *5*, 42. [CrossRef]
50. Kiambi, S.; Mwanza, R.; Sirma, A.; Czerniak, C.; Kimani, T.; Kabali, E.; Dorado-Garcia, A.; Eckford, S.; Price, C.; Gikonyo, S.; et al. Understanding Antimicrobial Use Contexts in the Poultry Sector: Challenges for Small-Scale Layer Farms in Kenya. *Antibiotics (Basel)* **2021**, *10*, 106. [CrossRef]
51. Jong, J.B.D.C. (National Director of Veterinary Directorate, Ministry of Agriculture and Fisheries, Timor-Leste). Personal Communication, 2021.

52. Democratic Republic of Timor-Leste. Decree-Law No. 3/2018 of March 14: About the Import Ban on Poultry and Poultry Products. Available online: http://extwprlegs1.fao.org/docs/pdf/tim187132.pdf (accessed on 19 February 2021).
53. Jong, J.B.D.C. Scavenging for protein and micronutrients: Village poultry in Timor-Leste. Available online: https://www.crawfordfund.org/wp-content/uploads/2017/04/CF-2016-Conference-Proceedings-Jong.pdf (accessed on 22 February 2021).
54. Conan, A.; Goutard, F.L.; Sorn, S.; Vong, S. Biosecurity measures for backyard poultry in developing countries: A systematic review. *BMC Vet. Res.* **2012**, *8*, 240. [CrossRef] [PubMed]
55. Coyne, L.; Patrick, I.; Arief, R.; Benigno, C.; Kalpravidh, W.; McGrane, J.; Schoonman, L.; Sukarno, A.H.; Rushton, J. The Costs, Benefits and Human Behaviours for Antimicrobial Use in Small Commercial Broiler Chicken Systems in Indonesia. *Antibiotics (Basel)* **2020**, *9*, 154. [CrossRef]
56. Kimera, Z.I.; Frumence, G.; Mboera, L.E.G.; Rweyemamu, M.; Mshana, S.E.; Matee, M.I.N. Assessment of Drivers of Antimicrobial Use and Resistance in Poultry and Domestic Pig Farming in the Msimbazi River Basin in Tanzania. *Antibiotics (Basel)* **2020**, *9*, 838. [CrossRef]
57. Lhermie, G.; Gröhn, Y.T.; Raboisson, D. Addressing Antimicrobial Resistance: An Overview of Priority Actions to Prevent Suboptimal Antimicrobial Use in Food-Animal Production. *Front. Microbiol.* **2017**, *7*, 2114. [CrossRef]
58. Ström, G.; Boqvist, S.; Albihn, A.; Fernström, L.L.; Andersson Djurfeldt, A.; Sokerya, S.; Sothyra, T.; Magnusson, U. Antimicrobials in small-scale urban pig farming in a lower middle-income country—Arbitrary use and high resistance levels. *Antimicrob. Resist. Infect. Control* **2018**, *7*, 35. [CrossRef]
59. Nhung, N.T.; Cuong, N.V.; Thwaites, G.; Carrique-Mas, J. Antimicrobial Usage and Antimicrobial Resistance in Animal Production in Southeast Asia: A Review. *Antibiotics (Basel)* **2016**, *5*, 37. [CrossRef] [PubMed]
60. Olatoye, O.; Afisu, B. Antibiotic Usage and Oxytetracycline Residue in African Catfish (Clarias gariepinus in Ibadan, Nigeria). *World J. Fish. Mar. Sci.* **2013**, *5*, 302–309. [CrossRef]
61. Aktas, I.; Yarsan, E. Pharmacokinetics of Conventional and Long-Acting Oxytetracycline Preparations in Kilis Goat. *Front. Vet. Sci.* **2017**, *4*, 229. [CrossRef]
62. Xu, J.; Sangthong, R.; McNeil, E.; Tang, R.; Chongsuvivatwong, V. Antibiotic use in chicken farms in northwestern China. *Antimicrob. Resist. Infect. Control* **2020**, *9*, 10. [CrossRef]
63. Carrique-Mas, J.J.; Trung, N.V.; Hoa, N.T.; Mai, H.H.; Thanh, T.H.; Campbell, J.I.; Wagenaar, J.A.; Hardon, A.; Hieu, T.Q.; Schultsz, C. Antimicrobial usage in chicken production in the Mekong Delta of Vietnam. *Zoonoses Public Health* **2015**, *62*, 70–78. [CrossRef] [PubMed]
64. Lekagul, A.; Tangcharoensathien, V.; Mills, A.; Rushton, J.; Yeung, S. How antibiotics are used in pig farming: A mixed-methods study of pig farmers, feed mills and veterinarians in Thailand. *BMJ Glob. Health* **2020**, *5*, e001918. [CrossRef] [PubMed]
65. Aidara-Kane, A.; Angulo, F.J.; Conly, J.M.; Minato, Y.; Silbergeld, E.K.; McEwen, S.A.; Collignon, P.J.; Group, W.H.O.G.D. World Health Organization (WHO) guidelines on use of medically important antimicrobials in food-producing animals. *Antimicrob. Resist. Infect. Control* **2018**, *7*, 7. [CrossRef] [PubMed]
66. Sommanustweechai, A.; Chanvatik, S.; Sermsinsiri, V.; Sivilaikul, S.; Patcharanarumol, W.; Yeung, S.; Tangcharoensathien, V. Antibiotic distribution channels in Thailand: Results of key-informant interviews, reviews of drug regulations and database searches. *Bull. World Health Organ.* **2018**, *96*, 101–109. [CrossRef]
67. Tufa, T.B.; Gurmu, F.; Beyi, A.F.; Hogeveen, H.; Beyene, T.J.; Ayana, D.; Woldemariyam, F.T.; Hailemariam, E.; Gutema, F.D.; Stegeman, J.A. Veterinary medicinal product usage among food animal producers and its health implications in Central Ethiopia. *BMC Vet. Res.* **2018**, *14*, 409. [CrossRef]
68. Carson, C.; Li, X.-Z.; Agunos, A.; Loest, D.; Chapman, B.; Finley, R.; Mehrotra, M.; Sherk, L.M.; Gaumond, R.; Irwin, R. Ceftiofur-resistant Salmonella enterica serovar Heidelberg of poultry origin—A risk profile using the Codex framework. *Epidemiol. Infect.* **2019**, *147*, e296. [CrossRef] [PubMed]
69. Sproston, E.L.; Wimalarathna, H.M.L.; Sheppard, S.K. Trends in fluoroquinolone resistance in Campylobacter. *Microb. Genom.* **2018**, *4*, e000198. [CrossRef]
70. Speksnijder, D.C.; Mevius, D.J.; Bruschke, C.J.; Wagenaar, J.A. Reduction of veterinary antimicrobial use in the Netherlands. The Dutch success model. *Zoonoses Public Health* **2015**, *62*, 79–87. [CrossRef] [PubMed]
71. Mouiche, M.M.M.; Moffo, F.; Betsama, J.D.B.; Mapiefou, N.P.; Mbah, C.K.; Mpouam, S.E.; Penda, R.E.; Ciake, S.A.C.; Feussom, J.M.K.; Kamnga, Z.F.; et al. Challenges of antimicrobial consumption surveillance in food-producing animals in sub-Saharan African countries: Patterns of antimicrobials imported in Cameroon from 2014 to 2019. *J. Glob. Antimicrob. Resist.* **2020**, *22*, 771–778. [CrossRef]
72. Simoneit, C.; Burow, E.; Tenhagen, B.A.; Käsbohrer, A. Oral administration of antimicrobials increase antimicrobial resistance in E. coli from chicken—A systematic review. *Prev. Vet. Med.* **2015**, *118*, 1–7. [CrossRef]
73. Van Cuong, N.; Nhung, N.T.; Nghia, N.H.; Mai Hoa, N.T.; Trung, N.V.; Thwaites, G.; Carrique-Mas, J. Antimicrobial Consumption in Medicated Feeds in Vietnamese Pig and Poultry Production. *Ecohealth* **2016**, *13*, 490–498. [CrossRef] [PubMed]
74. Schar, D.; Klein, E.Y.; Laxminarayan, R.; Gilbert, M.; Van Boeckel, T.P. Global trends in antimicrobial use in aquaculture. *Sci. Rep.* **2020**, *10*, 21878. [CrossRef]
75. Park, Y.H.; Hwang, S.Y.; Hong, M.K.; Kwon, K.H. Use of antimicrobial agents in aquaculture. *Rev. Sci. Tech.* **2012**, *31*, 189–197. [CrossRef] [PubMed]

76. Zellweger, R.M.; Carrique-Mas, J.; Limmathurotsakul, D.; Day, N.P.J.; Thwaites, G.E.; Baker, S.; Southeast Asia Antimicrobial Resistance Network. A current perspective on antimicrobial resistance in Southeast Asia. *J. Antimicrob. Chemother.* **2017**, *72*, 2963–2972. [CrossRef] [PubMed]
77. López-Angarita, J.; Hunnam, K.J.; Pereira, M.M.D.; Pant, J.; Teoh, S.J.; Eriksson, H.; Amaral, L.; Tilley, A. *Fisheries and Aquaculture of Timor-Leste in 2019: Current Knowledge and Opportunities*; WorldFish: Penang, Malaysia, 2019.
78. Food and Drug Administration. 2017 Summary Report on Antimicrobials Sold or Distributed for Use in Food-Producing Animals. Available online: https://www.fda.gov/media/119332/download (accessed on 22 February 2021).
79. Speksnijder, D.C.; Wagenaar, J.A. Reducing antimicrobial use in farm animals: How to support behavioral change of veterinarians and farmers. *Anim. Front.* **2018**, *8*, 4–9. [CrossRef] [PubMed]
80. Caudell, M.A.; Dorado-Garcia, A.; Eckford, S.; Creese, C.; Byarugaba, D.K.; Afakye, K.; Chansa-Kabali, T.; Fasina, F.O.; Kabali, E.; Kiambi, S.; et al. Towards a bottom-up understanding of antimicrobial use and resistance on the farm: A knowledge, attitudes, and practices survey across livestock systems in five African countries. *PLoS ONE* **2020**, *15*, e0220274. [CrossRef] [PubMed]
81. Vijay, D.; Bedi, J.S.; Dhaka, P.; Singh, R.; Singh, J.; Arora, A.K.; Gill, J.P.S. Knowledge, Attitude, and Practices (KAP) Survey among Veterinarians, and Risk Factors Relating to Antimicrobial Use and Treatment Failure in Dairy Herds of India. *Antibiotics (Basel)* **2021**, *10*, 216. [CrossRef]
82. Truong, D.B.; Doan, H.P.; Doan Tran, V.K.; Nguyen, V.C.; Bach, T.K.; Rueanghiran, C.; Binot, A.; Goutard, F.L.; Thwaites, G.; Carrique-Mas, J.; et al. Assessment of Drivers of Antimicrobial Usage in Poultry Farms in the Mekong Delta of Vietnam: A Combined Participatory Epidemiology and Q-Sorting Approach. *Front. Vet. Sci.* **2019**, *6*. [CrossRef] [PubMed]
83. Schar, D.; Sommanustweechai, A.; Laxminarayan, R.; Tangcharoensathien, V. Surveillance of antimicrobial consumption in animal production sectors of low- and middle-income countries: Optimizing use and addressing antimicrobial resistance. *PLoS Med.* **2018**, *15*, e1002521. [CrossRef] [PubMed]
84. Lekagul, A.; Tangcharoensathien, V.; Yeung, S. The use of antimicrobials in global pig production: A systematic review of methods for quantification. *Prev. Vet. Med.* **2018**, *160*, 85–98. [CrossRef] [PubMed]

www.ingramcontent.com/pod-product-compliance
Lightning Source LLC
LaVergne TN
LVHW070147100526
838202LV00015B/1908

MDPI
St. Alban-Anlage 66
4052 Basel
Switzerland
Tel. +41 61 683 77 34
Fax +41 61 302 89 18
www.mdpi.com

*Antibiotics* Editorial Office
E-mail: antibiotics@mdpi.com
www.mdpi.com/journal/antibiotics

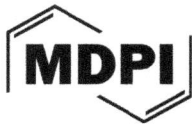